Multiparametric Ultrasound Diagnosis of Breast Diseases

Gennady T. Sukhikh
Alexander N. Sencha
Editors

Multiparametric Ultrasound Diagnosis of Breast Diseases

Springer

Editors
Gennady T. Sukhikh
Research Center for Obstetrics
Gynecology and Perinatology
Ministry of Healthcare of the
Russian Federation
Moscow
Russia

Alexander N. Sencha
Research Center for Obstetrics
Gynecology and Perinatology
Ministry of Healthcare of the
Russian Federation
Moscow
Russia

ISBN 978-3-319-75033-0 ISBN 978-3-319-75034-7 (eBook)
https://doi.org/10.1007/978-3-319-75034-7

Library of Congress Control Number: 2018941080

Printed on acid-free paper

This Springer imprint is published by the registered company Springer International Publishing AG part of Springer Nature.
The registered company address is: Gewerbestrasse 11, 6330 Cham, Switzerland

About the Book

This monograph summarizes our extensive experience in the application of new and promising ultrasound mammography technologies that have rapidly become integrated in clinical practice. Grayscale echography, various methods of Dopplerography, color-coded techniques, ultrasound elastography, and ultrasound contrast imaging are considered to be essential components of multiparametric studies of the breast. The book provides a comprehensive overview of current ultrasound techniques, including contrast-enhanced ultrasound, and the advantages and pitfalls of several imaging modalities. The role of innovative ultrasound technologies in the differential diagnosis of inflammatory breast diseases and benign and malignant tumors is discussed. Ways of integrating the ultrasound data with the Breast Imaging Reporting and Data System (BI-RADS) are also discussed. Close attention is paid to the early diagnosis of breast cancer.

The most important benign breast diseases are described, and are illustrated with high-quality images. Several chapters cover the age-related features of these diseases, including those in children and adolescents. A separate chapter deals with the problem of breast abnormalities in men. All aspects of lymph nodes, with a special focus on the differentiation of their lesions, are reviewed in detail. Ultrasound-guided breast interventions, imaging of breast implants, and postoperative follow-up are thoroughly discussed.

The book is intended for specialists in diagnostic ultrasound, radiologists, mammologists, oncologists, gynecologists, surgeons, pediatricians, and general practitioners, and is richly illustrated with a large number of echograms, Figures, schemes, and Tables.

Introduction

Each year dozens of new monographs, hundreds of articles, and thousands of scientific publications worldwide are devoted to the early detection and differential diagnosis of breast pathology with the use of radiological imaging. Multimillion dollar investments are being made in the search for new and effective technologies for the detection of breast cancer at earlier stages, and in monitoring the effectiveness of different types of treatment. Most of these activities are devoted to the possibilities and prospects of imaging techniques, X-ray, and ultrasound mammography in aiding the earlier detection of breast cancer.

Nevertheless, the urgency of the problem is obvious. According to the World Health Organization, in 2014, 14.1 million people worldwide were diagnosed with malignant breast tumors, and 8.2 million people died of the disease. In 2014, worldwide, 32.6 million people received regular medical check-ups in regard to breast cancer, and they had been having these check-ups for 5 years or more; 17 million of these people were citizens of developed countries and 15.6 million were citizens of developing countries. Despite the considerable progress that has been made in the significant optimization of healthcare systems, with increased diagnostic opportunities, the availability of highly effective diagnostic equipment at medical facilities, and the development of new diagnostic approaches, the proportion of patients whose disease is detected at an early stage remains low, especially in those with visually apparent tumors. Both the extent of preventive measures and practitioners' oncological alertness in the female population are still insufficient. There is a shortage of precise diagnostic equipment and highly qualified specialists, and the opinions and diagnostic strategies of various specialists often differ. The effectiveness of imaging techniques in the diagnosis of various types of breast pathology, the sequence of their use, and the complex analysis and approaches to the interpretation of the obtained results need further study, improvement, elaboration, and optimization.

Diagnostic strategies for a wide range of breast diseases are constantly being revised and improved with new developments in science and technology and the emergence of new methods and technologies in ultrasound, radiological imaging, and diagnostic equipment, as well as the expansion of their functional capabilities. In order to understand, analyze, and differentiate breast diseases, reach adequate medical conclusions, and suggest further strategies for treatment and monitoring, profound systematic knowledge of a large number of aspects of breast disease is absolutely necessary. Some of these aspects are:

- The indications and limitations of the imaging techniques employed
- Age-related breast changes
- Types of diffuse changes and focal lesions
- Peculiarities of normal breast vascularization and vascularization of neoplasms
- Topographic-anatomical relationships
- Neoplasm elasticity determined by quantitative and qualitative analysis of ultrasound elastography
- Contrast-enhanced ultrasound technologies
- Complex analysis of lymphatic drainage
- The state of other organs and systems.

Correct ultrasound evaluation of superficial organs requires profound and appropriate knowledge, the performance of complex analysis, certain experience and practical skills, the use of appropriate equipment and knowledge of its correct settings, and the effective implementation of ultrasound techniques. The availability of modern diagnostic equipment, high-level ultrasound scanners, and modern and innovative imaging technologies operated by highly specialized diagnosticians is an important component of timely and effective diagnosis and a specific issue in providing diagnostic services.

In the past 50 years, complex ultrasound diagnosis has taken a leading position in diagnoses of the pathology of the breast and other organs. Echography has advanced very rapidly and the quality of grayscale and color-coded images has significantly improved. Three-dimensional image reconstruction and multiplanar reconstruction and panoramic scanning have been introduced. Ultrasound compression elastography and elastometry and contrast-enhanced ultrasonography have found practical applications. However, many issues and unsettled problems have arisen during this period. Accurate and timely diagnosis involves the use of a set of methods and techniques and compliance with effective and efficient examination algorithms. Data on the complex use of the most advanced and innovative ultrasound technologies in the differential diagnosis of neoplasms and tumors requires elaboration and further study. The use of contrast agents in echography for the evaluation of neoangiogenesis and the differential diagnosis of focal lesions seems quite promising.

On the basis of the literature data, our own experience in scientific research, and the results of practical activities, we have attempted to analyze and summarize controversial and unresolved issues, problems, and prospects for the early differential diagnosis of various breast diseases. Undoubtedly, we have not solved all the problems of the ultrasound diagnosis of breast diseases, but we have provided the reader with the opportunity to analyze, criticize, reflect on, and comment on various aspects of the diagnosis of breast diseases, and to carry out further scientific and practical research in this field. This publication is a small contribution to solving a big problem, and it is believed that there are still many discoveries to be made and good prospects ahead for solving this problem.

The authors hope for a favorable reception from readers; remarks, clarifications, and suggestions will be gratefully accepted, analyzed, and taken into consideration in further practical activities, as well as in professional and scientific research.

Contents

Abbreviations

BPE	Background parenchymal enhancement
CDI	Color Doppler imaging
CEUS	Contrast-enhanced ultrasound
CNB	Core needle biopsy
CT	Computed tomography
3D	Three-dimensional
3DPD	Three-dimensional power Doppler imaging
4D	Realtime 3D
EDV	End diastolic velocity
FA	Fibroadenoma
FBD	Fibrocystic breast disease
FGT	Fibroglandular tissue
FNAB	Fine needle aspiration biopsy
IHC	Immunohistochemistry
ICC	Immunocytochemistry
MDCT	Multidetector computed tomography
MIP	Maximum intensity projection
MIM	Minimally invasive modality
MRI	Magnetic resonance imaging
MRM	Magnetic resonance mammography
PCV	Peak systolic velocity
PDI	Power Doppler imaging
PET	Positron emission tomography
PI	Pulsatility index
PW	Pulsed wave Doppler
RI	Resistive index
SLNB	Sentinel lymph node biopsy
SWE	Shear wave elastography (elastometry)
TIRM	Turbo inversion recovery magnitude
US	Ultrasound (sonography)

1 Current State of Diagnosis of Breast Diseases: Contribution of Medical Imaging Technologies

Alexander N. Sencha, Vladimir Bychenko, and Yury Patrunov

Abstract

Breast pathology is diagnosed in every fourth woman under the age of 30 and in 60% of older women. Accuracy of clinical examination in detecting benign and malignant tumors does not exceed 50–60%, sensitivity is 40–69%, and specificity is 88–95%. Digital mammography is the principle diagnostic method for breast pathology in women over 40 years of age. Ultrasound is now one of the most widespread and affordable imaging methods for diagnosis of breast pathology, early and differential diagnosis of breast masses, and guidance of minimally invasive modalities. US is more valuable for specification of cysts, fibroadenomas, lipomas, some malignant tumors, and duct ectasia. Both diagnostic methods would benefit from their combined use in the differential diagnosis of cysts, large benign soft tissue tumors, tumor-like masses, and malignant tumors. To assess the spread of the tumor, CT or MRI is strongly recommended. The risk of breast cancer increases with age. The basic concept of screening is the detection of the disease early enough to ensure optimistic prognosis and change of the "natural" clinical course. In female population, large-scale mammography screening can reduce mortality rate from breast cancer by 15–30%. The efficiency of mammography for screening has been tested in numerous randomized studies. In order to unify imaging findings description, a specialized BI-RADS lexicon was developed. Report categories in accordance with BI-RADS lexicon are presented. BI-RADS categories used in echography correspond to the categories used in other diagnostic procedures.

1.1 Imaging Techniques in the Diagnosis of Breast Diseases

Diagnosis of breast diseases is one important problem of women's health globally. Breast pathology is diagnosed in every fourth woman under the age of 30 and in 60% of older women; 50–95% of women suffer from diffuse fibrocystic breast disease (Rozhkova 1993; Radzinsky et al. 2016).

A. N. Sencha (✉)
Division of Visual Diagnostics, National Medical Research Center for Obstetrics, Gynecology and Perinatology named after Academician V.I.Kulakov of Ministry of Healthcare of Russian Federation, Moscow, Russia

V. Bychenko
Department of Radiology, National Medical Research Center for Obstetrics, Gynecology and Perinatology named after Academician V.I.Kulakov of Ministry of Healthcare of Russian Federation, Moscow, Russia

Y. Patrunov
Department of Ultrasound Diagnostics of Radiology Center, Yaroslavl Railway Clinic, Yaroslavl, Russia

G. T. Sukhikh, A. N. Sencha (eds.), *Multiparametric Ultrasound Diagnosis of Breast Diseases*,
https://doi.org/10.1007/978-3-319-75034-7_1

The issues of early detection of breast tumors remain relevant due to the high morbidity and mortality of the female population. Breast cancer takes one dominating malignancy in women around the world. According to the WHO, each year more than 1,300,000 new cases are detected globally. The incidence of cancer has also increased in the majority of countries in Europe and in the world over the past decades. In 2012, 1.67 million patients with breast cancer were registered worldwide. More than half of the breast cancer cases are registered in economically developed countries, where breast cancer occurs in 6% of the female population throughout life. Morbidity in the Russian Federation for the last 10 years is shown in Fig. 1.1 (Kaprin et al. 2017).

Over the past 10 years, the number of patients with malignant breast tumors (malignant tumors) in the Russian Federation has increased by 30%; the most dramatic growth (34%) was observed in women aged 19–39 years: 68,205 cases in 2016 (439 cases per 100,000 of population). In 2016, 642,720 women with breast cancer were registered in Russian oncologic dispensaries.

Despite the increasing incidence of the disease, there has been a significant increase in the 5-year survival rate in Russia for the last decade, which was 61.9% in 2016 (Fig. 1.2) (Kaprin et al. 2017).

Breast cancer amounts to 25.2% of all malignant tumors in the structure of oncological morbidity. It is the leading cause of cancer mortality among women. This is the result of late detection and, consequently, advanced stage at the time of diagnosis (Kaprin et al. 2017).

One important prognostic criterion for cancer is the extent of the tumor spread at the time of detection. An objective assessment of the changes in primary tumor size and regional lymph nodes in the process of preoperative systemic therapy is an essential part of the treatment (Semiglazov 2001). Decisions on the duration of preoperative treatment, the type of surgery, and the need for additional treatment methods depend on it.

High rates of morbidity and mortality from breast cancer force the development of new approaches to diagnosis. Early differential diagnosis of benign and malignant processes and evaluation of the severity and extent of malignancy are among the most burning problems. Despite the apparent availability and simplicity of breast examination, the incidence of detection of advanced disease was about 40%. In 2016, 24.7% of breast cancer were diagnosed in the first stage, 45% in the second stage, 21.5% in the third stage, and 8.2% in the fourth stage of the disease (Kaprin et al. 2017). 29.6% of cases of breast cancer were detected in late stages (III–IV); this is the evidence of low attention to obvious disease.

Nine hundred cases of breast carcinoma in situ were detected in Russia in 2016, which corresponds to 1.3 (2015—2.6) of cases per 100 of all newly diagnosed cases of cancer according to

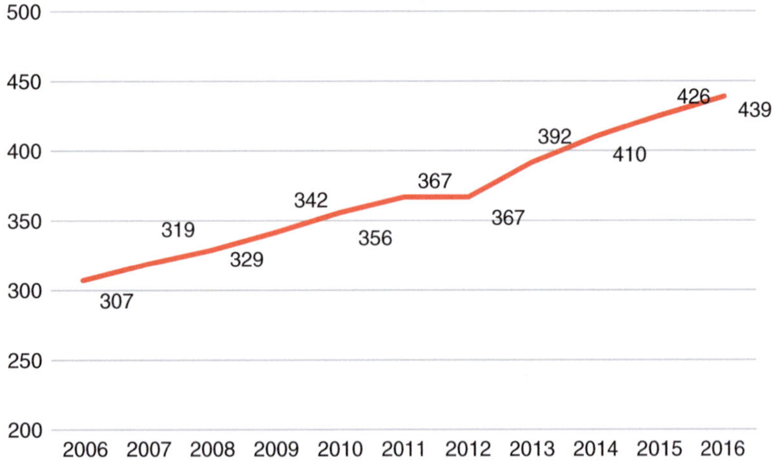

Fig. 1.1 The incidence of malignant breast tumors in Russia in 2006–2016. The number of patients is indicated per 100,000 of population

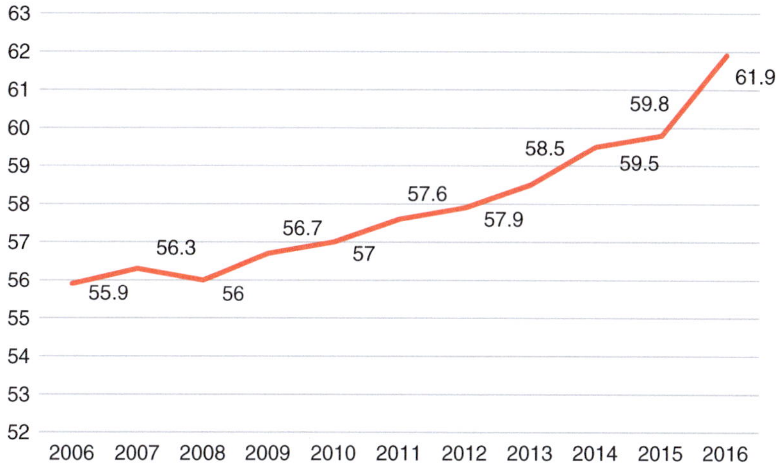

Fig. 1.2 Percentage of patients with breast cancer followed-up for ≥5 years in Russian oncologic facilities

Kaprin et al. (2017). Early detection of breast malignancies is a priority. In this regard, the issues of effective detection of breast cancer, especially in the preclinical stage, are urgent. Secondary cancer prevention, especially screening, involves tests aimed at earlier detection of the disease, i.e., before the onset of signs and symptoms, which makes patients apply for medical assistance. The value of early diagnosis is that early cancer stage is curable.

Over the last decade, the number of patients with breast cancer has increased by 76.7% in Russia (from 21.9 to 38.7%), primarily due to preventive mammography (Kaprin et al. 2017). Technical equipment of medical facilities provides opportunities for solving the problems of the so-called secondary prevention of breast cancer (screening) by means of preventive examination of asymptomatic women.

High efficacy of diagnosis of early breast cancer makes it possible to use a highly effective complex of treatment and perform breast-conserving operations in combination with optimized programs of radiation and chemical therapy.

Methods of Breast Cancer Diagnosis

1. Preoperative:

    Main:

    (a) Noninvasive:
    - Clinical examination (medical history, examination, palpation)
    - X-ray mammography
    - Ultrasound mammography

    (b) Invasive:
    - Stereotactic core needle biopsy with histological investigation of biopsy samples
    - US-guided FNA with cytological examination
    - Vacuum aspiration biopsy under ultrasound or X-ray control
    - Cytological evaluation of nipple discharge
    - Preoperative labeling of impalpable tumors by marking needles

    Supplementary (upon indication):
    - Ductography
    - MRI
    - CT
    - Scintigraphy
    - Others (electrical impedance tomography, radiothermometry, etc.)
2. Intraoperative:
    - Urgent histological investigation
    - X-ray study of removed breast sector
3. Postoperative:
    - Histological examination of a specimen

Asymmetry of breasts, areolas, and nipples and deformity and dimpling of the skin and nipple when the arm is raised are *clinical manifestations* of breast tumors. Palpation usually reveals dense immobile tumor with rough surface.

Ulceration may be observed in advanced stages. The skin and areola above the tumor are thickened (Krause symptom). Skin shrinkage and dimpling over the tumor or a symptom of "peau d'orange" are possible. Many breast diseases and tumors (benign and malignant) in the initial stages are asymptomatic.

Accuracy of the clinical examination in detecting benign and malignant tumors does not exceed 50–60%, sensitivity is 40–69%, and specificity is 88–95% (Shevchenko 1997; Korzhenkova 2004) (Fig. 1.3). Palpation also often fails to detect regional lymph nodes affection. The rate of errors in detection of metastatic lymph nodes reaches 32–45.8%.

Imaging techniques, particularly X-ray and ultrasound mammography, are essential in the diagnosis of breast pathology.

Mammography is a technology of obtaining a negative photographic image of the breast that reflects the projected attenuation of the X-ray radiation from mammography device passing through various tissues. First X-ray images of the breast were produced on amputated breasts by A. Salomon in 1913. Primary tumor with spread to the axillary lymph nodes was visualized. To now, the mammography is recognized worldwide as one of the most valuable diagnostic methods for a wide range of diseases, including breast tumors. Digital mammography is the principle diagnostic method for breast pathology in women over 40 years of age.

Mammography represents a two-dimensional image of the breast, which permits assessment of the thickness, glandular tissue density, and specification of the location, shape, borders, and size of focal lesions (Fig. 1.4). As a rule, mammography is performed in frontal (craniocaudal) and oblique (mediolateral) projections. Two projections provide imaging of the whole breast,

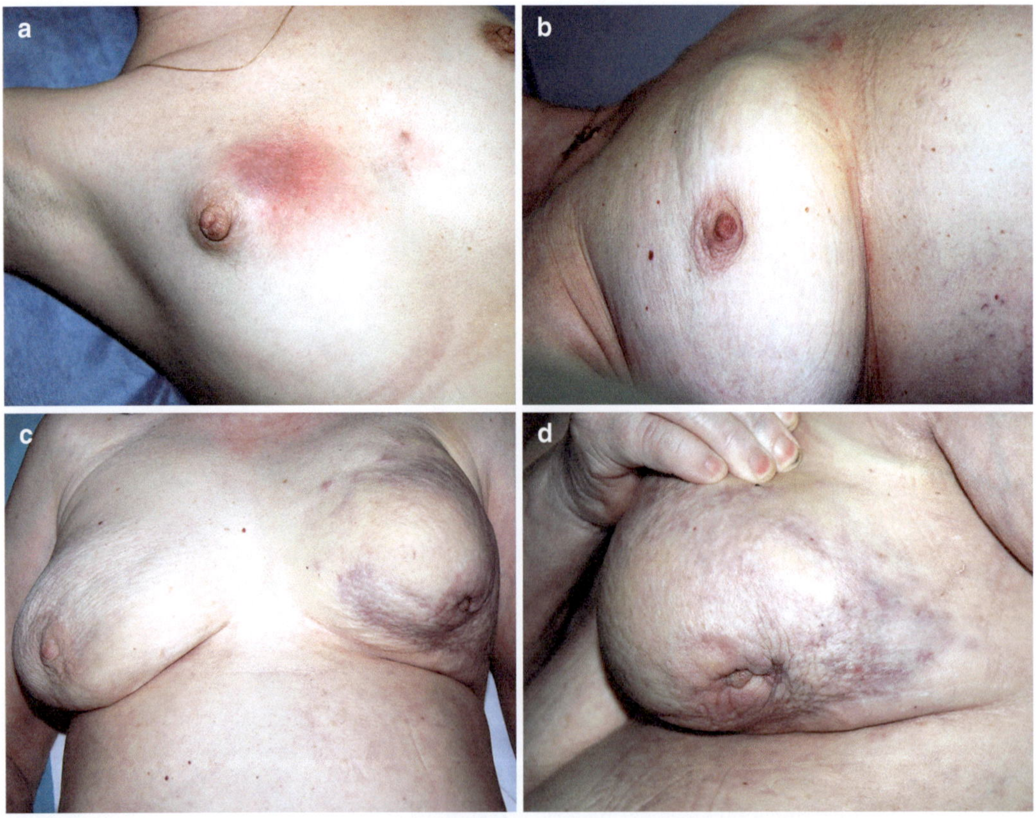

Fig. 1.3 (**a–d**) Visual inspection in patients with breast cancer

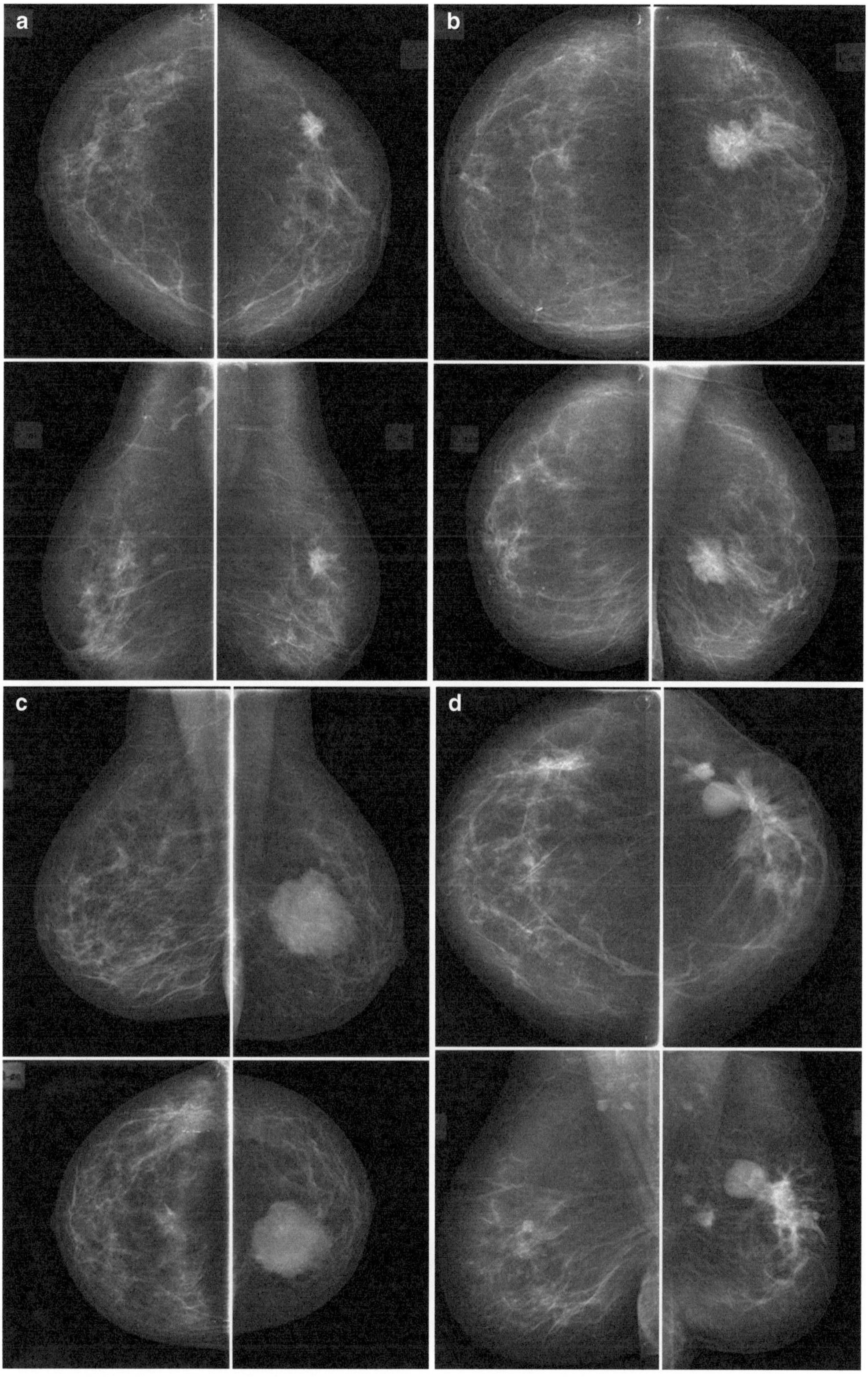

Fig. 1.4 (**a**–**h**) X-ray mammography. Breast cancer

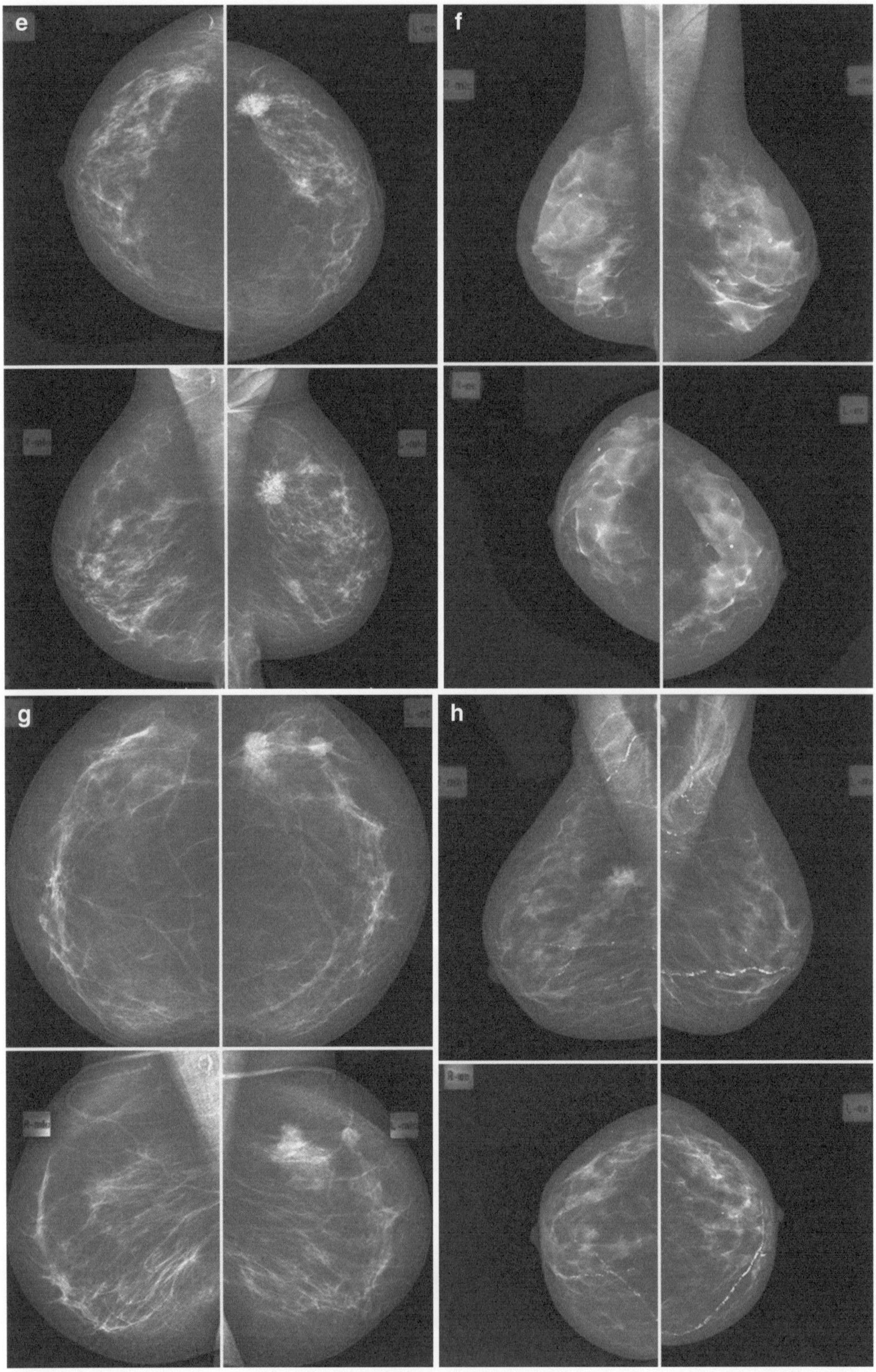

Fig. 1.4 (continued)

allowing to localize the pathological process and differentiate the palpable lesions from the areas with impaired architectonics. In some cases, additional lateral projection is used as a supplement, in order to clarify the lesion location.

Single projection mammography may miss 11–25% of tumors. The study of the sensitivity of mammography demonstrated the highest sensitivity (84%) in patients with correct breast positioning. Alternatively, if the images fail to display the whole breast (33.2%), the sensitivity decreased to 66.3%.

Modern X-ray equipment provides high-quality examination, since it has an automatic exposure system located on the surface of the digital detector, which is designed to recognize the characteristics of the target organ and to optimize contrast level of an image. High-contrast images are obtained owing to implementation of molybdenum (tungsten) anode and molybdenum filter with lower radiation load of the soft radiation spectrum. Adequate breast compression provides almost uniform thickness for achieving sharp mammogram images. Selective compression gives opportunity to estimate the delineation, density of the tumor, and reveal stellate structures, calcifications with a size of 50 μm. The quality of mammography is the result not only of technical characteristics of the equipment but also of the strict adherence to the technique of examination.

Mammography has the following advantages:

- Detection of impalpable breast lesions
- High diagnostic value
- Possibility of invasive and noninvasive diagnostic procedures
- Objective documented data accessible for dynamic analysis

Disadvantages of mammography are the following:

- Ionizing radiation
- Low value in dense and irregular structure of the breast
- Discomfort during the procedure due to breast compression

A patient is indicated for mammography in the following cases:

- Age of 40–50 years (with an interval of 2 years for preventive purposes)
- Age above 50 years (annually)
- Clinical signs or suspicion for breast carcinoma in any age

It should also be noted that standard mammography still has "blind" zones. For example, it is difficult to assess the axillary lymph nodes and the posterior-lateral segments of the breast that extend beyond the anterior axillary line.

Mammography is standardized, does not require any special training (except for studies with contrast agents), and has no contraindications (except for studies with contrast agents).

Tyurin (2011) reported that 2,936,212 mammographic examinations were performed in Russian Federation in 2009. Among them, 2,472,237 were screening mammograms. The sensitivity of mammography in breast cancer was 50–93%. Impalpable carcinomas can be detected with mammography in 76–82% of cases. The specificity of digital mammography in the differential diagnosis of impalpable lesions is 97.2–99.0%, the overall accuracy—98%. According to Rozhkova (1993), palpable breast tumor can be negative with mammography in 3.5–6% of cases.

Numerous randomized studies carried out in the USA by Shapiro, 1966, in Scotland by Alexander, 1999; in Canada by Morrison and Miller, 1992; in Sweden by Tabar, 1999 Andersson, 1997, and Nystrom, 2002; and in Finland by Hakama, 1997, demonstrated that 30–40% reduction in mortality from breast cancer was achieved due to introduction of mammographic screening. Depending on the age, which determines the condition of breast glandular tissue, there is a variability in the specificity and sensitivity of various screening tests. Mammographic screening of women over 50 years contributes to early breast cancer detection. The sensitivity of mammography in invasive breast cancer is lower in women of 40–49 years of age. It is 75% as compared with 93% in women of 50 years and older. This is associated with a greater proportion of fast-growing, more aggressive tumors in young women, resulting in appearance of interval breast cancer between regular screenings. About 8% of them are palpable by the time of mammography. It is believed that the tumor is local without metastases, if its size by the time of detection is smaller than 5–7 mm. The malignant tumors up to 1 cm in size are detected in 10–20% of cases. In fertile women, some tumors can grow up to 20–30 mm, remaining undetectable by mammography on the background of dense glandular tissue. Therefore, the use of other diagnostic methods (e.g., clinical examination) without mammography is useless in terms of early breast cancer detection.

Soft tissues of the axillary regions are rarely examined with radiography. The latter is replaced with mandatory ultrasound of regional lymph nodes, which exhibits high diagnostic value.

In recent years, mammography has undergone significant changes due to the introduction of tomosynthesis, contrast X-ray mammography, and their combinations. Introduction of these techniques eliminates the disadvantages of traditional X-ray mammography. However, they are also not perfect due to time consumption, high radiation exposure, the necessity for monitoring the biochemical indicators (creatinine), and the invasiveness of contrast procedures. It should be noted that due to introduction of tomosynthesis and contrast mammography the digital mammography method became multiparametric. Stereotactic biopsy with mammography is feasible, and impalpable lesions could be labeled under mammography control.

Utilization of new technologies in mammography and the combination of possibilities of analogue, digital, and 3D mammography are advantageous and open new prospects in diagnostics of breast malignancies (Rozhkova et al. 2008).

Digital tomosynthesis of the breast is a modern technology that implies the opportunities of 3D mammography. The breast undergoes a series of low X-ray exposures at different angles with subsequent conversion of obtained data into a series of tomograms with the use of a flat panel detector and the X-ray tube rotation.

Tomosynthesis allows to obtain three-dimensional images of breasts, to analyze each section, excluding the images of overlying or underlying tissues. Tomosynthesis has the following advantages over traditional mammography: it allows to significantly improve the diagnosis quality; reduces the number of additional examinations and biopsies due to improved imaging; increases breast cancer detection in patients with dense structure of breast tissue, FBD prostheses, and implants; reduces the time of examination; and makes the examination more comfortable due to breast compression.

The use of tomosynthesis in X-ray diagnostics increases the impalpable cancer detection, improves the differential diagnostics of the diseases associated with the glandular tissue restructuring by 4%, improves diagnosis of diseases accompanied by calcification by 5%, eliminates the need for additional studies (target mammography, additional settings), reduces the number of invasive interventions due to hyperdiagnosis, and raises the possibility of conservative surgery.

However, tomosynthesis has a higher radiation exposure than standard digital X-ray mammography and, therefore, extended monitoring intervals. Unfortunately, this method, as well as X-ray mammography, is often not effective in patients with dense breast tissue.

Breast MRI (*magnetic resonance imaging*), also known as MR mammography, implies T1- and T2-weighted images; complete magnetic resonance mammography (MRM) provides tomograms of pulse sequences in various planes (axial, sagittal, coronary) without any radiation load. The method allows noninvasive characterization of breast structure, detection of abnormal masses, differential diagnosis between benign and malignant tumors, and evaluation of nearby organs.

MRI is based on the analysis of proton behavior in hydrogen atoms. MR signal, which is captured by the HF coils, is generated due to the magnetization caused by the motion of protons in the transverse plane. Alterations of magnetic field intensity on the body cross sections provide spatial information. MRI allows to evaluate breast structure, to detect pathological lesions, to characterize their structure and the degree of homogeneity and margins, to reveal capsule, to specify invasion to the surrounding structures, and to visualize nearby lymph nodes. Dynamic MRI is a multiparameter technique that allows to detect and interpret minimal changes in breast based on a number of variables, which include different image characteristics (contrast, signal-to-noise ratio, resolution, time interval) and other parameters. At the same time, two important technical requirements are imposed for breast MRI: the use of special coils and contrast agents. According to Tyurin (2011), MRI of the breast constitutes up to 0.2% of the total number of tomography examinations.

The decision on breast MRI should be taken individually, depending on the specific clinical situation. The MRI method is not acceptable as a screening test. It is recommended to women with high-risk of breast cancer with BRCA 1 and BRCA 2 genes mutations.

MRI of the breast is often recommended in the following cases:

- Suspicious tumor in young women with dense breast tissue structure or at a genetic risk of breast cancer
- For determination of the disease extent
- For differential diagnosis of benign and malignant tumors
- For differential diagnosis of recurrent tumors and scarring in breast after previous surgery and radiation therapy (e.g., scar cancer)
- For staging, including assessment of adjacent areas and regional lymph nodes
- During dynamic monitoring of breast after reconstructive operations
- For adjuvant chemotherapy monitoring

MRM does not require special preparation; its contraindications are similar to those for MRI and to the administration of contrast agents.

Examination of breast by MRM takes 30–60 min. It is performed with a special coil, in the supine position. Certain attempts to shorten the duration of the procedure have been made. However, they have not achieved real success yet. Currently MRM is most frequently used for the assessment of breast implants and for the detection of malignant tumors. Specific pulse sequences allow to visualize silicone and to detect implant damage with practically 100% accuracy. Previously, this technical capability was used to detect silicone leaks after percutaneous breast plasty with gel. However, due to abandonment of this procedure, this issue is no longer relevant. For the detection of malignant tumors, the study is performed exclusively with bolus injection of contrast agent.

MRI has the following advantages (Serebryakova et al. 2011):

- High resolution and contrast of breast tissue
- Multiparameter evaluation of the detected changes (not only the image itself but also the cell density, the contrast agent kinetics, and even, if necessary, metabolites by MR spectroscopy are assessed)
- Possibility of simultaneous evaluation of both mammary glands and multiparametric analysis of an unlimited number of lesions
- Possibility of obtaining images in any random plane without mechanical repositioning, absence of "blind" zones
- Operator-independent procedure
- Noninvasiveness
- Absence of radiation load

Utilization of contrast agents (gadolinium-containing paramagnetics) significantly increases the diagnostic capabilities of MRI and allows to obtain better temporal and spatial resolution, differentiate malignant and benign breast tumors, and detect carcinomas up to 3 mm in size. Evaluation of contrast agent accumulation by an abnormal lesion with maximum intensity projection (MIP) reconstructions provides information of the tumor vasculature. Additional information is obtained by the analysis of contrast kinetics on T1-weighted images, such as contrast wash-in, washout, and time-intensity curves (Figs. 1.5, 1.6, and 1.7).

Dynamic studies make it possible to reliably differentiate lesions from normal tissue and to effectively detect extent, multifocality, and multicentricity of breast cancer. Sensitivity of

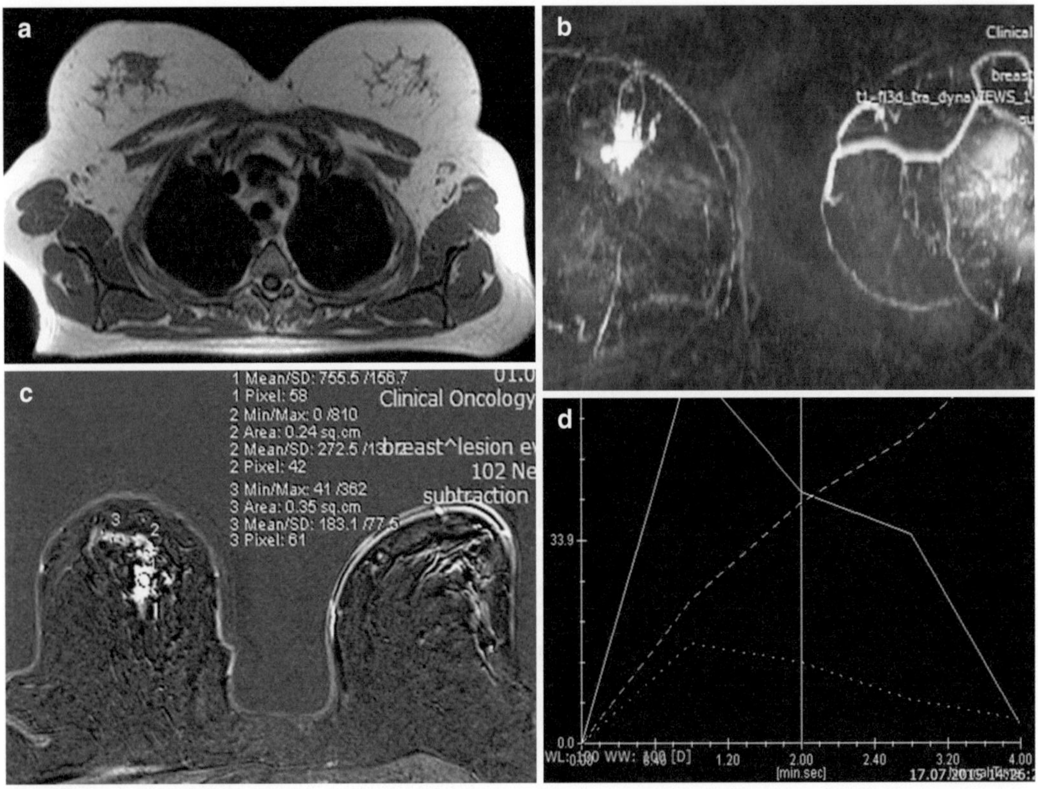

Fig. 1.5 Breast cancer. MRI. (**a**) T1WI. (**b**) MIP reconstruction. (**c**) TIRM (turbo inversion recovery magnitude). (**d**) Signal time-intensity curve

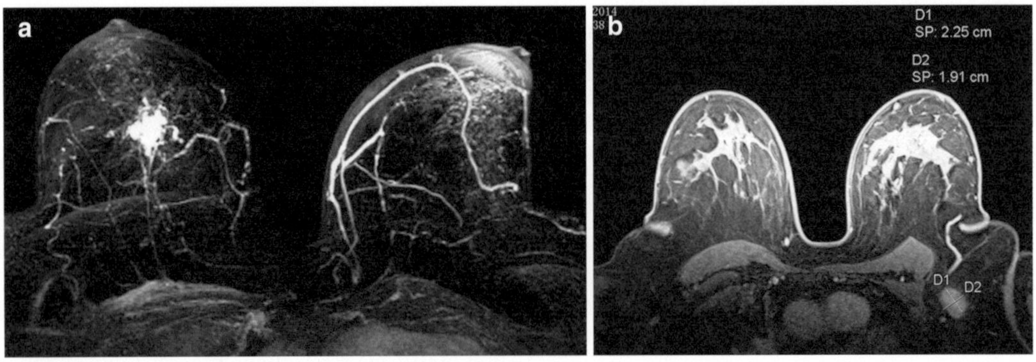

Fig. 1.6 Breast cancer. MRM. T1WI. (**a**) MIP. Coronal plane. Contrast accumulation in the central aspects of the right breast, deformation of vessel pattern. (**b**) Axial lymph node

contrast-enhanced MRM in the diagnosis of breast tumors is 83–100%, specificity—29–97% (Serebryakova et al. 2015). Berg et al. (2009) noted high diagnostic value of MRM in the detection of multifocality of breast cancer. Sensitivity of MRI in the diagnosis of breast cancer after augmentation mammoplasty is also high and reaches 85.7% with specificity of 98.2% (Savello and Shumakova 2014). High costs of MRI equipment make it reasonable to use the technology only in complicated diagnostic cases (Haylenko et al. 2005).

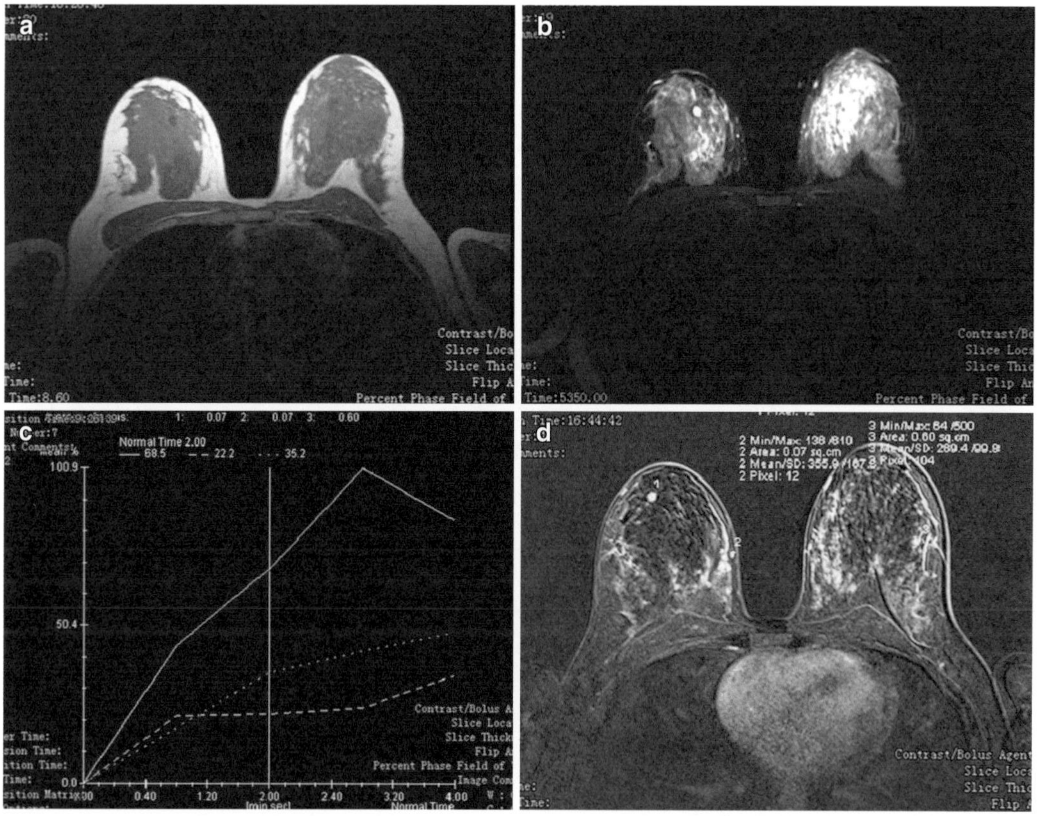

Fig. 1.7 Mammary fibroadenoma. MRM. T1WI: (**a**, **b**) TIRM (turbo inversion recovery magnitude). (**c**) Signal time-intensity curve. (**d**) MIP reconstruction

MRI allows detecting 2.7 times more tumors than X-ray mammography. A combination of these two methods increases detection of malignancies by 20% (Korzhenkova et al. 2006). MRI improves the detection of not only invasive tumors but also preinvasive ones, such as ductal carcinoma in situ and precancerous lesions (atypical ductal hyperplasia).

X-ray computed mammography (CT) is a modern radiological technology (Fig. 1.8). However, the technology is not a screening modality for breast carcinoma either. It is due to significant radiation, high cost of examination, and low throughput. CT practically has no advantages in early recognition of breast carcinoma as compared to mammography. However, the method is of great importance in assessment of cancer invasion and is indicated to detect spreading of the tumor to retromammary space, metastases in lymph nodes, and remote metastases. The diagnostic value of CT in detection of breast cancer is 60–62%, sensitivity is 100%, and specificity is 84% (Haylenko et al. 2005).

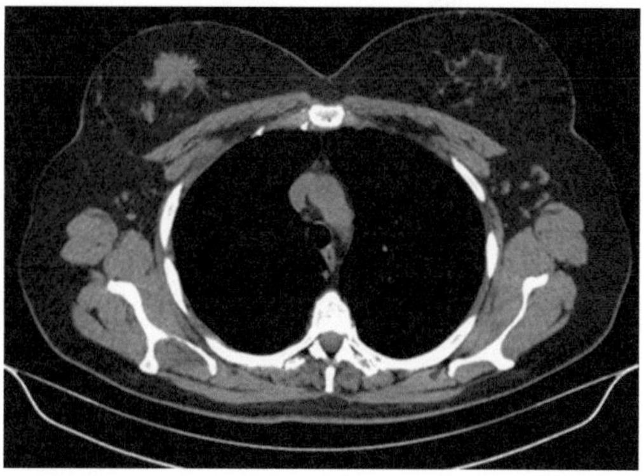

Fig. 1.8 Computed mammography. Breast cancer

The sensitivity and specificity of CT mammography with intravenous contrast enhancement in the diagnosis of recurrent breast cancer are 97.4% and 98.4%, in the diagnosis of metastases in regional lymph nodes—91.6% and 91.4%, respectively.

Mammoscintigraphy is a method of functional diagnostics of breast pathology, which is based on the assessment of distribution of radiopharmaceuticals in breast tissues (Fig. 1.9). ^{99m}Tc-MIBI,

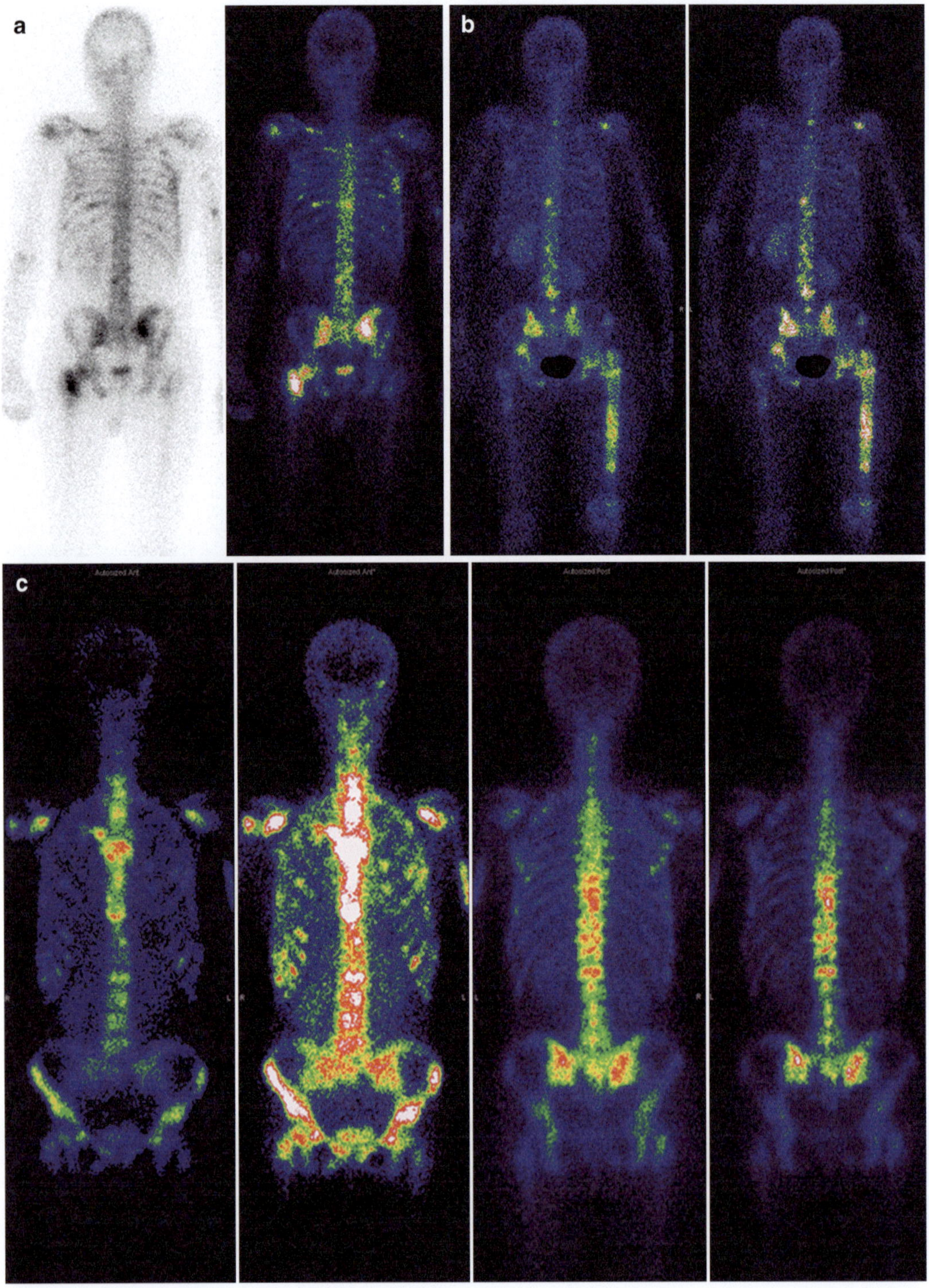

Fig. 1.9 Bone scintigraphy. (**a–d**) 500 mBq ^{99M}Tc Pyrfotech

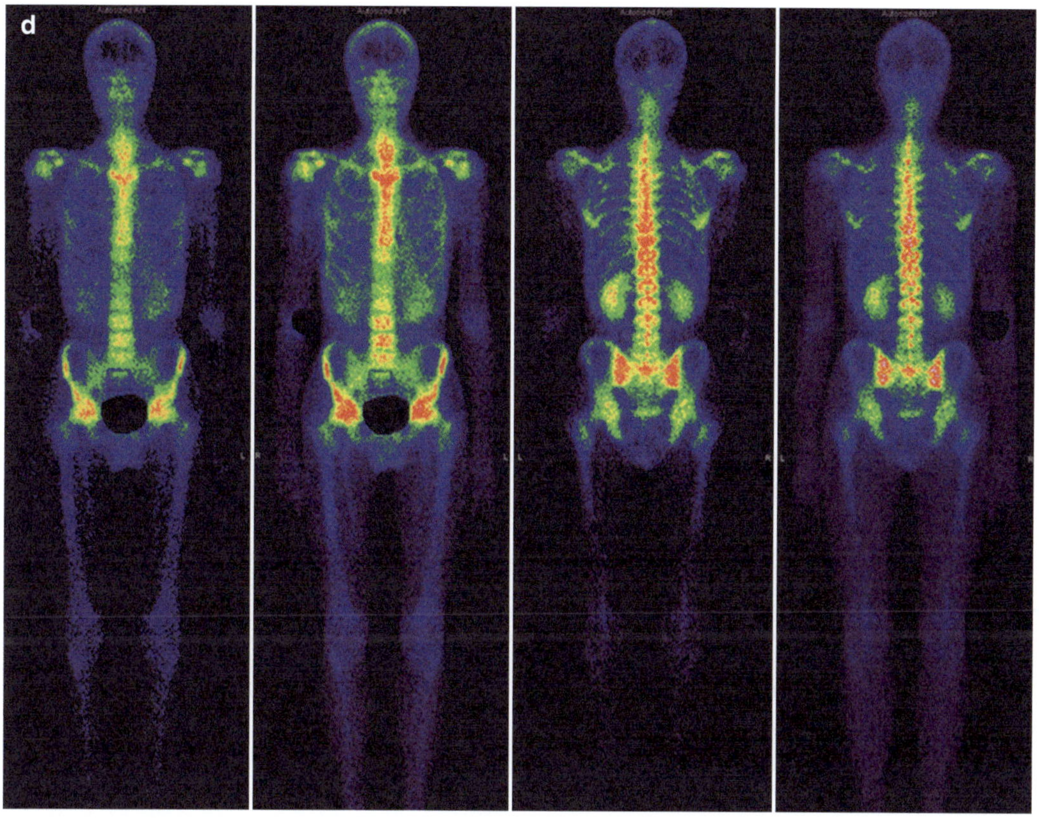

Fig. 1.9 (continued)

^{99m}Tc-tehnetril, ^{99m}Tc-teoksim, ^{99m}Tc-tetrofosmin, and others can be utilized for the examination. Mammoscintigraphy along with studying of the breast permits assessment of isotope distribution in other chest structures including axillary areas and other regions of possible metastases.

The technology can be performed in two varieties: with gamma chamber (planar scanning, emission gamma tomography) or positron-emission tomography. In those cases, it can be carried out as an isolated breast scintigraphy, a polypositional scintigraphy of the chest, or as a single-photon emission computed tomography of the breast area and thorax.

The overall sensitivity of breast scintigraphy in the diagnosis of breast diseases is 72.4%; in fibrocystic breast disease, fibrous adenoma, and duct ectasia, 52.5%; in glandular, mixed FBD with palpable masses, 79.9%.

Mammoscintigraphy with ^{99m}Tc-MIBI is not of great value in revealing primary breast carcinoma. Its sensitivity depends on the size of the lesion. The sensitivity differs in different cancer stages: at T1a (up to 0.5 cm), 26%; at T1b (up to 1 cm), 56%; at T1c (up to 2 cm), 95%; and at T2, 97%. The sensitivity of breast scintigraphy with ^{99m}Tc-technetryl in primary breast tumor is 62–96.7%, specificity 71–100% (Kharchenko and Rozhkova 2005). At the same time, ^{199}Tl is slightly less sensitive than ^{99m}Tc-MIBI the detection of regional lymph nodes metastasis.

SPECT with ^{199}Tl has a higher specificity (96.7%) compared to ^{99m}Tc-MIBI (90%). SPECT with ^{199}Tl and ^{99m}Tc-MIBI have higher sensitivity (98 and 98.5%, respectively) in detection of malignant breast tumors over 1 cm in size.

The sensitivity of scintigraphy in the detection of metastases of breast carcinoma in axillary lymph nodes is 51–85%, specificity is 91–93%, and diagnostic accuracy is 76–93% (Svensson et al. 2000).

In SPECT with ^{99m}Tc-technetryl, the sensitivity, specificity, and overall accuracy in the diagnosis of axillary lymph nodes lesions were 75%,

84%, and 81%, respectively. In SPECT/CT these indicators increased to 75%, 89%, and 84%, respectively. In absence of pathological changes at SPECT/CT images, the probability of metastasis to sentinel axillary lymph nodes does not exceed 6%. The use of SPECT/CT along with the administration of 555 MBq Tm-99m-technetryl (MIBI) allows a more detailed evaluation of the infiltrative-edematous breast cancer. The use of the technique is appropriate at the final stage of the diagnostic program as a clarifying method.

Positron-emission tomography (PET) is the nuclear medicine technology based on utilization of various agents (monosaccharides, fat acids, antibodies, peptides, etc.), marked with positron emitting radionuclides. A modified gamma chamber is applied. It permits detection of gamma photons, which result from annihilation of positron with electron. Since gamma photons are emitted in opposite directions, it is possible to localize the place of their formation. Short-lived radioactive tracer isotope, which is chemically incorporated into a biologically active molecule (more often 18F-fluordeoxyglucose), allows to detect areas with increased metabolic activity that is often the characteristic of malignant cells.

PET is not widely applied in diagnosis of breast carcinoma now. Nevertheless, it is quite a promising technology. Indications for PET are limited due to low diagnostic value in small cancers, which are smaller than 1 cm in size. However, PET surpasses all known anatomic imaging methods in the localization of centers of breast carcinoma in soft tissues. Its possibilities should be applied for individualization of therapy and monitoring, since tumor metabolism decreases much faster than tumor size with effective treatment. Alternatively, absence of changes in tumor metabolism after treatment predicts its inefficiency.

Some studies of preoperative staging of breast cancer have shown that the sensitivity of PET in the diagnosis of multifocal lesion was twice higher than the sensitivity of combined mammography and US. Sensitivity and specificity of PET in metastatic lesions of axillary lymph nodes are 79% and 92%, respectively.

Development of PET for the diagnosis of breast cancer has the following main trends: technological improvements (development of more efficient detectors, hybrid systems, hardware and software implementation), search for new radiopharmaceuticals for the diagnosis of specific tumors, and prediction of effects of chemo-, hormono- and radiotherapy.

Combined methods (hybrid PET technologies) are quite in demand in modern medicine. They allow simultaneous imaging of morphological and metabolic changes, thus increasing the accuracy of tumor specification, and assessment of the disease extent beyond the primary lesion (Fig. 1.10).

Currently, devices that combine PET with computed tomography and/or MRI (PET/CT, PET/MRI) are most common. Previously, PET and CT were regarded as complementary methods that were used consequently in the diagnosis of breast diseases. Combination of metabolic PET images and anatomical CT images required specific software. This problem was solved through the introduction of combined PET/CT. The first experimental scanner was created by Nutt and Townsend in 1998. Currently PET/CT is very important for detection of local recurrence of breast cancer, as well as regional and distant metastases.

PET/MRI is a recent achievement of hybrid radiology, and therefore this technology is still under study. According to the creators, this combined technology may be more sensitive in the diagnosis of some cancers and metastases than PET/CT. A great advantage of PET/MRI is significantly reduced radiation load in comparison with PET/CT and high contrast of soft tissues for MRI.

The importance of some other diagnostic methods for breast study (radiothermometry, electrical impedance computed tomography, laser mammography, microwave spectroscopy) is insignificant. Those technologies are rare and have limited clinical indications.

Electrical impedance tomography is a method of scanning of electrical impedance (full resistance) of breast tissues (Korzhenevsky 2003). It permits visual assessment of breast structure for

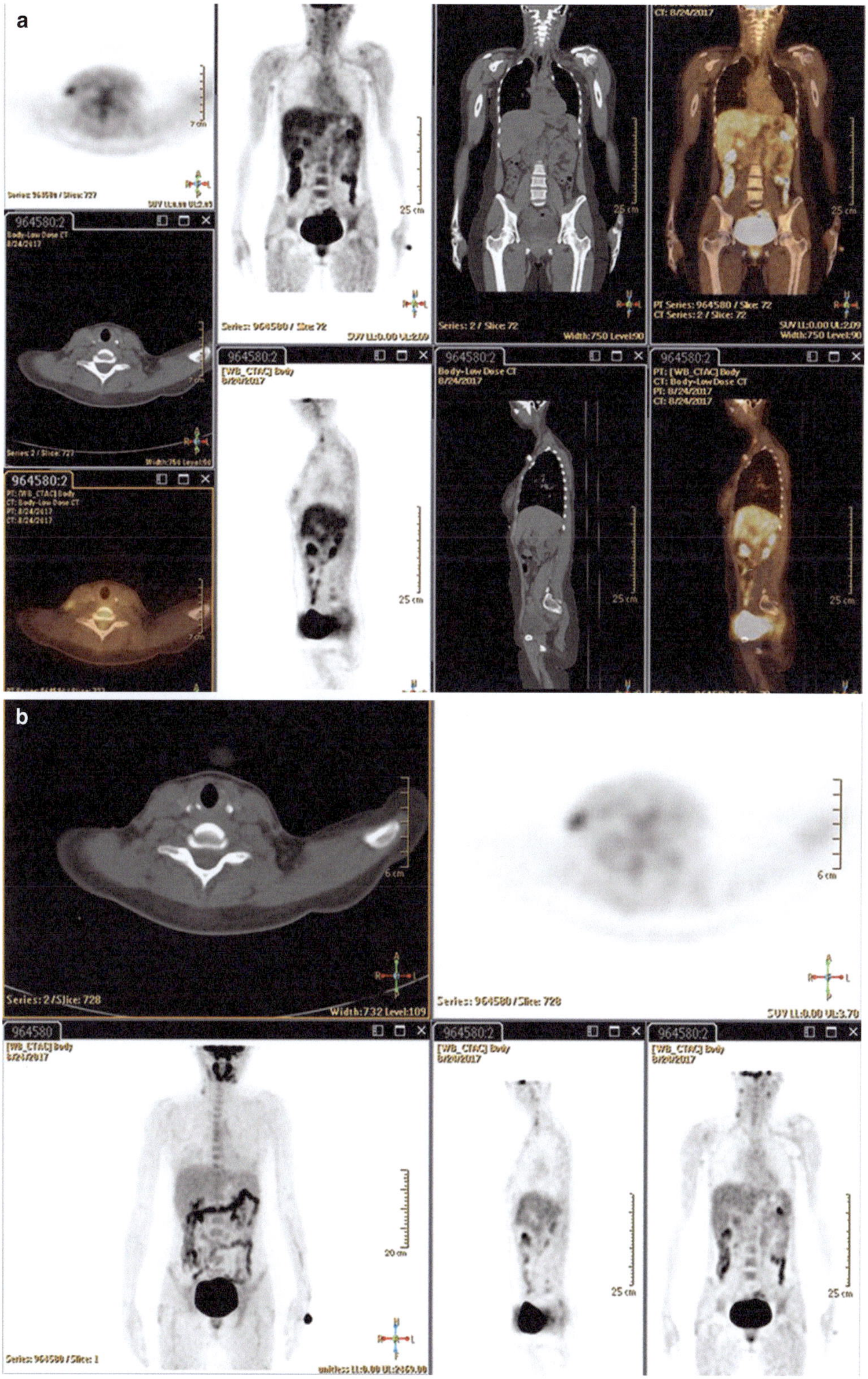

Fig. 1.10 (**a**, **b**) PET/CT. Distant metastases of breast cancer in bones and spine

differential diagnosis of various physiological conditions and changes, which accompany breast cancer. It analyzes distribution of electrical conductivity of breast tissues in several cross sections and detects pathological focus with abnormal value of electrical conductivity (Fig. 1.11).

According to Trohanova (2010), electrical impedance mammography is a simple and efficient method of screening of focal breast pathology in women of different ages. The sensitivity, specificity, and positive and negative prognostic values account for the following figures: for cysts, 91%, 99%, 93%, and 99%; for diffuse cystic breast disease, 98%, 97%, 95%, and 99%; and for breast carcinoma, 92%, 98%, 92%, and 98% (Trohanova 2010).

Radiothermometry is a modality, which permits noninvasive measurement of the temperature in deep tissues. It is based on remote registration of infrared radiation by means of special devices. The results of the examination are presented as a thermogram (temperature plot). The areas with increased temperature are suspicious for breast malignancy due to higher metabolism and good vascularity. The character of breast thermograms depends on the age. Besides, there are individual features of location of "cold" and "hot" areas that sometimes complicate correct interpretation of the results. Radiothermometry is not often used nowadays in diagnosis of breast cancer because of a large number of false-positive tests, which can exceed 25%. The specificity of radiothermometry in diagnosis of breast carcinoma is reported 85%, sensitivity 84%, and in combination with US 91% (Yemelyanov et al. 2011).

Evidence-based medicine forces to perform the most significant diagnostic tests to work out the strategy of treatment. It seeks to obtain the data about tumor morphology. The conclusion about tumor structure results from invasive diagnostic procedures.

Core needle biopsy of breast tumors implies a stereotactic X-ray device and special instruments—biopsy gun- and guillotine-type needles. The technique is intended for an accurate collection of biopsy material for pathologic study and is a definite procedure in the diagnosis of breast lesions (refer to Chap. 12). The sensitivity of stereotactic biopsy in breast cancer is 97.6%, specificity is 100%, and diagnostic accuracy is 98% (Kuplevatskaya 2004).

Vacuum-assisted breast biopsy with stereotactic mammography or ultrasound guidance is an ergonomic and highly effective method of obtaining cellular material for verification (refer to Chap. 12). It permits to obtain multiple samples of tissue via a single needle. The procedure can be carried out not only with diagnostic but also with the treating purpose.

Wide application of US as a navigation method permits targeted *fine needle aspiration biopsy* (FNAB), which is highly efficient in obtaining samples from pathological foci (refer to Chap. 12). Subsequent cytology allows to define cellular structures in the sample and to differentiate lesions of various natures. According to Sinyukova et al. (2007), US-guided FNAB of breast lesions in combination with mammography and routine breast US improves early detection of breast cancer (up to 95–98%).

Ultrasound (US) is now one of the most widespread and affordable imaging methods for diagnosis of breast pathology, early and differential diagnosis of breast masses, and guidance of minimally invasive modalities. High efficiency of US in breast cancer diagnosis is provided by high sensitivity and specificity (Table 1.1).

The sensitivity of US in diagnosis of different variants of breast carcinoma depends on the histological type of a neoplasm. If added to mammography, US increases the sensitivity in detection of early impalpable cancer.

Significant development of US equipment allows detecting minimal pathological changes of breast parenchyma (lesions from 1 to 2 mm) and registering pathognomonic signs for differentiation between benign and malignant processes. Modern US scanners in the majority of cases permit confirmation of mammographic conclusion of a breast carcinoma and allow to diagnose X-ray-negative tumors. According to Otto (1993), the rate of detection of mammography-negative breast malignancies reaches 62%.

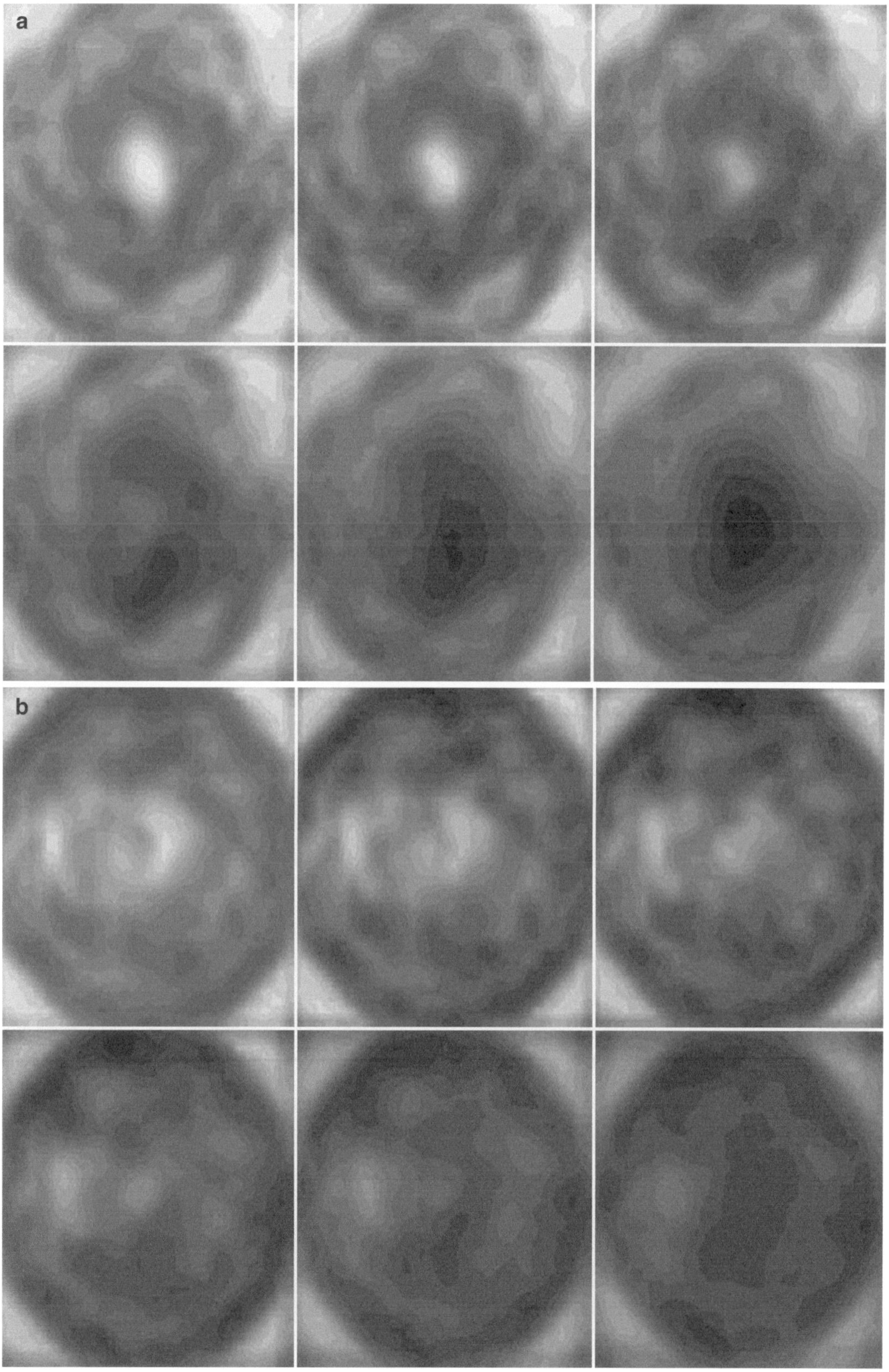

Fig. 1.11 Electrical impedance tomography. (**a**) Normal breast. (**b**) Breast carcinoma

Table 1.1 Diagnostic value of ultrasound in the diagnosis of breast cancer

Authors	Year	Sensitivity (%)	Specificity (%)
Skott	1992	59	98
Saitoh et al.	1994	95.2	83.6
Kuijpers et al.	1994	76	56
Lee et al.	1995	94.5	83.3
De Albertis et al.	1995	100	96
Schroeder et al.	1998	67	45
Elsamaloty	1999	86.9	99
Zabolotsky et al.	1999	94.1	95
Blohmer et al.	1999	95	80
Kook et al.	1999	77	76
Malur	2000	83	92
Sandrick	2001	89	76
Andrushenko	2001	56.2	87.5
Tsesarsky	2002	93.3	98
Houssami	2003	81.7	88.0
Yefremova et al.	2003	96	98
Sim et al.	2004	83.3	65.5
Kukhareva	2005	88.3	96.4
Myers et al.	2006	62	99
Kuklin	2006	58	80
Avramenko	2006	86.9	92.59
Grunwald et al.	2007	67.3	61.5
Korzhenkova	2007	83	86.1
Sinukova et al.	2007	83.6	86.9
Zikiryakhodzhaev	2007	85	90
Zabolotskaya	2009	90	82
Trufanov et al.	2009	92.3	84.1
Zubarev	2009	78.9	95.2
Rozhkova et al.	2010	73.3	92.8
Sencha et al.	2010	93.3	73.7
Khokhlova	2010	87.5	94.5
Yemelyanov et al.	2011	76	
Rozhkova et al.	2011	78.6	94.5
Fazylova et al.	2012	91.9	87.2
Sencha et al.	2015	94.4	91.6
Yevseeva	2015	76	57
Maksimiva	2015	97.6	86
Moon et al.	2017	90.4	94.7

US provides high accuracy of breast cancer diagnosis, including impalpable and X-ray negative neoplasms, in the cases with previous mammography. The role of US in evaluation of surrounding structures, especially regional lymph nodes, is also important (Table 1.2).

Advanced ultrasound technologies, such as color-coded modes, three-dimensional image reconstruction, multiplanar scanning, ultrasound elastography, and contrast-enhanced echography, provide new diagnostic solutions and advantages.

Improvement of diagnostic equipment and accessibility of modern mammography and ultrasound are urgent issues for differential diagnosis of benign and malignant breast tumors with simi-

Table 1.2 Diagnostic value of multiparametric ultrasound examination in the diagnosis of axillary lymph node metastases in breast cancer

Authors	Year	Sensitivity (%)	Specificity (%)	Diagnostic value (%)
Bonnemia	1988	87	56	
Harchenko et al.	1995	88		80
Fielder et al.	1997	87.5	56.9	
Stavros et al.	2005	91	72	57
Haylenko et al.	2005	91	72	57
Popli et al.	2006	86.3	41.6	73.3
Sinukova et al.	2007	91	57	72
Savelyeva	2014	92.9	79.2	

Table 1.3 Comparison of the diagnostic value of different techniques for benign and malignant breast diseases

	Techniques							
	Clinical examination		X-ray mammography		Ultrasound		Pathologic study	
Disease	$n = 4150$	Diagnostic value (%)	$n = 3952$	Diagnostic value (%)	$n = 4638$	Diagnostic value (%)	$n = 1011$	Diagnostic value (%)
Diffuse mastopathy	1298	99.5	1206	92.4	1278	98	104	8
Nodular mastopathy	1326	98.9	1268	94.6	1286	96	321	24
Cysts	318	56	204	36	560	98.9	2	0.4
Fibroadenoma	729	74	730	48	954	96.8	20	2
Impalpable breast cancer	0	0	76	100	74	97.3	73	96
Palpable breast cancer	479	84	468	82	468	94	491	86

lar or equivocal clinical or imaging data. Mammography is preferable in changes in the gland tissues, such as local fibrosis, microcalcifications, or subcentimetric tumors. US is more valuable for specification of cysts, fibroadenomas, lipomas, some malignant tumors, and duct ectasia (Table 1.3). In the diagnosis of tumors, breast US is more competitive than X-ray mammography. Both diagnostic methods would benefit from their combined use in the differential diagnosis of cysts, large benign soft tissue tumors, tumor-like masses, and malignant tumors (Sencha 2015; Evseeva 2015). To assess the spread of the tumor, CT or MRI is strongly recommended.

An effective breast examination flow integrates several imaging methods. This allows to increase the rate of detection of carcinomas at stage I from 13 to 80%. Information technologies that bring any specialty to a new level are actively integrated into mammology. A number of digital information technologies have been developed, such as CAD, computer-aided diagnostic system for screening; AWP, automated workplace of a radiologist-mammologist; radiology information system "IntegRIS"; and further on. These tools allow remote image reading and electronic archiving.

A system for integrated use of noninvasive and invasive diagnostic methods facilitates accurate timely diagnosis of breast diseases followed with individual management. The logistics of diagnostics and further tactics are demonstrated in Fig. 1.12).

Complex examination includes detection, differential diagnosis of diffuse and focal breast changes, and further selection of management tactics. In the case of suspected cancer, this should comprise a puncture with morphological verification, surgical treatment, and effective monitoring.

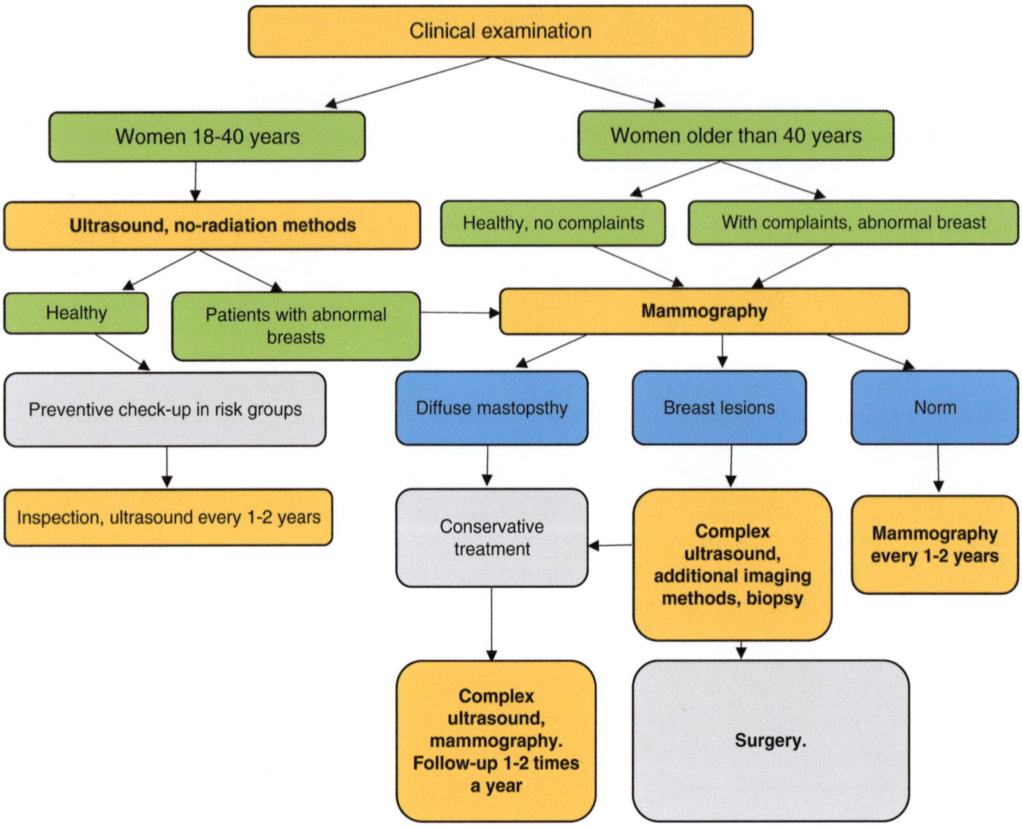

Fig. 1.12 Flowchart of breast examination in outpatients

1.2 Breast Cancer Screening

The risk of breast cancer increases with age. For a newborn girl, the risk of breast cancer is 3.5%, and the risk of dying from it is 1.8% (Korzhenkova 2004). The risk of developing breast cancer within 10 years is 1:72 for women 40–49 years old, 1:36 for women 50–64 years old, and 1:29 for women over 70 (Korzhenkova 2004). Unfortunately, there is no real way to prevent breast cancer. However, if breast cancer is detected at the preclinical stage with a tumor smaller than 1 cm^3, the probability of metastases is low and the majority patients can be cured. Therefore, practicing physicians should focus on the detection of tumors 1 cm^3 or smaller. According to some well-known model, the "natural history" of breast cancer lasts from the first hypothetical cancer cell till the death of the patient. The tumor reaches the size of 1 cm^3 in 30 cell doublings, i.e., within the period of 2–18 years depending on the rate of tumor doubling. The growth and metastatic spreading rate determine the "natural history" of the disease.

Populational health check-ups aimed at early detection of the disease is actually a screening program. The goal of the oncologic screening programs is an active detection of asymptomatic and early stages of cancer. Such programs should be implemented with regard to their reasonability for those cancer types that represent an important public health problem at the country or regional level because of high morbidity and mortality rate.

The screening program (for breast cancer, as well as for cancer of other organs) should meet the following requirements:

- Meet theoretical basis of screening studies
- Include a variety of tests of high sensitivity, specificity, and diagnostic accuracy
- To be noninvasive, if possible minimally (or absolutely) harmless

- Equipment should be accessible and easy to operate and maintain
- Affordable and cost-effective

The basic concept of screening is the detection of the disease early enough to ensure optimistic prognosis and change of the "natural" clinical course. Two parameters are essential in assessing the screening test quality: sensitivity and specificity. High specificity tests are more important for healthy population. They provide a minimum number of false-positive results thus allow to avoid unnecessary biopsies and sometimes excessive surgical treatment. The probability of breast cancer detection with screening depends on the length of time period when the tumor is detectable preclinically. The longer this interval, the greater the chance of tumor detection. The effect of applying better treatment methods, noted along with the introduction of screening programs, should not be confused with the role and impact of screening on morbidity and mortality in particular cancer types.

Breast cancer screening includes a massive preventive examination of healthy women to identify early-stage tumors. The value of any breast cancer screening method is a possibility to identify favorable in prognostic terms asymptomatic preinvasive and early invasive forms of the disease, which in most cases correspond to a tumor up to 1 cm in size.

Breast cancer screening methods:

1. Patient's self-examination
2. Medical examination, palpation of the breast and regional lymph nodes
3. Mammography
4. US
5. MRI
6. Laboratory study of hemostasis, immune and endocrine tests

About 80% of cases of breast cancer are self-detected, 10% detected by medical examination, and only 10% detected by mammography (Korzhenkova 2004).

Despite numerous publications on the importance of self-examination of mammary glands, its accuracy is not established. The sensitivity of the technique is about 26%, which is significantly less than in clinical examination and mammography. The decrease of sensitivity from 41% in women aged 35–39 to 21% among patients aged 60–74 years was observed. By now, there is no evidence of decrease in breast cancer mortality rate in self-examination group. According to various authors, the sensitivity of clinical breast examination is 40–69%, specificity—88–95%.

The main method of breast cancer screening is mammography. This method was a breakthrough in mammology as it was the first to supply an image of the breast structure and to detect impalpable neoplasms in a prompt and precise manner. Massive X-ray screening of healthy women for early breast cancer was proposed for the first time by Gohen in 1956 and was introduced into clinical practice by Frame and Carlson in 1975. Mammographic screening that is capable to detect a wide range of breast neoplasms is a typical example of successfully applied screening program in a number of European countries. The coverage of mammography screening in the USA was 70% in 2014. The highest coverage is reported by Scandinavian countries: in Finland, 90%, and in Sweden, 85%.

Tumor size is an important criterion for evaluation of the screening quality. The tumor of 0.5–1.0 cm in size is very difficult to detect clinically (Korzhenkova 2004). Mammography remains the best screening method for women with a "standard" risk of breast cancer (Semiglazov 2001). The efficiency of screening mammography is 77% in women 40–49 years of age and 95% in women over 50 years (Rasskazova and Rozhkova 2014). This is associated with two factors. First, in women under 50 years, fast-growing, aggressive neoplasms represent most cancer cases. In this group, the incidence of interval breast cancer is significantly higher. Second, the structure of breast tissue in fertile women makes it difficult to detect small malignant tumors. Positive screening tests indicate further examination (diagnostic mammography, US) in 2–22% of cases; diagnostic mammograms indicate biopsy in 12–78% (Korzhenkova 2004). Mammographic screening can reduce mortality from breast cancer by 30% in 5–7 years from the first screening and by 20% in 15–20 years from the first screening (Semiglazov 2001).

Efficiency of preventive mammography examination depends on the factors mentioned below:

- Standards compliance
- The quality of mammography equipment
- Qualification of the personnel
- Experience in conducting massive examinations

In order to conduct an effective screening, there is a need for trained personnel at mammography facilities to properly assess the inevitable (in 4–12% of cases) X-ray-negative breast tumors, as well as interval tumors, detected (in 15–25% of cases) in the intervals between cancer screening examinations (Semiglazov 2001).

The sensitivity of mammography is 77–95% with the specificity of 94–97%. It depends on the woman's age, breast density, the quality of examination, etc. In women with dense mammary glands (young age, hormone replacement therapy), with low quality of mammography, or insufficient radiologist's skills the diagnostic value of mammography may be low. Early detection of breast cancer reduced the mortality rate in women of 50–69 years to one-third.

However, mammography as a screening method has a number of drawbacks:

- "Interval" breast cancer occurs in 15–25% of cases; this is not the drawback of mammography itself but of screening programs in general.
- X-ray negative breast cancer occurs in 5–12% of cases. It is diagnosed with other methods.
- False-negative mammography results (5–25%).

Different countries use different intervals between screening mammography studies. It is, as a rule, 1–2 years, which are needed to reduce both costs and radiation exposure. Many authors report that interval cancer is usually detected at early stage and does not significantly affect the survival rate in this group of patients.

True X-ray-negative breast cancer occurs not so often (no more than in 12%). The majority of diagnostic mistakes are associated with high mammographic density of the mammary gland. The diagnostic accuracy of mammography in patients under 40 years is significantly lower than the same of US due to large glandular component. Alternatively, it is higher, as compared with US, in patients over 50 years with fatty involution of mammary glands.

A number of cases appear false negative at both mammography and clinical examination. This can result from a variety of factors, such as the quality of equipment, personnel's skills, or breast anatomical features (e.g., density, scars). It leads to delayed diagnosis and late treatment. Some women refuse further examination and monitoring. Up to 25% of cases of invasive breast cancer are missed with mammography in patients aged 40–49 years, in comparison with 10% cases in patients aged 50–59 years. Therefore, it is necessary to use additional methods, possibly self-examination, MRI, or US in 40–49 year old women (Korzhenkova 2004).

Although MRI allows effective tumor detection in high-risk women with a mutation in the BRCA 1 or BRCA 2 gene, the MRI screening is unacceptable as a screening test due to high cost and lack of consistent standard approaches to its performance. MRI of the breast is less accessible for a patient. It is characterized by high sensitivity, but not specificity, thus producing a large number of false-positive results, which, in turn, can lead to unreasonable biopsy.

In daily practice of a mammologist-oncologist, US, as a rule, is not regarded as a breast cancer screening method. This is a consequence of the fact that US in outpatient facilities has limited value due to middle class equipment with low resolution and high dependence on the skills and experience of US specialist. However, in the last decade, advanced ultrasound equipment and new options (Doppler modes, 3D reconstruction, elastography, contrast enhancement, high-frequency probes up to 12–18 MHz) significantly expanded the diagnostic capabilities of US (Rybnikova et al. 2017). This method has a number of advantages that can compensate the drawbacks of mammography and make it appropriate for mass examinations in young female population.

Table 1.4 Comparison of sensitivity of screening test for breast cancer in patients with family history of breast cancer

%	Mammography	US	Mammography + US	MRM	MRM + US	MRM + mammography
Sensitivity	33	37	48	93	93	100
Specificity	93	98	98	98	99	98
PPV	39	36	33	48	50	40
NPV	99	99	99	99	99	100

Table 1.5 Comparison of sensitivity of screening test for breast cancer in patients at high genetic risk of breast cancer

%	Mammography	US	Mammography + US	MRM	MRM + US	MRM + mammography
Sensitivity	50	52	63	91	93	93
Specificity	99	99	98	97	97	97
PPV	74	77	65	62	60	59
NPV	98	98	98	97	99	99

Echography is accessible and widely used, easy enough to perform, and effective in early and differential diagnosis of breast cancer and in assessment of surrounding tissues and regional lymph nodes (Sencha et al. 2017).

Differentiation of palpable breast cancer, diffuse fibrocystic breast disease, fibroadenoma, and lipoma is efficient with US screening. On the contrary, certain types of breast pathology, such as local fibrosis, adenosis, noninvasive breast cancer in situ, edematous-infiltrative, and some other types of breast cancer, are more effectively detected by X-ray method. US, in contrast to mammography, does not detect microcalcifications. Breast focal changes, which do not exclude malignant process, are detected with US and X-ray methods almost with the same rate. Diagnostic capabilities of US, mammography, and MRI are mostly determined by women's age-specific features, necessitating complex use of these methods in breast pathology screening.

Laboratory screening of breast cancer selects patients of risk groups based on blood coagulation indicators and immune and endocrine tests (Adamyan et al. 1989). Various cancer markers (CA 15-3, CA 27-29, cancer embryonic antigen) are being used in modern oncology. At the same time, their use for screening is associated with significant expenses and technical limitations.

Since the sensitivity of mammography in the diagnosis of malignant tumors in dense breast is limited, it seems more efficient to use either a combination of mammography with US/MRI or just multiparametric mammography. It is especially valuable in patients with dense breast and/or scarring, for detection of metastatic lymph nodes, and in follow-up of high-risk patients. An effective examination system integrates mammography, US, MRI, and MDCT. This increases the detection of the stage I carcinomas from 13% to 80% (Semiglazov 2001).

The statistics on the detection of breast malignancies is different in patients of risk group (with familial or genetic risks of breast cancer) (Tables 1.4 and 1.5).

The sensitivity of mammography as a screening test in high-risk groups does not exceed 50%. However, additional use of the second screening method significantly increases its sensitivity. Nevertheless, WHO does not recommend using MRM and MDCT for screening purposes.

The population coverage is an important aspect for the success of screening program. In case of low turnout for routine screening (below 60%), its final effect will be minimal (Semiglazov 2001). The motivation of the population to undergo a screening test is based on permanent education and information through mass media, presentations, booklets, journal articles, and movies about the main risk factors of breast cancer development, methods of its detection, diagnosis, and treatment. High-quality mammographic screening finally results in significant (up to 30%) decrease in mortality rate. Women, who do not participate in mammographic screening for various reasons, should be aware that other methods (physical examination, self-examination) fail to reduce mortality rate from this disease.

In female population, large-scale mammography screening can reduce mortality rate from breast cancer by 15–30%. The efficiency of mammography for screening has been tested in numerous randomized studies in the USA, Scotland, Canada, Sweden, and Finland. The results have demonstrated significance of mammography, clinical breast examination, and self-examination.

Breast cancer screening, as a rule, consists of three stages:

- Stage 1. A city outpatient clinic, which supplies screening among the female population in assigned area, makes active calls and referrals for examinations. It also documents the screening results. Each outpatient clinic compiles lists of women aged 40–60 years, who live in the assigned area.
- Stage 2. A facility with mammograph equipment that performs the exams for the patients assigned to several different outpatient clinics.
- Stage 3. In case of pathological changes in mammograms, the patient is referred for the third screening stage to the district mammological department to specify the diagnosis. If cancer or benign mass is detected, the patient is referred for treatment to an oncological facility.

Early diagnosis of breast cancer contributes to reduction in treatment costs due to the following factors:

- Reduction of the volume of surgery from a mastectomy to a sector resection reduces the length of inhospital stay.
- Breast conserving treatment reduces the period of temporary disability and rehabilitation.
- There is no need for reconstructive surgery and prosthetic repair.
- In the absence of lymph node involvement, treatment can be curative without expensive chemotherapy (with a tumor up to 1 cm in diameter, T1a-1bN0M0).

The success of screening mammography is not limited with the reduction of mortality rate. It facilitates detection of neoplasms in early stages that results in less aggressive treatment and better cosmetic results. Mammographic screening initially leads to rapid increase in breast cancer incidence with subsequent decrease in the detection of common types of breast cancer in women, who undergo screening. Screening decreases the incidence of invasive breast cancer and mortality rate. According to WHO, a retrospective analysis of mortality trends following the development of screening programs for breast cancer in 30 European countries has demonstrated the following facts. During the period 1989–2006, breast cancer mortality rate decreased on the average by 19%, ranging from a 45% decrease in Iceland to a 17% increase in Romania. Different rates of mortality were noted in different age groups. In women under 50, the decrease was observed on average by 37% (ranging from 76 to 14%). In the age group of 50–69 years, the decrease was 21% (ranging from 40 to 14%). Average decrease in women of 70 years and older was only 2% (ranging from 42 to 80%). Continuing increase in mortality rates was registered in 17 countries concurrently.

The analysis of X-ray screening results in Finland in 1985–2004 has shown that screening activities contribute to the detection of 20% of new breast cancer cases. The neoplasms detected with screening were smaller. They were detected in earlier stages, with a 10-year survival rate of 90%, in comparison with 70% in the cases detected out of screening program ($p = 0.003$). A meta-analysis of seven randomized studies, which involved 500,000 women, who participated in mammography screening, demonstrated a 25% reduction in breast cancer mortality rate in the group of patients, who underwent screening. An in-depth analysis carried out by the experts group has revealed a 30–35% reduction in mortality rate in women aged 50–69 as a result of mammography screening. Mammography screening in Norway in 1996–2004 demonstrated a statistically insignificant 11% decrease in breast cancer mortality rate, while 40% of women underwent routine mammography examination before introduction of organized mammography screening.

The problem of the benefits and possible adverse aspects of breast cancer screening remains debatable. First of all, such doubts are associated with the problem of hyperdiagnosis, i.e., detection of breast cancer, which most likely will not be identified throughout the life span. The analysis of the results of 11 randomized screening programs conducted in the UK has shown that the problem of hyperdiagnosis really exists, but it is not possible to accurately estimate its significance. Rough calculations provide the following indicators: according to the forecast for women aged 50–52 subject to annual screening, 1% of the breast cancer hyperdiagnosis can be expected in the next 20 years. The analysis of the results of screening programs implemented in seven European countries has demonstrated that the percentage of hyperdiagnosis ranged from 10 to 20%.

Currently, it is recommended to inform all women about possible adverse aspects of mammographic screening, when they are invited for screening. The issue of favorable outcomes and possible risks of mammographic screening for women aged 40–49 years remains debatable. A meta-analysis of publications in MEDLINE for the period 1996–2005, as well as the data of the Cochrane Central Register of Controlled Trials, has been conducted. The analysis of the studies has shown a 7–23% reduction in breast cancer mortality rate in women from the age group of 40–49 years, who underwent mammographic screening. Screening with mammography is associated with an increased risk of mastectomy and a reduced risk of adjuvant chemotherapy and hormonal therapy. The risk of breast cancer mortality because of radiation exposure during mammography screening is very low and not comparable to the indicators of breast cancer mortality rate decrease due to early diagnosis. False-positive results have an insignificant impact on psychological state of women and their attitude to subsequent screening stages. Although many women complain of pain during mammography, few regard pain as a deterrent to subsequent examinations. According to the recommendations of US Preventive Services Task Force (USPSTF) of 2009, the mammography screening should be started in women from the age of 50 and should be conducted every other year. It is expected that in the future a comprehensive genetic study of breast tumors will make it possible to detect tumors with a potential for progress.

Taking into account the large number and a variety of specialists involved in diagnosis of breast pathology and screening examinations, it is important to introduce a unified terminology, which describes breast abnormalities. It should also be considered that during various diagnostic procedures, the breast is positioned in different aspects related to the body, and this can complicate anatomical description of the lesion localization.

In order to unify imaging findings description, a specialized BI-RADS lexicon was developed. Currently the fifth version of 2013 is in use (hereinafter freely available ACR version is given).

The structure of X-ray (mammographic) report includes:

1. Indications for examination
2. Description of the breast structure
3. Description of important findings according to the lexicon
4. Comparison with the previous tests (if available)
5. Assessment
6. Recommendations

1. Indication for Examination
   Provide a brief description of the indication for examination. This may be screening for an asymptomatic woman, recall of the finding detected by screening, evaluation of a clinical finding (specify the finding and its location), or follow-up of either a probably benign lesion or cancer treated with breast conservation. If an implant is present, both standard and implant-displaced views should be performed, and this should be stated in the mammography report.
2. Succinct Description of the Overall Breast Composition
   This is an overall assessment of the volume of attenuating tissues in the breast, which helps to indicate the relative possibility that a

lesion could be obscured by normal tissue and that the sensitivity of examination thereby may be compromised by dense breast tissue. A few coalescent areas of dense tissue may be present in breasts with as little as 10% dense tissue, whereas primarily fatty areas may be present in breasts with as much as 90% dense tissue. Since mammography does not depict all breast cancers, clinical breast examination is a complementary element of screening. Findings at clinical breast examination should not be ignored and may have increased importance in the dense breast. The available data do not support the use of mammographic breast density for determining screening frequency. The following four categories of breast composition are defined by the visually estimated content of fibroglandular-density tissue within the breasts. Please note that the categories are listed as *a*, *b*, *c*, and *d* so as not to be confused with the numbered BI-RADS® assessment categories. If breasts are not of apparently equal density, denser breast should be used to categorize breast density. The sensitivity of mammography for noncalcified lesions decreases as the BI-RADS® breast density category increases. The denser the breast, the larger the lesion(s) that may be obscured. There is considerable intra- and interobserver variation in visually estimating breast density between any two adjacent density categories. Furthermore, there is only a minimal and insignificant difference in the sensitivity of mammography between the most dense breast in a lower-density category and the least dense breast in the next-higher-density category. These factors limit the clinical relevance of breast density categorization for the individual woman.

Breast composition category is estimated the following way:

(a) The breasts are almost entirely fatty.
(b) There are scattered areas of fibroglandular density.
(c) The breasts are heterogeneously dense, which may obscure small masses.
(d) The breasts are extremely dense, which lowers the sensitivity of mammography.

(*a*) *The breasts are almost entirely fatty.* Unless an area containing cancer is not included in the image field of the mammogram, mammography is highly sensitive in this setting (Fig. 1.13).

(*b*) *There are scattered areas of fibroglandular density* (historically, there are scattered fibroglandular densities). It may be helpful to distinguish breasts in which there are a few scattered areas of fibroglandular-density tissue from those in which there are moderate scattered areas of fibroglandular-density tissue. Note that there has been a subtle change in the wording of this category, to conform to BI-RADS® lexicon use of the

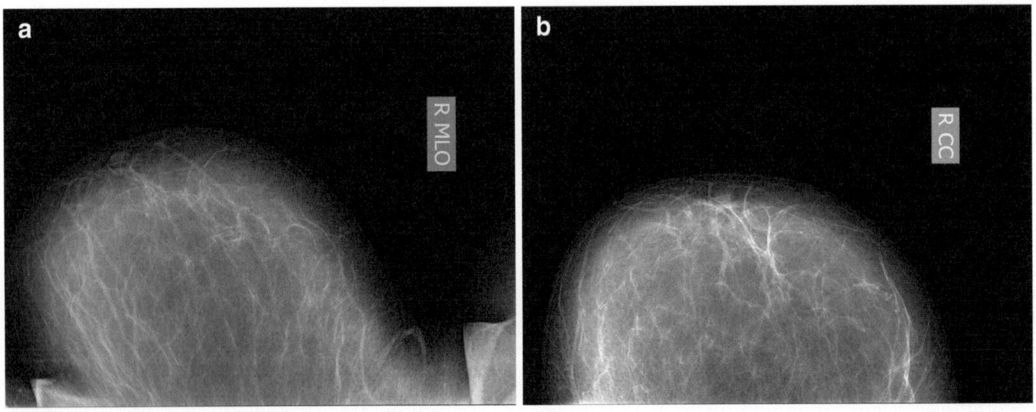

Fig. 1.13 (**a**, **b**) Mammography. The breasts are almost entirely fatty

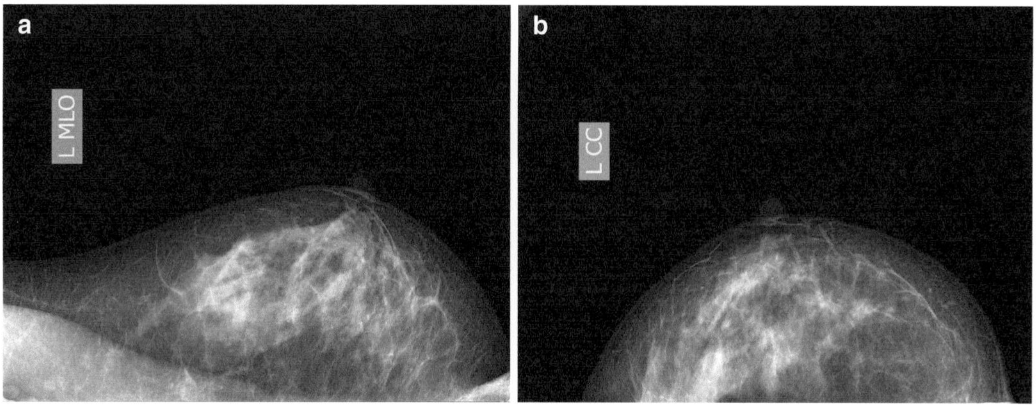

Fig. 1.14 (**a**, **b**) Mammography. Scattered areas of fibroglandular density

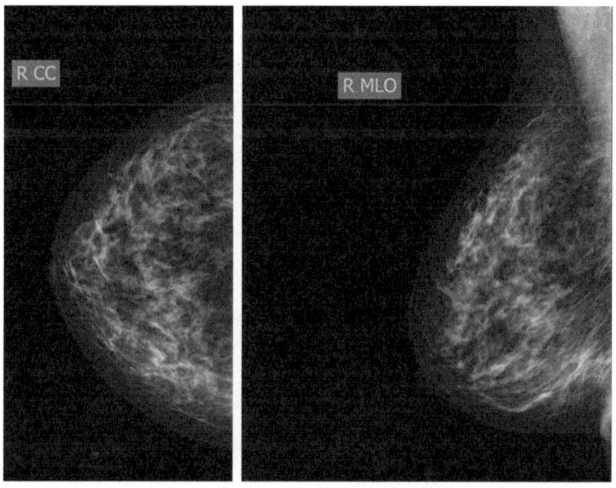

Fig. 1.15 Mammography. The breast is heterogeneously dense, which may obscure small masses

term "density" to describe the degree of X-ray attenuation of breast tissue but not to represent discrete mammographic findings (Fig. 1.14).

(*c*) *The breasts are heterogeneously dense, which may obscure small masses.* It is not uncommon for some areas in such breasts to be relatively dense, while other areas are primarily fatty. When this occurs, it may be helpful to describe the location(s) of the denser tissue in a second sentence, so that the referring clinician is aware that these are the areas in which small noncalcified lesions may be obscured. Suggested wordings for the second sentence include: "The dense tissue is located anteriorly in both breasts, and the posterior portions are mostly fatty." "Primarily dense tissue is located in the upper outer quadrants of both breasts; scattered areas of fibroglandular tissue are present in the remainder of the breasts" (Fig. 1.15).

(*d*) *The breasts are extremely dense, which lowers the sensitivity of mammography.* The sensitivity of mammography is lowest in this density category. The fourth edition of BI-RADS®, unlike previous editions, indicated quartile ranges of percentage dense tissue (increments of 25% density) for each of the four density categories, with the expectation that the assignment of breast density would be distributed more evenly across categories than the historical distribution of 10% fatty, 40% scattered, 40% heterogeneously, and 10% extremely dense (Fig. 1.16). However, it has since been demonstrated in clinical practice that there has been essentially no change in this historical distribution across density categories, despite the 2003 guidance provided in the BI-RADS® Atlas.

3. Clear description of any important findings
   It is assumed that most important findings are either of concern at screening, inherently suspicious, new, or seen to be larger/more extensive when compared to previous examination.
   (a) *Mass*:
      - Size
      - Morphology (shape, margin)
      - Density
      - Associated calcifications
      - Associated features
      - Location

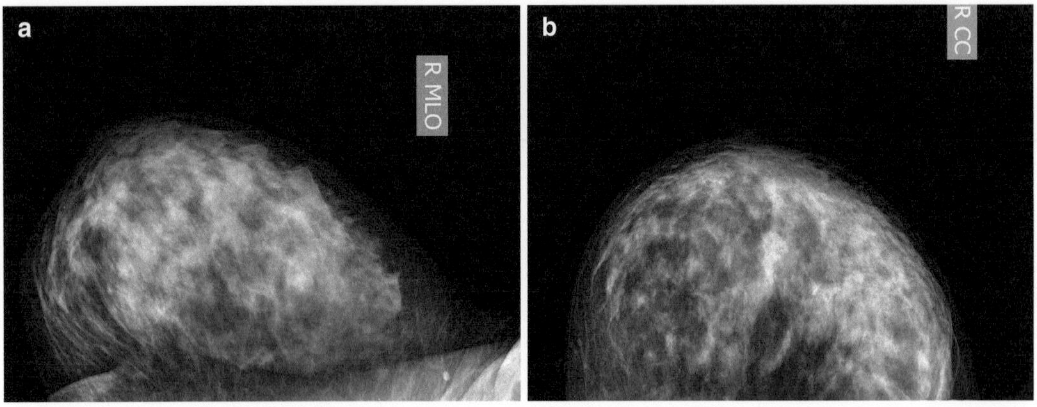

Fig. 1.16 (**a**, **b**) Mammography. The breast is extremely dense, which lowers the sensitivity of mammography

Margins and shape are estimated in accordance with Fig. 1.17.

Pathological lesion localization is described in accordance with Fig. 1.18 (applied to all imaging methods).

(b) *Calcifications*:

Morphology—describes typical benign type or describes shape of particles

Distribution (may not be appropriate for typical benign calcifications)

Associated features

Location

- Typical benign:
  - Skin calcifications.
  - Vascular calcifications.
  - Popcorn calcifications (involutional calcinated fibroadenomas).
  - Large (>1 mm) rod-shaped calcifications (sometimes may be branching) correspond to calcium deposition in dilated ducts.
  - Round calcifications, less than 1 mm in size, often multiple and grouped (deposits of calcium within acini).
  - Spherical, with clarification in the center, from 1 mm to 1 cm in size, with even, clear contours.
  - Ring-shaped or "egg shell" type.
  - "Milk of calcium" corresponds to deposits of calcium within cysts).
  - Calcifications within cutaneous scar (after surgical interference).
  - Dystrophic calcifications (usually after a trauma or radiation therapy). Generally of irregular shape, more than 0,5 mm in size.
- Atypical calcifications: it is impossible to diagnose as unambiguously benign, usually small calcifications with vague or poorly identified contours that cannot be referred to a certain group.
- Calcifications suspicious for malignant tumors:
  - Pleomorphic or granular, of various shapes and size, generally less than 0.5 mm in size
  - Small linear, punctate, or branching calcifications, in the form of a broken (or dotted) line less than 1 mm thick. Correspond to the filling of the affected ducts with calcium salts

(c) *Architectural Distortion*:
- Associated calcifications
- Associated features
- Location

(d) **Asymmetries** (asymmetry, global asymmetry, focal asymmetry, developing asymmetry):
- Associated calcifications
- Associated features
- Location

(e) **Intramammary lymph node** (rarely important):
- Location

(f) **Skin lesion** (rarely important):
- Location

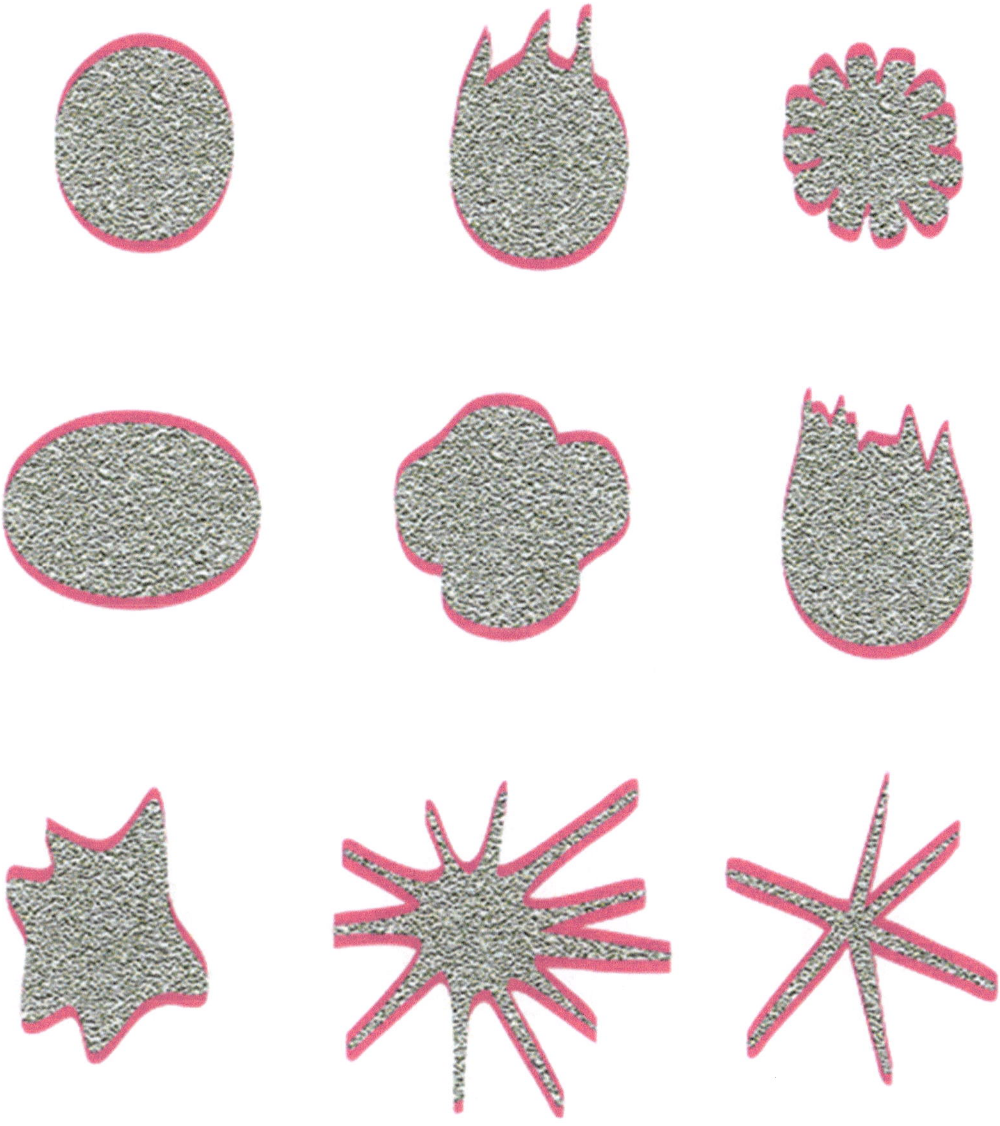

Fig. 1.17 (**a**, **b**) Estimation pattern of the lesion shape and margins for description applying BI-RADS lexicon is used regardless of X-ray examination

(g) **Solitary dilated duct** (rarely present):
  - Location

4. Assessment
   The incorporation of an assessment category in the overall summary of the mammography report is mandated by the Food and Drug Administration, Quality Mammography Standards, Final Rule. Whereas FDA-mandated assessments are not linked to management recommendations, BI-RADS® assessment categories are designed to be concordant with specific management recommendations. The linking of assessment categories with concordant management recommendations further enhances sound medical practice.

   All final assessments (BI-RADS® categories 1, 2, 3, 4, 5, and 6) should be based on thorough evaluation of the mammographic

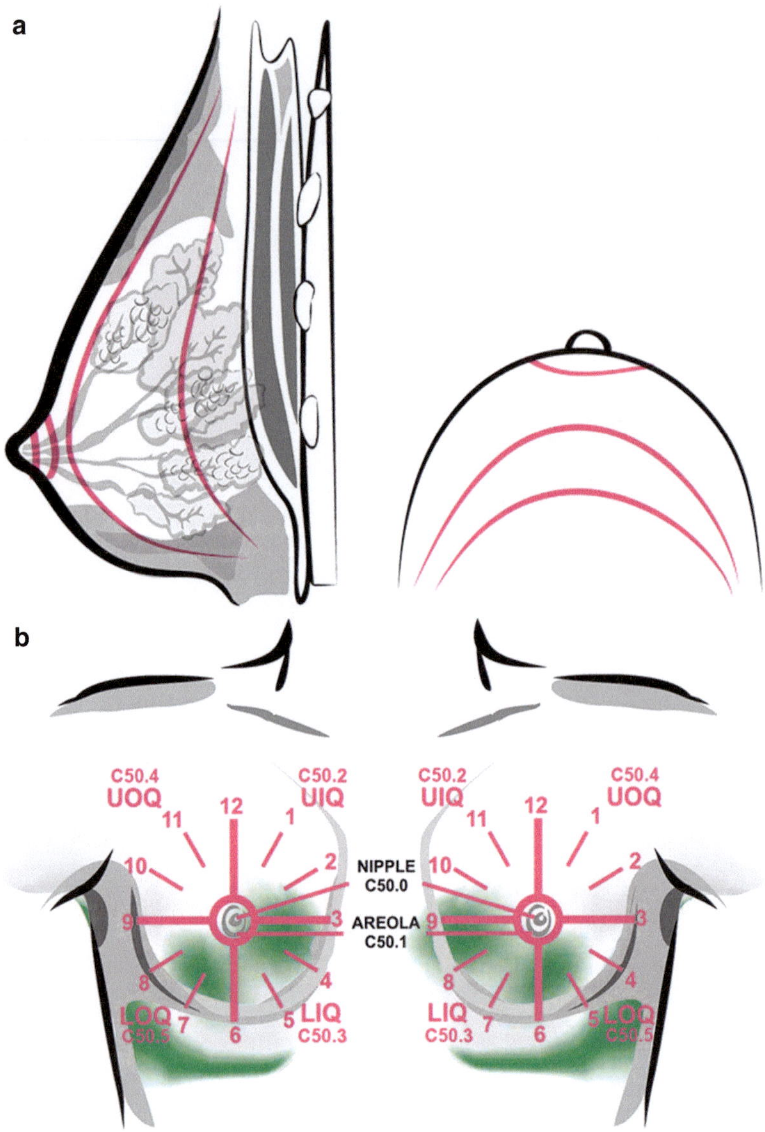

Fig. 1.18 (**a**) Segmentation of mammary gland regions to describe lesion localization. Used regardless of X-ray diagnostics method. Lateral projection (sagittal plane) and anteroposterior projection (axial plane). (**b**) Frontal projection

features of concern or after determination that an examination is negative or benign.

An incomplete (category 0) assessment is usually given for screening examinations when additional imaging evaluation is recommended before it is appropriate to render a final assessment. There may be rare situations in the screening setting in which a category 4 or 5 assessment is used, but this practice is discouraged because it may compromise some aspects of outcome analysis. A recall (category 0) assessment should include specific suggestions for the next course of action (spot compression magnification views, US, etc.).

Report categories in accordance with BI-RADS lexicon are presented in Table 1.6 (applied to all imaging methods).

(a) Mammographic Assessment Is Incomplete

Category 0: Incomplete—Need Additional Imaging Evaluation and/or Prior Mammograms for Comparison. For this assessment category, the text may be shortened to “Incomplete—Need

Table 1.6 BI-RADS categories (applied to all imaging methods)

Conclusion	Recommendations	Probability of malignant tumors
Category 0: incomplete—need additional imaging evaluation and/or prior mammograms for comparison	Recall for additional imaging and/or comparison with prior examination(s)	N/A
Category 1: negative	Routine mammography screening	Essentially 0% likelihood of malignancy
Category 2: benign	Routine mammography screening	Essentially 0% likelihood of malignancy
Category 3: probably benign	Short-interval (6-month) follow-up or continued surveillance mammography	>0% but ≤2% likelihood of malignancy
Category 4: suspicious	Tissue diagnosis	>2% but <95% likelihood of malignancy
Category 4A: low suspicion for malignancy		>2% to ≤10% likelihood of malignancy
Category 4B: moderate suspicion for malignancy		>10% to ≤50% likelihood of malignancy
Category 4C: high suspicion for malignancy		>50% to <95% likelihood of malignancy
Category 5: highly suggestive of malignancy	Tissue diagnosis	≥95% likelihood of malignancy
Category 6: known biopsy-proven malignancy	Surgical excision when clinically appropriate	N/A

Additional Imaging Evaluation" or "Incomplete—Need Prior Mammograms for Comparison," as appropriate. There is a finding for which additional imaging evaluation is needed. This is almost always used in a screening situation. Under certain circumstances, this assessment category may be used in a diagnostic mammography report, such as when US equipment or personnel are not immediately available or when the patient is unable or unwilling to wait for completion of a full diagnostic examination. A recommendation for additional imaging evaluation includes the use of spot compression (with or without magnification), special mammographic views, and US. Category 0 should not be used for diagnostic breast imaging findings that warrant further evaluation with MRI. Rather, the interpreting physician should issue a final assessment in a report that is made before the MRI examination is performed.

In most circumstances and when feasible, if a mammography examination is not assessed as negative or benign, the current examination should be compared with prior examination(s). The interpreting physician should use judgment on how vigorously to attempt obtaining prior examinations, given the likelihood of success of such an endeavor and the likelihood that comparison will affect the final assessment. In this context, it is important to note that comparison with previous examination(s) may be irrelevant when a finding is inherently suspicious for malignancy. Category 0 should be used for prior image comparison only when such comparison is required to make a final assessment. When category 0 is used in the context of awaiting prior examinations for comparison, there should be in place a tracking procedure guaranteeing with 100% reliability that a final assessment will be made within 30 days (preferably sooner) even if prior examinations do not become available. Some mammography practices may reasonably choose never to use category 0 in the context of awaiting prior examinations simply because they do not have a 100% reliable tracking procedure. If a mammography examination is assessed as category 0 in the context of awaiting prior examinations and then the prior examinations do become available, an addendum to the initial mammography report should be issued, including a revised assessment. For auditing purposes, the revised assessment should replace the initial assessment (see the Follow-up and Outcome Monitoring section).

(b) Mammographic Assessment Is Complete—Final Assessment Categories

Category 1: Negative. There is nothing to comment on. This is a normal examination.

Category 2: Benign. Like category 1, this is a normal assessment, but here the interpreter chooses to describe a benign finding in the mammography report. Involuting calcified fibroadenomas, skin calcifications, metallic foreign bodies (such as core biopsy and surgical clips), and fat-containing lesions (such as oil cysts, lipomas, galactoceles, and mixed-density hamartomas) all have characteristically benign appearances and may be described with confidence. The interpreter may also choose to describe intramammary lymph nodes, vascular calcification, implants, or architectural distortion clearly related to prior surgery while still concluding that there is no mammographic evidence of malignancy. On the other hand, the interpreter may choose not to describe such findings, in which case the examination should be assessed as negative (category 1). Note that both category 1 and category 2 assessments indicate that there is no mammographic evidence of malignancy. Both should be followed by the management recommendation for routine mammography screening. The difference is that category 2 should be used when describing one or more specific benign mammographic findings in the report, whereas category 1 should be used when no such findings are described (even if such findings are present).

Category 3: Probably Benign. A finding assessed using this category should have a $\leq 2\%$ likelihood of malignancy but greater than the essentially 0% likelihood of malignancy of a characteristically benign finding. A probably benign finding is not expected to change over the suggested period of imaging surveillance, but the interpreting physician prefers to establish stability of the finding before recommending management limited to routine mammography screening. There are several prospective clinical studies demonstrating the safety and efficacy of periodic mammographic surveillance instead of biopsy for specific mammographic findings. Three specific findings are validated as being probably benign (noncalcified circumscribed solid mass, focal asymmetry, and solitary group of punctate calcifications). All the previously cited studies emphasize the need to conduct a complete diagnostic imaging evaluation before making a probably benign (category 3) assessment; hence, it is recommended not to render such an assessment in interpreting a screening mammography examination. The practice of rendering category 3 assessments directly from screening examination also has been shown to result in adverse outcomes: (1) unnecessary follow-up of many lesions that could have been promptly assessed as benign and (2) delayed diagnosis of a small number of cancers that otherwise may have been smaller in size and less likely to be advanced in stage. Also, all the previously cited studies exclude palpable lesions, so the use of a probably benign assessment for a palpable lesion is not supported by robust scientific data, although there are two single-institution studies that do report successful outcomes for palpable lesions. Finally, because evidence from previously cited studies indicates the need for biopsy rather than continued surveillance when a probably benign finding increases in size or extent, it is not prudent to render a category 3 assessment when a finding that otherwise meets "probably benign" imaging criteria is either new or has increased in size or extent. While the vast majority of probably benign findings are managed with an initial short-interval follow-up (6 months) examination followed by additional examinations until long-term (2- or 3-year) stability is demonstrated, there may be occasions in which a biopsy is done instead (patient preference or overriding clinical concern).

Category 4: Suspicious. This category is reserved for findings that do not have the classic appearance of malignancy but are sufficiently suspicious to justify a recommendation for biopsy. The ceiling for category 3 assessment is a 2% likelihood of malignancy, and the floor for category 5 assessment is 95%, so category 4 assessments cover the wide range of likelihood of malignancy in between. Thus, almost all recommendations for breast interventional procedures will come from assessments made using this category. By subdividing category 4 into 4A, 4B, and 4C, as recommended in Guidance chapter and using the cut points indicated therein, it is hoped that patients and referring clinicians will more readily make informed decisions on the ultimate course of action.

Category 5: Highly Suggestive of Malignancy. These assessments carry a very high probability (≥95%) of malignancy. This category initially was established to involve lesions for which 1-stage surgical treatment was considered without preliminary biopsy, in an era when preoperative wire localization was the primary breast interventional procedure. Nowadays, given the widespread acceptance of imaging-guided percutaneous biopsy, 1-stage surgery is rarely, if ever, performed. Rather, current oncologic management almost always involves tissue diagnosis of malignancy via percutaneous tissue sampling to facilitate treatment options, such as when sentinel node biopsy is included in surgical management or when neoadjuvant chemotherapy is administered prior to surgery. Therefore, the current rationale for using a category 5 assessment is to identify lesions for which any nonmalignant percutaneous tissue diagnosis is automatically considered discordant, resulting in the recommendation for repeat (usually surgical) biopsy.

Category 6: Known Biopsy-Proven Malignancy. This category is reserved for examinations performed after biopsy proof of malignancy (imaging performed after percutaneous biopsy but prior to complete surgical excision), in which there are nomammographic abnormalities other than the known cancer that might need additional evaluation.

BI-RADS terminology for MRM also differs from the terminology for mammography and US. The report of MRM results should have the following structure:

1. Indication for examination
2. MRI technique
3. Succinct description of the overall breast composition (screening only)
4. Clear description of any important findings
5. Comparison to previous tests
6. Composite reports
7. Assessment
8. Management

1. Indication for Examination
   Provide a brief description of the indication for examination. For example, this may be high-risk screening, follow-up of a probably benign lesion, follow-up of cancer treated with neoadjuvant chemotherapy, or evaluation of the newly diagnosed cancer patient. As background parenchymal enhancement can be affected by cyclical hormonal changes, it may be helpful to include menstrual history. If the patient is pre-menopausal, the week of the menstrual cycle may be important information to aid in interpretation. Current therapy (neoadjuvant, adjuvant, hormonal, or radiation therapy) for breast cancer treatment in the pre- or postsurgical setting may be important information and may inform exam interpretation. The indication for examination should contain a concise description of the patient's clinical history, including:
   (a) Reason for performing the exam (e.g., screening, staging, problem solving)
   (b) Clinical abnormalities, including size, location, and duration:
      - Palpable finding
      - Nipple discharge
      - Other pertinent clinical findings or history
   (c) Previous biopsies:
      - Biopsy type
      - Biopsy location
      - Benign or malignant pathology (cytology or histology)
   (d) Hormonal status if applicable:
      - Pre- or postmenopausal
      - Menstrual cycle phase (second week or other) or last menstrual period
      - Peripartum
      - Exogenous hormone therapy, tamoxifen, aromatase inhibitors, or other hormones or medications/herbs/vitamins that might influence MRI

2. MRI Technique
   Give a detailed description of the technical factors of how the MRI examination was obtained. At a minimum, a bright-fluid sequence of both breasts should be obtained. Pre- and post-gadolinium T1-weighted images should be obtained, preferably with fat suppression, simultaneously of both breasts. Subtraction imaging may be desired as well as other as processing techniques and parametric analysis. Elements of this description routinely include:
   (a) Right, left, or both breasts
   (b) Location of markers and their significance (scar, nipple, palpable lesion, etc.)
   (c) Weighting:
      - T1 weighted
      - T2 weighted
      - Fat saturation
      - Scan orientation and plane
      - Other pertinent pulse sequence features
   (d) Contrast dose:
      - Name of contrast agent
      - Dosage (mmol/kg) and volume (in cc)
      - Injection type: bolus or infusion
      - Timing (relationship of bolus injection to scan start time and scan length)
      - If multiple scans: number of post contrast scans and acquisition techniques of each (how fast, how many slices, and slice thickness)
   (e) Post-processing techniques as applicable:
      - MPR/MIP
      - Time/signal intensity curves
      - Subtraction
      - Other techniques
3. Succinct description of overall breast composition
   This should include an overall description of the breast composition, including:
(a) The amount of FGT that is present:
   Breast Tissue—Fibroglandular Tissue (FGT) (Figs. 1.19, 1.20, 1.21, and 1.22)
      - Almost entirely fat
      - Scattered fibroglandular tissue
      - Heterogeneous fibroglandular tissue
      - Extreme fibroglandular tissue

The four categories of breast composition are defined by the visually estimated content of FGT within the breasts. If the breasts are not of apparently equal amounts of FGT, the breast with the most FGT should be used to categorize breast composition. Although there may be considerable variation in visually estimating breast composition,

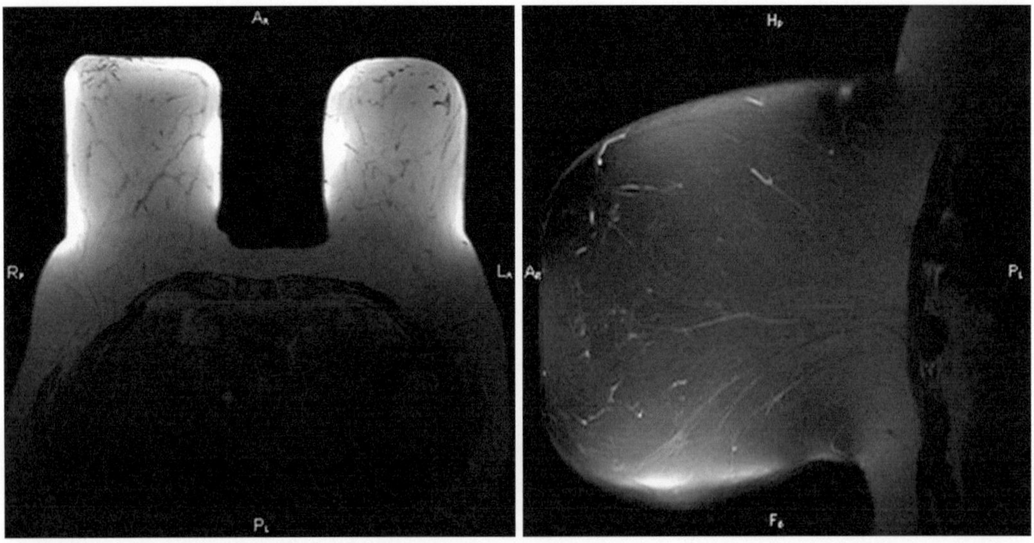

Fig. 1.19 Example of FGT assessment. T1-weighted MR image in axial plane and T2-weighted MR image with fat suppression in sagittal plane. Almost entirely fat

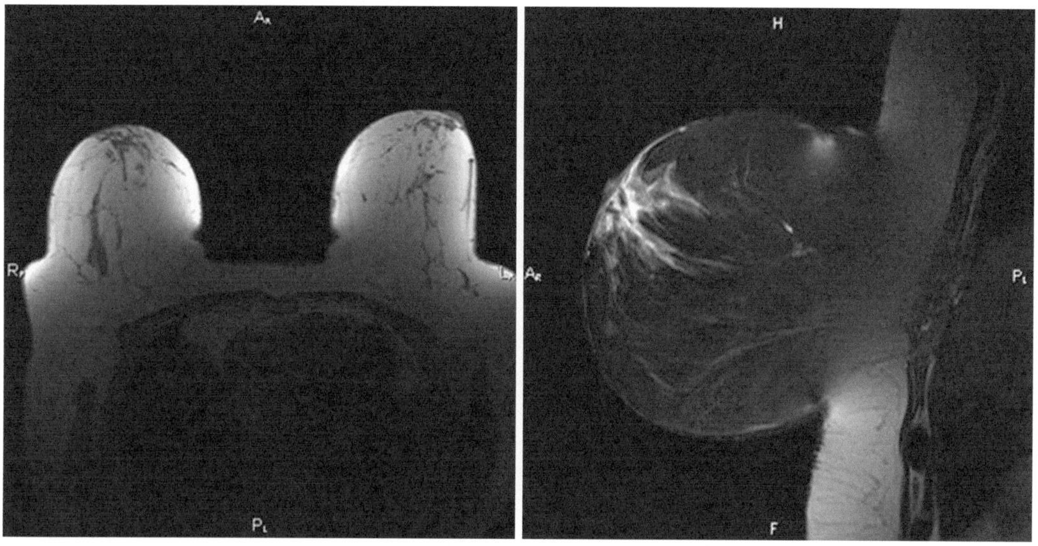

Fig. 1.20 Example of FGT assessment. T1-weighted MR image in axial plane and T2-weighted MR image with fat suppression in sagittal plane. Scattered fibroglandular tissue

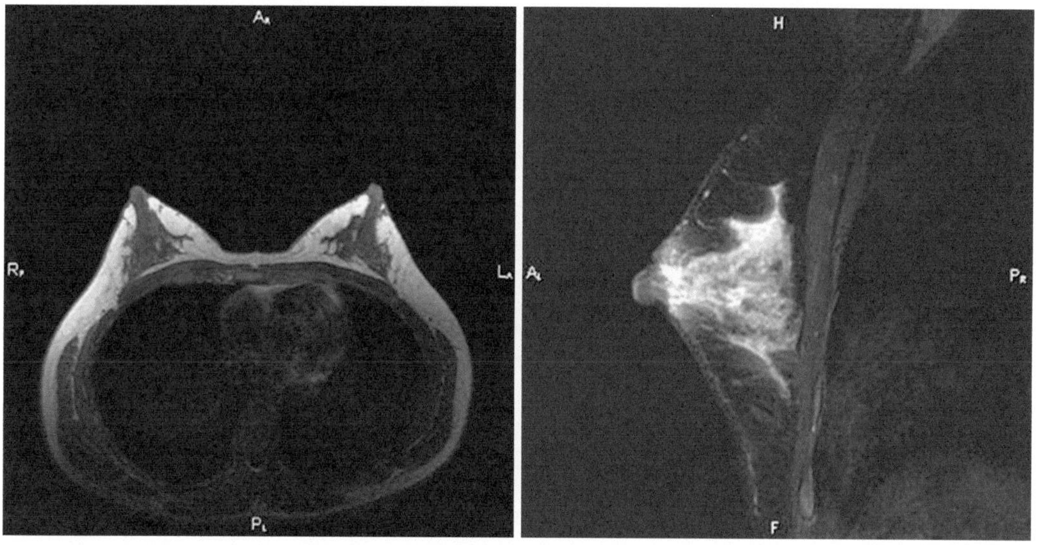

Fig. 1.21 Example of FGT assessment. T1-weighted MR image in axial plane and T2-weighted MR image with fat suppression in sagittal plane. Heterogeneous fibroglandular tissue

categorizing based on percentages (and specifically into quartiles) is not recommended. We recognize that quantification of breast FGT volume on MRI may be feasible in the future, but we await publication of robust data before endorsing percentage recommendations. We urge the use of BI-RADS® terminology instead of numbers to classify breast FGT in order to eliminate any possible confusion with the BI-RADS® assessment categories, which are numbered.

(b) The amount of background parenchymal enhancement in the image:

Breast Tissue—Background Parenchymal Enhancement (BPE) (Fig. 1.23)

- Minimal
- Mild

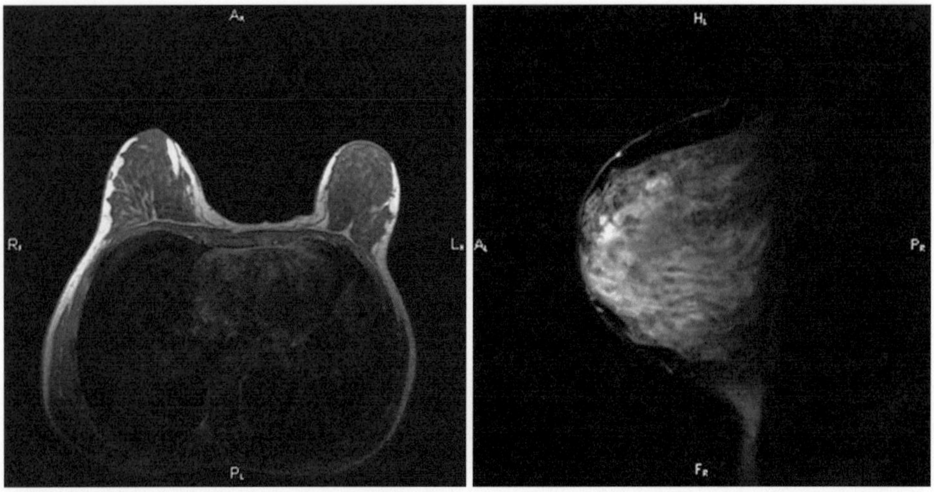

Fig. 1.22 Example of FGT assessment. T1-weighted MR image in axial plane and T2-weighted MR image with fat suppression in sagittal plane. Extreme fibroglandular tissue

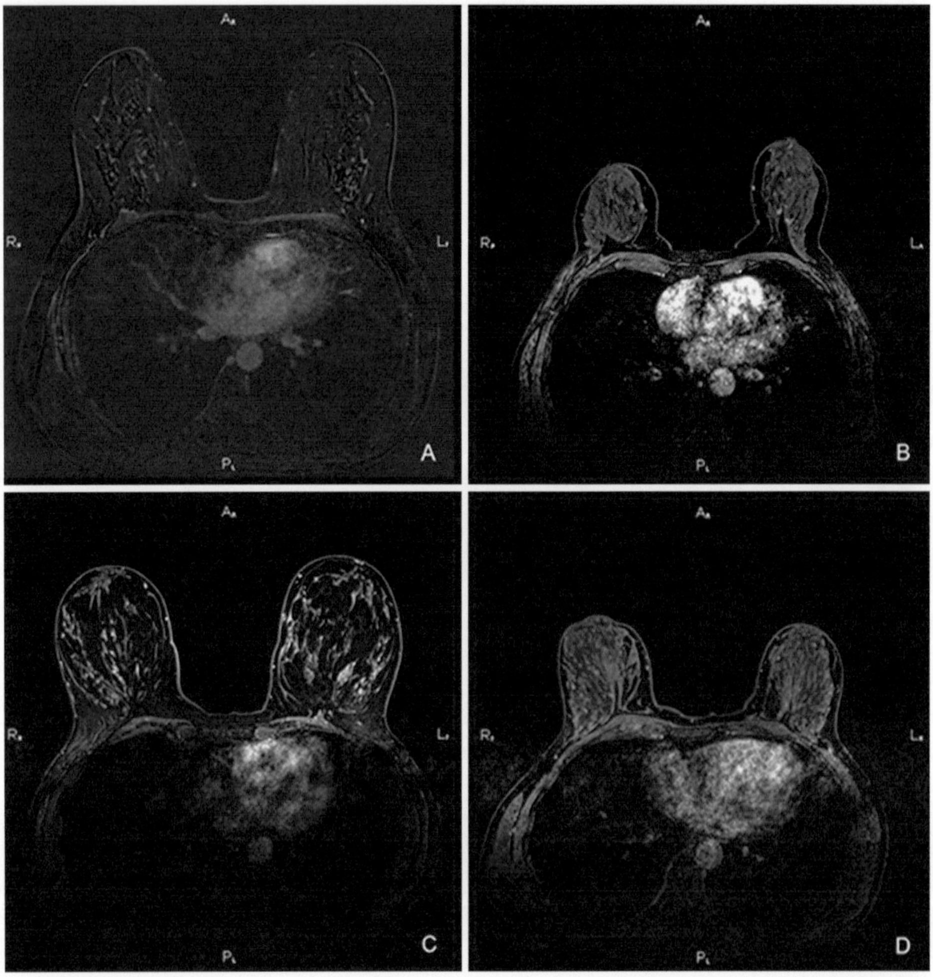

Fig. 1.23 Example of BPE assessment. T1-weighted MR images with fat suppression and contrast enhancement. Axial plane. *A* minimal, *B* mild, *C* moderate, *D* marked

- Moderate
- Marked

The four categories of BPE are defined by the visually estimated enhancement of the FGT of the breast(s). If the breasts are not of apparently equal amounts of BPE, the breast with the most BPE should be used to categorize BPE. In the event that treatment has altered BPE in one or both breasts, this can be reported. Although there may be considerable variation in visually estimating BPE, categorizing based on percentages (and specifically into quartiles) is not recommended. Quantification of BPE volume and intensity on MRI may be feasible in the future, but we await publication of robust data on that topic before endorsing percentage recommendations. We recognize that there are variations in BPE distribution and morphology. However, we defer on recommending descriptions of distribution or morphology until additional data are available. Currently, BPE refers to the volume of enhancement and the intensity of enhancement. For consistency, BPE should be included for all patients.

On bilateral scans, describe whether the pattern is asymmetric or symmetric, if appropriate. Asymmetric denotes more significant enhancement in one breast than in the other. Symmetric enhancement is mirror image.

(c) Whether implants are present if an implant is present, it should be so stated in the report. Information should include its composition (saline, silicone, or others) and the number of lumens (single or multiple).

4. Clear description of any important findings
   Abnormal enhancement is unique and separate from BPE. Its description should indicate the breast in which the abnormal enhancement occurs, the lesion type, and modifiers. The clinical location of the abnormality as extrapolated from the MRI location (based on clock-face position and quadrant location) should be reported. It should be recognized that there may be variation in location of a clinically detected lesion (patient is upright or supine), a lesion detected by mammography (patient is upright and compressed), a lesion detected by sonography (patient is supine or supine oblique), and an MRI-detected lesion (patient is prone) based on positional differences. A more consistent measurement is the distance from the nipple. It is encouraged that distance from the nipple for a lesion be reported in order to facilitate correlation between modalities, although it should be understood that one should expect some difference in distance from the nipple among the breast imaging modalities. For bilateral axial examinations, the breasts should be pointing up, following the cross-sectional imaging convention. The descriptors should include:
   (a) Size
   (b) Location:
      - Right or left
      - Breast quadrant and clock-face position (or central, retroareolar, and axillary tail descriptors)
      - Distance from the nipple, skin, or chest wall in centimeters (if applicable)

Descriptors for abnormal enhancement:

(c) Findings associated with abnormal enhancement include:
   - Artifacts that affect interpretation
   - Focus: a tiny dot of enhancement that does not clearly represent a space-occupying lesion or mass and does not clearly show a mass on precontrast imaging.
   - Masses: space-occupying lesions, usually spherical or ball-like, may displace or retract surrounding breast tissue. Descriptors—modifiers describing a mass:
     – Shape: describes the overall morphology of the enhancement:
        Oval (includes lobulated)
        Round
        Irregular
     – Margin: describes the borders:
        Circumscribed
        Not circumscribed:

        - Irregular
        - Speculated
    - Internal enhancement characteristics:
        - Homogeneous
        - Heterogeneous
        - Rim enhancement
        - Dark internal septations
- Non-mass enhancement (NME): modifiers describing enhancement patterns with a specific MRI pattern:
    - Distribution:
        - Focal
        - Linear
        - Segmental
        - Regional
        - Multiple regions
        - Diffuse
    - Internal enhancement patterns (for all other types):
        - Homogeneous
        - Heterogeneous
        - Clumped
        - Clustered ring
- Intramammary lymph node (rarely important)
- Skin lesion (rarely important)
- Non-enhancing findings:
    - Ductal precontrast high signal on T1W
    - Cyst
    - Postoperative collections (hematoma/seroma)
    - Post-therapy skin thickening and trabecular thickening
    - Non-enhancing mass
    - Architectural distortion
    - Signal void from foreign bodies, clips, etc.
- Associated features:
    - Nipple retraction
    - Nipple invasion
    - Skin retraction
    - Skin thickening
    - Skin invasion:
        - Direct invasion
        - Inflammatory cancer
    - Axillary adenopathy
    - Pectoralis muscle invasion
    - Chest wall invasion
    - Architectural distortion:
- Fat-containing lesions
    - Lymph nodes:
        - Normal
        - Abnormal
    - Fat necrosis
    - Hamartoma
    - Postoperative seroma/hematoma with fat
- Stability: describe how the enhancement changed (if new, stable, or changed in size from previous examination)
- Kinetic curve assessment (if applicable):
    - The fastest enhancing portion of the lesion or the most suspicious washout curve pattern in the lesion should be assessed:
        - Sample fast enhancing areas
        - Sample for and report on the worst looking kinetic curve shape
    - Signal intensity/time curve:
        - Initial enhancement phase—describes the enhancement pattern within the first 2 min or when the curve starts to change:
        - Slow
        - Medium
        - Fast
        - Delayed phase—describes the enhancement pattern after 2 min or after the curve starts to change:
        - Persistent
        - Plateau
        - Washout
- Implants:
    - Implant material and lumen type:
        - Saline
        - Silicone:
            - Intact
            - Ruptured
    - Other implant materials (such as soy oil, polypropylene, polyurethane, and sponges; includes direct injections)
    - Lumen type
    - Implant location:
        - Retroglandular
        - Retropectoral
    - Abnormal implant contour:

Focal bulge
- Intracapsular silicone findings:
  Radial folds
  Subcapsular line
  Keyhole sign (teardrop, noose)
  Linguine sign
- Extracapsular silicone:
  Breast
  Lymph nodes
- Water droplets
- Peri-implant fluid

Also, we recognize that other techniques may be used in the evaluation of breast lesions. Newer and evolving techniques are constantly being introduced. Findings from other techniques, such as diffusion-weighted imaging or MR spectroscopy, should be reported if clinically important.

5. Comparison to Previous Examination(s)
   Include a statement indicating that the current examination has been compared to previous examination(s) with specific date(s). If this is not included, it should be assumed that no comparison has been made; however, it is preferable to indicate explicitly that no comparison was made. Comparison to a previous examination may assume importance if the finding of concern requires an evaluation of change or stability. Comparison is less important when the finding has characteristically benign features. Comparison may be irrelevant if the finding is inherently suspicious for malignancy. Information in this area should include:
   (a) Previous MRI—date of examination
   (b) Other imaging studies (mammogram, US, nuclear medicine examination, others) and date of examination
6. Assessment
   This is a description of an overall summary of MRI findings, including assessment. Incorporating an assessment category in the overall summary of the breast MRI report is sound medical practice. All final impressions should be complete with each lesion fully categorized. An incomplete assessment (category 0) is used when full diagnostic imaging has not been performed and should be given only when additional imaging or clinical evaluation is recommended to establish the benignity of a finding (e.g., a possible intramammary lymph node or fat necrosis at MRI may require additional mammography and/or US examination). Interpretation is facilitated by recognizing that almost all MRI examinations may be classified into a few assessment categories, listed in the section on Assessment Categories.
7. Management
   This is a description of patient management recommendations, as appropriate. If an incomplete assessment (category 0) is rendered, a specific suggestion for the next course of action should be given (physical examination, diagnostic mammography, targeted diagnostic US, etc.). Note that an incomplete assessment (category 0) should not be rendered when recommending targeted US in order to determine the feasibility of performing biopsy using sonographic guidance; such a scenario requires the use of a category 4 or 5 assessment (suspicious or highly suggestive of malignancy). If a suspicious abnormality is detected, the report should indicate that a biopsy should be performed in the absence of clinical contraindication. This means that the radiologist has sufficient concern that a biopsy is warranted; the term "clinical contraindication" indicates that there may be reasons why the patient and her physician might wish to defer the biopsy.

1. Assessment is incomplete
   Category 0: Incomplete—Need Additional Imaging Evaluation. Use this for a finding that needs additional imaging evaluation. This may be used for a technically unsatisfactory scan or when more information is needed to interpret the scan. A recommendation for additional imaging evaluation might involve a repeat MRI with satisfactory technique or obtaining information with other imaging modalities (mammographic views, US, etc.). The radiologist should use judgment in how vigorously to pursue previous studies.

Every effort should be made not to use category 0. The reason for this is that almost always there is enough information on the initial breast MRI examination to provide a management recommendation. In general, the decision to biopsy or not may be made on the basis of the existing MRI study. A situation in which a final assessment of 0 may be helpful is when a finding on MRI is suspicious, but demonstration that the finding is characteristically benign on an additional study would avert biopsy. For example, if a small mass is suspicious on MRI but there is a possibility that it may represent a benign finding, such as an intramammary lymph node, then a category 0 assessment may be made, with the recommendation for targeted US (that might demonstrate characteristically benign features) to possibly avert biopsy. Another example would be a suspicious finding at MRI that may represent fat necrosis, with the recommendation for diagnostic mammography (that might demonstrate characteristically benign features) to possibly avert biopsy. If a category 0 assessment is rendered at MRI, detailed recommendations should describe the subsequent diagnostic imaging workup and the level of suspicion (pertinent in case the additional imaging does not establish benignity). When additional studies are completed, a final assessment is rendered. If the additional studies are described in the same report, separate paragraphs indicating the pertinent findings from each imaging study will contribute to the final integrated assessment that takes all the findings into consideration.

2. Assessment is Complete—Final Assessment Categories
   Category 1: Negative. There is nothing to comment on. This is a normal examination. No abnormal enhancement was found; routine follow-up is advised. There is nothing to comment on. The breasts are symmetric, and no enhancing masses, architectural distortion, or suspicious areas of enhancement are present. Category 1 includes a normal description of breast composition (amount of FGT) and the degree of BPE. It should be emphasized that BPE is a normal finding, and short-term follow-up is not necessary to assess BPE for stability.
   Category 2: Benign. Like category 1, this is a normal assessment, but here the interpreter chooses to describe a benign finding in the breast MRI report. The interpreter may describe a benign finding such as intramammary lymph node, implants, metallic foreign bodies (such as core biopsy and surgical clips), enhancing and non-enhancing fibroadenomas, cysts, old non-enhancing scars or recent scars, postoperative collections, and fat-containing lesions (such as oil cysts, lipomas, galactoceles, and hamartomas). On the other hand, the interpreter may choose not to describe such findings, in which case the examination should be assessed as negative (category 1). Both category 1 and 2 assessments indicate that there is no evidence of malignancy. The difference is that category 2 should be used when describing one or more specific benign MRI findings in the report, whereas category 1 should be used when no such findings are described (even if such findings are present). The committee supports a directive for annual follow-up MRI and mammography after either a category 1 or 2 screening MRI assessment, in line with established guidelines for high-risk screening.
   Category 3: Probably Benign. A finding assessed using this category should have a ≤2% likelihood of malignancy but greater than the essentially 0% likelihood of malignancy of a characteristically benign finding. A probably benign finding is not expected to change over the suggested period of imaging surveillance, but the interpreting physician prefers to establish stability of the finding before recommending management limited to routine breast screening. Although data are becoming available that shed light on the efficacy of short-interval follow-up for selected MRI findings, at the present time, such management recommendations are based on limited data. The use of a probably benign (category 3) assessment is reserved for specificfindings that are separate from the BPE and are very likely benign. The use of a category 3 assessment has been intuitive in the past; however, there are several studies that specifically address rates of

malignancy and, to a very limited extent, types of lesions. Although these studies examined different populations of patients, several of them were able to demonstrate a ≤2% malignancy rate, demonstrating the feasibility of using category 3 assessments at MRI. However, none of the studies provided PPVs for specific types of lesions, so the use of category 3 assessment at MRI remains intuitive for radiologists who lack extensive (audited) personal experience with any given specific type of lesion. Currently, this is an evolving area that needs the support of robust data before an unqualified endorsement is made to use category 3 assessments at MRI.

As at mammography, if a probably benign finding is smaller or less prominent (i.e., less contrast enhancement) on follow-up examination, the finding should be assessed as benign (category 2), eliminating the need for continued surveillance imaging. When a finding that otherwise meets probably benign imaging criteria is either new or has increased in size, extent, or conspicuity, then a recommendation for biopsy would be prudent and a recommendation for follow-up should not be rendered. BPE, a benign finding on nearly all MRI examinations, should not be the reason for a probably benign assessment. However, if findings cannot be ascribed to normal variation of BPE and there is a question about whether observed enhancement could be transient and related to the hormonal status of the patient, then a probably benign (category 3) assessment with a recommendation to return for very-short-interval follow-up (2–3 months) may be appropriate. Because a benign hormonal enhancement can vary from cycle to cycle, a category 3 assessment may be used for the menstruating patient who was scanned in a suboptimal phase of her cycle; a follow-up MRI examination should be scheduled for the optimal (week 2) phase of her cycle. Additionally, a category 3 assessment may be used for the postmenopausal patient who is on hormone replacement therapy (HRT) and in whom probable hormonal enhancement is observed. Stopping HRT for several weeks and repeating the scan may be warranted in this scenario. It should be emphasized that unexplained areas of enhancement that are demonstrated to be due to HRT are uncommon. As with mammography, if the finding is smaller or less prominent (i.e., less contrast enhancement) at follow-up examination, the finding is benign. Recommendations will likely undergo future modifications as more data accrue regarding the validity of using category 3 assessments at MRI, the follow-up interval required, and the type of findings that should be followed.

Follow-Up of Foci

Foci are defined as small dots of enhancement that are unique and stand out from the BPE. They are too small to be accurately assessed with respect to margin or internal enhancement. Indeed, if margin or internal enhancement can be assessed, the finding should be considered a small mass and not a focus. New foci or foci that have increased in size should be viewed with suspicion and carefully evaluated. Correlation with bright-fluid imaging (T2W imaging or STIR imaging) can be helpful in the evaluation of a focus. If a correlate is uniformly very high in signal intensity or if cyst-like features are identified, the focus may be assessed as benign. (Most of these foci represent lymph nodes or small myxomatous fibroadenomas.) However, if the focus does not have a very high signal correlate on bright-fluid imaging, then the focus may or may not be benign. These foci may be followed or biopsied. In certain cases (if the finding is new or increased in size), the focus always should be biopsied. Note that malignant foci may be brighter than the surrounding FGT, although they do not usually appear cyst-like.

Follow-Up of Masses

Masses that enhance and are identified on an initial MRI examination should undergo assessment based on morphology and kinetics. It has been documented that occasionally malignancy may demonstrate benign-appearing MRI features, such as an oval or round shape with a circumscribed margin and homogeneous internal enhancement. Therefore, in a scenario in which the stability of the finding is unknown, periodic surveillance imaging may be appropriate, depending on various factors that affect the prior probability of malignancy (age, cancer risk, etc.) as well as the patient's willingness to accept surveillance imaging as an alternative to biopsy, given less than robust data that support a watchful-waiting approach. If surveillance imaging is undertaken, an increase in size of the mass should prompt immediate biopsy.

Follow-Up of NME

NME that is unique and separate from the overall background enhancement should undergo assessment based on morphology and kinetics. Bright-fluid imaging sequences can be helpful in these instances to demonstrate any associated cysts, which may support a diagnosis of focal fibrocystic change and a benign (category 2) assessment. However, limited data on linear, clumped, and segmental enhancement indicate that these findings should not be followed, as the malignancy rate appears to be greater than 2%. 4 At this time, the literature is not sufficiently robust to endorse the use of a category 3 assessment for NME.

Timing of Follow-Up

Final assessment category 3 is best used for a unique focal finding and managed with an initial short-interval follow-up (6 months) examination followed by additional examinations until long-term (2- or 3-year) stability is demonstrated. For category 3 assessments, the initial short-term follow-up interval is usually 6 months, involving the breast(s) containing the probably benign finding(s). Assuming stability at this 6-month examination, a category 3 assessment again will be rendered with a management recommendation for a second short-interval follow-up examination in 6 months but now involving both breasts if the opposite breast will be due for routine annual screening. Again assuming stability at this second short-interval follow-up, the examination is once more assessed as category 3, but now the recommended follow-up interval usually is lengthened to 1 year due to the already-observed 12-month stability. The recommended 2- or 3-year follow-up in these cases is 6 months, 6 months, 1 year, and, optionally, 1 more year to establish stability. After 2–3 years of stability, the finding should be assessed as benign (category 2). It should be emphasized that this approach is borrowed from mammography. While the vast majority of probably benign findings are managed with follow-up, there may be occasions in which biopsies are done instead (patient preference or overriding clinical concern). As with any interpretive examination, a less experienced reader may conclude that a finding such as benign BPE, for example, should be classified as category 3. A more experienced reader may recognize this as normal or benign at 6 or 12 months and classify it as category 1 or 2. With a properly worded report, the assessment category may then be changed to one that the current reader feels is appropriate, even though long-term stability has not been demonstrated.

It is imperative that surveillance imaging does not alter the stage at diagnosis or prognosis of the few patients with malignancies who are given category 3 assessments. Because this has not yet been demonstrated for MRI, as it has been for mammography, careful auditing of the use of category 3 assessments is necessary, and publication of outcomes data is strongly recommended. Although the data are not robust, it appears the ≤2% malignancy rate already demonstrated at mammographic follow-up also may be achieved at MRI. Several publications have demonstrated that focal lesions assigned to category 3 had a ≤2% malignancy rate, albeit without use of specific BI-RADS® MRI descriptors for the lesions included in the studies. Publication of outcomes data for specific category 3 lesions, using BI-RADS® MRI, is strongly recommended. It should be noted that a ≤2% malignancy rate may be difficult to achieve due to the high-risk population that usually is studied by MRI (higher than average prior probability of cancer).

A desirable goal for the frequency of making category 3 assessments at MRI is less than 10%. Over time, this rate should decrease to the point that a mature program should demonstrate a rate much closer to the approximately 1%–2% rate currently achieved at mammography, especially as the availability of previous examination(s) increases. A decrease in the frequency of category 3 assessments and false-positive outcomes has been demonstrated in the breast MRI literature as experience is gained.

Category 4: Suspicious. This category is reserved for findings that do not have the classic appearance of malignancy but are sufficiently suspicious to justify a recommendation for biopsy. The ceiling for a category 3 assessment is a 2% likelihood of malignancy, and the floor for a category 5 assessment is 95%, so category 4 assessments cover the wide range of likelihood of malignancy in between. Thus, almost all recommendations for breast interventional procedures will come from assessments made using this assessment category. In breast MRI, assessment category 4 is not currently divided into subcategories 4A, 4B, and 4C. Category 4 is used for the majority of findings prompting breast intervention, which can be performed by percutaneous biopsy, by US or stereotactic guidance, or by MRI guidance for lesions not visible at either US or mammography. As cysts rarely pose a problem in interpretation at MRI, diagnostic aspiration is not commonly performed. In many patients with a suspicious abnormality at MRI, targeted US will identify a corresponding abnormality so that US-guided biopsy can be performed. US-guided biopsies are faster, more comfortable for the patient, and more cost effective than MRI-guided biopsies. There are no established guidelines on who should undergo targeted US. However, in general, patients with masses larger than 5 mm should be examined by targeted US if the MR appearance is suspicious. Areas of NME may be evident on US as well, thus bringing the radiologist's judgment into play. Factors that may limit visibility at US include fatty breasts, extremely complex breasts with multiple cysts, very large breasts, and very deep lesions. If there is any question about whether a presumed sonographic correlate actually is the same as the suspicious MRI lesion, MR-guided biopsy is advised.

Category 5: Highly Suggestive of Malignancy. These assessments carry a very high probability (≥95%) of malignancy. This category initially was established to include lesions for which 1-stage surgical treatment was considered without preliminary biopsy, in an era when preoperative wire localization was the primary breast interventional procedure. Nowadays, given the widespread acceptance of imaging-guided percutaneous biopsy, 1-stage surgery rarely if ever is performed. Rather, current oncologic management almost always involves tissue diagnosis of malignancy via percutaneous tissue sampling. This facilitates treatment options, such as when sentinel node biopsy is included in surgical management or when neoadjuvant chemotherapy isadministered prior to surgery. Therefore, the current rationale for using category 5 assessment is to identify lesions for which any nonmalignant percutaneous tissue diagnosis is considered discordant, resulting in a recommendation for repeat (usually surgical) biopsy. No single MRI descriptor is sufficiently predictive of malignancy to produce the ≥95% probability required for a category 5 assessment. Just as in mammography and US, an appropriate combination of suspicious findings is needed to justify a category 5 assessment at MRI. It is recommended that category 5 assessments be audited separately to verify a ≥95% PPV, thereby validating that the assessment is not being overused.

Category 6: Known Biopsy-Proven Malignancy. This category is reserved for examinations performed after biopsy proof of malignancy (imaging performed after percutaneous biopsy) but prior to surgical excision, in which there are no abnormalities other than the known cancer that might need additional evaluation. That is, a cancer diagnosis has already been established, a lesion is depicted at MRI, and this lesion corresponds to the previously biopsied cancer. A category 6 is not appropriate following successful lumpectomy or mastectomy (margin of resection free of tumor). The rationale for establishing category 6 is exclusion of these cases from auditing, because additional malignancy is frequently found such that auditing these cases would inappropriately skew overall outcomes. In the event that the breast with known cancer has a separate suspicious MRI finding that requires biopsy for diagnosis, the appropriate category 4 or 5 assessment should be rendered, and this would be the overall assessment because it leads to more prompt intervention.

BI-RADS lexicon *for echography* is a little bit different from the lexicon for mammography, thus the US report should have the following structure:

1. Indication for examination
2. Statement of scope and technique of breast US examination
3. Succinct description of the overall breast composition (screening only)
4. Clear description of any important findings
5. Comparison to previous examination(s), including correlation with physical, mammography, or MRI findings
6. Composite reports
7. Assessment
8. Management

1. Indication for Examination
   The reason for performing the examination should be stated briefly at the beginning of the report. The most common indications for breast US are confirmation and characterization of a palpable mass or mammographic or MRI abnormality, guidance of interventional procedures, and as the initial imaging technique for young, pregnant, or lactating patients. Additional applications are listed in the ACR Practice Guideline for the Performance of the Breast Ultrasound Examination and include the extent of disease evaluation supplementing mammography in high-risk women who are not candidates for breast MRI or who have no easy access to MRI and in breast imaging practices that provide the service, supplementary whole-breast screening in order to increase cancer detection in asymptomatic women with mammographically dense breasts.
2. Statement of Scope and Technique of Breast US Examination
   The scope of examination and technique used should be stated, for example, whether the examination was directed or targeted to a specific location or whether it was performed for supplementary screening. It is important, since US is a real-time examination, to indicate who performed the examination (sonographer, sonographer and physician, physician alone) or whether an automated whole-breast scanning system was used. If a lesion was evaluated with color or power Doppler or with strain or shear wave elastography, observations relevant to the interpretation should be reported. In certain situations, it may be beneficial to describe the position of the patient during the examination (e.g., "The breasts were imaged in both supine and lateral decubitus position" or "The patient was imaged in seated position, the position in which she feels the left breast thickening best").

   Automated whole-breast scanners that acquire in 3D are available for clinical use and can be formatted in three planes. These scanners depict the entire breast in coronal, transverse, and sagittal planes, with the coronal view similar to the coronal MRI view. Reporting of these studies continues to evolve, but where possible the interpretation structure outlined previously and the reporting procedures described earlier in this section should be followed.
3. Succinct Description of the Overall Breast Composition (Screening Only)
   Tissue composition patterns can be estimated more easily in the large FOVs of automated US scans but can also be discerned in the small FOV of a handheld US scan. The three US descriptors for tissue composition described earlier in the US lexicon, "homogeneous background echotexture-fat," "homogeneous background echotexture-fibro glandular," and "heterogeneous background echotexture" (below), correspond loosely to the four density descriptors of mammography and the four fibroglandular tissue descriptors of MRI. At US, breast tissue composition is determined by echogenicity. Subcutaneous fat, the tissue relative to which echogenicity is compared, is medium gray and darker than fibroglandular tissue, which is light gray. Heterogeneous breasts show an admixture of hypoechoic and more echogenic areas. Careful real-time scanning will help differentiate a small hypoechoic area of normal tissue from a mass.
   (a) Homogeneous background echotexture-fat
   (b) Homogeneous background echotexture -fibroglandular
   (c) Heterogeneous background echotexture
4. Clear Description of Any Important Findings

The description of important findings should be made, in order of clinical relevance, using lexicon terminology, and should include:

(a) Characterization of a mass using the morphological descriptors of shape, margin, and orientation. Note should be made of the lesion's effect on the surrounding tissue, such as architectural distortion. Feature categories, such as posterior features and echogenicity, and techniques, such as color or power Doppler and elastography, may contribute information to the analysis, but only pertinent positives need to be described. Recognition of special case findings, such as simple and complicated cysts, clustered microcysts, intramammary lymph nodes, and foreign bodies, should simplify interpretation. In reporting screening examinations in asymptomatic women, as in mammography, characteristically benign findings may be reported (assessment category 2), but it is not obligatory, and the appropriate assessment would then be negative (assessment category 1).

(b) For important findings, lesion size should be given in at least two dimensions; three dimensions are preferable, especially if the volume of a mass is compared with one or more previous examinations. It is not necessary to report the measurements of every small simple cyst, and if numerous cysts are present, especially in both breasts, location and measurements of the largest cyst in each breast will suffice. If a mass is measured, images should be recorded with and without calipers. Marginal characteristics are one of the most important criteria to be applied in assessing the likelihood of malignancy of a mass, and, particularly with small masses, caliper markings may obscure the margin, hindering analysis.

(c) Location of the lesion(s) should be indicated using a consistent and reproducible system, such as clock-face location and distance from the nipple. When more than one mass or abnormality is located in the same scan frame or in the same locale, measurement of the distance from the skin to the center of the mass or its anterior aspect may help to differentiate one lesion from another. This measurement may be particularly useful when one mass is singled out for biopsy and others are depicted in the field. There may be variability within breast imaging practices, and members of a group practice should agree upon a consistent policy for documenting lesion location on subsequent examinations. In some practices, for all examinations that follow the initial US study, the lesion location annotation will be repeated without change. Other breast imagers may report a different location to signify the same lesion but indicate in their reports that the lesion is now seen at another clock-face position and distance from the nipple (these differences are often related to positioning and technique).

(d) As at mammography, multiple bilateral circumscribed masses usually are assessed as benign (category 2) unless one mass has different imaging features than all the others. In the unusual circumstance in which the interpreting physician chooses to describe multiple benign-appearing masses individually within the US report, the masses should be listed by breast, by location within in the breast, and by size. The reader of the report will be less confused, and, if surveillance is suggested as management, the performer of the subsequent examination will appreciate a list rather than verbose text. For bilateral findings, describe all the findings in each breast in a separate paragraph.

5. Comparison to Previous Examination(s), Including Correlation with Physical, Mammography, or MRI Findings
Breast US should be correlated with physical findings, mammography, MRI, or other imaging studies, if performed. If no statement of comparison is included in the US report, it

will be assumed that no comparison was made. Note that some report templates include a "comparison" heading, in which the word "none" (if appropriate) may be entered. When correlating US findings with those seen at mammography and/or MRI, the operator performing handheld scanning should correlate the size and location of lesions and match the type and arrangement of tissues surrounding the lesion in order to reduce the likelihood of misregistration (identifying a different lesion or lesions at different imaging modalities). In doing this, allowance for positional changes should be made going from upright with mammography and prone with MRI to supine or supine-oblique with US. If it is determined that a sonographic finding corresponds to a palpable abnormality or to a mammographic or MRI finding, this should be stated explicitly in the US report. If the US finding is new or has no correlate, this should also be stated in the report. If the US examination was performed as part of a surveillance protocol to assess a previously identified finding, or if the finding was reported on a previous examination, the current report should describe any changes. An increase of 20% or more in the longest dimension of a probably benign solid mass within 6 months may prompt biopsy. 1 An increase of only 1–2 mm in lesion size may be related to differences in scanning technique or patient positioning.

6. Composite Reports
When more than one type of examination is performed concurrently (on the same day), it is preferable that the examinations be reported together. The findings for each examination should be described in separate paragraphs with an overall assessment and management recommendations for the combined examinations. In general, when the assessments for two examinations differ, the overall assessment (and concordant management recommendations) should reflect the more abnormal of the individual assessments (whatever management is expected to come first, supplemented by likelihood of malignancy), according to the following hierarchy of increasing abnormality: categories 1, 2, 3, 6, 0, 4, and 5 (Table 1.7). Exceptions to this rule occur when the characteristically benign features of a given imaging finding on one examination supersede the less specifically benign features of the same finding on the other examination. An example is that of a partially circumscribed, noncalcified mass at mammography, superseded by simple cyst at US.

Table 1.7 Abnormality hierarchy

BI-RADS assessment category	Degree of abnormality
1	Lowest
2	↓
3	
6	
0	
4	
5	Highest

7. Assessment
The report should conclude with a concise summary of pertinent US findings with a final assessment using BI-RADS® US categories 1–6 and the phrases associated with them. If report of a US examination is integrated with that of a concurrently performed mammography examination, the combined final assessment should reflect the highest likelihood of malignancy assessed at the two examinations. Clear and consistent communication is a goal that can be achieved for breast US by using the same assessment categories and similar wording described in the BI-RADS® Mammography section. In some cases, the interpreting physician may render an incomplete assessment (category 0) in order to request additional examination(s), such as mammography, comparison with previous but currently unavailable examinations, or additional physician-performed real-time scanning after either a sonographer-produced, real-time, or automated whole-breast screening US examination.

BI-RADS categories used in echography analysis corresponds to the categories used in other diagnostic procedures (Sect. 6.6 in Chap. 6).

(a) Assessment Is Incomplete

Category 0: Incomplete—Need Additional Imaging Evaluation and/or Prior Images for Comparison. There is a finding for which additional imaging evaluation is needed. This is almost always used in a screening situation. In this context, additional imaging evaluation includes the recording of (nonstandard) US images to supplement the standard images recorded for a screening examination. Note that this does not include repeat real-time scanning by the interpreting physician and/or colleague as long as additional images are not recorded. This respects the unique real-time nature of US and does not penalize its use. Under certain circumstances, assessment category 0 may be used in a diagnostic US report, such as when equipment or personnel are not immediately available to perform a needed concurrent diagnostic mammography examination or when the patient is unable or unwilling to wait for completion of a full diagnostic examination. Category 0 should not be used for diagnostic breast imaging findings that warrant further evaluation with MRI. Rather, the interpreting physician should issue a final assessment in a report that is made before the MRI examination is performed. In most circumstances and when feasible, if a screening US examination is not assessed as negative or benign, the current examination should be compared to prior examination(s), if any exist.

The interpreting physician should use judgment on how vigorously to attempt obtaining prior examinations, given the likelihood of success of such an endeavor and the likelihood that comparison will affect the final assessment. In this context, it is important to note that comparison to previous examination(s) may be irrelevant when a finding is inherently suspicious or malignant. Category 0 should be used for prior image comparison only when such comparison is required to make a final assessment. When category 0 is used in the context of awaiting prior examinations for comparison, there should be in place a tracking system guaranteeing with 100% reliability that a final assessment will be made within 30 days (preferably sooner), even if prior examinations do not become available. Some breast imaging practices may reasonably choose never to use category 0 in the context of awaiting prior examinations simply because they do not have a 100% reliable tracking system. If an US examination is assessed as category 0 in the context of awaiting prior examinations and then the prior examinations do become available, an addendum to the initial US report should be issued, including a revised assessment. For auditing purposes, the revised assessment should replace the initial assessment. A need for previous studies to determine appropriate management might also temporarily defer a final assessment.

(b) Assessment Is Complete—Final Categories

Category 1: Negative. There is nothing to comment on. This is a normal examination.

Category 2: Benign. As with category 1, this is a "normal" assessment, but here the interpreter chooses to describe a benign finding in the US report. For example, the interpreter may choose to describe one or more simple cysts, intramammary lymph nodes, postsurgical fluid collections, breast implants, or complicated cysts/probable fibroadenomas that are unchanged for at least 2 or 3 years while still concluding that there is no sonographic evidence of malignancy. On the other hand, the interpreter may choose not to describe such findings, in which case the examination should be assessed as negative (category 1). Note that both category 1 and category 2 assessments indicate that there is no sonographic evidence of malignancy. Both should be followed by the management recommendation for routine age-appropriate screening. The difference is that category 2 should be used when describing one or more specific benign sonographic findings in the report, whereas category 1 should be used when no such findings are described (even if such findings are present).

Category 3: Probably Benign. Category 3 assessment, probably benign, is not an indeterminate category for use simply when the radiologist is unsure whether to render a benign (BI-RADS® category 2) or suspicious

(BI-RADS® category 4) assessment, but one that is reserved for specific imaging findings known to have >0% but ≤2% likelihood of malignancy. For US, there is robust evidence that a solid mass with a circumscribed margin, oval shape, and parallel orientation (most commonly fibroadenoma), and an isolated complicated cyst have a likelihood of malignancy in the defined (≤2%) probably benign range, for which short-interval (6-month) follow-up sonography and then periodic sonographic surveillance may represent appropriate management. Similar data have been reported for clustered microcysts, but these data are less strong because they involve many fewer cases. The use of category 3 assessment for sonographic findings other than these three should be considered only if the radiologist has personal experience to justify a watchful-waiting approach, preferably involving observation of a sufficient number of cases of an additional sonographic finding to suggest a likelihood of malignancy within the defined (≤2%) probably benign range. This edition of the BI-RADS® Atlas also emphasizes the recommendation that a category 3 assessment should not be made at screening; rather, this should be done only after completion of a full diagnostic breast imaging examination. This recommendation is appropriate for screening mammography, for which batch interpretation usually is utilized, because in this setting there is no opportunity to complete the diagnostic workup before interpreting the screening examination. However, screening US almost always is interpreted online, so a full diagnostic examination also is completed while the patient remains in the breast imaging facility, and a single breast imaging report may be issued that combines the findings of both screening and diagnostic components of the examination. Hence, there is no purpose in recommending against category 3 assessment at screening US because the diagnostic workup would be completed simultaneously. Note that for auditing purposes, the screening component of a category 3-assessed screening US examination will be audit-positive, not only because additional nonstandard (diagnostic) images will be recorded but also because a category 3 assessment at screening is defined as being audit-positive. For category 3 assessments, the initial short-term follow-up interval is usually 6 months, involving the breast(s) containing the probably benign finding(s). Assuming stability at this 6-month examination, a category 3 assessment again is rendered with a management recommendation for a second short-interval follow-up examination in 6 months. Again assuming stability at this second short-interval follow-up, the examination is once more assessed as category 3, but now the recommended follow-up interval usually is lengthened to 1 year due to the already-observed 12-month stability. Note that although the 1-year follow-up coincides with the routine screening interval in the USA, a category 3 assessment is rendered, to indicate that the period of imaging surveillance is still underway. As with surveillance using mammography, after 2–3 years of stability, the final assessment category should be changed to benign (BI-RADS® category 2). A benign evaluation may also be rendered before completion of category 3 analysis if, in the opinion of the interpreter, the finding has no chance of malignancy and is thus a category 2.

Category 4: Suspicious. This category is reserved for findings that do not have the classic appearance of malignancy but are sufficiently suspicious to justify a recommendation for biopsy. The ceiling for category 3 assessment is a 2% likelihood of malignancy, and the floor for category 5 assessment is 95%, so category 4 assessments cover the wide range of likelihood of malignancy in between. Thus, almost all recommendations for breast interventional procedures will come from assessments made using this category. By subdividing category 4 into 4A, 4B, and 4C, as recommended in and using the cut points indicated in the Guidance chapter, it is hoped that patients and referring clinicians will more readily make informed decisions on the ultimate course of action. An example of separating the BI-RADS assessment category from the management recommendation (new to fifth edition—see Follow-up and Outcome Monitoring section) occurs when a simple cyst, correctly assessed as BI-RADS 2, undergoes cyst aspiration for pain control.

Category 5: Highly Suggestive of Malignancy. These assessments carry a very high probability (≥95%) of malignancy. This category initially was established to involve lesions for which 1-stage surgical treatment could be considered without preliminary biopsy in an era when preoperative wire localization was the primary breast interventional procedure. Nowadays, given the widespread acceptance of imaging-guided percutaneous biopsy, 1-stage surgery rarely if ever is performed. Rather, current oncologic management almost always involves tissue diagnosis of malignancy via percutaneous tissue sampling to facilitate treatment options, such as when sentinel node imaging is included in surgical management or when neoadjuvant chemotherapy is administered prior to surgery. Therefore, the current rationale for using a category 5 assessment is to identify lesions for which any nonmalignant percutaneous tissue diagnosis is considered discordant, resulting in the recommendation for repeat (usually vacuum-assisted or surgical) biopsy. Also note that whereas the fourth edition simply indicated that "appropriate action should be taken" as management for category 5 assessments, the fifth edition provides the more directed management recommendation that "biopsy should be performed in the absence of clinical contraindication." This new text unequivocally specifies tissue diagnosis as the interpreting physician's management recommendation for category 5 assessments, appropriately and effectively transferring the burden of establishing a contraindication to this recommendation to the referring clinician.

Category 6: Known Biopsy-Proven Malignancy. This category is reserved for examinations performed after biopsy proof of malignancy (imaging performed after percutaneous biopsy but prior to surgical excision), in which there are no abnormalities other than the known cancer that might need additional evaluation.

The use of the BI-RADS system, with X-ray, ultrasound, and MR imaging, facilitates communication between radiologists and clinicians resulting in increased accuracy of diagnosis and better treatment outcomes.

The following breast cancer screening algorithm is recommended (Fig. 1.24):

1. In order to timely detect breast pathology, US is mostly used as a supplementary test in women aged ≤49 years.
2. During preventive medical check-ups aimed at timely diagnosis of breast pathology, annual breast US should be performed in 20–39-year-old women in addition to physical examination.
3. In 40–49-year-old women, mammography should be performed every other year. Breast US is carried out in the intervals between mammography.
4. In women of the age 50 years and older, as a rule, mammography is performed every other year.

Inclusion of the ultrasound method in the complex breast cancer screening algorithm will make it possible to balance out the drawbacks of the X-ray method in women with dense breast and to conduct a complete breast examination in women under the age of 40. This will allow the detection of not only malignant tumors but also benign proliferative breast diseases, which may cause breast cancer development in many cases.

Imaging techniques became very important for early and differential diagnosis of breast diseases. Successful implementation of screening programs and reasonable combination of traditional and innovative technologies facilitate the work of radiologists, mammologists, oncologists, surgeons, and endocrinologists and permit detection of a wide range of breast diseases at early stages, to choose effective treatment methods, specify prognosis, and determine rational terms of follow-up.

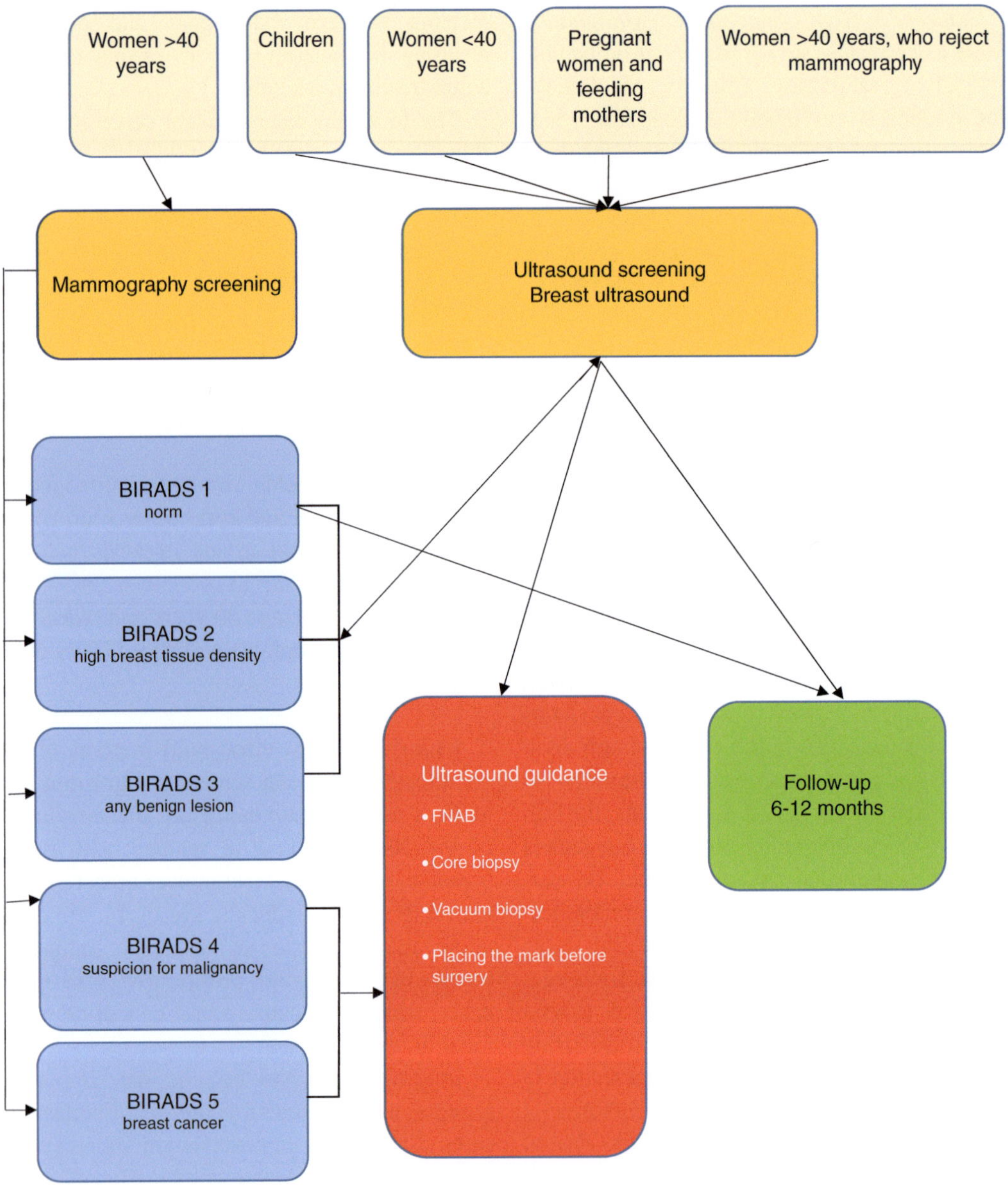

Fig. 1.24 The flowchart of screening programs with US

Breast Ultrasound Technology

2

Alexander N. Sencha, Mikhail Pykov, and Ekaterina Sencha

Abstract

The role of US is great in definition of breast masses in the areas that are technically difficult to examine with other imaging methods (e.g., on the margin of medial quadrants near the breastbone, in aberrant mammary lobes). US is unique for the analysis of the whole-breast vascularity and vascular pattern of its lesions. Additionally, US precisely characterizes abnormal lymph nodes. Breast US is performed with linear probes with the frequency of 5–12 MHz. Retromammary space is better examined with a 5.0 MHz probe and the nipple and areola with 10 MHz or higher frequency probe. The most common causes of errors in the diagnosis of breast cancer are small tumor size, tumor development on the background of diffuse adenosis, fibrous stellate bands, multiple small cysts with dense contents, perifocal inflammation, etc. Lymph nodes, which are adjacent to the breast, often cause difficulties in correct diagnosis. The conclusion of breast lesion is only permitted in the case of its clear demonstration at least in two perpendicular projections. Auxiliary methods, such as lifting of patient's arms, turns of the body to one or another side, and change of body position, are important for differential diagnosis. Correct diagnosis sometimes requires long follow-up or application of other diagnostic methods.

A. N. Sencha (✉)
Division of Visual Diagnostics, National Medical Research Center for Obstetrics, Gynecology and Perinatology named after Academician V.I.Kulakov of Ministry of Healthcare of Russian Federation, Moscow, Russia

M. Pykov
Department of Ultrasound Diagnostics in Neonatology and Pediatrics, National Medical Research Center for Obstetrics, Gynecology and Perinatology named after Academician V.I.Kulakov of Ministry of Healthcare of Russian Federation, Moscow, Russia

E. Sencha
Department of Ultrasound Diagnostics, Federal State Budget Hospital "9 Treatment and Diagnostic Center" of the Ministry of Defense of the Russian Federation, Moscow, Russia

2.1 Methodology and Technique of Breast Ultrasound

Breast ultrasound (US) is an effective and highly informative method of examination, screening, detection, and differential diagnosis of various breast conditions.

US exhibits the following advantages in diagnosis of breast pathology:

- High resolution of modern US equipment and high diagnostic value.
- It is relatively simple to perform, fast, and cost-effective.

G. T. Sukhikh, A. N. Sencha (eds.), *Multiparametric Ultrasound Diagnosis of Breast Diseases*,
https://doi.org/10.1007/978-3-319-75034-7_2

- Noninvasive and painlessness.
- Can be done without any preparation of a patient.
- Has no contraindications.
- Harmless and safe for the patient, hence possible to be used for children, pregnant women and feeding mothers, and patients with serious accompanying pathology and perform multiple repeated examinations.
- Permits differential diagnosis based on complex analysis of grayscale, Doppler modes, 3D reconstruction, and other options.
- Supports objective follow-up by means of digital archiving.
- Permits computer processing, archiving of US data in an objective form suitable for delayed analysis, and digital transfer with virtual consultations via telemedicine systems and the Internet.
- Supplies precise guidance for minimally invasive manipulations.

US demands certain skills, detailed knowledge of the anatomy and physiological changes of the breast, correlations of findings with clinical signs, results of mammography, and other diagnostic methods. US is thought to be inappropriate for screening of breast cancer. This opinion is based on several disadvantages, as follows:

- Impossibility to image the breast as a whole
- Low diagnostic value in cases of fatty involution
- Subjective interpretation
- Impossibility of detection of noninvasive intraductal neoplasms in the form of calcifications without tumoral mass

US is a primary method of examination in the following cases:

- Pregnant women and nursing mothers
- Dense breast background in young women
- Differential diagnosis between solid and cavitary lesions
- Early assessment of the breast after trauma or acute inflammation
- Detection of regional and peripheral lymph nodes
- Guidance of biopsies
- Assessment of the condition of silicone implants

The role of US is great in definition of breast masses in the areas that are technically difficult to examine with other imaging methods (e.g., on the margin of medial quadrants near the breastbone, in aberrant mammary lobes). US is unique for the analysis of the whole-breast vascularity and vascular pattern of its lesions. Additionally, US precisely characterizes abnormal lymph nodes.

Due to the fact that the ultrasound method is harmless, noninvasive, accessible, and quite effective in diagnosis of a wide range of breast conditions, it is often performed without special indications, often for preventive purposes.

Indications for breast US are the following:

- Complaints and symptoms, which are often associated with breast pathology, such as the change in shape, pulling in of the nipple, discomfort or pain, and hyperemia
- Pathological discharge from the nipples
- Palpable lesions within the breast, in axillary, subclavian, or parasternal areas
- Breast pathology revealed by other diagnostic methods
- Chronic diseases of female reproductive system
- Follow-up of the patients treated for breast diseases
- Postoperative period
- Annual preventive examination

Breast US does not demand special preparation of the patient. The optimum period for examination is the first phase of menstrual cycle in fertile women.

Breast US is performed with linear probes with the frequency of 5–12 MHz, more often 7.5–10 MHz. Retromammary space is better examined with a 5.0 MHz probe and the nipple and areola with 10 MHz or higher frequency probe. The patient is positioned supine with the hands under the head.

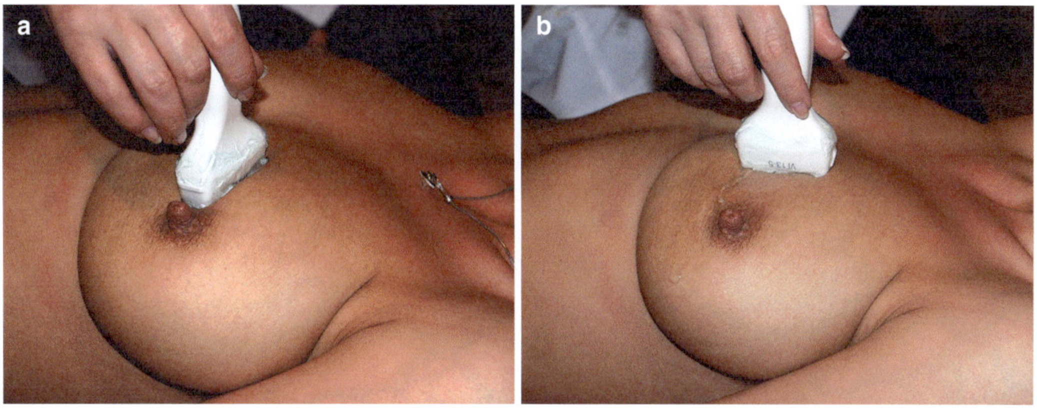

Fig. 2.1 Breast US. (**a**, **b**) Position of US probe

In the case of large breast, it is reasonable to carry out the examination with the patient on her back, on the right and left side, and in sitting position with her hands under the head. The probe is positioned perpendicularly to the breast skin. The compression should be limited (Fig. 2.1).

Examination is carried out in a multiprojection, multipositional manner. Ultrasonography should be performed as systematically and technologically accurate as possible. It should be comprehensive, understandable, and reproducible for the clinician. Comfort, painlessness, and quick performance are main criteria for the patient.

While describing the location of pathological process, the breast is conventionally divided into four quadrants: upper (superior)-outer (lateral), upper (superior)-inner (medial), lower (inferior)-inner (medial), and lower (inferior)-outer (lateral). Subareolar area (central portion) and the nipple are mentioned separately. The terminology of "clock positions" is appropriate as additional subsite descriptor to indicate the exact location of abnormality (Fig. 2.2).

The examination, as a rule, begins with the intact breast or at any side in cases of no complaints. The direction of scanning does not matter. Breast US more often begins with the upper-outer quadrant of the right breast and follows clockwise with the probe movements in radial direction from the periphery to the nipple area along the course of lactiferous ducts. The examination of the left breast often starts with the upper-inner quadrant proceeding clockwise. For more detailed examination, the scans are repeated in a clockwise circular direction from periphery to nipple area. Special attention is paid to subareolar and nipple areas, since the acoustic shadow from the nipple can hide various pathological processes. Finally, most painful site is examined one more time.

The following instances should be assessed during breast US:

1. The breast as a whole:
    - Location, symmetry
    - Echodensity
    - Echostructure, the ratio of fatty and glandular tissue
    - Condition of lactiferous ducts
    - Nipple area and areola
    - Blood vessels of the parenchyma (symmetry and intensity of vascularization)
2. Changes within the breast:
    - Character of changes (diffuse, focal)
    - Number of lesions
    - Location (quadrants, sectors)
    - Sizes of lesions (three dimensions in mutually perpendicular planes)
    - Echodensity
    - Echostructure of lesions
    - Contours (even/rough, distinct/vague)
    - Mobility of the lesion, discomfort, and change in shape with compression
    - Vascularity

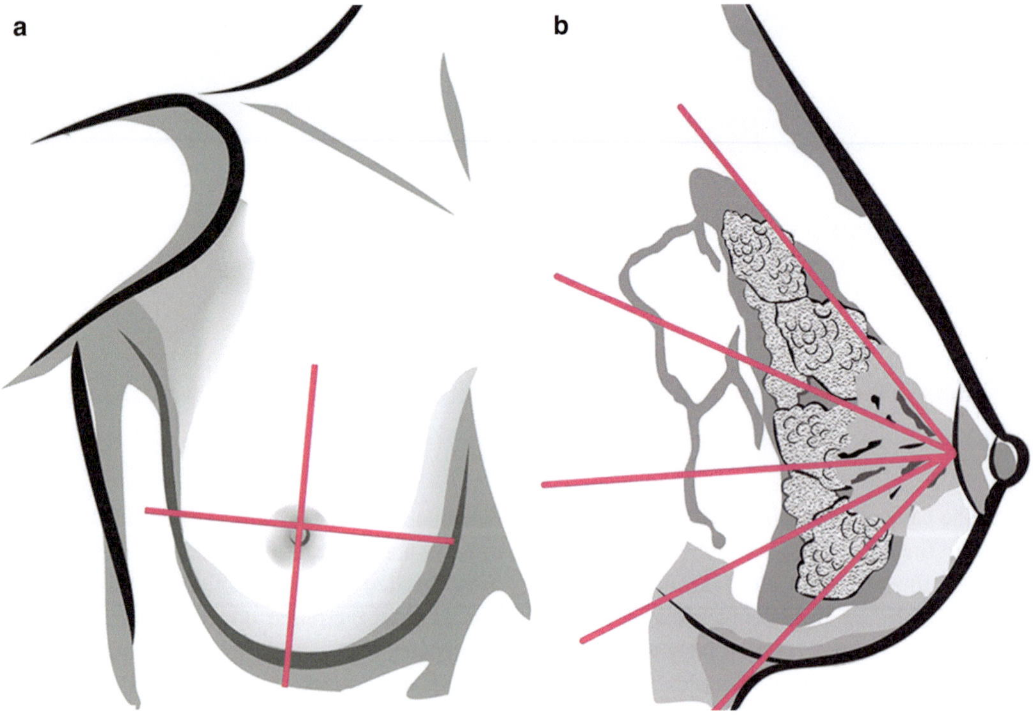

Fig. 2.2 The scheme of breast areas. (**a**) O'clock positions and quadrants of the breasts. (**b**) Sectors

3. Relations of breast lesion with surrounding structures (assessment of invasion of breast carcinoma into surrounding tissues)
4. Condition of regional lymph nodes

If an area suspicious for pathological process is detected within the breast, moderate compression with the probe is applied. This aims to assess the mobility of the lesion against the surrounding tissues, its density (deformation), and to decrease US artifacts resulting from connective tissue elements (e.g., lateral acoustic shadows). Ultrasound image of this area should be compared with a similar area of the other breast.

2.2 Main Challenges and Pitfalls in Breast Ultrasound

Precise and efficient echography requires certain skills, detailed knowledge of breast anatomy and physiological changes, and an ability to compare clinical data, history, mammographic findings, and results of other tests.

Diagnostic errors and misinterpretation that result in wrong management are not rare. The most common causes of errors in the diagnosis of breast cancer are small tumor size, tumor development on the background of diffuse adenosis, fibrous stellate bands, multiple small cysts with dense contents, perifocal inflammation, etc.

The causes of mistakes at breast US can be divided into the following groups:

1. Objective
   - Anatomic, physiological, and constitutional features of the patient that decrease the quality of breast imaging
   - Limitations of the equipment (class of US scanner, characteristics of probes, etc.)
2. Subjective
   - Lack of experience of personnel
   - Inadequate or incomplete technique of the examination

Low reproducibility of breast US is often a consequence of the differences in the class of equipment and qualification of the doctor. Rare breast pathology can be misinterpreted because of insufficient experience of US specialist that results in diagnostic errors. Psychological predilection to bring the detected abnormalities under standards also affects the quality of diagnosis.

At the same time, there are cases of hyperdiagnostics of pathology in the normal breast, when normal breast structures are interpreted as lesions. This especially concerns the structures located on the periphery of the breast, in retromammary space, and in subareolar area.

Differentiation of malignant and benign tumors and tumor-like and non-tumoral processes of the breast requires special attention. Correct diagnosis of local tumors, such as breast carcinoma with expansive growth, requires certain experience and efforts. Breast carcinoma without nodular structure and prominent diffuse or local infiltration is also difficult for differential diagnosis. The minimum changes in a kind of local clump of ducts (dilated or not dilated), in association with their chaotic distribution, especially in peripheral parts of the breast can be a sign of ductal breast carcinoma. Differentiation of sclerosing adenosis from breast carcinoma is extremely important, since this borderline breast disease is associated with high incidence of malignancy. Sclerosing adenosis can hide early signs of breast carcinoma due to the number of identical US features (excessive fibrosis, calcifications, heterogeneity of breast structure). Hence, only the examination targeted to the search of characteristic features for malignant neoplasm results in the correct diagnosis.

Lymph nodes, which are adjacent to the breast, often cause difficulties in correct diagnosis. It is necessary to use the highest possible frequency of US probe to achieve detailed image and to pay attention to specific features of lymph nodes, such as the shape, echostructure with differentiation of the cortex and hilum, and typical pattern of blood flow in the hilum. Alternatively, there are mistakes, when breast lesions are interpreted for lymph nodes. The conclusion of breast lesion is only permitted in the case of its clear demonstration at least in two perpendicular projections. Correct diagnosis sometimes requires long follow-up or application of other diagnostic methods.

Auxiliary methods, such as lifting of patient's arms, turns of the body to one or another side, and change of body position, are important for differential diagnosis.

Following the methodology of the examination is extremely valuable. Breast structure can be assessed only with linear probes with the frequency of 7.5 MHz or higher. Convex probes for abdominal examinations can be used additionally for the measurement of large breast lesions. The use of a convex probe alone for breast examination results in multiple severe errors and discredits the field of sonography.

Color Doppler mapping also requires special regimens (packages), optimum choice of technologies for improving the color image quality, small region of interest, correct Doppler angles, minimization of noises, high-quality preprocessing and averaging, and minimum values of color Doppler scale to improve the obtained data.

At US elastography (analysis of qualitative parameters and calculation of quantitative indications of breast elasticity) the methodology, experience and skills of the operator, and a comprehensive analysis of the obtained results are extremely important.

Undoubtedly, such factors as definition of indications, contraindications, correct execution of the procedure, precise dosage, and injection of an echocontrast (if CEUS is applied) are extremely important. Correct visualization, ultrasound scanner settings, adequate choice of the contrast and its dose, the complex analysis of qualitative and quantitative indicators, and the experience of operator largely determine the effectiveness of CEUS.

The recommended terms for breast US are the following:

- Normal breast for preventive purposes—once in 2 years
- Benign diffuse and nodular changes for assessment of the disease development—one to two times a year
- Postoperative breast—once in 6 months

Dynamic observation of newly diagnosed breast lesions with no definite pathognomonic signs of malignancy with a 6-month interval may be a reasonable alternative to aggressive surgical tactics.

Due to the safety and availability of US the monitoring of breast pathology can be performed with shorter intervals if relevant indications arise.

Ultrasound Image of the Normal Breast

3

Mikhail Pykov, Alexander N. Sencha, and Elena Philipova

Abstract

US image of the normal breast is quite variable and depends on the age of the patient and the phase of menstrual cycle in fertile women. Parenchyma normally looks like a layer with slightly decreased echodensity and irregular echostructure. Pregnancy and lactation are associated with significant enlargement of the thickness of glandular tissue, which reaches 25–30 mm. In patients older than 40 years, the number of glandular lobes decreases; adipose tissue starts to prevail over the glandular one. Accessory mammary glands (polymastia), accessory nipples (polythelia), or other variants of ectopic breast tissue are a rather rare anomaly, occurring in 1–6% of cases. Breasts in newborn boys and girls have similar structure. The breasts enlarge by the 7th to 8th day of life in 60% of newborns (crisis genitalis neonatorum). It is a normal physiological transitory condition. Primary breast growth in girls older than 3 years of age requires differential diagnosis with precocious puberty. At later age, there are two periods of increase in the number of breast glandular structures at 4 and 9 years. Normally, distinct breast enlargement is also observed at the age of 11–13 years. The arising pathologies in children form the following groups: breast anomalies (amastia, polythelia, polymastia, aberrant lobes), age-related disturbances (premature or late development), disturbance of symmetric growth of the right and left breasts, hypo- or hypermastia, inflammatory processes and trauma, mastopathy, cysts, ductectasia, and benign tumors (fibroadenoma, hamartoma, etc.). It is necessary to remember about the restrictions for biopsies in children.

3.1 Anatomical Features of the Breast at Different Ages

Echographic image of the breast is rather complex for interpretation. This is not only due to anatomical features, which depend on the age and physiological state of a woman, but also due to endocrine state and genital diseases. It is necessary to know and take into account the anatomical features of the normal breast, zones of regional

M. Pykov (✉) · E. Philipova
Department of Ultrasound Diagnostics in Neonatology and Pediatrics, National Medical Research Center for Obstetrics, Gynecology and Perinatology named after Academician V.I.Kulakov of Ministry of Healthcare of Russian Federation, Moscow, Russia

A. N. Sencha
Division of Visual Diagnostics, National Medical Research Center for Obstetrics, Gynecology and Perinatology named after Academician V.I.Kulakov of Ministry of Healthcare of Russian Federation, Moscow, Russia

G. T. Sukhikh, A. N. Sencha (eds.), *Multiparametric Ultrasound Diagnosis of Breast Diseases*,
https://doi.org/10.1007/978-3-319-75034-7_3

lymph drainage, and physiological features of the breast at the time of examination.

The breast (mammary gland) is a paired organ of the apocrine type of glands that has evolved as modification of the sweat glands. It produces milk after the childbirth. It is located on the front surface of the chest, on the fascia of the large pectoral muscle between the parasternal and anterior axillary line. The nipple is located along the midclavicular line.

The place of breast attachment to the thorax is within the segment from ribs II to VI along the median-clavicular line. The breast size and shape are variable and can change with age. The diameter of the breast attachment site varies from 12 to 15 cm. The normal breast volume is 200–300 cm^2. As a rule, the body of the breast consists of 15–20 separate conical segments (lobes) located radially around the nipple and separated by interlayers of connective tissue. Each lobe consists of larger and smaller lobules. Each lobule consists of alveoli with a diameter of 0.05–0.07 mm. The nipple consists of the muscle and epithelial tissue and is surrounded by the areola—pigmented patch of the skin with a large number of sweat glands.

The breast consists of adipose, glandular, and connective tissues, bordered by anterior and posterior layers of the split superficial fascia of the thorax (Fig. 3.1).

Adipose tissue is defined as a subcutaneous layer in superficial to the glandular tissue. Its thickness depends on the age and constitutional features of a woman. There are also inclusions of adipose tissue surrounded by fibrous connective tissue.

Breast capsule is formed by connective tissue that produces septa (Cooper's ligaments), thus forming the breast "skeleton" and maintaining structural integrity. In places of fixation of Cooper's ligaments to glandular tissue, there appear prominences called crests of Duret. Connective tissue is also included into the structure of fibrillar tissue between glandular elements and in the walls of lactiferous ducts. With years, along with the beginning of involution, Cooper's ligaments become denser and surround areas of fatty tissue, thus forming fatty lobes.

The glandular tissue located separately from the main breast parenchyma may make an additional glandular lobe. More often, additional lobes are found in the axillary regions, less often along the parasternal line of the subclavicular area.

Beast parenchyma consists of alveolar-tubular complexes, the latter united in lobules, and then in lobes, which tend to integrate together locating radially in relation to the nipple. Terminal duct lobular units are the basic functional units of the breast that produce milk. During pregnancy and

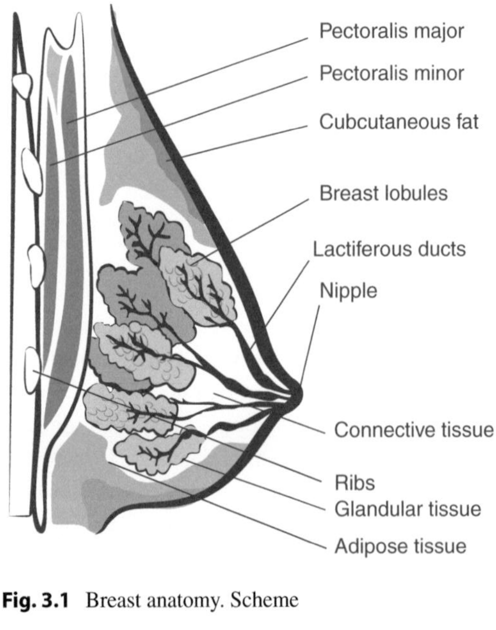

Fig. 3.1 Breast anatomy. Scheme

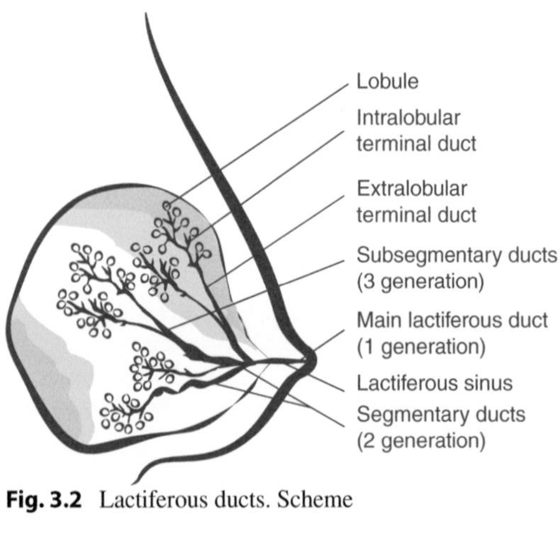

Fig. 3.2 Lactiferous ducts. Scheme

lactation, the terminations of ducts develop acinar structures, which produce milk, and atrophy by the end of feeding period. There are several generations of lactiferous ducts ending with subsegmentary and segmentary ducts and lactiferous sinus (Fig. 3.2).

Terminal ducts starting from every lobule run into ducts of the second generation (intralobar) the latter running into the ducts of the third generation (central ducts located in subareolar area). Before draining to the nipple, the major ducts form lactiferous sinus, in which supposedly milk accumulates between breastfeeding sessions.

The breast is highly vascular and is supplied by the branches of the internal thoracic, subclavian, axillary, and intercostal arteries that form the rete of anastomoses predominantly in subareolar area (Fig. 3.3). The venous rete accompanies corresponding arteries and arterioles.

Breast innervation is provided by the branches of thoracic, humeral, intercostal nerves.

The lymphatic system is presented by intramammary and abducent lymph ducts and regional lymph nodes, the latter conferring axillary, subclavian, supraclavicular, pectoral, and substernal groups (see Chap. 8). Intramammary lymph ducts form a complex rete with anastomoses and plexuses. There are some outflow lymph tracts from the breast: axillary (more than 90%), subclavian, parasternal, retrosternal, intercostal, epigastric, and cross way to the other side (Trufanov et al. 2009).

3.2 Types of Ultrasound Image of the Normal Breast

US signs of breast abnormalities are a consequence of certain morphological changes. US image of the normal breast is quite variable and depends, first of all, on the age of the patient and the phase of menstrual cycle in fertile women. Variability of US picture also is the result of anatomic and constitutional features of women, interrelation of fatty, glandular, and connecting tissues.

Zabolotskaya and Zabolotsky (2000) distinguish several types of breast structure at ultrasonography: juvenile, early reproductive, premenopausal, postmenopausal, and during pregnancy and lactation.

In fertile women US, as a rule, assesses the status of the following breast structures (Fig. 3.4):

- Subcutaneous adipose layer
- Superficial leaf of the fascia
- Parenchyma (glandular tissue)
- Lactiferous ducts
- Cooper's ligaments
- Nipple
- Back leaf of the fascia
- Vascular pattern of the breast (vascularity)
- Retromammary space
- Regional lymph nodes

The possibility to assess the condition of the breast skin depends on the frequency of US probe and the class of US scanner.

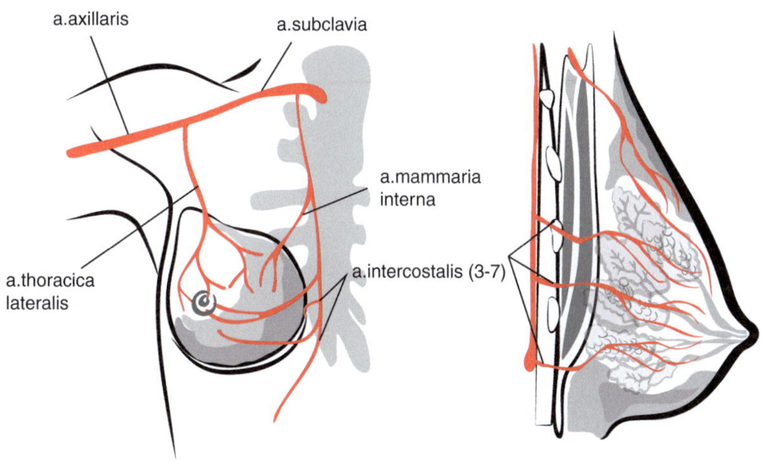

Fig. 3.3 Blood supply to the breast. Scheme

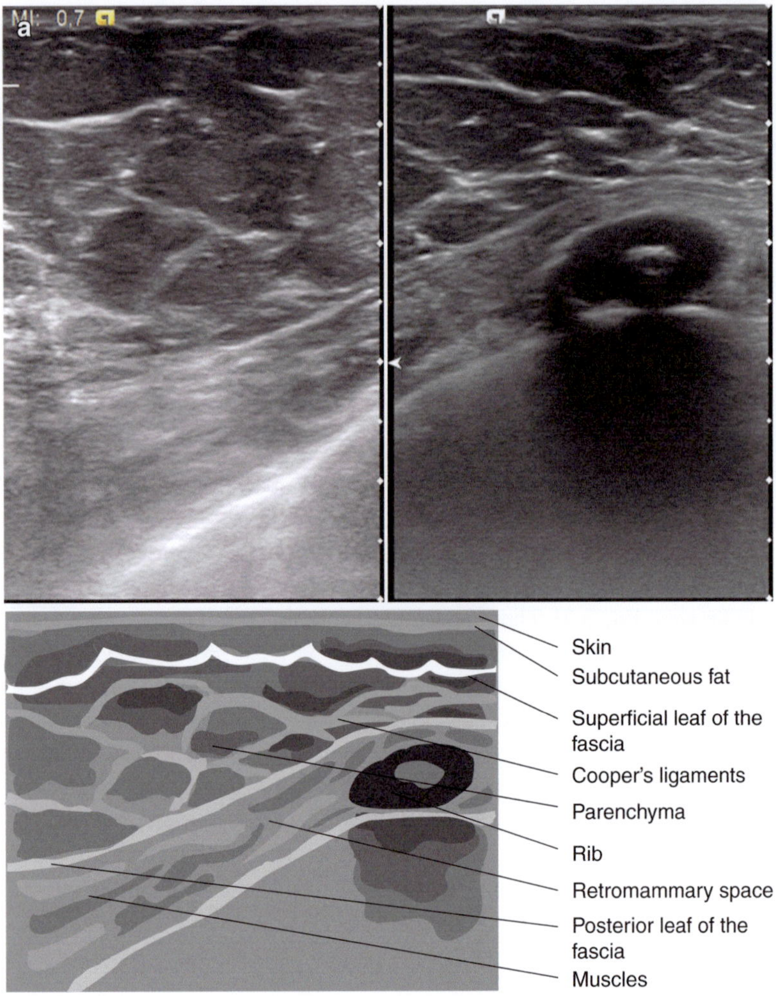

Fig. 3.4 Normal breast US. (**a**) Grayscale US. (**b**) Graphic

The normal skin is imaged as homogeneous echogenic layer of 0.5–7 mm thickness. Prior to puberty and in early fertility, the thickness of the skin usually ranges from 0.5 to 2 mm. The skin thickness reaches 2–4 mm in premenopause, postmenopause, pregnancy, and lactation.

Inflammatory process, condition after radiation therapy, and postoperative edema are accompanied with thickening and rough echostructure of the skin. The echodensity, as a rule, decreases. Irregular anechoic fluid collections may be observed in some cases. The margin between the skin and subcutaneous fat is not always possible to differentiate with 5–7.5 MHz probe. On the contrary, the probes with the frequency of 10 MHz and higher permit clear differentiation of superficial and profound surfaces of derma of the breast skin.

Subcutaneous fat. Adipose tissue is characterized with decreased or normal echodensity, homogeneous enough structure with linear echogenic incorporations, which often exhibit vague acoustic shadows (Fig. 3.5). The thickness of the adipose layer depends on patient's constitution but, as a rule, increases with age.

In young women the adipose tissue is presented by a thin layer between the skin and glandular tissue. With age, after pregnancies and childbirths the thickness of this adipose layer increases accompanied with a little increase in echodensity. In postmenopause with the beginning of mammary involution, the adipose tissue

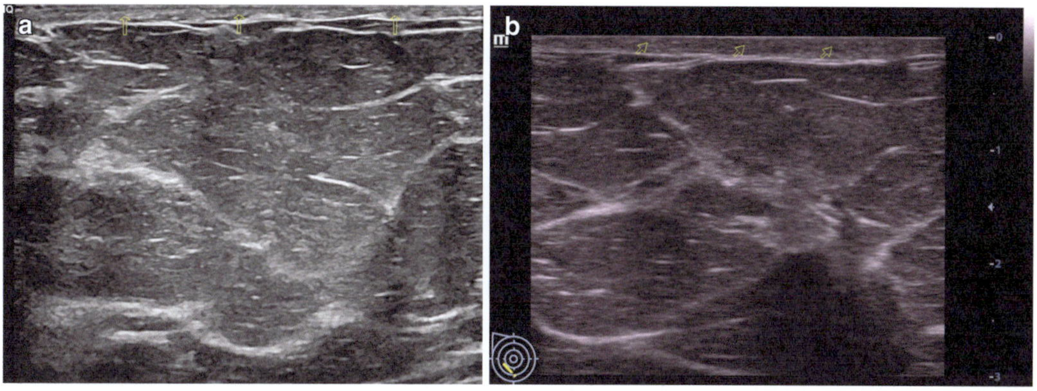

Fig. 3.5 (**a**, **b**) Normal breast. Subcutaneous adipose layer. Grayscale US

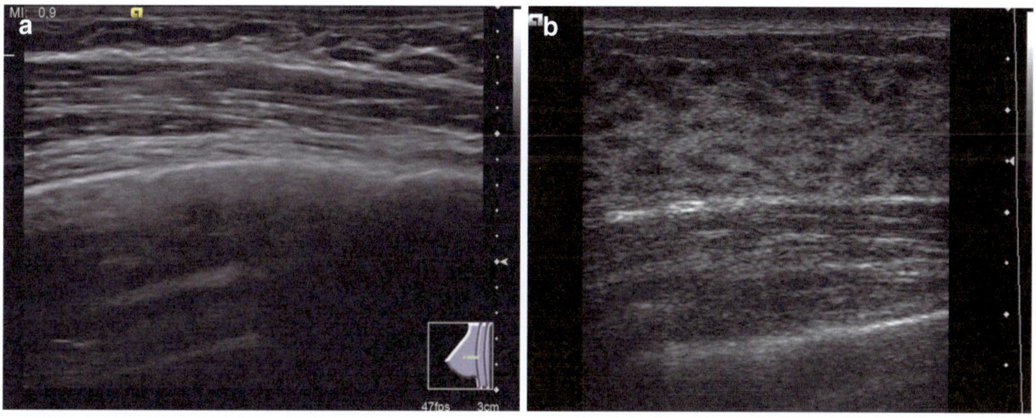

Fig. 3.6 (**a**, **b**) Normal breast. Anterior (superficial) leaf of fascia. Grey scale US

becomes more irregular due to the development of connective tissue, which is defined as echogenic linear structures. Cooper's ligaments become thicker and often form adipose lobules with lateral acoustic shadows. Fibrous and involutional changes in the breast with large number of these acoustic shadows negatively affect the quality of imaging of deep structures and detection of abnormalities, especially small-sized lesions.

The anterior (superficial) leaf of the fascia is often distinctly observed as an echogenic line that separates subcutaneous fat from breast parenchyma (Fig. 3.6).

Parenchyma (glandular tissue) normally looks like a layer with slightly decreased echodensity and irregular echostructure. The anterior contour of breast parenchyma in fertile women has protrusions in the places of fixation of Cooper's ligaments.

In anatomical terms, glandular lobule and glandular lobe are distinguished. Nevertheless, owing to the fact that glandular lobules and lobes have no actual capsule, US fails to differentiate them.

Depending on the age, endocrine status, and ratio of glandular and adipose tissues in the patient, the echodensity of glandular tissue can vary from decreased to increased. The echodensity of parenchyma can also change depending on the phase of menstrual cycle. Proliferative processes decrease the echodensity of glandular tissue.

In young women glandular tissue is usually isoechoic or slightly hyperechoic and is observed as a relatively homogeneous uniform layer.

Connective tissue fibers have small amount of collagen and are practically invisible against the basic layer. Only in the second phase of menstrual cycle there can arise granularity due to echogenic fields of glandular tissue against hypoechoic lactiferous ducts (Fig. 3.7a).

In reproductive age the ratio of parenchyma and stromal component is individual and depends mainly on constitutional features, endocrine status, numbers of pregnancies, childbirths, and the duration of lactation. The greatest thickness of glandular tissue is registered, as a rule, in upper-outer quadrants and, the least, in the inner quadrants.

With aging, after pregnancies and lactation periods, the thickness of glandular layer decreases. There appear hypoechoic adipose lobes and echogenic fields of fibrous tissue against glandular tissue, the latter being of increased echodensity (Fig. 3.7b).

During lactation the ductal ectasia of various degree is usually defined (Fig. 3.7c). Pregnancy and lactation are associated with significant enlargement of the thickness of glandular tissue, which reaches 25–30 mm, and grainy structure of the parenchyma.

In patients older than 40 years, the number of glandular lobes decreases; adipose tissue starts to prevail over the glandular one.

In women at the age of 45–50 years, due to the onset of menopause, involutive changes in the breast evolve. The alveolar parts disappear, their epithelium becomes atrophic, the stroma grows and undergoes fibrosis and hyalinosis, and the amount of adipose tissue increases. After 3–5 years of menopause, the only glandular elements are large excretory ducts surrounded by the hyalinized connective tissue and fat.

In a postmenopause the glandular tissue becomes thin. Its thickness, as a rule, does not exceed 4 mm. The major part of the breast is usually presented by multiple adipose lobes, detected as homogeneous structures of decreased echodensity surrounded with echogenic rims of connective tissue fibers (Fig. 3.8).

The presence of fully formed *accessory mammary glands (polymastia), accessory nipples (polythelia), or other variants of ectopic breast tissue* is a rather rare anomaly, occurring in 1–6% of cases. Accessory mammary glands can be located anywhere on the milk line, but their most common location is the anterior margin of the axilla. They may also be bilateral. The following classification of polymastia and polythelia is often used:

Type I—fully formed accessory breast with the areola and the nipple

Type II—accessory breast with the nipple only

Type III—accessory breast with the areola only

Type IV—ectopic or aberrant breast tissue

Type V—"false breast" consisting of adipose tissue but having the areola and the nipple

Type VI—polythelia (additional nipples)

Type VII—only accessory areolas (polythelia areolaris)

At ultrasound, an accessory breast does not differ from the normal glandular tissue, with lobules of parenchyma, which are hypoechoic, heterogeneous, surrounded by Cooper's ligaments, and hypovascular (Fig. 3.9a, b).

Often, the ectopic accessory breast lobe shows vascularization and vascular enhancement pattern at CEUS, which are similar to the typically located breast lobules (Fig. 3.9c, d). Thus, CEUS, along with grayscale and color-coded modes, may be used in differential diagnosis of accessory breast tissue (accessory lobe) and other parenchymal masses.

Less often an accessory lobe may simulate pathological changes and neoplasms.

Cooper's ligaments are connective tissue septa, which derive from fascia and follow on perpendicularly to the anterior surface of the skin. They appear on the US image as thin echogenic linear structures (Fig. 3.10).

They surround adipose lobules and can produce lateral acoustic shadows, hence imitate breast lesions. The structure of Cooper's ligaments becomes denser with aging with more expressed acoustic shadows. Differentiation of such areas from breast pathology is possible with polypositional examination.

The image of *lactiferous ducts* depends on the patient's age, the phase of menstrual cycle,

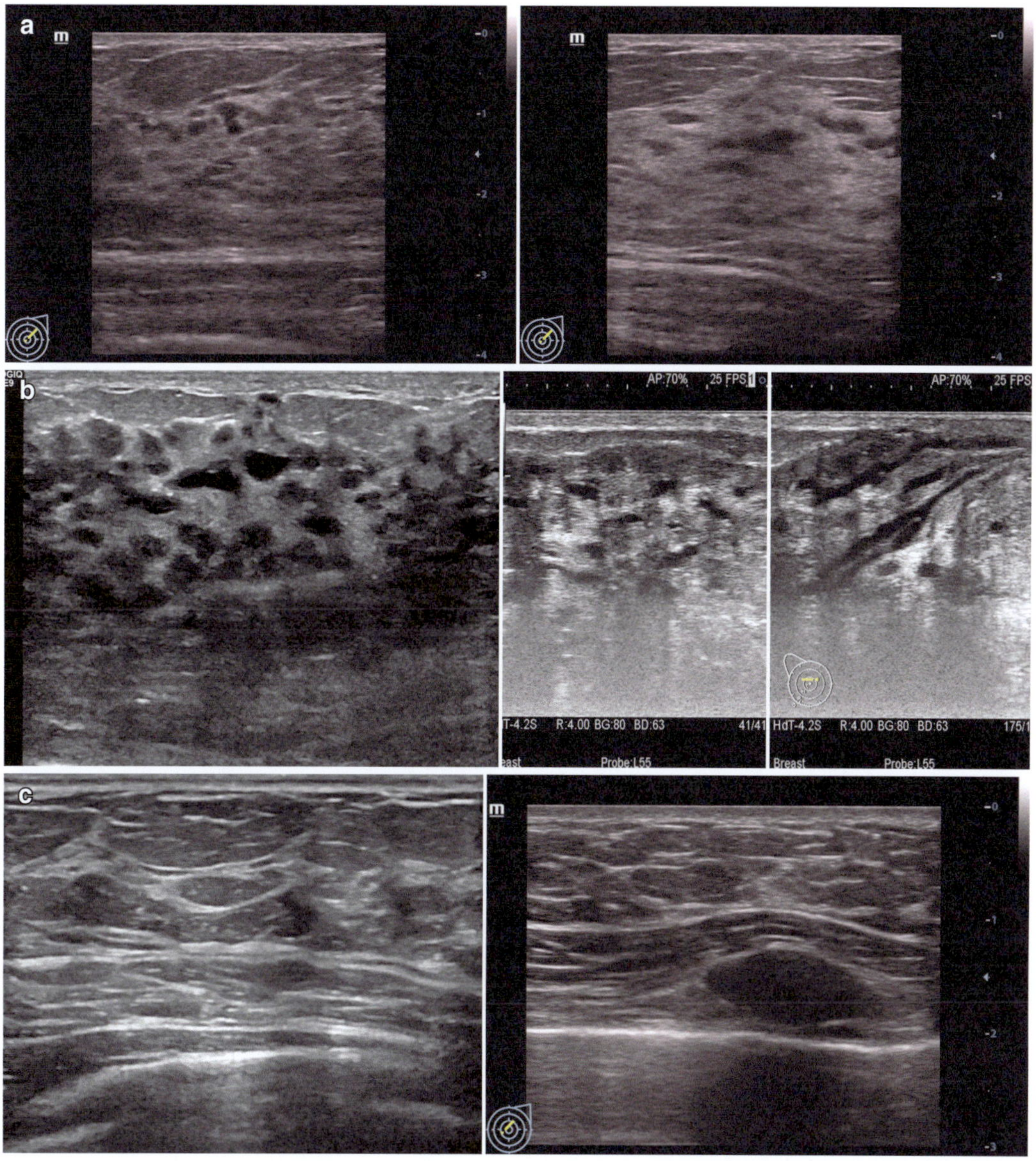

Fig. 3.7 Breast parenchyma. Grayscale US. (**a**) Reproductive age. (**b**) Menopause. (**c**) Lactation period

and the frequency of US probe. Breast US with linear 5.0–7.5 MHz probe in the first phase of menstrual cycle normally detects terminal and interlobar ducts smaller than 2 mm in caliber or fails to differentiate them. The caliber of ducts in subareolar area can reach 3–5 mm. Probes with the frequency of 10–12 MHz practically always permit detection of interlobar ducts in the first phase of menstrual cycle, in spite of their diameter which does not exceed 1 mm.

In the second phase of menstrual cycle, the ducts are usually imaged as an- or hypoechoic tubular structures directed to subareolar area. Their caliber, as a rule, is larger than 2 mm (Fig. 3.11a, b). Some days before menses, the echodensity of ducts decreases to anechoic that gives the opportunity to differentiate interlobar and main lactiferous ducts.

During pregnancy the ducts can be easily imaged, and their caliber exceeds 2 mm. During lactation period the diameter of ducts can reach

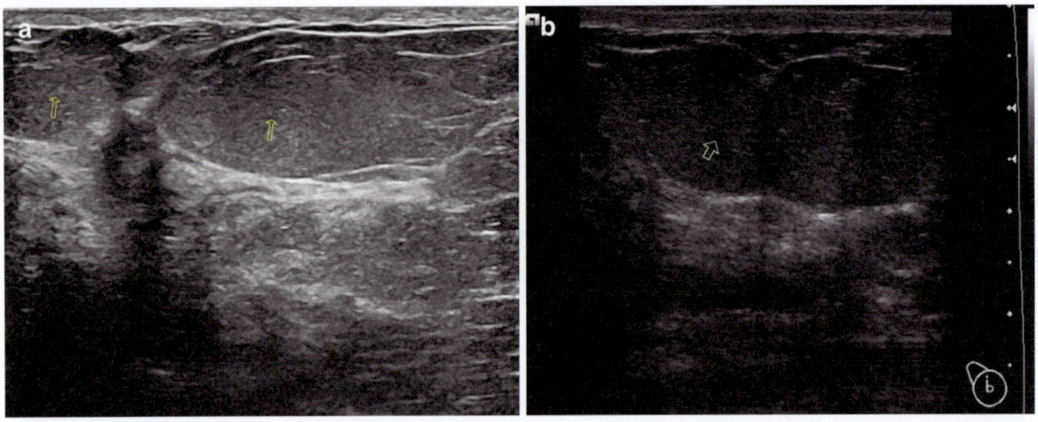

Fig. 3.8 (**a**, **b**) Normal breast. Adipose lobes. Grayscale US

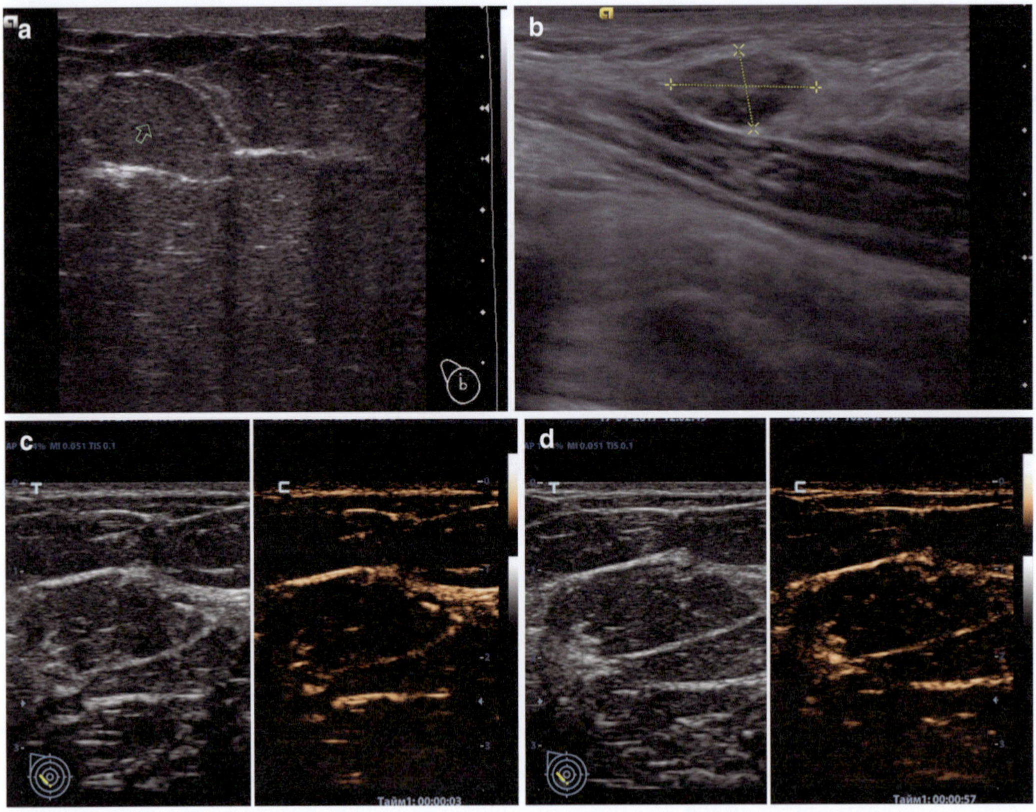

Fig. 3.9 Normal breast. Accessory breast lobules. (**a**, **b**) Grayscale US. (**c**, **d**) Contrast-enhanced US of breast parenchyma. SonoVue, 2.4 mL. Single contrast enhancement loci in the accessory lobule and in breast parenchyma

3.5–4 mm. They can be observed as hypoechoic or anechoic tubular structures that sometimes get colored in CDI and PDI modes (Fig. 3.11c, d).

Main lactiferous duct may exhibit four patterns of branching: magistral (21%), scattered (67.1%), duplicated (7%), and looped (4.9%) (Rozhkova 1993).

In connection with the changes in endocrine status of a woman with age and in cases of hormone replacement therapy, the difference

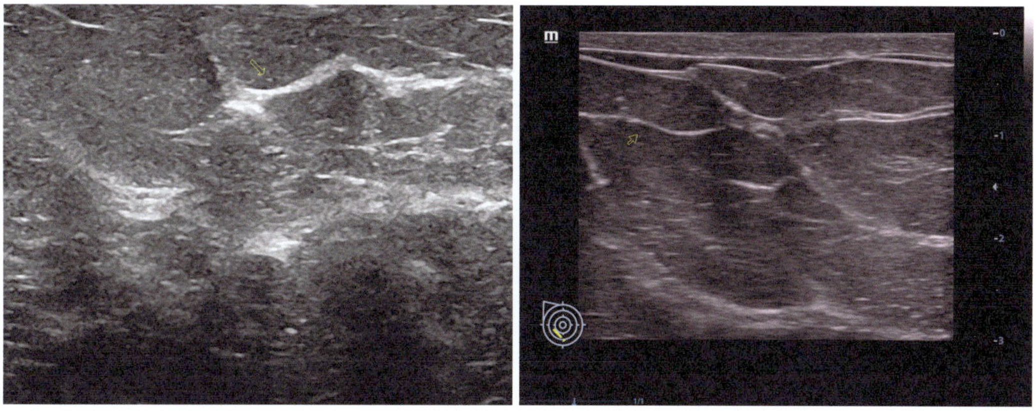

Fig. 3.10 Normal breast. Cooper's ligaments. Sonograms. Grayscale US

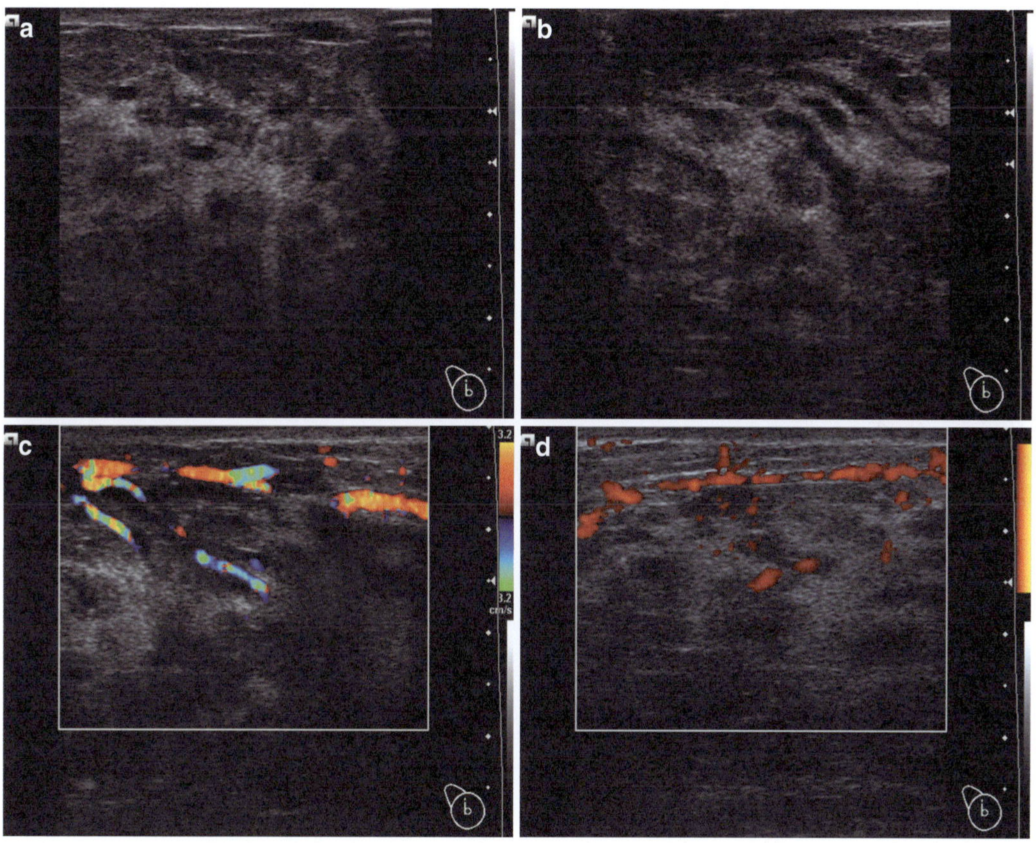

Fig. 3.11 Lactiferous ducts of the normal breast. (**a**, **b**) Grayscale US. (**c**) CDI. (**d**) PDI

between US images of ducts in the first and the second phases of menstrual cycle decreases.

The back leaf of the fascia borders the breast from retromammary space and is imaged as thin homogeneous echogenic linear structure (Fig. 3.12).

The retromammary space contains retromammary adipose tissue (as a rule of decreased echodensity and irregular echostructure), the pectoralis major and minor muscles, intercostal muscles, and pleura (Fig. 3.13).

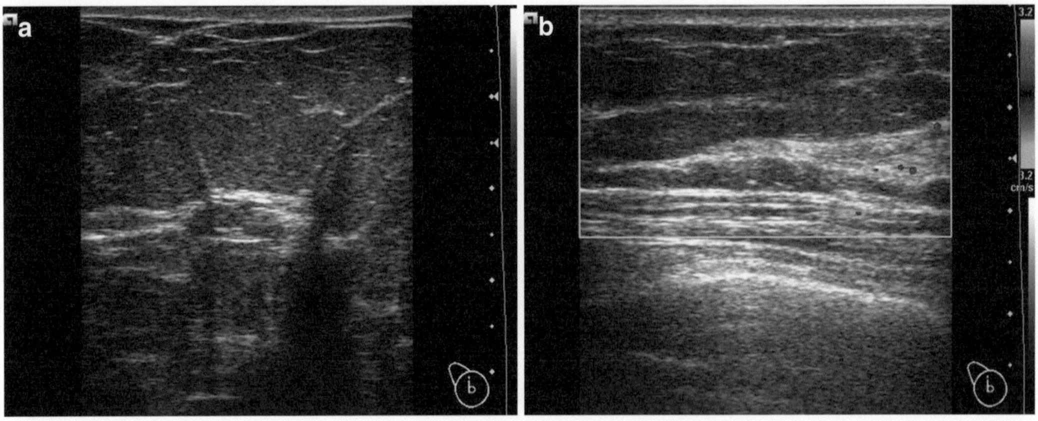

Fig. 3.12 Normal breast. The back leaf of the fascia. (**a**) Grayscale US. (**b**) CDI

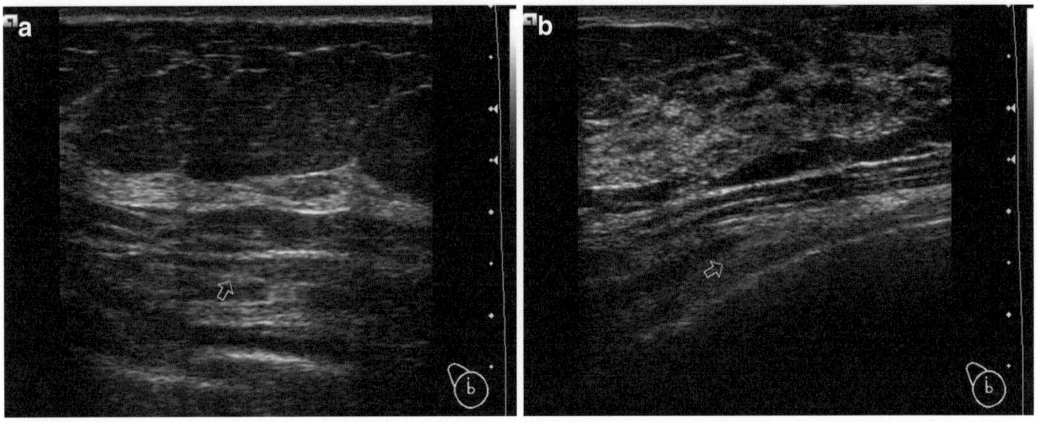

Fig. 3.13 (**a**, **b**) Normal breast. Retromammary space. Grayscale US

It is not always possible to differentiate the structures of retromammary space. It mainly depends on the class of US scanner, the frequency of probes, and the experience of US specialist.

Pectoralis major and minor muscles are defined as hypoechoic structures isolated with septa. The echostructure of ribs depends on the amount of osteal and cartilaginous component. Therefore, the echodensity and uniformity of their structure may vary.

The nipple normally is defined as a roundish structure of average or decreased echodensity with comparatively homogeneous structure and accurate even contours (Fig. 3.14).

Sometimes the nipple is accompanied by the posterior acoustic shadow, which results from connective tissue structures. It dictates the necessity to examine subareolar area polypositionally to rule out abnormalities in this area, especially in cases of inverted or retracted nipples.

Vessels of the normal breast are often impossible to detect with CDI, PDI, or 3DPD (Fig. 3.15). They sometimes may be observed as individual color spots with linear orientation in longitudinal scans. Blood flow with pulsed Doppler is characterized by the following parameters: PSV, 10–13 cm/s; EDV, 3–6 cm/s; PI, 1.20; RI, 0.59 (Harchenko et al. 1993).

Internal and lateral (external) mammary arteries are not always easily visualized in healthy women and under pathological conditions. This is often due to the constitution, the breast size, and the class of the ultrasound scanner. In asthenic women with small breasts, visualization of these vessels in grayscale and color US modes is more effective. The blood flow velocity is sym-

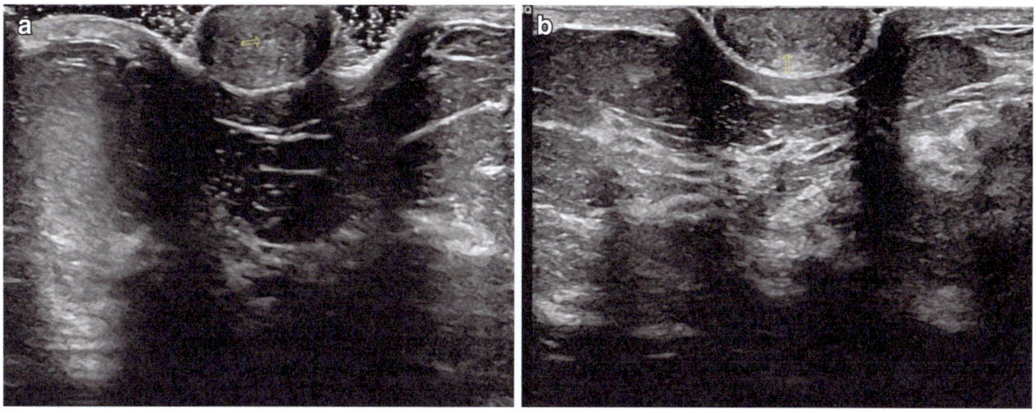

Fig. 3.14 (**a**, **b**) Normal breast. The nipple. Grayscale US

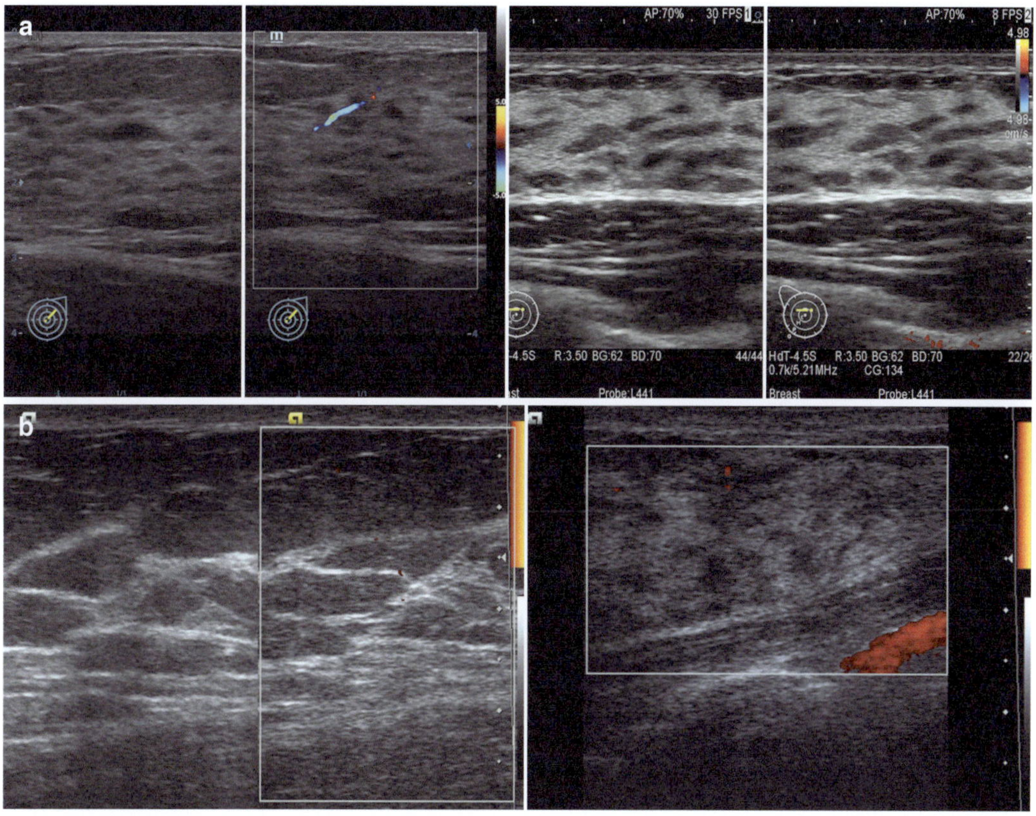

Fig. 3.15 Normal breast US. (**a**, **b**) CDI. (**c**, **d**) PDI

metric in the vessels of both breasts. Systolic and diastolic blood flow velocity in the internal thoracic artery (mean V_{max}, 29.2 ± 0.85 cm/s) is 1.6–2.2 times higher than in the lateral thoracic artery (mean V_{max}, 13.2 ± 0.9 cm/s) and 2.2–3.0 times higher than in parenchymal arteries (mean V_{max}, 9.8 ± 0.35 cm/s) (PI, 3.78 ± 0.14; 2.8 ± 0.4; 2.7 ± 0.42; RI, 0.63 ± 0.07; 0.59 ± 0.08; 0.64 ± 0.18, respectively).

Multislice, panoramic scanning and 3D reconstruction of ultrasound images allow detailization of spatial relation of breast components, precise evaluation of minor physiological and pathological changes, and correlation of US images with mammography, MDCT, and MRI (Fig. 3.16).

The normal breast has rather symmetric, homogeneous fine- or medium-grained staining with compression US elastography (Fig. 3.17a). As a rule, not the whole breast needs compression; elasticity is evaluated only in the areas that are suspicious of pathological changes. Strain ratio in these areas is approximately 1–1.5 higher as compared with elasticity of closely located unchanged parts of breast parenchyma. Young modulus 18–24 kPa is specific for normal breast (Fig. 3.17b).

Contrast-enhanced US in the arterial phase reveals single asymmetrically located vessels within the unchanged parenchyma (Fig. 3.18).

Normal breast pattern with ultrasound is quite variable and depends on a number of factors (Zabolotskaya and Gavrilenko 2015).

The juvenile type of breast is typical for girls in the postpubertal period. With ultrasound

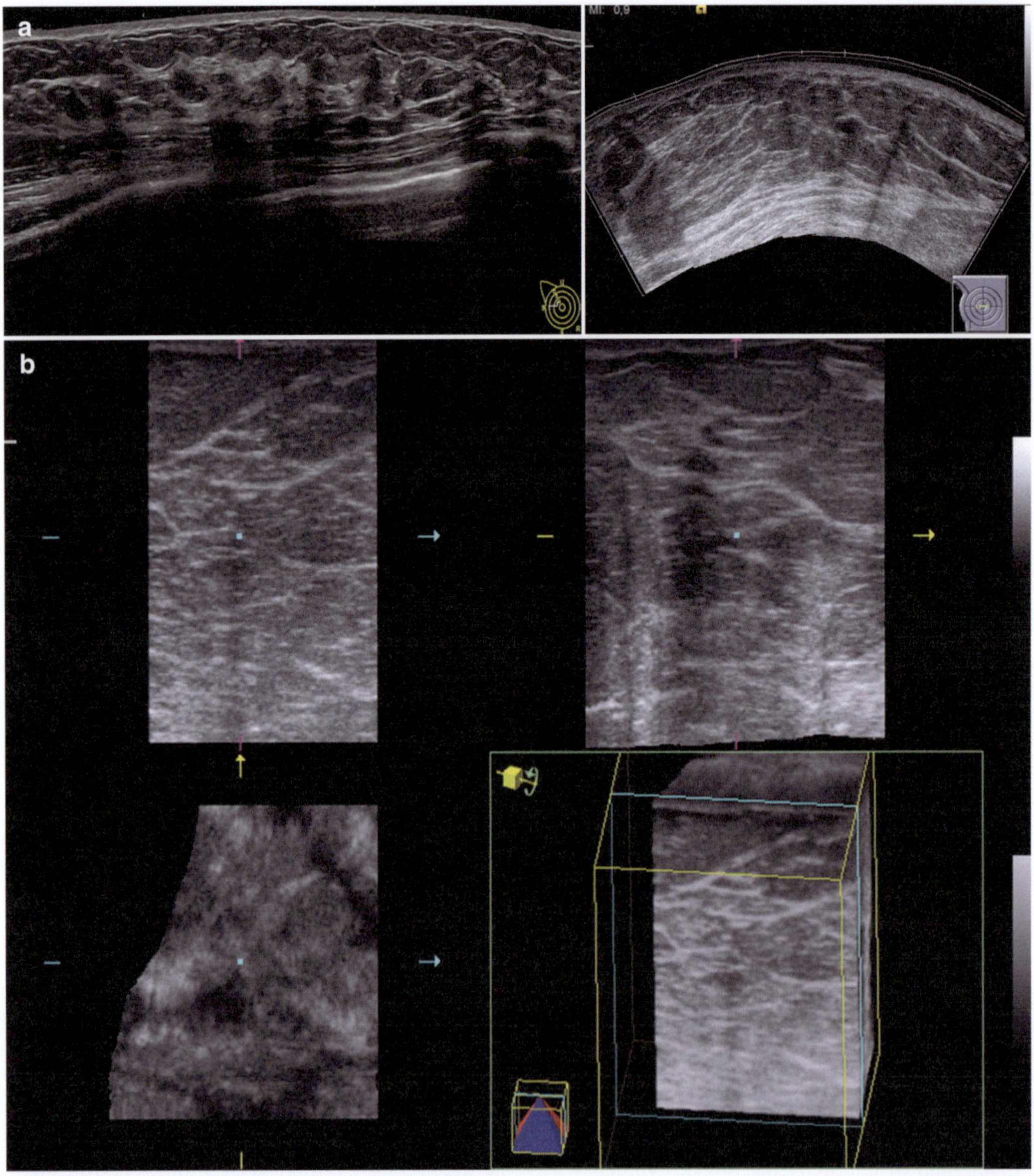

Fig. 3.16 Normal breast. Echograms. (**a**) Panoramic scan. (**b**) 3D. (**c**) Multislice view

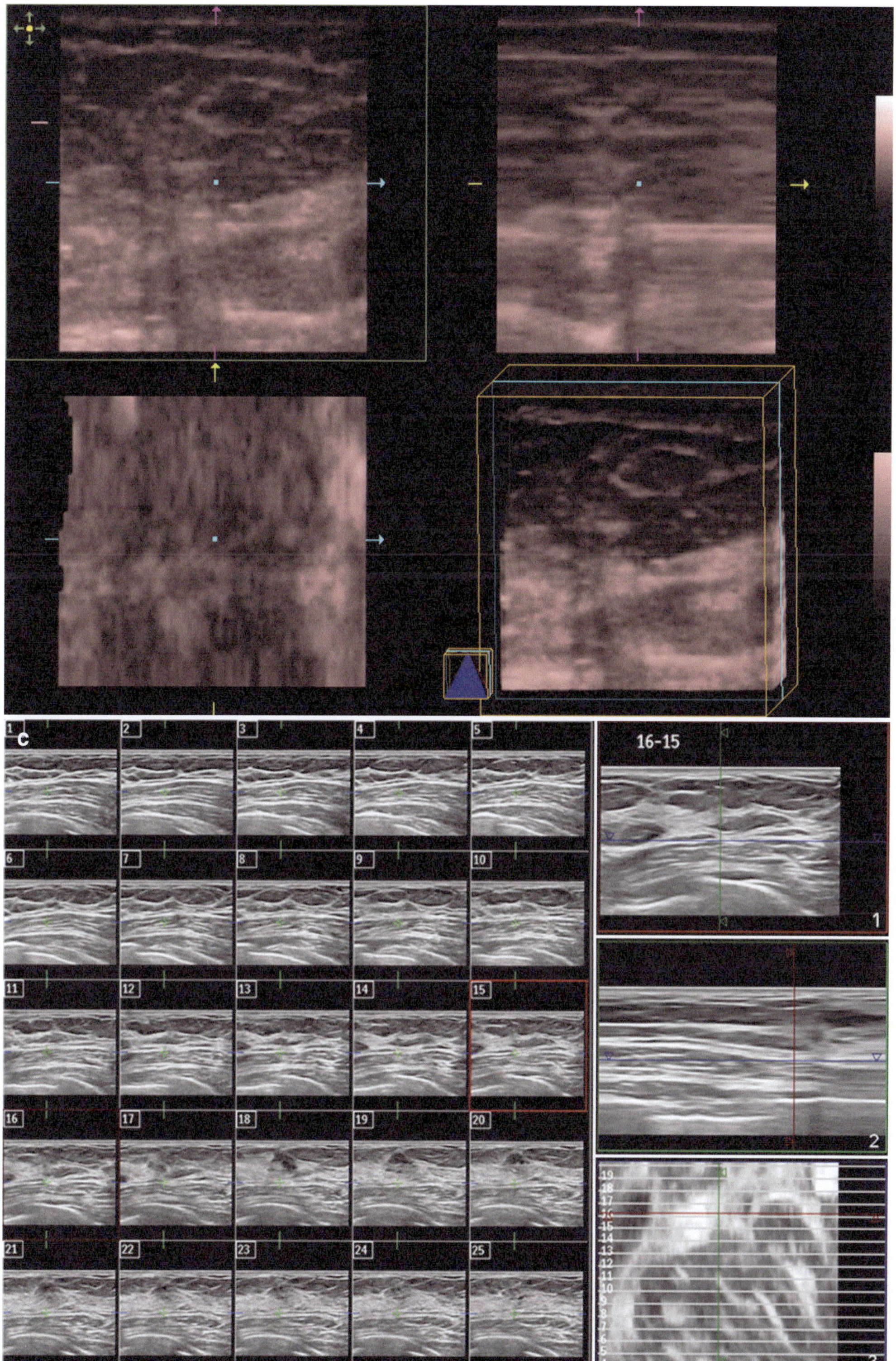

Fig. 3.16 (continued)

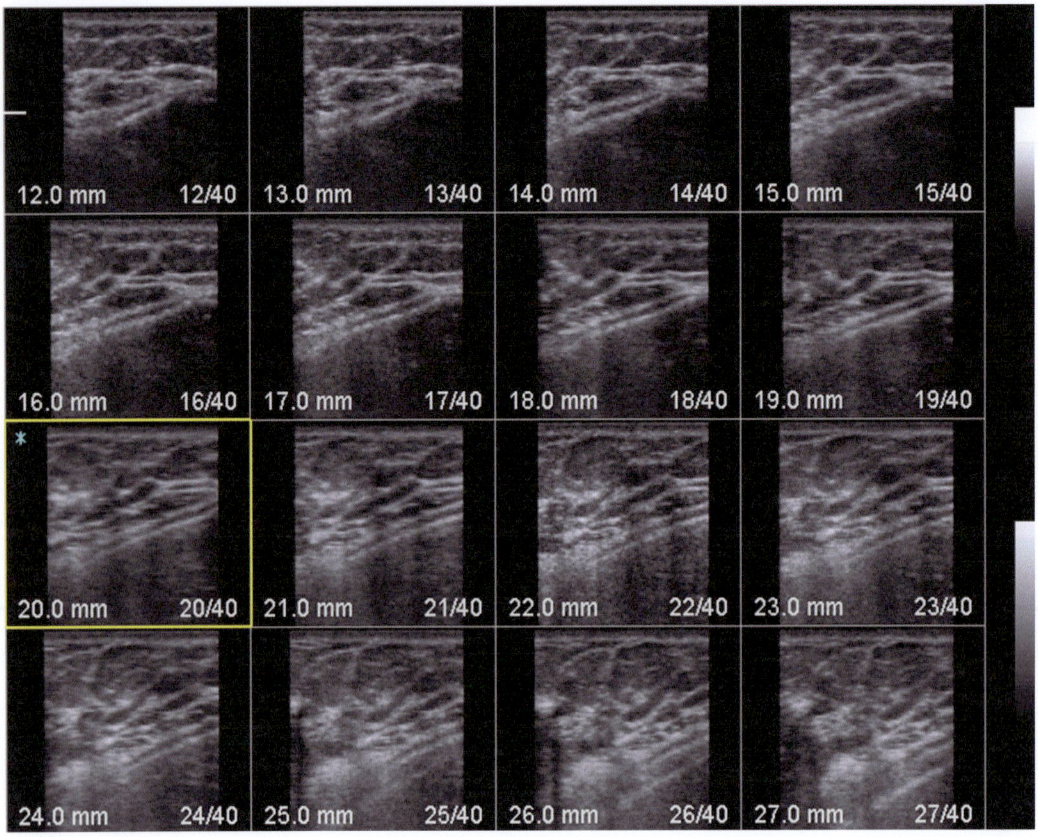

Fig. 3.16 (continued)

examination the skin is visualized as a thin hyperechoic line with thickness up to 2 mm, which is thinner in the inner quadrants of the breast. The breast tissue has mainly isoechoic fine-grained structure (Fig. 3.19). Subcutaneous fat is thin or practically invisible. The nipple is visualized as a round mass of medium echodensity with acoustic shadow. Connective tissue structures are not clearly visualized. Pectoral muscles look like hypoechoic striated structures with the shadows from the ribs behind them.

The breast of reproductive type (beyond and during pregnancy and lactation) is more characteristic for women of 18–49 years. On the 10–12th day after menses, the skin is visualized as a hyperechoic strip 2–3 mm thick, subcutaneous fat—as a hypoechoic layer 1.5–2.5 cm thick. The thickness of the latter may vary depending on the age and constitution. The glandular tissue is imaged as a fine-grained hyperechoic layer containing vessels and lactiferous ducts, bordered by connective tissue septa (Fig. 3.20).

In the second phase of the menstrual cycle, echography may reveal physiologically dilated ducts as thin parallel lines (longitudinal scan) or fine round structures (transverse scan) up to 3 mm in diameter. During this period, the breast connective tissue elements are poorly differentiated. The base of the breast is clearly bordered from the thorax by thin hypoechoic layer of retromammary space with thickness up to 3 mm. Muscular layer of the chest appears heterogeneous and hypoechoic with hyperechoic inclusions. The ribs show as a hyperechoic rim with posterior acoustic shadow.

The US pattern of the *pre- and menopausal type of the breast* is characterized by larger amount of subcutaneous fat. It is visualized as hypoechoic layer just under the skin. Its thickness varies depending on the constitution and

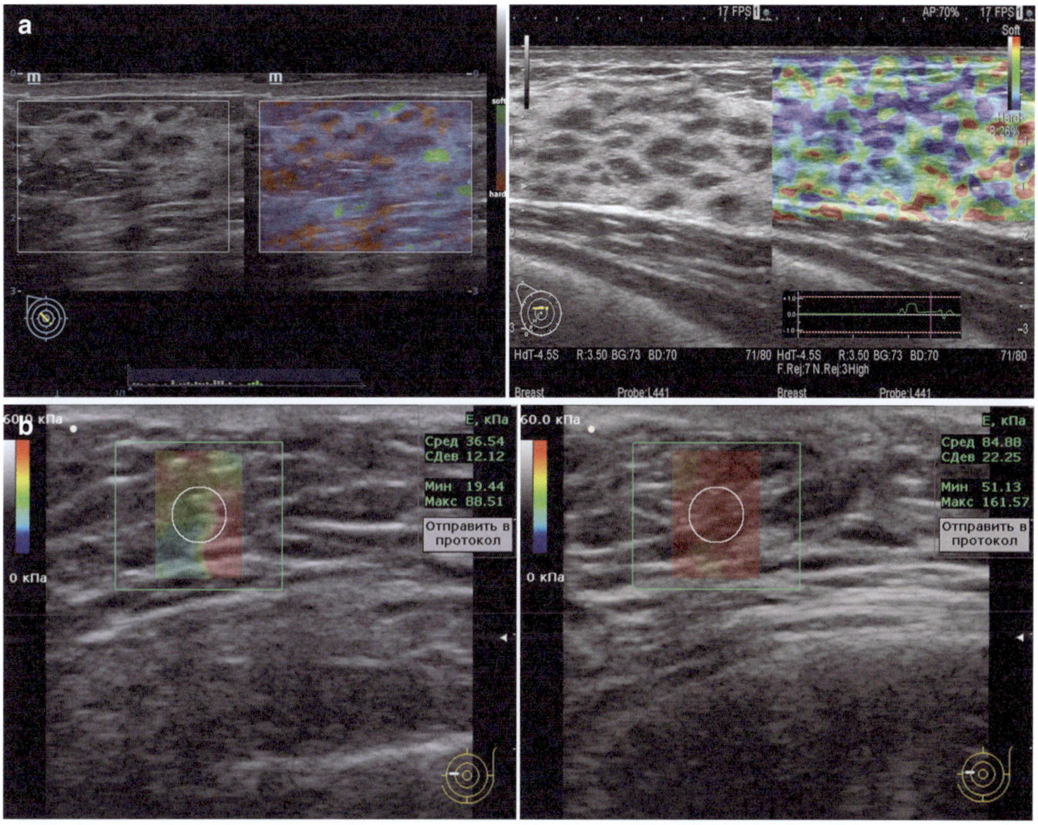

Fig. 3.17 (**a**) Compression soloelastography. Fine-grained, symmetric, homogenous breast pattern. (**b**) Measurement of quantitative indices of breast parenchyma

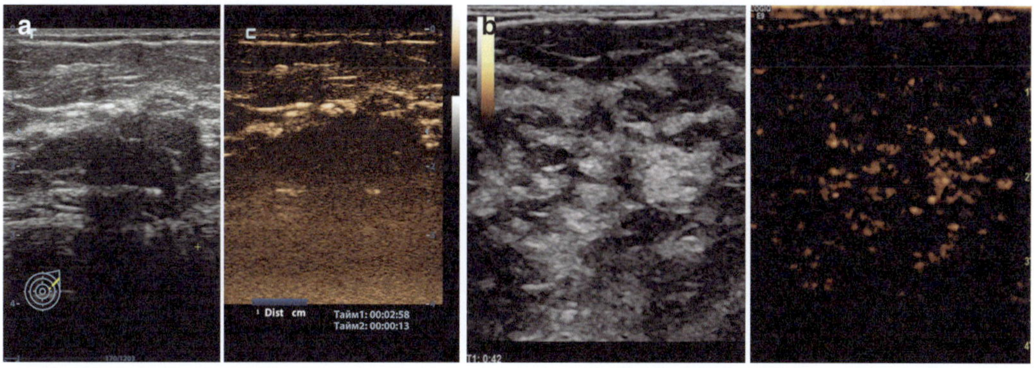

Fig. 3.18 (**a**, **b**) Contrast-enhanced US of normal breast parenchyma. SonoVue, 2.4 ml. Single contrast enhancement loci in breast parenchyma

age. This type of image is typical for women aged 40–55 years. Components of adipose tissue start to dominate in breast structure.

In postmenopausal women, the glandular tissue of the breast is replaced with fat. It is possible to see a small number of fat lobules in the retromammary space. In this period, Cooper's ligaments can be well differentiated. They show as hyperechoic cords attached to the inner layer of the skin (Fig. 3.21). That is why the anterior

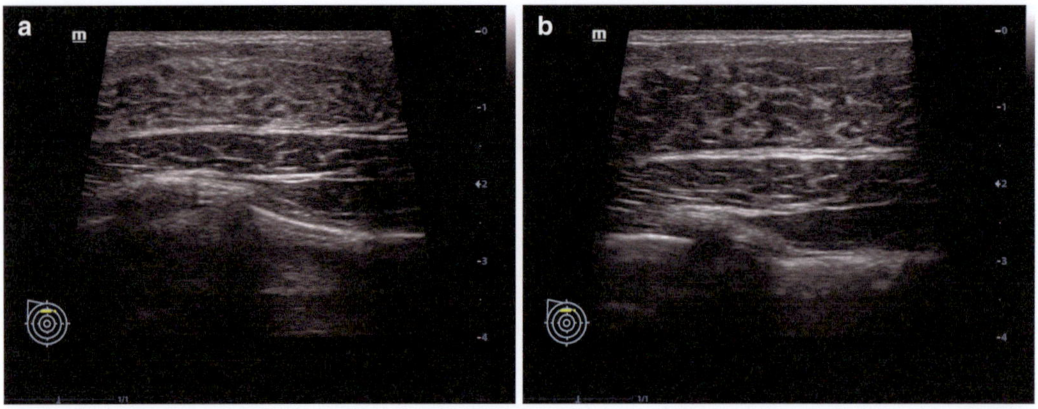

Fig. 3.19 (**a**, **b**) Normal breast. Juvenile type. Grayscale US

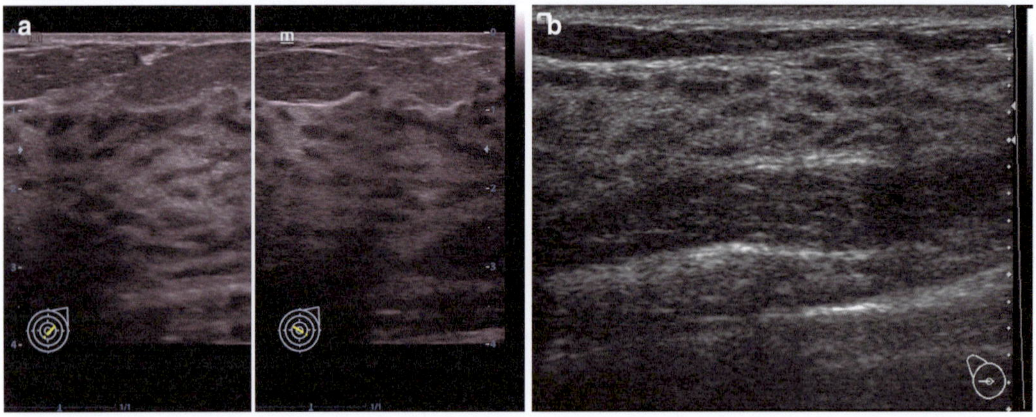

Fig. 3.20 Normal breast. Reproductive type. (**a**, **b**) Grayscale US

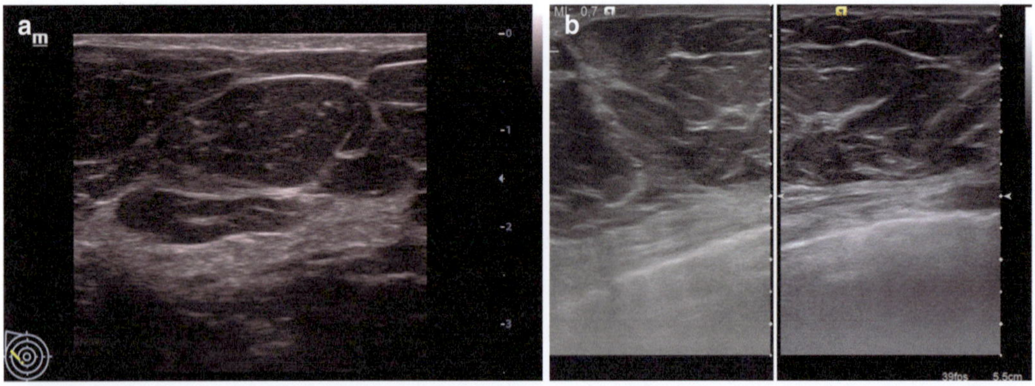

Fig. 3.21 Normal breast. Postmenopause. (**a**, **b**) Grayscale US

margin of the glandular parenchyma becomes indulating.

During breast US it is necessary to compare the structures of the right and left breasts and assess dynamic changes in US picture in the current cycle phase and in a certain time interval (2–3 months) in the corresponding phase of menstrual cycle. Complete and correct information about the breast condition can be obtained only taking into account all features, such as the age, phase of menstrual cycle, functional, and endocrine status.

The doctor in the conclusion can recommend repeated US in a specific phase of menstrual cycle or after a certain period of time to analyze the changes in pathological process or differentiate it from physiological features.

The example of US report in normal breast:

First name, middle initial, last name:

Age:

Patient's record:

Date:

The 1st day of last menses:

The breasts are of reproductive type, mainly presented with adipose tissue. The thickness of glandular tissue up to 20 mm. Fibrous tissue is moderately expressed in all regions. Lactiferous ducts are not dilated; the caliber up to 2 mm. Cystic and solid lesions are not detected.

Axillary, supraclavicular, and subclavian lymph nodes are not enlarged.

Conclusion: Normal breast US. US BI-RADS 1.

3.3 Specific Features of Ultrasound Image of the Breast in Children

The psychoemotional and hormonal status and regulation of the hypothalamus, thyroid, adrenals, ovaries, and other organs affect the breast structure in different ages.

Indications for breast US in children and adolescents are as follows:

- Underdevelopment or rapid breast growth caused by hormonal changes
- Palpable breast mass
- Trauma

The technique of echography in children and adolescents is the same as in adults. Clinical examination and palpation should precede the study. In girls, the examination is appointed in the first phase of the menstrual cycle.

Breasts are examined in patient's supine position with the arms behind the head or, if necessary, lying on the right or left side for better visualization of the outer quadrants. To avoid acoustic artefacts, the breast skin should be lubricated with acoustic gel.

Taking into account the leanness of the glandular tissue and the considerable thickness of the subcutaneous fat in children, the frequency of the linear probe over 7.5–10.0 MHz is most appropriate. The study is performed by fan-shaped movements from the breast periphery to the areolar zone. After this the areolar zone should be examined. Comparison of symmetrical areas of both breasts facilitates the examination.

Each age group has specific anatomical features and pathologic conditions of the breast.

It is important to be aware that abnormal breast conditions may occur in a child. One abnormality is the presence of glandular tissue at inappropriate age. This condition is not due to the pathological state of the breast tissue itself, but to abnormal hormonal status of the child in different ages, both in boys and girls. Other abnormalities confer pathological changes of breast structure, which are more typical for children in puberty.

Embryology. At 4–6 weeks of gestation, mammary-specific progenitor cells may be observed. About day 35 of gestation, proliferation of paired areas of epithelial cells in the epidermis of the thoracic region occurs. These discrete areas of proliferation extend in a line between the fetal axilla and inguinal region and form two ridges called the mammary crests or milk lines.

The primary bud subsequently begins growth downward as a solid diverticulum into the underlying dermis during the 7th week. By the 10th week, the primary bud begins to branch, yielding secondary buds by the 12th week, which eventually develop into the mammary lobules of the adult breast.

Later these structures turn into acini and remain only in the chest area. On the 5th month, the rudimentary epithelial structures begin to branch at the ends, and the sinus of the nipple is being formed.

The nipples are formed in the prenatal period (after the 22nd week of gestation) as a result of the growth of the mesenchyme underlying the areola. In newborns of both sexes, the nipples are located in small grooves. Soon after birth, they acquire their normal appearance due to proliferation of the surrounding connective tissue.

Breasts in newborn boys and girls have similar structure. In the first 1–2 days of life, US clearly depicts the skin as a thin hyperechoic line up to 1 mm thick, as well as subcutaneous fat and gentle connective tissue. The area of the nipple is not differentiated. The thickness of subcutaneous fat and its structure vary depending on the gestational age and the weight at birth. The posterior border of the breast shows as the hyperechoic line of the split thoracic fascia and the anterior fascia of the pectoral muscles. The breast parenchyma is absent. Lactiferous ducts are not differentiated. The retromammary area contains pectoral muscles, ribs, intercostal muscles, and pleura (Fig. 3.22).

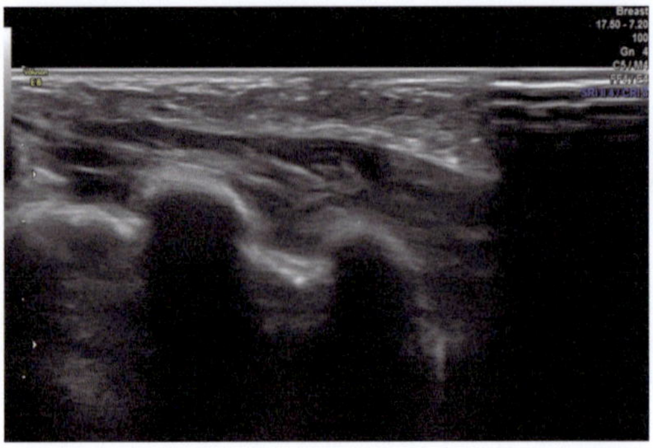

Fig. 3.22 The breast in a girl on the 2nd day of life. Grayscale US

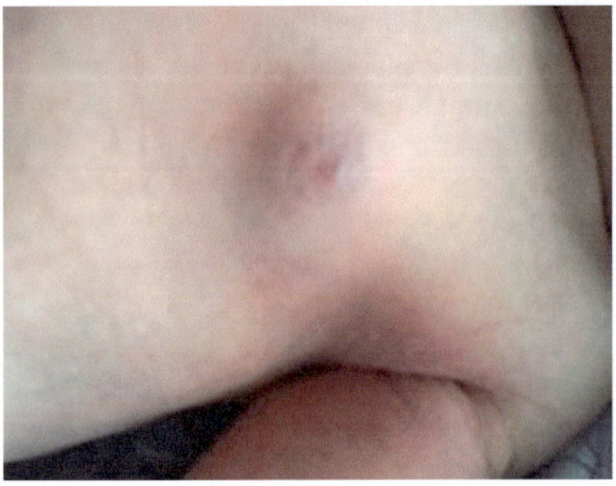

Fig. 3.23 Breast of a girl on the 6th day of life. General appearance

The breasts enlarge by the 7th to 8th day of life in 60% of newborns (both in girls and boys). This condition is called *crisis genitalis neonatorum* and is a normal physiological transitory condition. It is caused by quick decrease of the estradiol level (obtained from the mother) and simultaneous stimulating effect of the baby's prolactin on the epithelium of the mammary glands. Clinical manifestations of this condition are the breast induration and possible galactorrhea (Fig. 3.23).

Echography demonstrates a round or polycyclic hypoechoic area with distinct contours behind the nipple, which results from the ductal system stimulation (Fig. 3.24). Parenchyma of the gland is not visible.

In some cases, with a prolonged sexual crisis, the ducts may be dilated, and a bloody nipple discharge appears. This condition is also transitory. Clinical and US monitoring is necessary in all cases. Invasive diagnostic methods are not applicable because of high risk of damage to immature glandular tissue. The follow-up tactics for newborn babies and children at puberty with nipple discharge differs. Ultrasonography exhibits tubular structures with an- or hypoechoic contents behind the nipple (Fig. 3.25).

In case of massive desquamation of the epithelium and obturation of immature ducts in the posterior nipple area, small cystic inclusions appear, as a complication of the crisis genitalis neonatorum. The size of the cysts may vary from few millimeters to several centimeters. The cysts are asymptomatic in the absence of inflammation. Sometimes the cystic inclusions are accompanied by nipple discharge. The cysts in children are always localized in the sub- or periareolar region. They may be palpable as a soft elastic mass or as a dense inclusion, clearly delineated from the

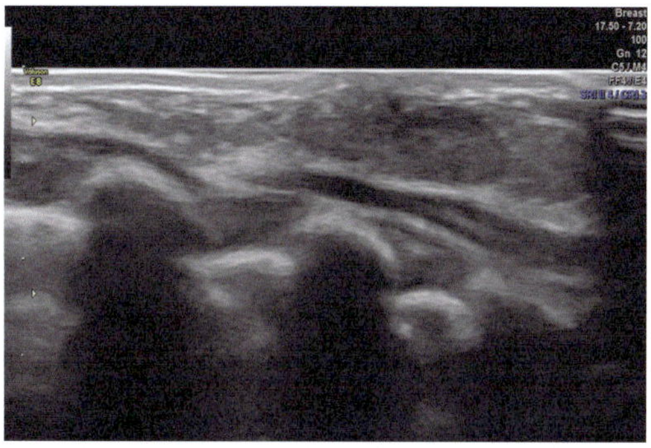

Fig. 3.24 Breast of a girl on the 6th day of life. Crisis genitalis neonatorum. Grayscale US

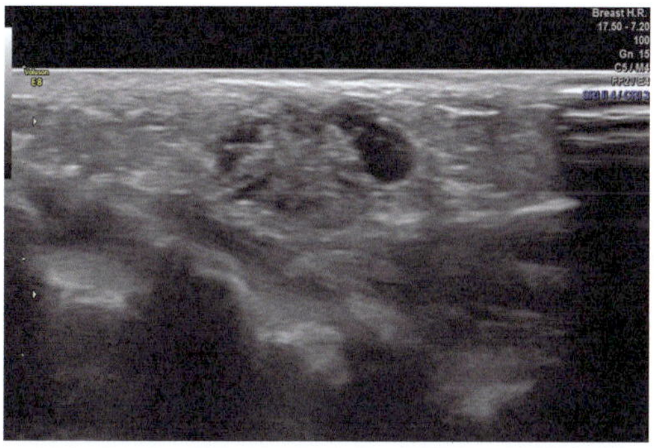

Fig. 3.25 Breast of a boy on the 20th day of life. Grayscale US. Dilatation of a lactiferous duct behind the nipple

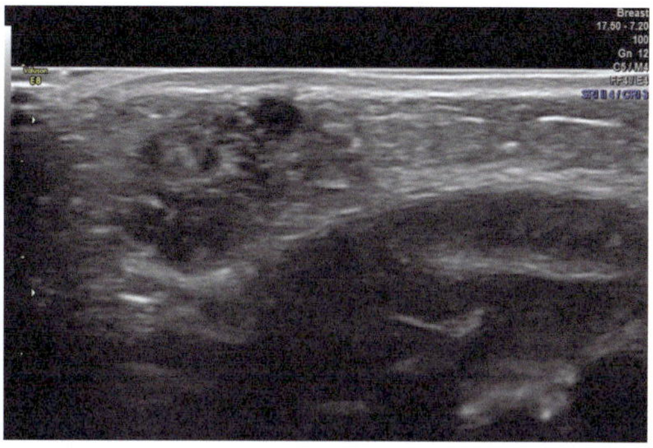

Fig. 3.26 Breast of a girl on the 25th day of life. Grayscale US. Small cystic inclusions behind the nipple

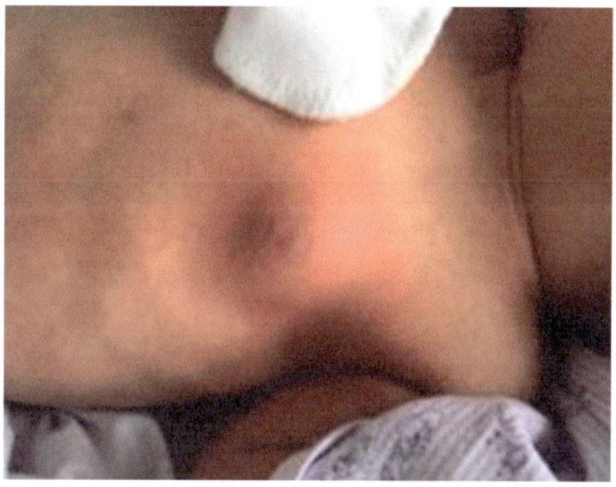

Fig. 3.27 Breast of a girl on the 20th day of life. Mastitis. General appearance of the breast

surrounding tissue. Ultrasonography helps to differentiate a cyst from the glandular tissue in the posterior nipple area (Fig. 3.26).

A more serious complication of the prolonged crisis genitalis neonatorum is *mastitis in a newborn* (Fig. 3.27). The diffuse form of mastitis is specific for newborns, but not for children in puberty. Clinically, this condition manifests with worsening of the general health condition, breast enlargement, pain, and hyperemia. In a newborn's diffuse form of mastitis, US defines thickening of the skin and subcutaneous tissue with increased echodensity and fluid (anechoic) linear layers.

In the case of breast abscess, US demonstrates the area of decreased echodensity that corresponds to fluid and pus collection. Mastitis should be differentiated from physiological breast induration, hemangiomas, and lymphangiomas, which often occur in infants in the 1st year of life (Faden 2005).

In the infants of both sexes, mini-pubertal manifestations occur in the 1st year of life. This is a physiological phenomenon caused by transitory stimulation of the hypothalamic-pituitary axis. In boys, the luteinizing hormone and testosterone levels increase. The cavernous bodies and the scrotum are the target organs. The mammary glands are not affected. In girls, isolated pulse secretion of follicle-stimulating hormone occurs. This leads to stimulation of the ovary and the estrogen synthesis. The breast is the target organ for estrogens. Clinically, this manifests with thelarche.

Breast enlargement in the 1st year of life may be associated with excessive development of adipose tissue. Ultrasound examination allows to make a differential diagnosis and to define the exact volume of glandular tissue and the degree of its development. In the posterior nipple area, in addition to the rudiment of the ductal system (hypoechoic region), the parenchyma appears. It is a segment of the glandular tissue—coarse-grained tissue of moderate or high echogenicity and heterogenous structure (Figs. 3.28 and 3.29).

These breast changes can be observed in children aged 2.5–3 years. By the end of the mini-pubertal period, the stimulating hormonal effect declines and the glandular tissue formation stops. Clinically, the breast induration resolves. Ultrasound registers the decrease in the volume of glandular tissue. The ductal system is not differentiated.

Primary breast growth in girls older than 3 years of age requires differential diagnosis with precocious puberty. Usually, US findings are non-specific. The area of areola is enlarged, and differentiated glandular tissue and lactiferous ducts are defined behind the nipple (Fig. 3.29).

The isolated breast enlargement in a child before puberty is subject for oncologic examination. Approach to examination and treatment of breast conditions in children differs in many aspects from that in adults, including differential diagnosis.

At later age, there are two periods of increase in the number of breast glandular structures at 4 and 9 years (Fig. 3.30). Normally, distinct breast enlargement is also observed at the age of 11–13 years.

In a number of cases, in the absence of clinical and laboratory evidence for precocious puberty, breast enlargement in girls aged 7–9 years is defined as a premature isolated thelarche. From the age of 10–11 years, the breast grows more intensively. Often the stromal component develops much faster than the glandular tissue.

Estrogens stimulate the growth and development of the ducts and the adipose tissue. Progesterone stimulates proliferation of alveoli and promotes the formation of lobes and lactocytes. Estrogens and progesterone cause cyclic changes in the glandular tissue, both in the breast and in the uterus. The greatest activity of mammogenesis is registered with activation of growth and development of a female organism at the age

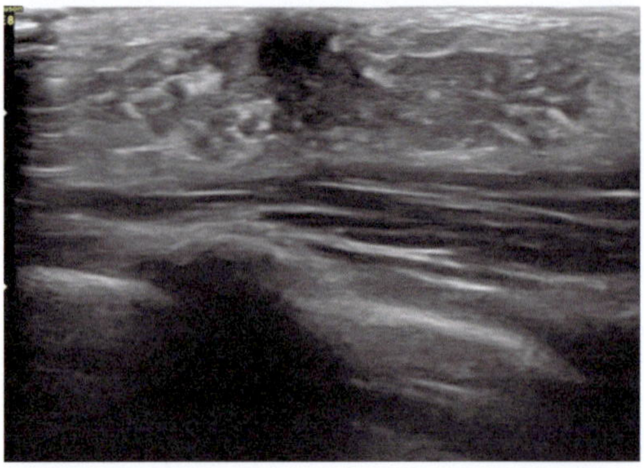

Fig. 3.29 Breast in a girl at the age of 4 years. Precocious puberty. Grayscale US

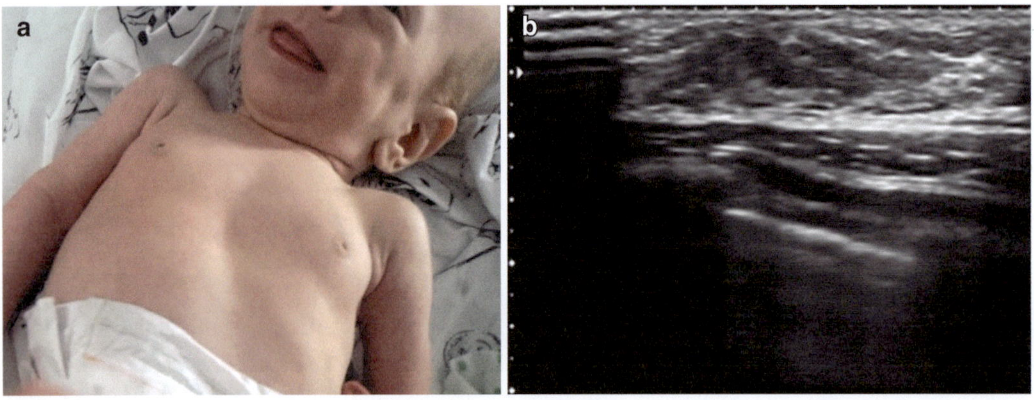

Fig. 3.28 Breast of a girl at the age of 10 months. Thelarche. (**a**) General appearance. (**b**) Grayscale US. A segment of glandular tissue is defined behind the nipple

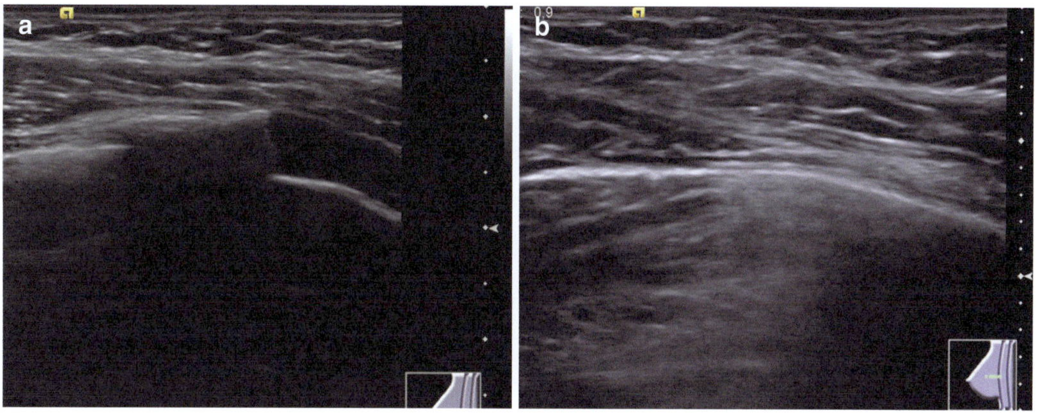

Fig. 3.30 (**a**, **b**) Normal breast. An 8-year-old girl before menarche. Grayscale US

from 11 until 25 years. The first wave of breast development comes at 12–14 years; the second, 2–3 years later; and then, last, 5–7 years later.

In puberty, fibrous and adipose stroma starts to develop earlier than glandular tissue. It confers two types: supporting stroma and periglandular stroma. Breast enlargement in girls of 11–13 years (prior to menarche) is accompanied with significant changes in its structure. US reveals layers of low echodensity of 0.1–0.3 cm thick, which alternate with thin layers of high echodensity.

The layers of low echodensity merge in subareolar area and form a region of irregular shape. Therefore, US fails to differentiate glandular tissue from periglandular stroma in most cases. The expression of periglandular stroma corresponds to the development of glandular tissue.

Development of lactiferous ducts, alveoli, and acini occurs at the age of 10–12 years. The stroma confers two aspects: the labile (periductal) part, which surrounds the glandular elements, and the part with stable supporting stromal cells. In the premenarche girls, secretion of the epithelium increases with mucoid edema of the labile part of stroma. After menarche, the decrease of epithelial secretion and of stromal thickness, resolvement of mucoid edema, and collagenization of fibers are observed. During puberty (12–16 years), the breast continues to grow along with formation and development of the glandular tissue. In girls under 10–12 years of age, the breast structure stays "dormant" and the breasts do not grow. Most part of the breast in this period consists of stroma and subcutaneous fat (Fig. 3.31).

In girls, further development of the breast rudiment occurs at the age 10–12 years with menarche, when a clear correlation between the changes in the mammary glands and the ovarian hormonal function is established. Not only ovarian estrogens are of great importance but also the activity of the hypothalamic-pituitary system and the balance between the estrogens and progesterone. The breast development and its function are under the complex influence of several hormones produced by the ovaries, the pituitary gland, the adrenals, and the thyroid. Each of the hormones has its own specific action. The growth of the ducts depends on estradiol, while the alveolar parts develop under the influence of progesterone. However, both these hormones act only in presence of pituitary hormones. The secretory activity of the breast occurs under the influence of the luteotropic, pituitary hormone (prolactin) after cessation of the action of the placental hormones. The neuro-reflectory mechanisms play an important role in milk production and secretion.

The menstrual cycle throughout the entire reproductive period is a manifestation of the cyclic physiological morphofunctional changes. In puberty, at 11–16 years of age, the breasts continue to develop glandular tissue. The morphological feature of mammary glands in girls of 14–16 years is the formation of new structures—tubular lobules. Breasts in girls of this age after

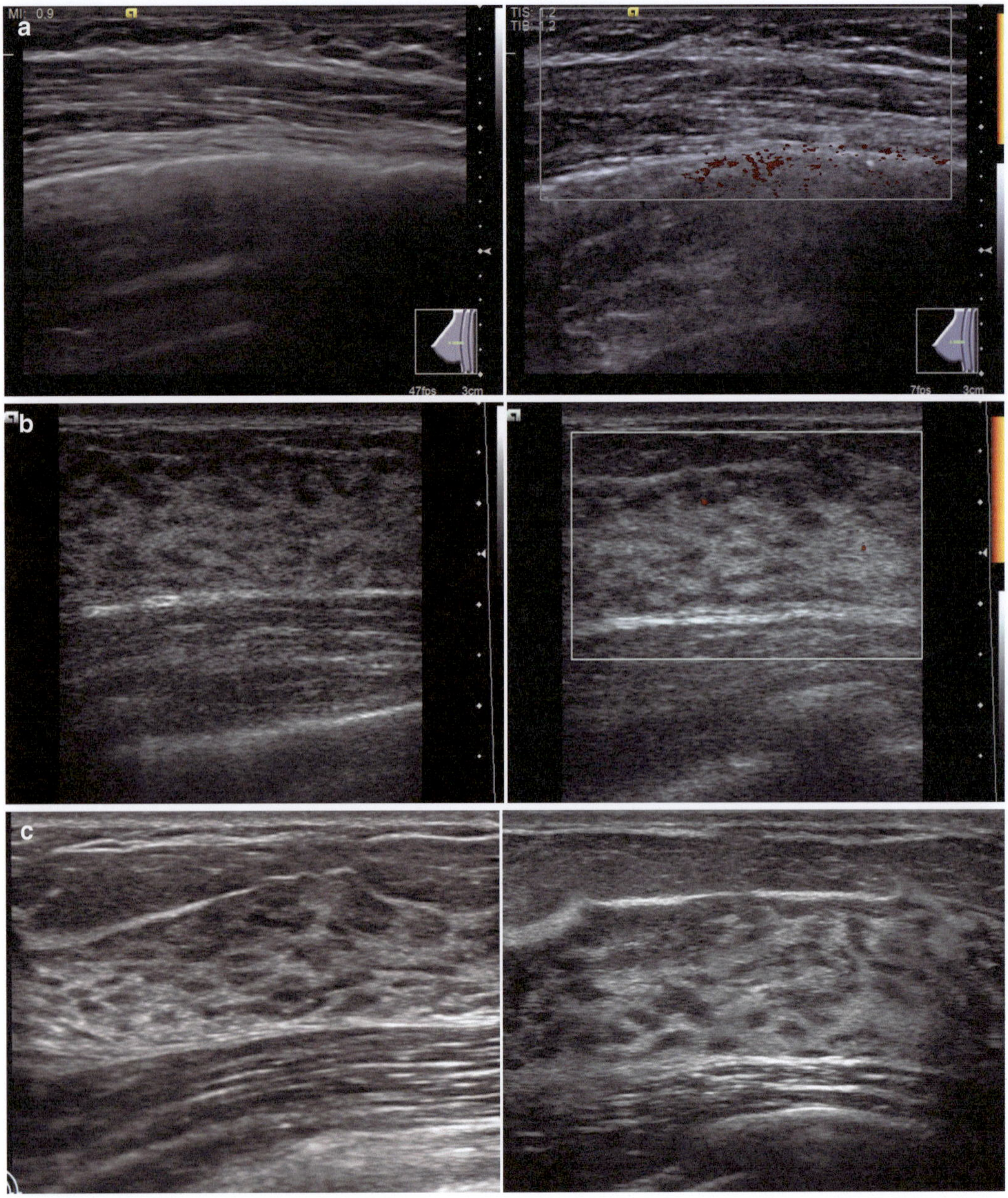

Fig. 3.31 Normal breast. (**a**) A 12-year-old girl. Grayscale US and PDI. (**b**) Adolescent girl, aged 15 years. Grayscale US and PDI. (**c**) An 18-year-old girl. Grayscale US

menarche exhibit "reticular" structure with US. Transverse scanning demonstrates areas of decreased echodensity of 0.1 cm in size (small-cell type), 0.2 cm (middle-cell type), or 0.3 cm (large-cell type) surrounded with layers of high echodensity. Longitudinal scanning of these areas reveals their elongated shape. They are thought to represent glandular lobules (the shape and size are identical), while the surrounding layers of high echodensity correspond to the supporting stroma. Such reticular pattern of mammary glands is associated with their complete structural development.

Individual adipose lobules in the form of elongated fields of decreased echodensity with horizontal "striation" are sometimes defined with US in breast structure, mainly in inner quadrants, in girls of this age group. Girls of 15 and older have larger number of glandular elements with tubular lobules, especially on the periphery of the glands.

The relation of glandular and adipose components in fully developed breast is variable and depends on the loss or increase of body weight. The process of formation of lobules is complex and is influenced by many factors, including hereditary, constitutional, and physiological features.

Pathologic conditions of mammary glands in children. Most publications on the echography and the diagnosis of breast diseases in pediatrics refer to children aged 5–7 years. However, there are many pathological processes, which cause a non-age-related enlargement of the breast in a child, as well as pathological changes in children's breast before puberty. This may be due to complicated pregnancy, assisted reproductive technologies, or hormonal treatment. The percentage of prematurely born children increases. They often have brain injuries affecting hypothalamic-pituitary-gonadal axis, leading to preterm release of gonadotropic hormones. Hormonal disorders in puberty can induce the appearance of breast pathology in teenagers. The great value has an imbalance between estrogen and progesterone.

The arising pathologies form the following groups:

- Breast anomalies (amastia, polythelia, polymastia, aberrant lobes)
- Age-related disturbances (premature or late development)
- Disturbance of symmetric growth of the right and left breasts
- Hypo- or hypermastia
- Inflammatory processes and trauma
- Mastopathy, cysts, ductectasia
- Benign tumors (fibroadenoma, hamartoma, etc.)

All variants of breast anomalies and malformations are divided into the following groups:

- Abnormal number of breasts, nipples, and areolas
- Abnormalities of the breast position, shape, and size

Both unilateral and bilateral anomalies or malformations are possible.

Breast dysplasia in children is either hyperplasia or hypoplasia. Hyperplasia is echographically characterized with the increase in stromal and ductal components and of subcutaneous fat layer (false gynecomastia).

Hypoplasia is a result of the disruption in the development of anatomical structures under insufficient production of sex hormones.

Aplasia is a complete underdevelopment of the breast. It is a rare condition. A small areola with an underdeveloped nipple is present on the skin.

Amastia is a complete absence of the breast, including the nipple-areolar complex. It may be unilateral or bilateral and occurs very rarely. It is usually diagnosed at birth.

Monomastia is the absence of one breast. Anisomastia is a compensatory hyperplasia of the second breast.

Athelia is the absence of nipples in normal breast development. It occurs extremely rarely.

An excessive number of breasts (*polymastia*) and an increased number of nipples (*polythelia*) are more common conditions. As a rule, additional breasts and nipples are located along the lactiferous lines, more often in axillary and submammary areas. There are rare cases of localization of additional breasts not only at milk points but also on the face, ear, neck, hip, or back.

Ectopia is a congenital displacement of the breast. Ectopic breast can be morphologically and functionally underdeveloped or completely developed.

Breast asymmetry is more common in girls in puberty and rare in boys. By the end of puberty, the asymmetry becomes less expressed. However, this anomaly, if severe, may cause great discomfort and be a serious cosmetic challenge.

Underdevelopment of the breast (including in men) is often a part of complex syndromes caused by severe genetic or chromosomal diseases. In these situations, pathological changes of reproductive organs are also present. Similar pathological conditions develop on the background of disrupted production of gonadotropic hormones or other disturbances of hypothalamic-pituitary system.

Premature breast development is associated with an increase in the blood estrogens levels or the increased sensitivity of the breast to estrogens. Delayed breast development is more often observed under estrogen deficiency.

Hyper- or macromastia occurs rarely. This is caused by proliferation of the lactiferous ducts, hyperplasia of ductal epithelium, and proliferation of connective tissue. As a rule the hormonal background is normal.

Hypomastia occurs more often. The height of the breast (the distance from the nipple to the base of the breast) is less than 4–5 cm in girls aged 16–18 years.

Among malformations of the nipple-areolar complex, the nipple *invagination* and *enlarged areola* occur rarely. The nipple invagination may be congenital and acquired and may occur both independently and due to hypertrophy of the breast.

In recent years, the incidence of oncological diseases in children has increased: congenital tumors (germinogenous ovarian tumors, prolactinomas, embryonic tumors of the hypothalamus (hamartoma), pineal gland tumors).

The majority of pathological processes in children's breast are benign. It should be noted that pathological changes in subcutaneous fat, ducts, parenchyma, breast stroma, and the surrounding (underlying) tissues are among the most common breast diseases in the juvenile and early reproductive period.

Lipoma is a benign tumor of fatty tissue with expansive growth. It has its own capsule. In children, it is often visualized as a hypoechoic 2.0–2.5 cm mass of round or oval shape, with distinct and even hypoechoic contour located in the subcutaneous fat, rarely in retromammary space. It is often located in the subareolar region, in the upper-external quadrants.

Breast cysts are found in 6% of girls. Their incidence is the same both in healthy girls of prepubertal and pubertal age and in girls with abnormal levels of sex hormones. Echographic characteristics (echogenicity, structure, borders, vascularization) do not differ from those in adult women.

Hemangioma is a rare benign breast lesion in younger children. The capillary type develops as a bright red spot and consists of normal capillaries. Often hemangioma is detected immediately after birth or in the 1st year of life. The size of the spot and the depth of the lesion are determined with ultrasound.

Fibroadenoma (FA) is a hormone-induced hyperplastic tumor. It often occurs in the adolescent age (16–18 years). FA is often a single, one-sided, elastic, mobile tumor located in the upper-external quadrant of the breast. It grows horizontally with displacement of the surrounding tissues to the periphery. Multiple and bilateral masses occur less often. Fibroadenomas are variable in size, from small (0.5 cm) to large (more than 6 cm). Large juvenile fibroadenomas are mostly found in girls and young women and are characterized by large-cell structure and rapid growth. The ultrasound picture depends on the size and the shape of the mass. As a rule, FA is visualized as an oval, round, or irregular delineated mass of low echogenicity with clear, even contours.

According to literature data, breast cancer rarely occurs in children. There are only single reports on secretory ductal adenocarcinoma and phyllodes tumor (Valeur et al. 2015).

Considering high incidence of breast pathology in children and adolescents, it is necessary to conduct examination, palpation, and breast ultrasound in all girls, who are referred to gynecologists for consultation. Breast abnormalities are diagnosed clinically. Liquid-containing and soft tissue breast masses are subject to imaging and follow-up. Complex echography permits highest precision and efficiency for that.

It is necessary to remember about the restrictions for biopsies in children, which in some cases is vitally necessary, but may lead to damage of the developing breast tissue.

4 Multiparametric Ultrasound in Benign Breast Diseases (Inflammatory, Diffuse Degenerative)

Alexander N. Sencha and Ekaterina Sencha

Abstract

The incidence of breast diseases in fertile women is 10–65%. All breast changes can be divided into two basic groups: tumoral and non-tumoral processes. Diffuse mastopathy is the most widespread disease that accounts for 30–60% of the total number of breast diseases. Fibroadenomas, cysts, intraductal papillomas, and nodular mastopathy are less frequent (1–5%). Mastitis is an inflammatory nonspecific processes in the breast. It is divided into lactational (up to 90%) and non-lactational types. Ultrasonography is valuable in breast trauma with hematomas. Fibrocystic breast disease is characterized with abnormal ratio of epithelial and connective tissue components, wide range of proliferative and regressive breast changes. Nodular type of fibrocystic breast disease is a pathological condition with one or several dense foci within the breast. US permits precise differentiation of cysts in 100% of cases. Intraductal papilloma is a benign, mostly solitary fibroepithelial tumor located within a lactiferous duct (cystadenopapilloma) or in a cyst, often in the subareolar region. Galactocele is a retention breast cyst, single- or multi-chambered, formed during pregnancy and/or lactation and filled with milk. Ultrasound findings in duct ectasia and sclerosing adenosis are usually nonspecific and depend on the stage. Focal fibrosis, radial scar, and gigantomastia are also discussed.

A. N. Sencha (✉)
Division of Visual Diagnostics, National Medical Research Center for Obstetrics, Gynecology and Perinatology named after Academician V.I. Kulakov of Ministry of Healthcare of Russian Federation, Moscow, Russia

E. Sencha
Department of Ultrasound Diagnostics, Federal State Budget Hospital "9 Treatment and Diagnostic Center" of the Ministry of Defense of the Russian Federation, Moscow, Russia

The incidence of breast diseases in fertile women is 10–65% (Sencha 2015). All breast changes can be divided into two basic groups: tumoral and non-tumoral processes. The diagnosis of breast diseases should always implicate oncologic concern. Breast carcinoma is differentiated with the big group of benign focal and diffuse breast changes.

Benign breast changes are observed most often. They confer abnormalities with various clinical, morphological, and etiological features. There are several types of classifications. For example, the following classification is used for practical purposes in Russia since 1985:

1. Diffuse mastopathy
   (a) With prevalence of a glandular component (adenosis)
   (b) With prevalence of a fibrous component

G. T. Sukhikh, A. N. Sencha (eds.), *Multiparametric Ultrasound Diagnosis of Breast Diseases*,
https://doi.org/10.1007/978-3-319-75034-7_4

   (c) With prevalence of a cystic component
   (d) Mixed type
2. Nodular mastopathy
3. Benign tumors and tumor-like processes
   (a) Adenoma
   (b) Fibroadenoma
   (c) Intraductal papilloma
   (d) Cyst
4. Special types
   (a) Phyllodes tumor

Benign breast pathology is diagnosed, as a rule, in patients with characteristic clinical signs or with screening tests. Diffuse mastopathy is the most widespread disease that accounts for 30–60% of the total number of breast diseases. Fibroadenomas, cysts, intraductal papillomas, and nodular mastopathy are less frequent (1–5%) (Radzinsky et al. 2016; Rybnikova et al. 2017). A comparative analysis of the incidence of breast diseases with mammography and ultrasonography is given in Table 4.1.

Comparative analysis of this data shows the superiority of ultrasonography over mammography in detecting most breast diseases, except for local fibrosis. Differential diagnosis of nodular mastopathy, which has radiographic and ultrasound characteristics similar to malignant neoplasms, is difficult. Equivocal ultrasound and mammography findings, insufficient for differentiation of benign and malignant masses, are the reason to recommend magnetic resonance mammography. MRM is not routinely used to diagnose benign breast diseases, because of the high cost of the study.

Non-tumoral breast pathology confers pathological processes of different etiology and pathogenesis. About 30% of them associate with hyperplasia of ductal and/or lobular epithelium (Trufanov et al. 2009).

Mastitis is an inflammatory nonspecific processes in the breast. It is divided into lactational (up to 90%) and non-lactational types. The inflammatory process can be acute or chronic. Acute mastitis exhibits the following phases of development: serous inflammation, infiltration, and abscess.

Mastitis has the following US features (Fig. 4.1):

- Thickening of the skin over the area of inflammation (it exceeds the same of healthy areas and the other breast)
- Increase in echodensity of subcutaneous fat
- Indistinct margin between the deep layer of derma and adjacent structures (fat or glandular tissue)
- Poor differentiation of the structure of breast parenchyma
- One or several hypoechoic areas with distinct or vague margins within breast parenchyma
- Underlined connective tissue component
- Cystic cavities and/or dilatations of lactiferous ducts
- Regular vascular pattern of breast parenchyma, uniform reduction of vessel caliber with CDI or PDI
- Enlargement of axillary lymph nodes

Table 4.1 The breast diseases detection rate with ultrasonography and mammography among women over 40 years, as per 100 women surveyed

	Ultrasonography			X-ray mammography		
Age	40–49	50 and older	Total	40–49	50 and older	Total
Diffuse FBD	26.5	23.8	25.4	8.8	15.5	11.4
Diffuse fibrous breast disease	16.2	33.3	22.7	6.6	21.4	12.3
Diffuse mixed breast disease	5.9	7.4	6.3	31.2	35.6	33.2
Adenosis	1.5	0.6	1.1	0.9	0.4	0.7
Nodular FBD	0.4	0.7	0.5	0.9	1.2	1.1
Local fibrosis	0.6	0.4	0.5	3.2	2.8	3.1
Cyst	11.0	14.3	12.3	4.8	5.6	6.3
Lipoma	13.2	16.7	14.5	9.5	10.7	10.0
Fibroadenoma	6.1	5.7	5.9	4.4	4.7	4.5
Other focal changes	0.7	0.9	0.8	0.7	1.2	0.9
Total	82.9	104.9	90.9	72.5	100.7	85.0

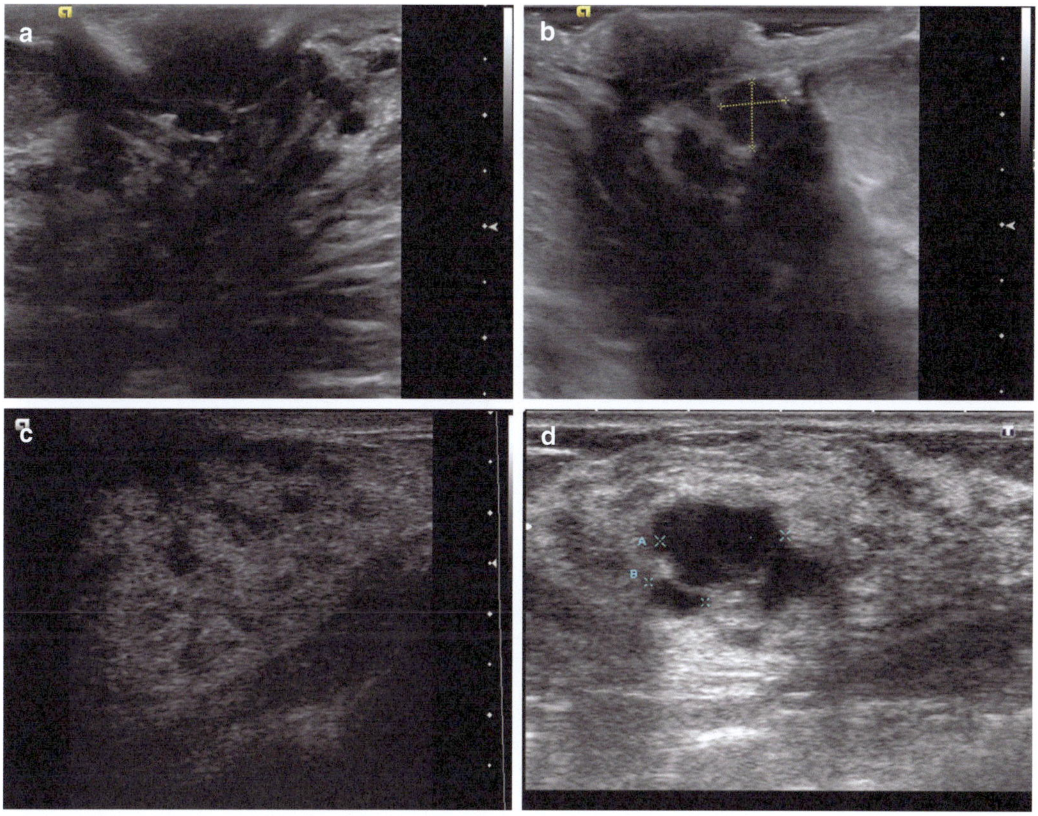

Fig. 4.1 (**a**–**d**) Acute mastitis. Grayscale US. Differentiation of breast tissue is difficult due to an increase in overall echogenicity, structural heterogeneity, and dilated lactiferous ducts

The expression of US features directly depends on clinical symptoms. Early diagnosis with optimal combination of clinical, imaging, and other tests is extremely important.

Contact of an ultrasound probe with the skin in the area of inflammation often causes pain or severe discomfort. In these cases, it is advised to warm up (37–38 °C) the US gel or use warm water as a lubricant. Mastitis, depending on the form, shows specific dynamics of echographic changes.

Proliferative phase with US is characterized with skin thickening by more than 3 mm and decrease in echodensity in comparison with healthy areas. During this period, the echogenicity of subcutaneous tissue and parenchyma of the gland is increased, and they lack differentiation.

Further development of the inflammatory process promotes the appearance of single or multiple heterogeneous areas within breast parenchyma. One echographic feature of acute mastitis is the spread of the pathological process along the intraparenchymal lymphatic pathways and the appearance of secondary hypo- and anechoic sites in other quadrants of the mammary gland.

Differential diagnosis of diffuse mastitis with inflammatory type of breast cancer is often difficult. A detailed history, characteristic signs of the inflammatory process, especially with abscess, and effective treatment with antibiotics facilitate correct diagnosis.

In some cases, such as late or inadequate treatment, the inflammation develops from serous infiltration to diffusive purulent stage with fine foci of purulent fusion of the parenchyma, which aggregate and form abscesses. Breast abscesses can be classified in accordance with their location into subcutaneous, subareolar, intramammary, and retromammary. In the majority of cases, the infection enters the breast tissue through the damaged skin of the nipple, areola, or epithelium of lactiferous ducts. However, the infection may develop due to weak immune response with hematogenic or lymphogenous contamination.

Breast abscess is sonographically characterized with a mass of heterogeneous structure due to anechoic necrotic foci and echogenic debris, which is accurately boarded by echogenic pseudocapsule (Fig. 4.2). Abscess can show mainly hypoechoic or anechoic structure. It is avascular with CDI and PDI and often surrounded with the zone of increased vascularity.

Follow-up of the patients with acute mastitis with appropriate conservative treatment generally reveals the normalization of skin thickness and breast tissue structure (decrease in the number and size of hypo- and anechoic areas, disappearance of reactive lymph nodes) and the decrease in the number of visualized vessels in the inflammation zone.

In cases of difficulties in the differentiation of acute mastitis and diffuse type of breast carcinoma, special care should be paid to case history, clinical data, and mammographic and US features. The biopsy of the breast and abnormal lymph nodes with cytology or histology is of great benefit. Core biopsy in cases of expressed inflammatory process is often impossible and in diffuse type of breast carcinoma appears not informative.

Specific inflammatory lesions (tuberculosis, syphilis) are rare enough and do not have a specific ultrasound pattern. In these cases, the diagnosis is based on the patient's history, laboratory tests, and pathology of the punctate.

Small breast trauma, bruises, and abrasions may exhibit only the edema of subcutaneous fat with US. Cystic or solid posttraumatic lesions are absent in these cases (Fig. 4.3).

Ultrasonography is valuable in breast trauma with hematomas (Fig. 4.4). *Posttraumatic breast*

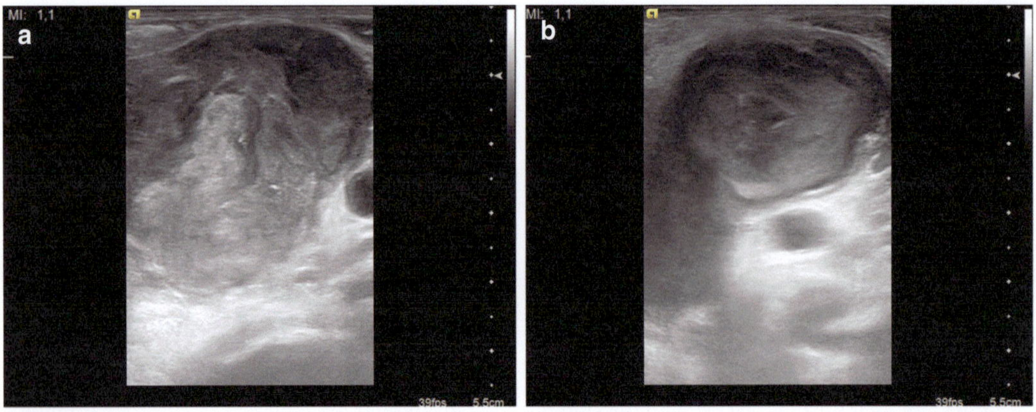

Fig. 4.2 (**a**, **b**) Breast abscess. Grayscale US

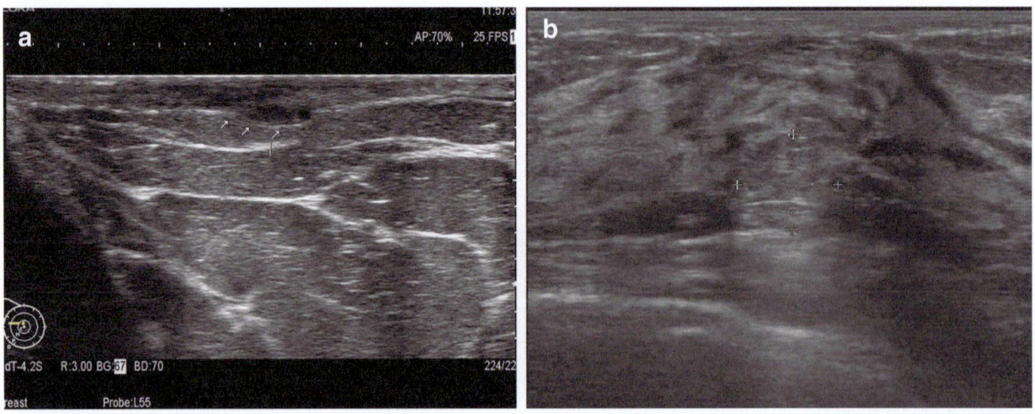

Fig. 4.3 (**a**, **b**) Contusion of the breast. Grayscale US

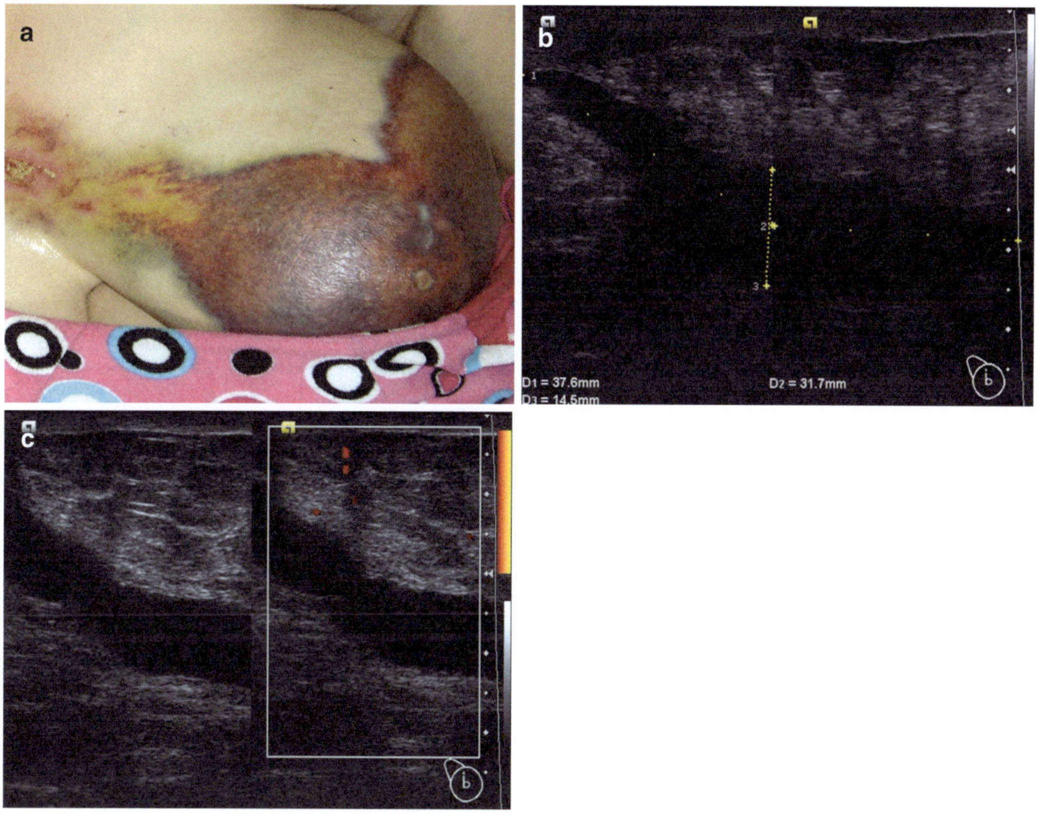

Fig. 4.4 Posttraumatic breast hematoma. (**a**) Photo. (**b**) Grayscale. (**c**) PDI

hematomas are blood accumulations in soft tissues and/or parenchyma of the mammary gland. They confer the following periods: acute, the first 4–7 days; intermediate, up to 2 weeks; and late, the term within a year and longer after the trauma. Division into the periods is necessary for correct interpretation of sonographic and clinical signs. During the first days and weeks, hematoma is detected with US as anechoic incorporations of roundish or irregular shapes of various sizes, as a rule located superficially. Breast hematoma demands special attention as it can be the first sign of a malignant tumor, considering neoangiogenesis (vessels within a malignant neoplasm have no muscular layer, are fragile, and easily damaged).

Hematoma undergoes slow resorption and/or organization. Breast trauma can also induce breast fat necrosis, which is defined as hypoechoic or echogenic breast fields of irregular shape with indistinct or accurate margins, often with posterior acoustic shadow. Architectonics of surrounding tissues is quite often affected. Further, there appear coarse calcifications, which exhibit irregular shape or correspond to roundish margins of the lesion. The location of such masses corresponds to the place of former trauma or hematoma. Surgical interventions, inflammatory processes, local ischemia, and other conditions also can lead to such lesions. They need to be differentiated with breast malignancies.

Breast trauma or surgery in patient's history and absence of malignant signs with US and mammography suggest lipogranuloma. It is necessary to remember about the possibility of recurrent breast carcinoma in the scar. FNAB and cytology assist in correct diagnosis. Breast MRI and excision biopsy may be indicated in most ambiguous cases.

Breast condition is associated with female sex hormones. Nevertheless, one important mechanism of pathological influence is considered the depression of progesterone against superfluous (relative or absolute) level of estrogens. The changes in breast structure and function are named fibrocystic breast disease (FBD).

Fibrocystic breast disease is characterized with abnormal ratio of epithelial and connective tissue components, wide range of proliferative and regressive breast changes. There are many synonyms of this condition, such as diffuse cystic breast disease, chronic cystic mastitis, fibrocystic breast disease, mammary dysplasia, Reclus-Schimmelbusch disease, and others. FBD is the most widespread benign breast disease that affects 30–63% of women. Diffuse mastopathy is observed in 29.4–42.6% of women more often at the age of 30–50 years. It accounts for 29–95% in fertile women with gynecologic disorders. Breast carcinoma arises 3–5 times more often against benign diseases, especially in the cases of nodular type of FBD with epithelial proliferation (30–40 times more often than in normal breast tissue) (Sinyukova et al. 2007). The diagnosis of different types of mastopathy is important, because these processes can hide clinical signs and complicate breast imaging of carcinoma.

Clinical symptoms are nonspecific and confer general symptoms, such as pain, palpable breast lesions, and discharge from nipples. The disease exhibits hyperplasia of ductal epithelium and sclerosis of connective tissue with histology that results in the development of cysts.

US features of diffuse FBD (Fig. 4.5) are the following:

- Irregular dilation of lactiferous ducts
- Dense Cooper's ligaments
- Fine-grained highly echoic glandular tissue
- Multiple anechoic incorporations (cysts)
- Poor asymmetric vascular pattern of breast parenchyma in color coded modes
- Grainity increase (from fine-grained to moderate- and coarse-grained), irregular, asymmetric coloring with compression US elastography

For adequate FBD treatment, it is crucial to determine the following aspects:

- Individual or complex factors that induced the disease
- Type of fibrocystic breast disease

Therefore, precise echographic specification of the type of FBD is necessary, for example:

- Diffuse FBD with predominance of glandular component
- Diffuse FBD with predominance of fibrous component
- Diffuse FBD with predominance of cystic component
- Mixed type

Specification of the type of the disease determines further treatment and follow-up.

The opinions about the changes in blood flow in the vessels within the abnormal area and outside of it are ambiguous. Smirnova (1995) and Vetshev et al. (1997) report that PSV in the fields of mastopathy does not exceed 0.09 m/s (as compared to the norm of 0.13–0.16 m/s).

Ultrasound criteria help to assess the effectiveness of the treatment of the diffuse FBD. It registers the decrease in thickness of glandular tissue and Cooper's ligaments, cysts size and number, decrease in duct ectasia, normalization of echodensity, and structure of glandular tissue. A negative ultrasound dynamics can be regarded as a recurrent or progressive course of diffuse FBD, which requires monitoring, repeated courses of complex therapy, or correction of the treatment.

Breast cancer develops 3–5 times more often on the background of benign diseases and 30–40 times more often in cases of nodular mastopathy with epithelial proliferation (Sinyukova et al. 2007). FBD can mask clinical symptoms and image of breast cancer, especially at early stages. The risk of malignancy in nonproliferative types of FBD is 0.9% and in cases of expressed proliferation 2–3% (Korzhenkova 2004).

The sensitivity of US in diagnosis of FBD accounts for 77.8% with specificity of 99.5% and diagnostic accuracy of 93.2% (Sencha et al. 2013).

Nodular mastopathy (nodular type of FBD) is a pathological condition with one or several dense foci within the breast. It is, first of all, a clinical concept. There is a wide range of diseases that hide behind the mask of nodular mastopathy, such as local fibrosis (45%), cyst (22%),

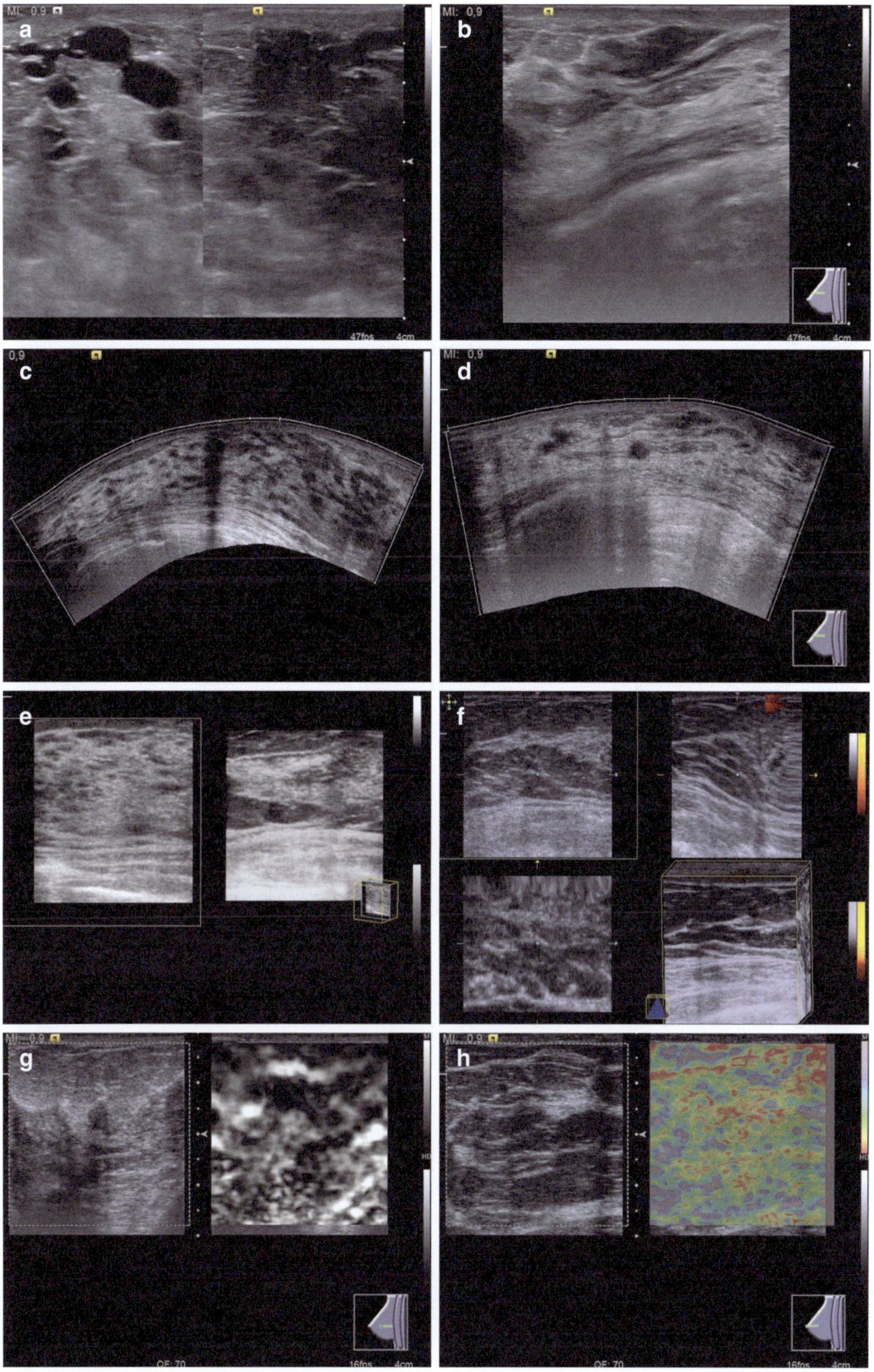

Fig. 4.5 Diffuse fibrocystic breast disease. (**a**, **b**) Grayscale US. (**c**, **d**) Panoramic scan. (**e**) 3D US. (**f**) 3DPD. (**g**, **h**) Compression US elastography

fibroadenoma (17%), lipoma (10%), breast carcinoma, oleogranuloma, cystadenopapilloma, etc. (Korzhenkova 2004).

Pathological examination of the fields of nodular mastopathy detects hyperplasia of glandular lobules, cysts, fibrosis, proliferation of cellular elements of cysts and ducts lumen, and other changes. Atypia of epithelium is regarded a precancer.

US features of nodular mastopathy are listed below (Fig. 4.6):

- Solitary or multiple fields of decreased echodensity
- Various dimensions
- Irregular shape
- Indistinct borders
- A- or hypovascularity with CDI, PDI, and 3DPD
- Asymmetric rough- or moderate-grained type of coloring with compression US elastography

According to Sinyukova et al. (2007), CDI more often reveals linear vessels in nodular mastopathy without any change in its intensity. The average PSV is 0.16–0.50 m/s; EDV, 0.65–0.07; PI, 0.63–1.2; and RI, 0.65–1.2. Contrast enhancement reveals asymmetric vascularization at the end of the arterial and the beginning of the venous phase; a perfusion defect in the affected area sometimes can be seen.

As a rule, altered parenchyma more often exhibits asymmetric rough- or medium-grained pattern with compression US elastography in nodular FBD as compared with diffuse FBD. At elastometry, different parts of the parenchyma may have significant differences in the stiffness (Fig. 4.6).

US picture of nodular mastopathy often does not differ from the early stage of a breast carcinoma; therefore all kinds of nodular hyperplasia should have morphological verification. Microscopic substrate, which represents the clinical syndrome of FBD, confers all structural elements of the mammary gland—lobules, cystically transformed ducts, and fibrous and adipose tissues. Lobules, ducts, or cystic lesions may prevail, but fibrous tissue is always presented in significant amount. Dilation of lactiferous ducts and ductal cysts in diffuse and nodular mastopathy often results from excessive fibrosis of parenchyma with local compression of lactiferous ducts.

Cystic lesions are the most frequent feature of FBD. The mechanism of appearance of cysts implicates on one hand excessive fluid secretion by epithelial cells, which undergo apocrine metaplasia, and disturbance of fluid absorption in ducts on the other. Cysts are palpated as individual or multiple elastic movable lesions, often painful with compression. They can be individual, multiple (more often), unilateral, bilateral, simple, or complex. US permits precise differentiation of cysts in 100% of cases, while they are clinically defined as palpable lesions and mammographically detected as foci of average intensity within the glandular triangle, which are accurately bordered or merging with surrounding breast structures.

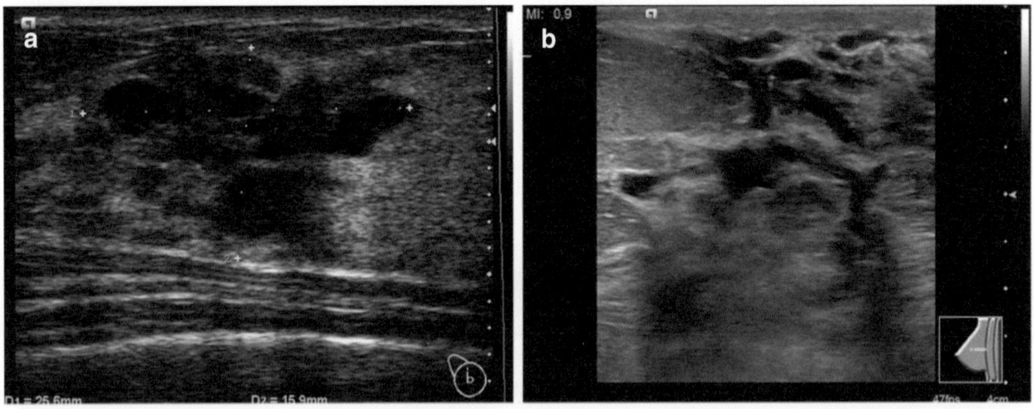

Fig. 4.6 FBD. Nodular type. (**a–d**) Grayscale US. (**e**) CDI. (**f, g**) Panoramic scan. (**h**) Compression US elastography. (**i, j**) CEUS. SonoVue, 2.4 mL. A slight asymmetric increase in contrast enhancement at the end of the arterial phase

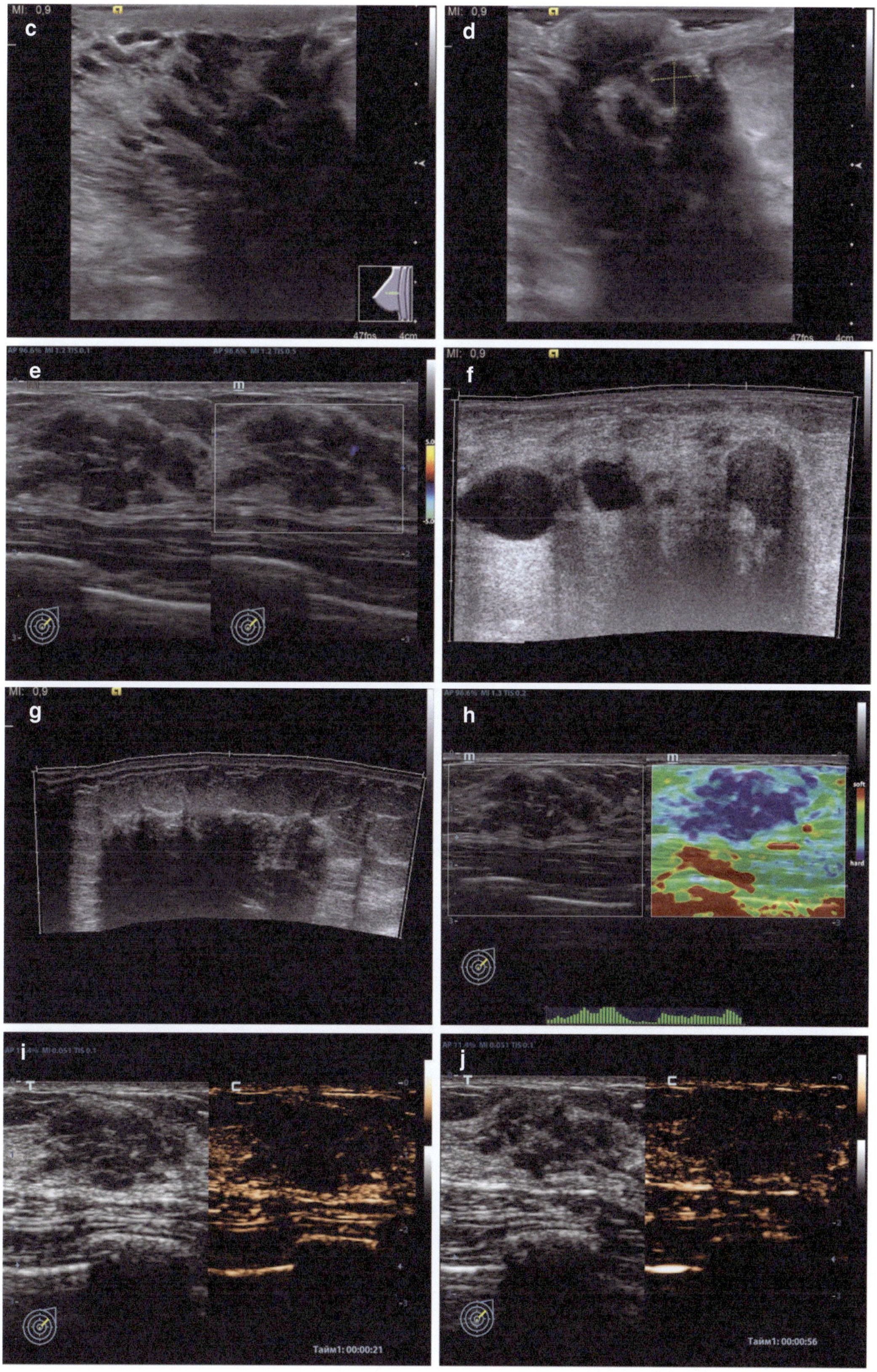

Fig. 4.6 (continued)

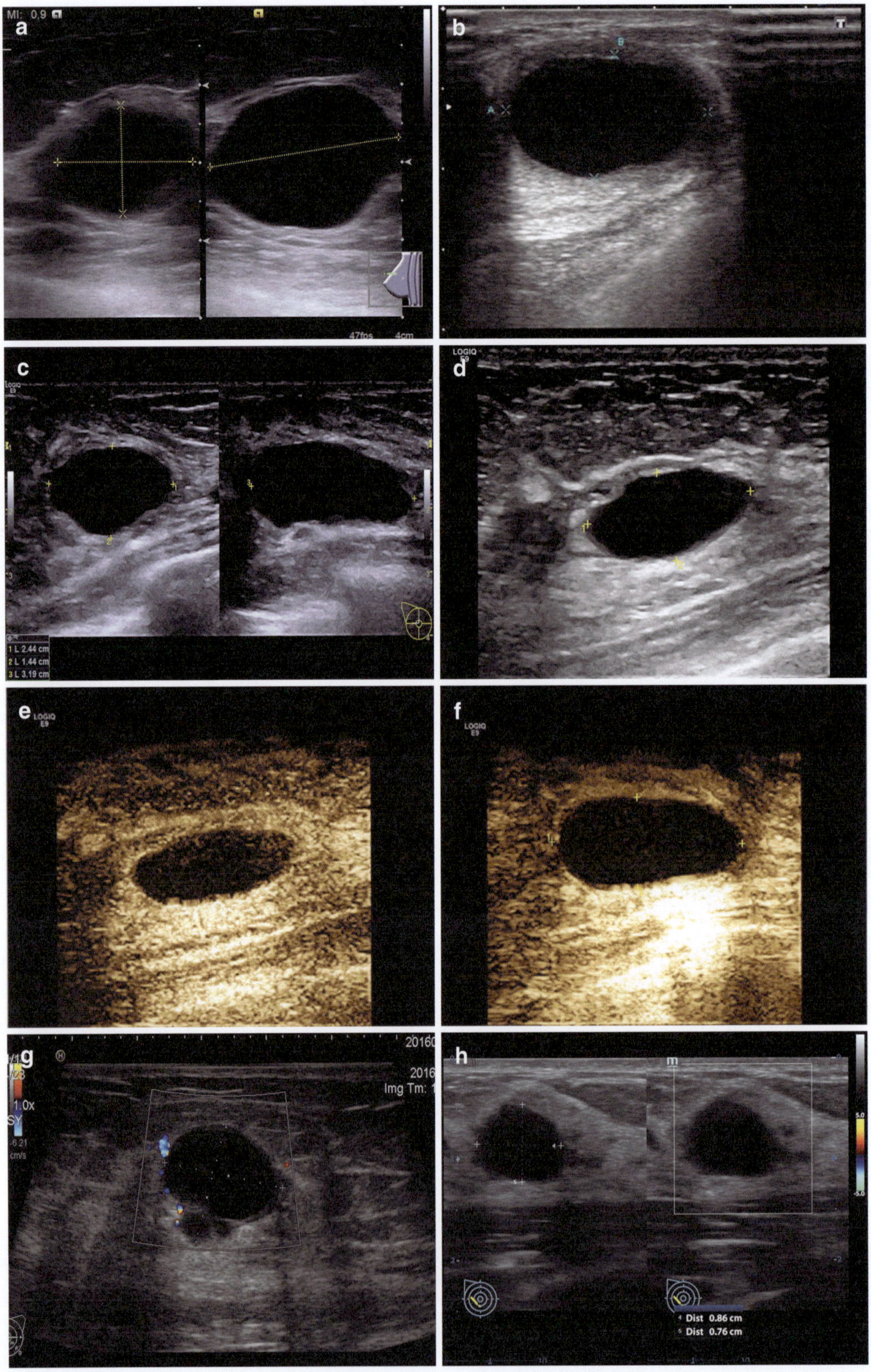

Fig. 4.7 A simple breast cyst. (**a–d**) Grayscale US. (**e**, **f**) B-flow. (**g–i**) CDI. (**j**) PDI. (**k**) Panoramic scan. (**l**) 3DPD. (**m–p**) Compression US elastography. (**q**, **r**) CEUS. SonoVue 2.4 mL. Perfusion defect

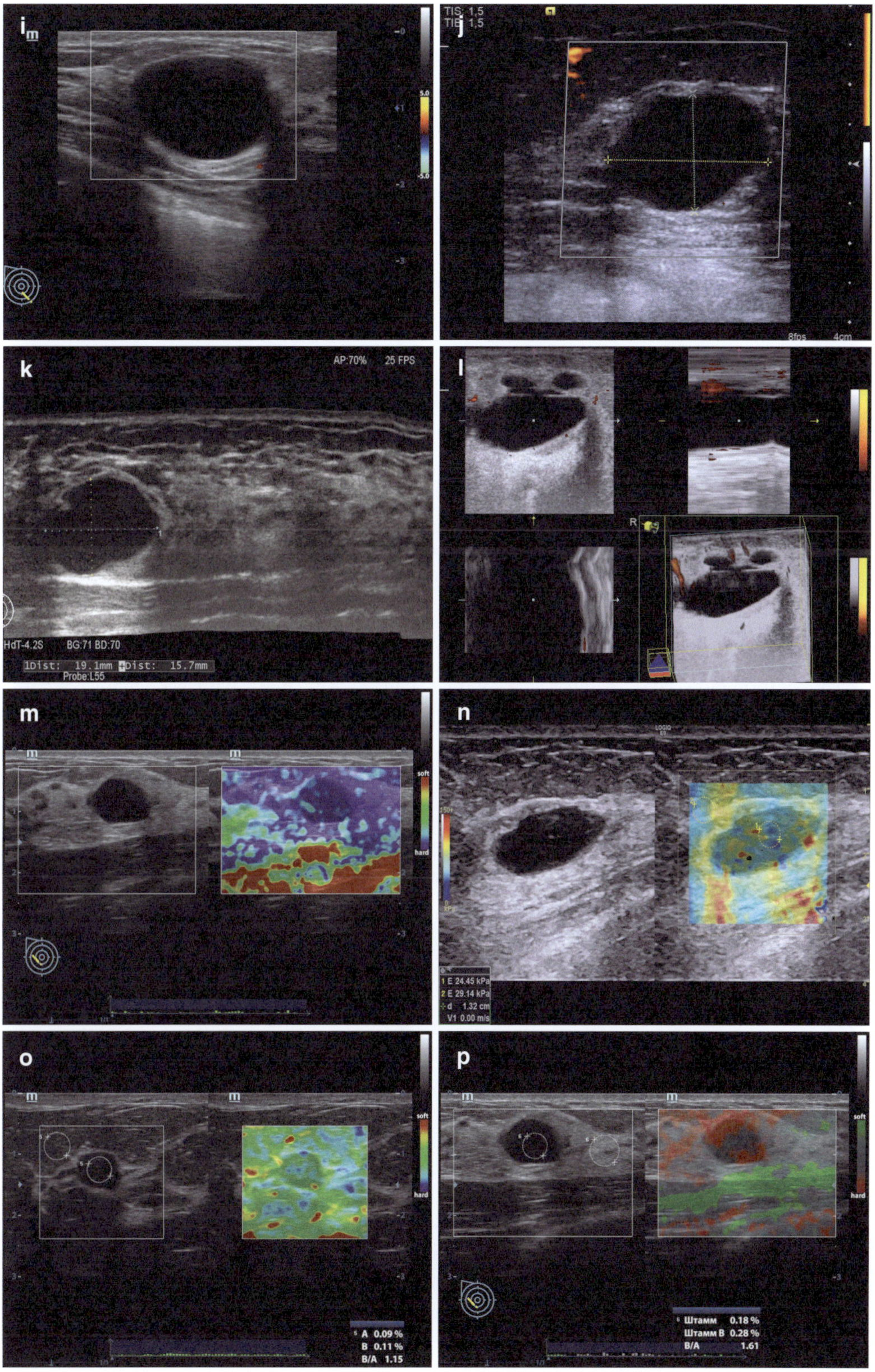

Fig. 4.7 (continued)

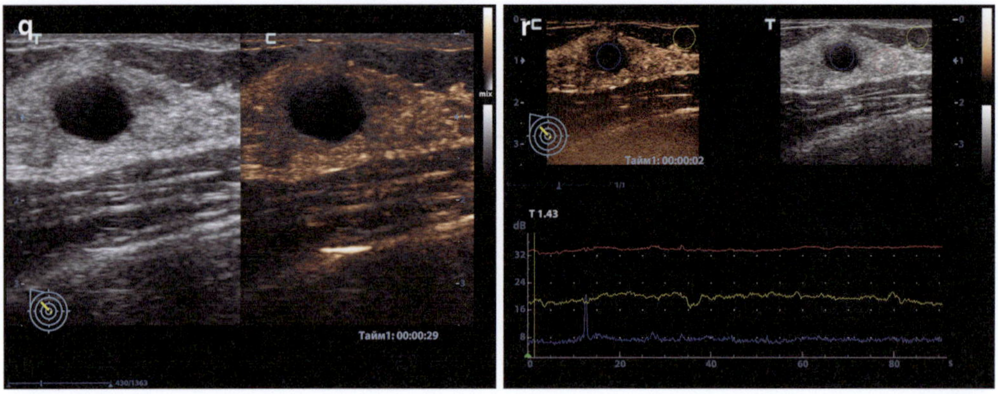

Fig. 4.7 (continued)

The majority of breast cysts exhibit typical US features (Fig. 4.7), as follows:

- Anechoic structure.
- Homogeneous structure.
- Roundish or oval shape.
- Distinct accurate margins.
- Posterior echo enhancement.
- Easy deformation and painlessness with compression.
- Avascularity with CDI, PDI, and 3DPD.
- The absence of color pattern within the lesion with US elastography.
- The elasticity index, as a rule, is within the range of 1.0–1.5.
- Perfusion defects, lack of contrast enhancement with CEUS.

Up to 95% of breast cysts have no solid component on the capsule (Korzhenkova 2004). Such cysts are characterized as simple (typical) and uncomplicated. There are also breast microcysts (with the size of 1–2 mm) and macrocysts (simple and multilocular), individual and multiple (Trufanov et al. 2009).

Breast cysts in some cases may not exhibit such a characteristic symptom as posterior echo enhancement. This happens more often in small cysts, the cysts surrounded by dense structures, near to the thorax, or in cysts with expressed fibrous capsule.

In color-coded modes, up to 95–100% of cysts do not have any vascular pattern. In compression US elastography mode, simple breast cysts, as a rule, are not colored or colored similar to the surrounding structures, since they often have similar elasticity with the surrounding parenchyma. CEUS reveals no contrast enhancement—a typical perfusion defect (Fig. 4.7q, r). Many experts do not advise to use contrast ultrasound for the diagnosis of breast cysts, except for the cases when they are complex and simulate a solid mass with echogenic content. In these cases, contrast echography can prove the cystic nature of the lesion by demonstrating no contrast enhancement.

Simple cysts are easily diagnosed with echography. Infected cysts, according to echography, in contrast to simple cysts, have thick, irregular margins, and heterogeneous structure (Fig. 4.8). The surrounding structures and parenchyma show the features typical for acute mastitis with enlargement of regional lymph nodes. Color Doppler mapping detects the increase in the number of vessels in surrounding tissues. Elastography reveals a slight change in elasticity.

Acute lactation abscesses are often defined as single-chamber (73.1%) or multi-chamber (26.9%) lesions of anechoic structure, with fine suspension (46.2%) and hyperechoic capsule (23.1%), often with distinct, uneven contours (65.4%). Fluctuation of abscess contents can be observed in 80.8% of cases and absence of blood flow in necrotic cavity with peripheral hypervascularization in 73.1% of cases. Lactiferous ducts in the infiltrate can be detected in 38.5% of cases. In 100% of cases, US signs of acute mastitis were visualized on the periphery of the abscess with

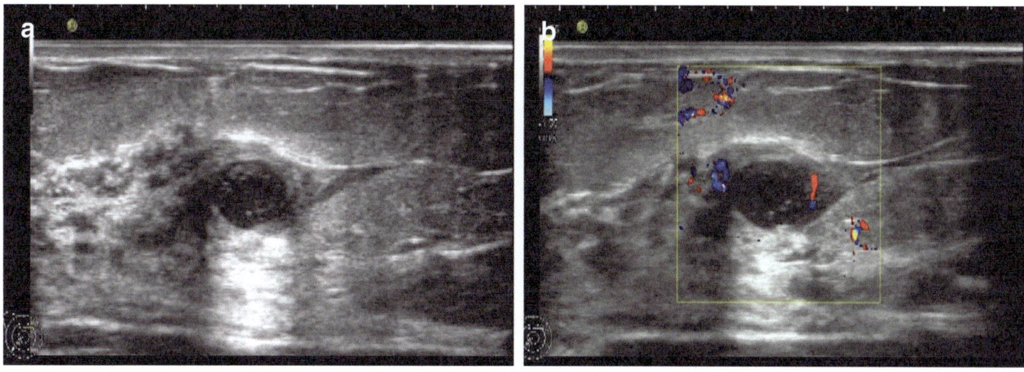

Fig. 4.8 Infected breast cyst. (**a**) Grayscale US. (**b**) CDI

infiltration and thickening of the skin over the abscess. Reactive axillary lymph nodes on the side of the abscess with hypervascular, hypoechoic structure and preserved differentiation of the cortex and hilum arise in the majority of cases. It is very important not to confuse abscessed breast cysts and cystic type of cancer. Cancer in a cyst exhibits indistinct, irregular margins, debris in the cavity, and hypoechoic mural solid component with chaotic vascularity with color/power Doppler modes. Solid component of carcinoma is characterized with stiff color pattern with compression US elastography and high strain ratio. The sensitivity of ultrasound in the diagnosis of breast abscesses is 89.6%, with specificity of 100%, and diagnostic accuracy of 96.8%.

If ultrasound findings are confusing, a puncture of the suspected breast abscess is advised, with both diagnostic and therapeutic purposes.

Atypical cysts may be sometimes observed among fluid breast lesions. They confer long existing, recurrent cysts, and the cysts with inflammation.

US features of atypical cysts are listed below (Fig. 4.9):

- Thick cystic walls
- Contents with inclusions
- Solid component with different types of vascularization
- Various vascularization of solid component in color-coded modes
- Different stiffness of the wall and solid component with compression US elastography
- Increased vascularity of the solid component with CEUS

Atypical US images of cysts in up to 2% of cases can be the result of intracavitary growth originating from the cystic wall (Korzhenkova 2004). Seventy-five percent of them are papillomas of benign nature.

Intraductal papilloma is a benign, mostly solitary fibroepithelial tumor located within a lactiferous duct (cystadenopapilloma) or in a cyst, often in the subareolar region. It constitutes up to 1.0–1.5% of all breast tumors (Trufanov et al. 2009). Single tumors, as a rule, are not prone to malignancy. Multiple papillomas are often located at the periphery of the breast and have a high potential for malignancy (Haylenko et al. 2005). Intraductal papilloma is usually defined with US as a homogeneous solid mass of moderate or low echogenicity with distinct, even margins within a larger fluid-containing anechoic avascular cavity (Fig. 4.10).

Twenty percent of intracystic masses are papillary cancer (Figs. 4.11 and 4.12). Any growth inside the cyst or lactiferous duct along with heterogeneity of the solid component in association with hypervascularization are always suspicious for cystadenocarcinoma (cancer in the cyst) and require US-guided puncture with cytology.

Complex cysts with vascularized septa, papillary vegetations, and solid component must be differentiated from other lesions. Such cysts with hyperechoic septa may be a challenge, since neither grayscale nor color Doppler imaging can specify solid tumor growth. A valuable option is contrast enhanced sonography. It permits identification of invasive tumor growth within cysts

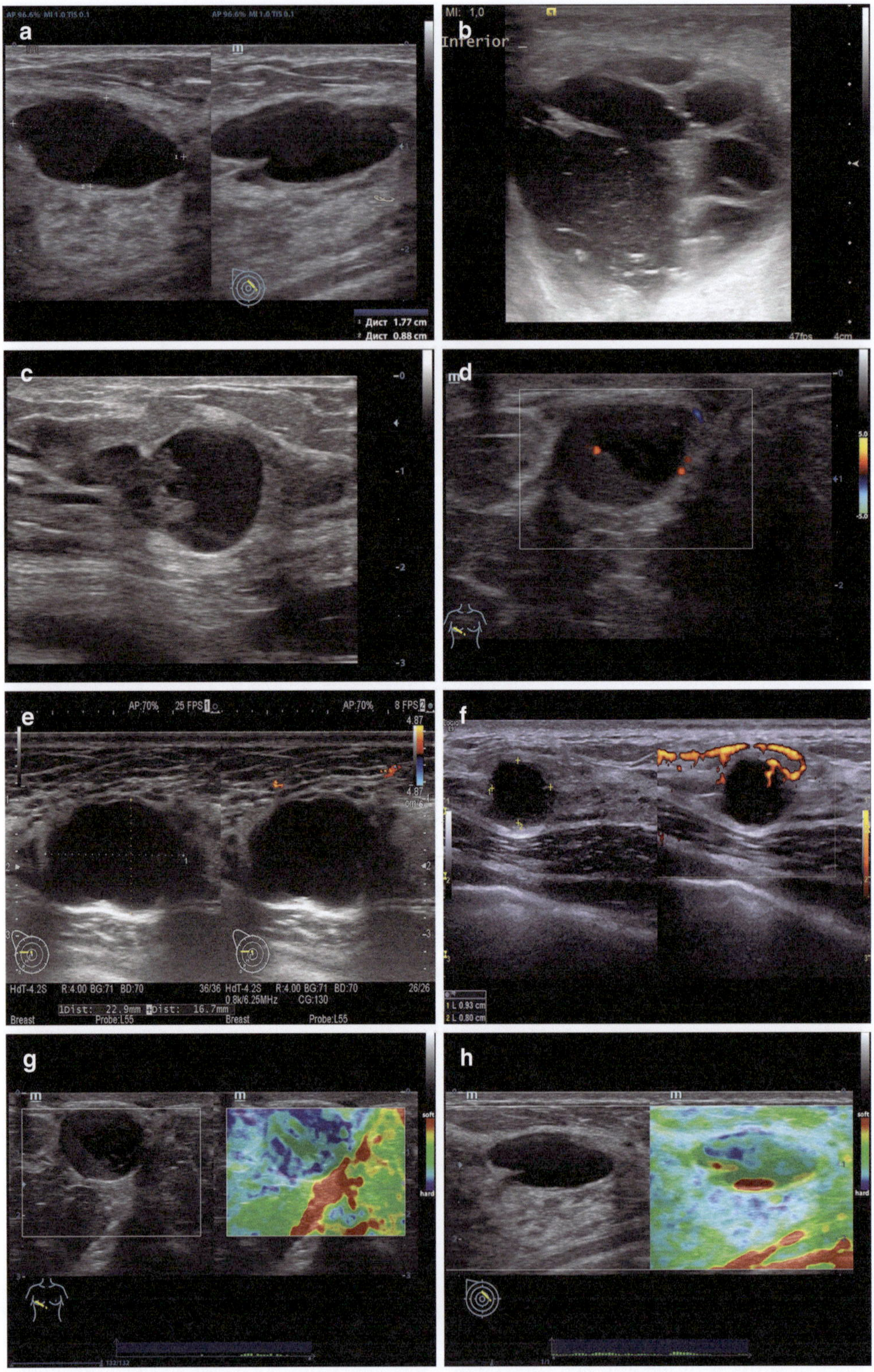

Fig. 4.9 A complex breast cyst. (**a–c**) Grayscale US. (**d**, **e**) CDI. (**f**) PDI. (**g**, **h**) Compression US elastography

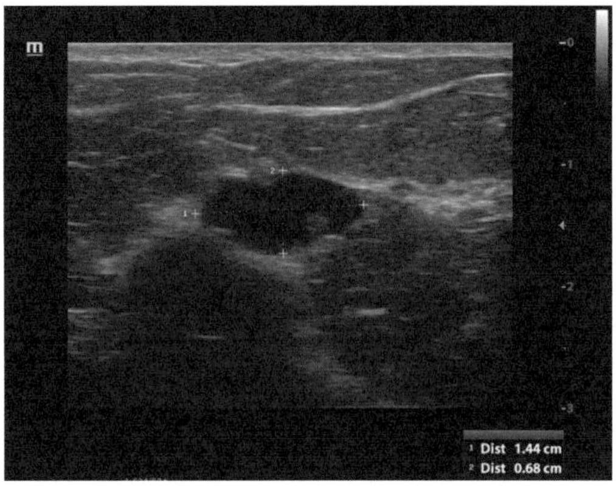

Fig. 4.10 Intraductal papilloma. Grayscale US

based on heterogeneous contrast enhancement (Fig. 4.13). US-guided biopsy of the lesion is still necessary.

Complex ultrasound imaging can detect breast cysts and precisely specify their location, size, inner structure, elasticity, and vascularity with sensitivity up to 92%, specificity up to 95%, and diagnostic accuracy up to 95–100% (Shevchenko 1997).

Galactocele is a retention breast cyst, single- or multi-chambered, formed during pregnancy and/or lactation and filled with milk. Galactocele is also possible in newborns and children of the younger group (children's galactocele).

Galactocele appears with US as a retroareolar hypo- or anechoic oval or round lesion well delimited from nearby tissues, with a thin (up to 1 mm) capsule of increased echogenicity. Its structure is often heterogeneous due to dense pieces ("dairy crumbs") and fluid component (refer to Chap. 7).

It is often difficult to differentiate galactocele from simple and complex cysts and multiple cysts of small size, especially with background FBD, dilatation of the lactiferous ducts, and local duct ectasias (Fig. 4.14).

Duct ectasia (periductal mastitis, plasma cell mastitis) can develop progressively. Clinically, it manifests with a local induration, which varies periodically in size, accompanied by pain and regional lymph node enlargement. Echographically periductal mastitis and local duct ectasia may be difficult to differentiate from the edematous-infiltrative breast cancer.

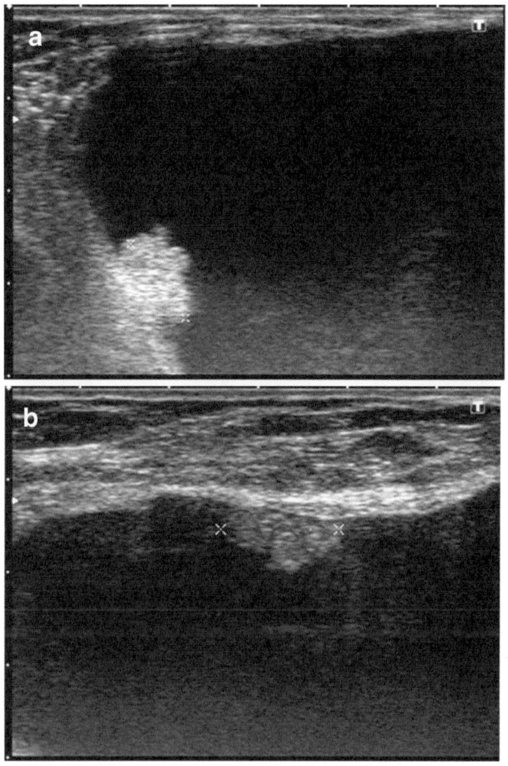

Fig. 4.11 (**a**, **b**) Breast cystadenocarcinoma. Grayscale US

Local duct ectasia is not always easy to differentiate from focal adenosis (localized fibroadenomatosis) basing on ultrasound alone. Isolated foci of adenosis are detected in 3.7% of women. According to the current WHO classification, sclerosing adenosis is a benign neoplasm. A focal, diffuse, sclerosing, apocrine, and microglandular types of adenosis are specified.

Ultrasound findings are often nonspecific and depend on the stage of sclerosis. At echography, the areas of decreased echogenicity, heterogeneous structure, irregular shape, and indistinct, uneven contours are most common (Fig. 4.15).

Differential diagnostics of *sclerosing adenosis* (a variety of diffuse non-tumoral breast pathology) is often complex. Adenosis is a borderline condition. It is normal for young women, while considered abnormal in women over 22–25 years. It occurs in 5% of women. It accounts for about 28% of all benign breast changes.

The disease is characterized with breast pain (especially before menses), swelling, and indura-

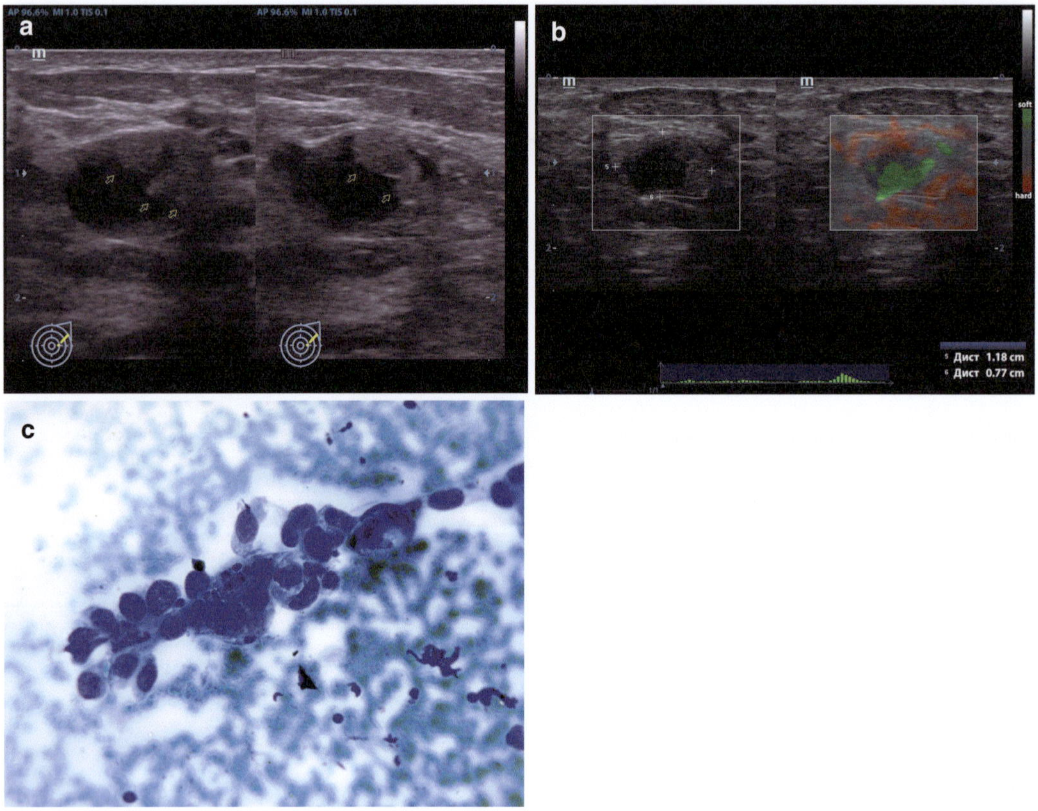

Fig. 4.12 Infiltrative ductal carcinoma. (**a**) Grayscale US. (**b**) Compression US elastography. (**c**) Pappenheim-stained smears, original magnification, ×400

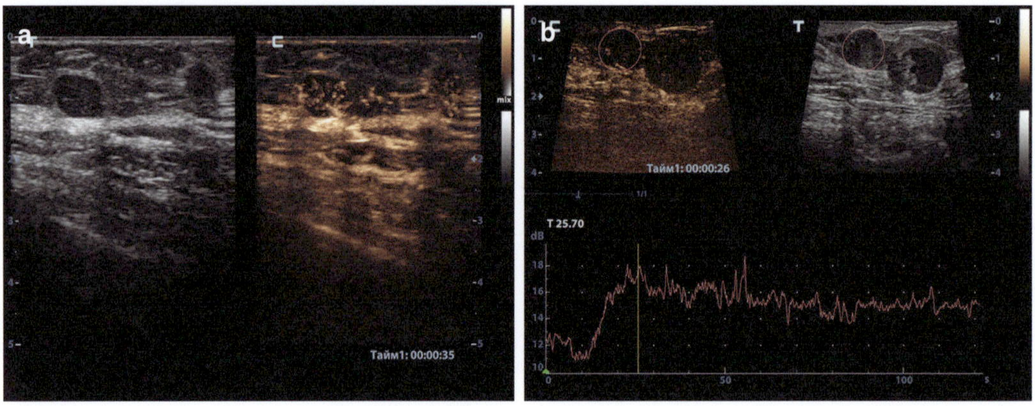

Fig. 4.13 A complex breast cyst. CEUS. Sonovue, 2.4 mL. (**a**, **b**) Enhancing of the solid component. (**c**) Avascular of solid component

tion but in some cases can be asymptomatic. The breasts are dense with palpation, with separately located nodules, not clearly delineated from the surrounding tissues. Differential diagnosis with early cancer, diffuse, and nodular FBD is difficult. The condition is a risk factor for breast cancer.

Ultrasound criteria (as well as X-ray criteria) are usually nonspecific and depend on the stage of sclerosis. At ultrasound image, adenosis

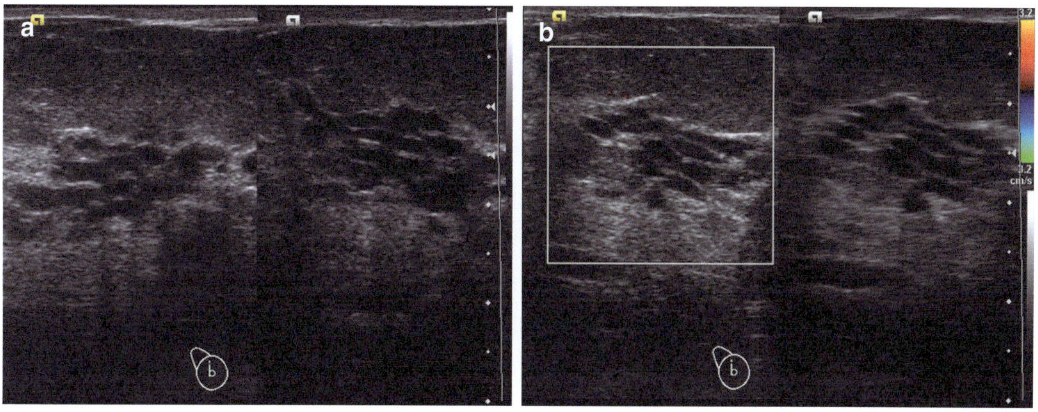

Fig. 4.14 Local duct ectasia. (**a**) Grayscale US. (**b**) CDI

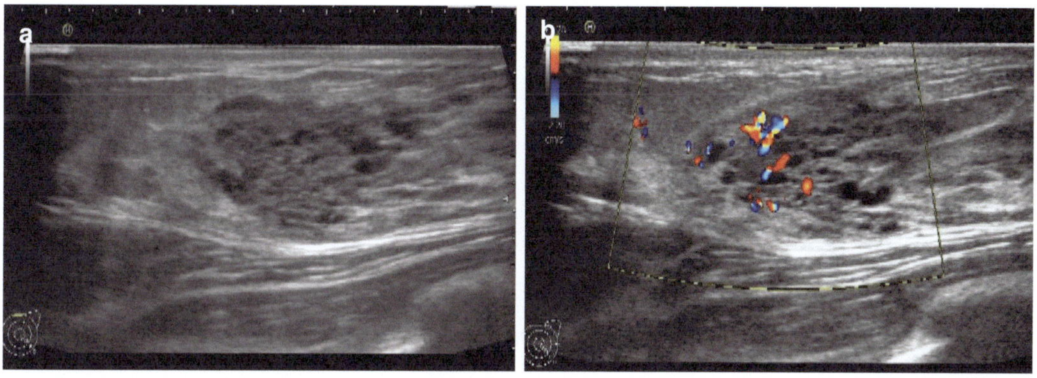

Fig. 4.15 Focal adenosis. (**a**) Grayscale US. (**b**) CDI

usually shows, with dense glandular tissue, rich fibrous component with diffuse calcifications (hyperechoic incorporations of 0.1–0.3 cm), sometimes with acoustic shadows in the thickened fibro-glandular breast complex (Fig. 4.16). Stromal fibrosis of lobules is defined as multiple dense foci (3–5 mm). This condition requires morphological diagnosis with CNB and pathological examination.

Focal fibrosis is a focal proliferation of breast stroma with atrophic surrounding parenchyma. This condition can result from inflammation associated with FBD. Less often it is a form of normal involution or a hormone-dependent condition. It is observed in 50% of women aged 40–49 years, in 38% of women aged 30–39 years, and less often in other age groups. The incidence does not exceed 4–8% (Trufanov et al. 2009).

Focal fibrosis is hardly diagnosed and differentiated with US from adenosis, nodular type of FBD, and early nodular breast cancer. It is characterized by nonspecific increase of parenchyma density in some areas, which are usually hypovascular, with indistinct, uneven contours and heterogeneous structure, sometimes with posterior acoustic shadowing and increased stiffness with compression US elastography (Fig. 4.17).

Radial scar is a condition that is often associated with lobular or ductal preinvasive cancer or tubular carcinoma. The risk of infiltrative cancer is high. The condition is difficult to differentiate from tubular cancer. CNB is recommended. If there is no evidence of malignancy with stereotactic biopsy, follow-up is recommended. If foci of atypical hyperplasia or preinvasive cancer are detected, resection of the mammary gland is carried out.

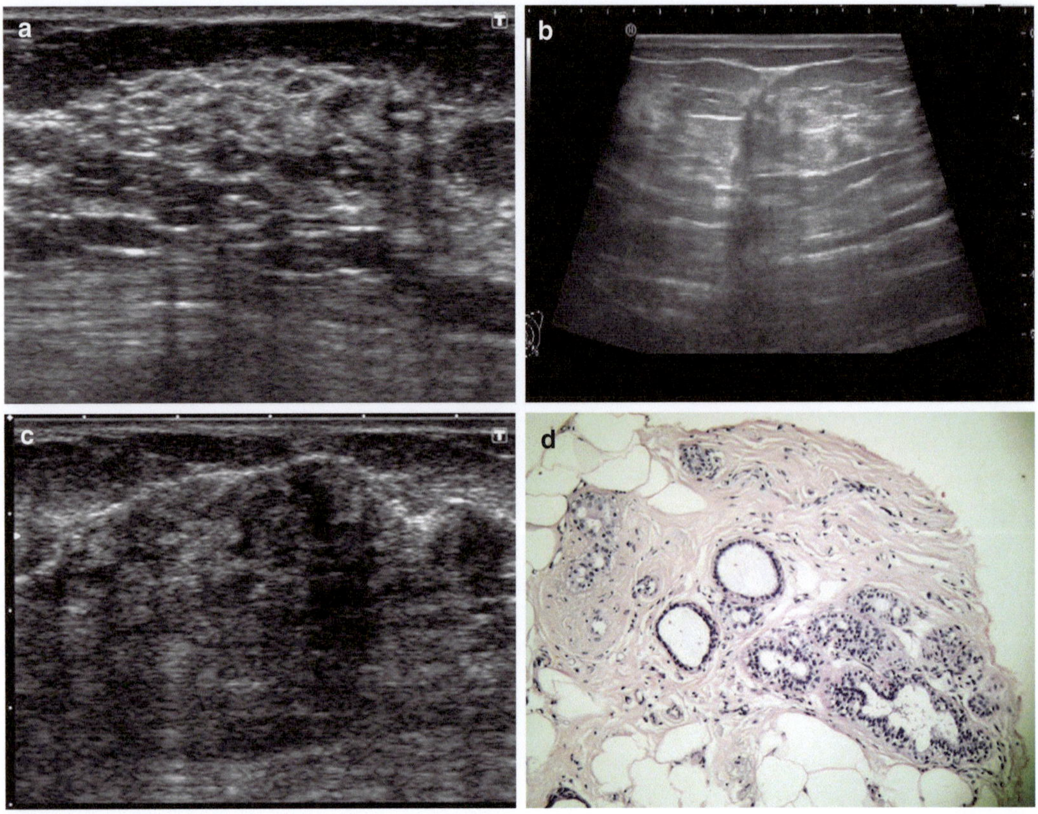

Fig. 4.16 Sclerosing adenosis of the breast. (**a–c**) Grayscale US. (**d**) H&E-stained image of a section; original magnification, ×100

Gigantomastia (macromastia, megalomastia) is a benign condition with fast, rapidly progressing symmetrical breast enlargement. The disease can occur in puberty, and early reproductive age (juvenile gigantomastia), and during pregnancy (gestational gigantomastia) (for more details, refer to Chap. 9). Gigantomastia is characterized with the weight of the breasts higher than 3% overall body weight. Some authors consider gigantomastia as the increase in breast volume more than 1500 cm^3. The breast enlargement in true gigantomastia is associated with the increase in glandular tissue amount. False gigantomastia results from excessive adipose tissue.

Exact etiology and pathogenesis of gigantomastia is still unclear. Juvenile gigantomastia is an extremely rare pathology. Clinically, juvenile gigantomastia is characterized by rapid (usually within 6–12 months), unrestrained, and extreme breast enlargement from the time of their formation with continuing growth in adolescent and early reproductive age (Fig. 4.18). Gigantomastia is often accompanied with severe pain, breast ulcers, necrosis, or hemorrhage. Without appropriate treatment, a secondary infection (mastitis, pyogenic abscesses) and other complications may join.

Gigantomastia leads to physical discomfort and suffering, often emotional disorders, depression, and social phobia. It may be also associated with fibrocystic mastopathy (19% of cases), mastitis (17% of cases), thyroid diseases (17% of cases), and myasthenia gravis (7.1% of cases).

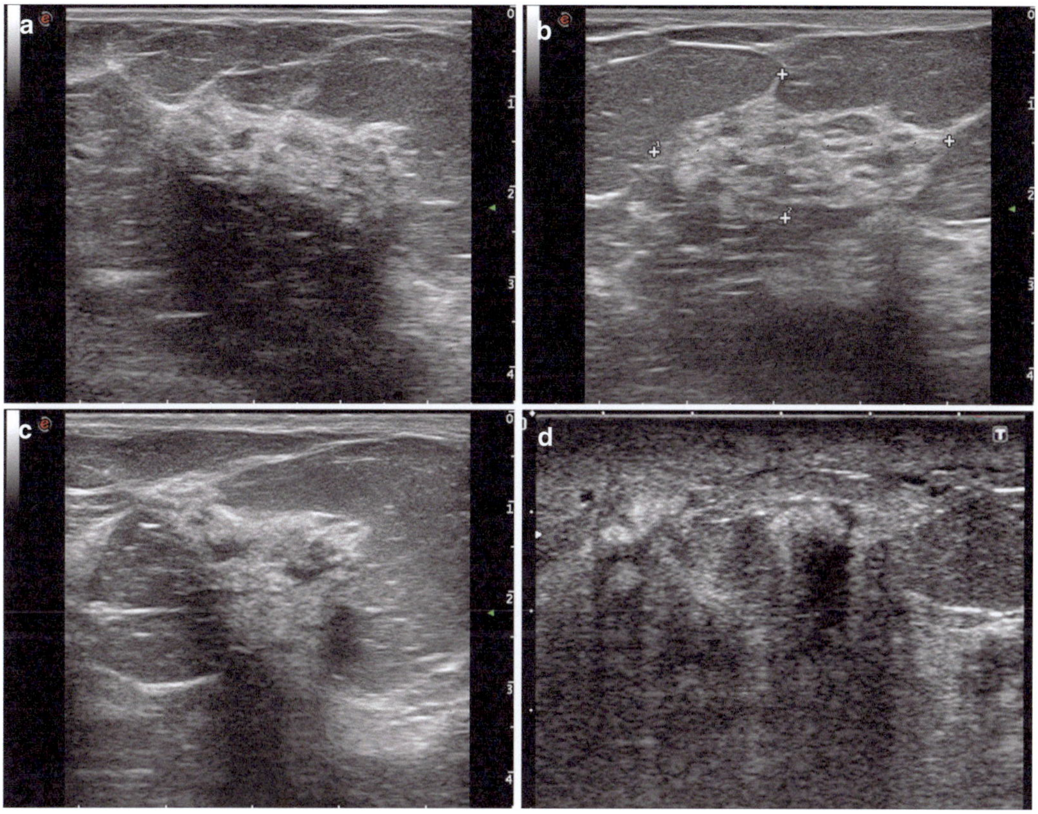

Fig. 4.17 Focal breast fibrosis. (**a**–**d**) Grayscale US

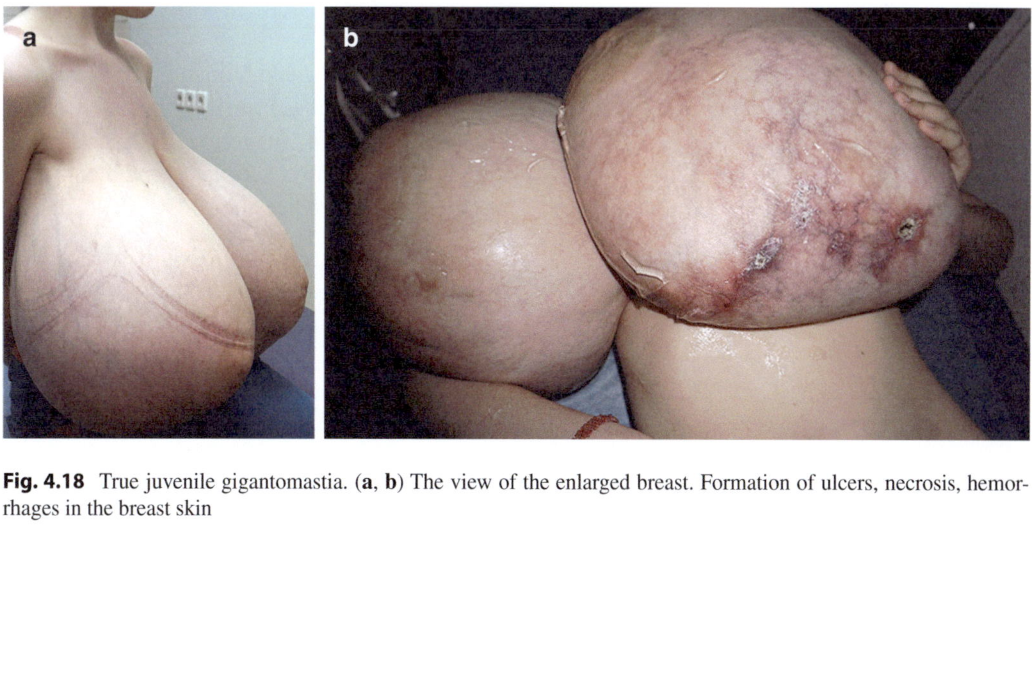

Fig. 4.18 True juvenile gigantomastia. (**a**, **b**) The view of the enlarged breast. Formation of ulcers, necrosis, hemorrhages in the breast skin

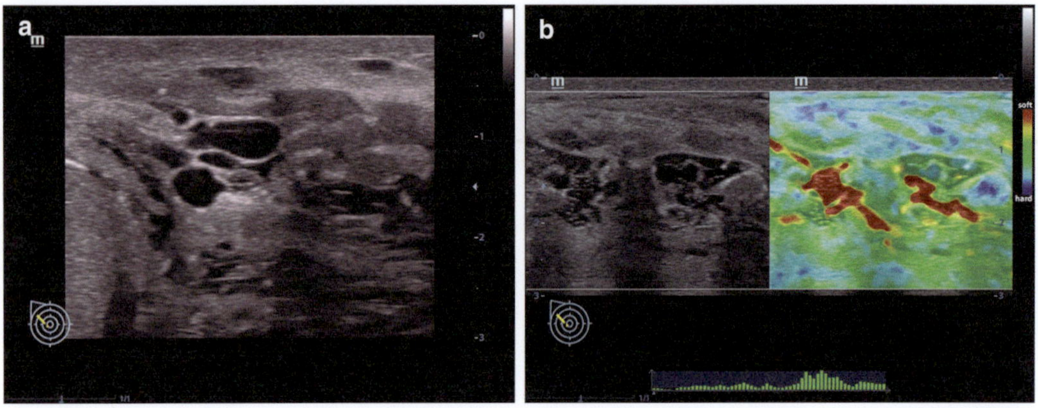

Fig. 4.19 True juvenile gigantomastia. (**a**) Grayscale US. Heterogeneous parenchyma, dilatation of lymphatic ducts and superficial veins. (**b**) Compression US elastography

US signs of juvenile gigantomastia (Fig. 4.19), besides breast enlargement, are listed below (Sencha et al. 2017):

- Edema with decreased echogenicity and heterogeneous structure of the skin and subcutaneous fat.
- Dilated lymphatic vessels.
- Heterogeneous parenchyma.
- Irregular duct ectasia, both in pregnant and nonpregnant women.
- Dilated superficial varicose veins (with the symptom of "spontaneous contrasting" of the blood flow), colored in color-coded modes.
- Irregular stiffness of parenchyma with compression US elastography.
- Average strain ratio may reach 1.8–2.1.
- Indifferent regional lymph nodes.

Differential diagnosis of juvenile gigantomastia with mastitis (non-lactational), juvenile breast hypertrophy, benign breast conditions (such as FBD or fibroadenoma), Hodgkin's lymphoma, and infiltrative breast cancer should be carried out.

Sometimes, juvenile breast fibroadenoma can be detected on the background of degenerative changes of parenchyma in juvenile gigantomastia. It is visualized as a homogeneous hypoechoic mass up to 5–10 cm in size with distinct borders, with poor blood flow in color-coded modes (Fig. 4.20).

Treatment of gigantomastia is still a debatable issue. Various options from drug therapy to surgical correction are suggested. In most cases, surgery (mastectomy or reduction mammoplasty) is the method of choice.

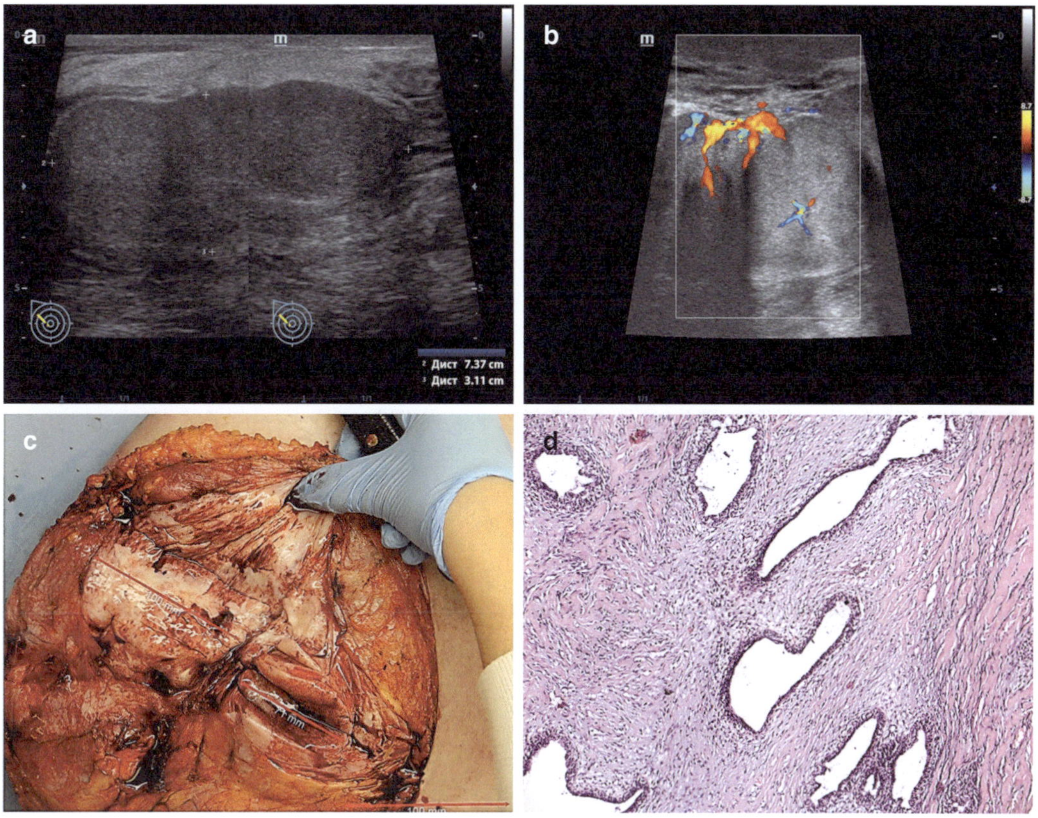

Fig. 4.20 Juvenile fibroadenoma on the background of true juvenile gigantomastia. (**a**) Grayscale. (**b**) CDI. (**c**) Macroscopic view of the removed mammary gland. Section shows gray-pink, round of 4–10 cm. (**d**) H&E-stained image of a section; original magnification, ×100

5 Ultrasound Diagnosis of Benign Tumors

Alexander N. Sencha, Yury Patrunov, Ella Penyaeva, and Ekaterina Sencha

Abstract

Fibroadenoma is a benign tumor of the mammary gland, which belongs to a group of mixed connective tissue and epithelial tumors. It constitutes up to 95% of all benign breast masses. Phyllodes tumor (phyllodes fibroadenoma, intracanalicular fibroadenoma with a cell stroma) is a mixed connective tissue and epithelial tumor. It demonstrates the incidence not exceeding 0.5–2% of all breast lesions and 2.5–5.4% of all fibroadenomas. Juvenile (giant, cellular) fibroadenoma is a benign fibroepithelial tumor with enlarged convoluted ducts, usually with papillary-cribose proliferation of the epithelium and stroma, with edema and/or desmoplasia. Lipoma is a benign tumor originating from adipose tissue. It accounts for 9% of all breast lesions. True lipoma consists of mature adipose tissue surrounded with a capsule. Intraductal papilloma is represented with a lesion that grows within the lumen of lactiferous ducts. Solitary or multiple lesions may arise. Intraductal papilloma is associated with abnormal discharge from the nipples. Atheroma is retention cyst of the sebaceous gland located in the benign skin and subdermal tissues, which occurs by increased sweating of the sebaceous gland, occlusion of its duct, and forming of a capsule around the fatty content.

Fibroadenoma (FA) is a benign tumor of the mammary gland which belongs to a group of mixed connective tissue and epithelial tumors. It constitutes up to 95% of all benign breast masses. It is a well-delineated nodule displaceable against the surrounding tissues. Most often, FA occurs in reproductive age (20–45 years). Tumor dimensions may be different, but usually do not exceed 3 cm. Usually, FA is a single nodule; in 20% of cases masses are multiple, in 10%—bilateral (Korzhenkova 2004). Sometimes they are characterized by rapid growth, especially during puberty and after abortion. With age, FA tends to regress. Involution is accompanied by hyalinosis and calcification of the stroma.

Microscopically, FA nodes are characterized by a variable combination of epithelial and connective tissue components. Malignant

A. N. Sencha (✉)
Division of Visual Diagnostics, National Medical Research Center for Obstetrics, Gynecology and Perinatology named after Academician V.I.Kulakov of Ministry of Healthcare of Russian Federation, Moscow, Russia

Y. Patrunov · E. Penyaeva
Department of Ultrasound Diagnostics of Radiology Center, Yaroslavl Railway Clinic, Yaroslavl, Russia

E. Sencha
Department of Ultrasound Diagnostics, Federal State Budget Hospital "9 Treatment and Diagnostic Center" of the Ministry of Defense of the Russian Federation, Moscow, Russia

G. T. Sukhikh, A. N. Sencha (eds.), *Multiparametric Ultrasound Diagnosis of Breast Diseases*,
https://doi.org/10.1007/978-3-319-75034-7_5

transformation of FA is rare (1–5%); lobular carcinoma in situ arises most often in these cases (Haylenko et al. 2005; Sinyukova et al. 2007).

Depending on histological structure, fibroadenoma can have several types: intracanalicular, pericanalicular, mixed, and juvenile.

Fibroadenoma usually demonstrates the following US features (Fig. 5.1):

- Solid breast lesion of decreased or usual echodensity
- Homogeneous structure (rare cases of heterogeneous structure result from fluid incorporations, calcifications, or echogenic fibrous structures)
- Always accurate contours
- Smooth or lobulated borders, which depend on histological type
- Sometimes with posterior echo enhancement
- Mobile at compression the US probe
- A- or hypovascular in CDI, PDI, and 3DPD

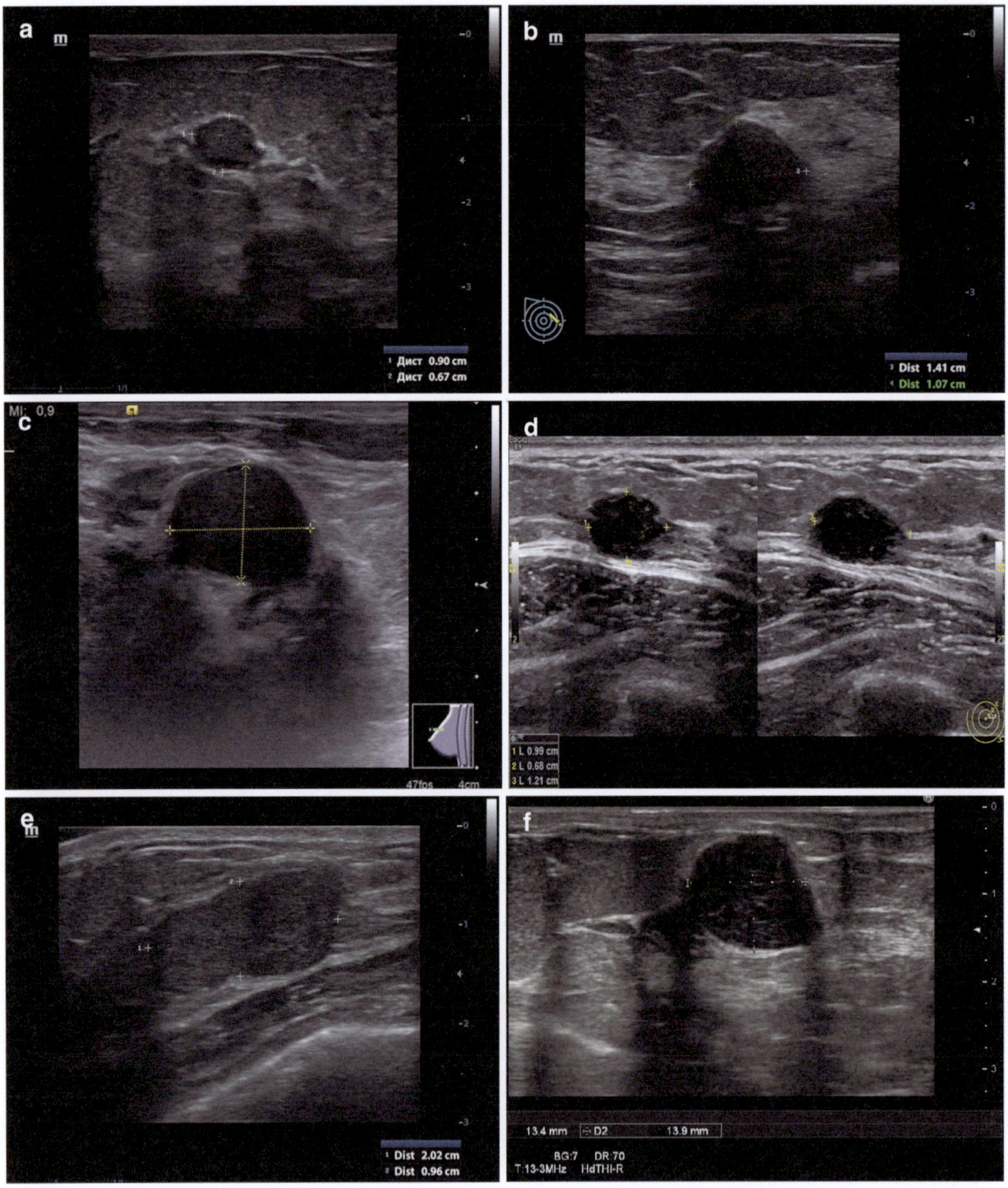

Fig. 5.1 Breast fibroadenoma. (**a–i**) Grayscale US. (**j**) Pappenheim-stained smears, original magnification, ×1000

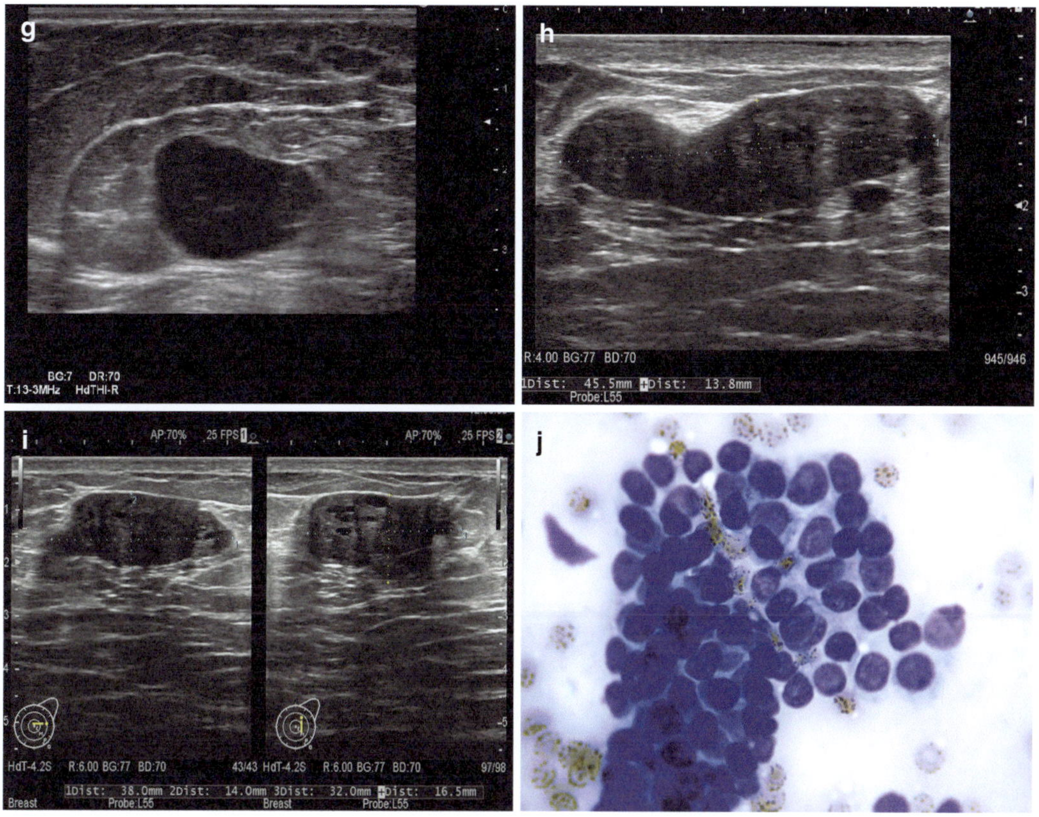

Fig. 5.1 (continued)

- Irregular mosaic staining with compression US elastography
- Strain ratio above 2.5

Fibroadenoma exhibits different US features depending on the size. Nodules smaller than 1 cm often are characterized with roundish shape, homogeneous structure, decreased echodensity, and smooth or irregular contours. Fibroadenoma of more than 2 cm in size more often has regular spherical or oval shape with accurate and smooth or irregular contours. Surrounding tissues, normally, do not change. Well-outlined isolated adipose lobules can imitate fibroadenoma. The most important is to differentiate between fibroadenoma and nodular breast carcinoma expansive growth.

According to Haylenko et al. (2005) and Sinyukova et al. (2007), US usually fails to detect the vessels in fibroadenoma, especially in subcentimeter nodules (Fig. 5.2). Rarely, one to two normal vessels with low velocities can be imaged: PSV, 0.19–0.2 m/s; EDV, 0.06–0.1 m/s; RI, 0.63–0.79; and PI, 1.21–1.65. Zabolotskaya and Zabolotsky (2000) reported hypervascularization with CDI and PDI in 36% of fibroadenomas.

With color-coded modes, benign breast tumors usually display poor vascular network mostly at the periphery of the mass, with uniform and sparse branching of the vessels. In some cases, it is possible to visualize a feeding or draining vessel. In most cases, vascular pattern in the adjacent tissues is not enhanced, which is different from breast cancer.

As a rule, compression US elastography shows intensive irregular coloring of FA (Fig. 5.3).

A characteristic feature of breast fibroadenoma with CEUS is peripheral enhancement (Fig. 5.4). Combination of peripheral contrast enhancement and prolonged washout is observed in 80% of histologically confirmed fibroadenomas.

Fibroadenomas may exhibit longer time to peak of contrast enhancement (30 s and more)

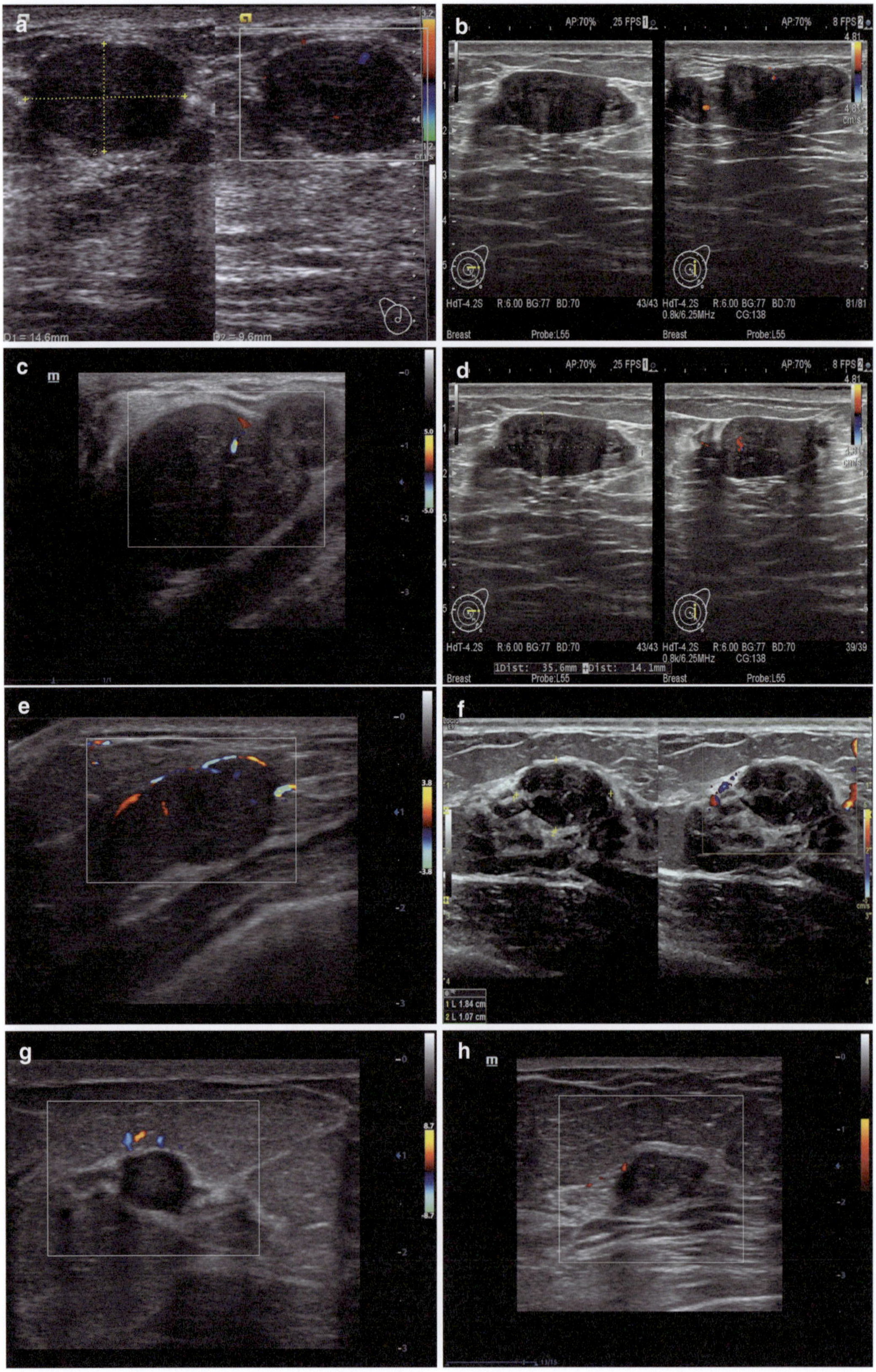

Fig. 5.2 Breast fibroadenoma. (**a**–**g**) CPI. (**h**) PDI

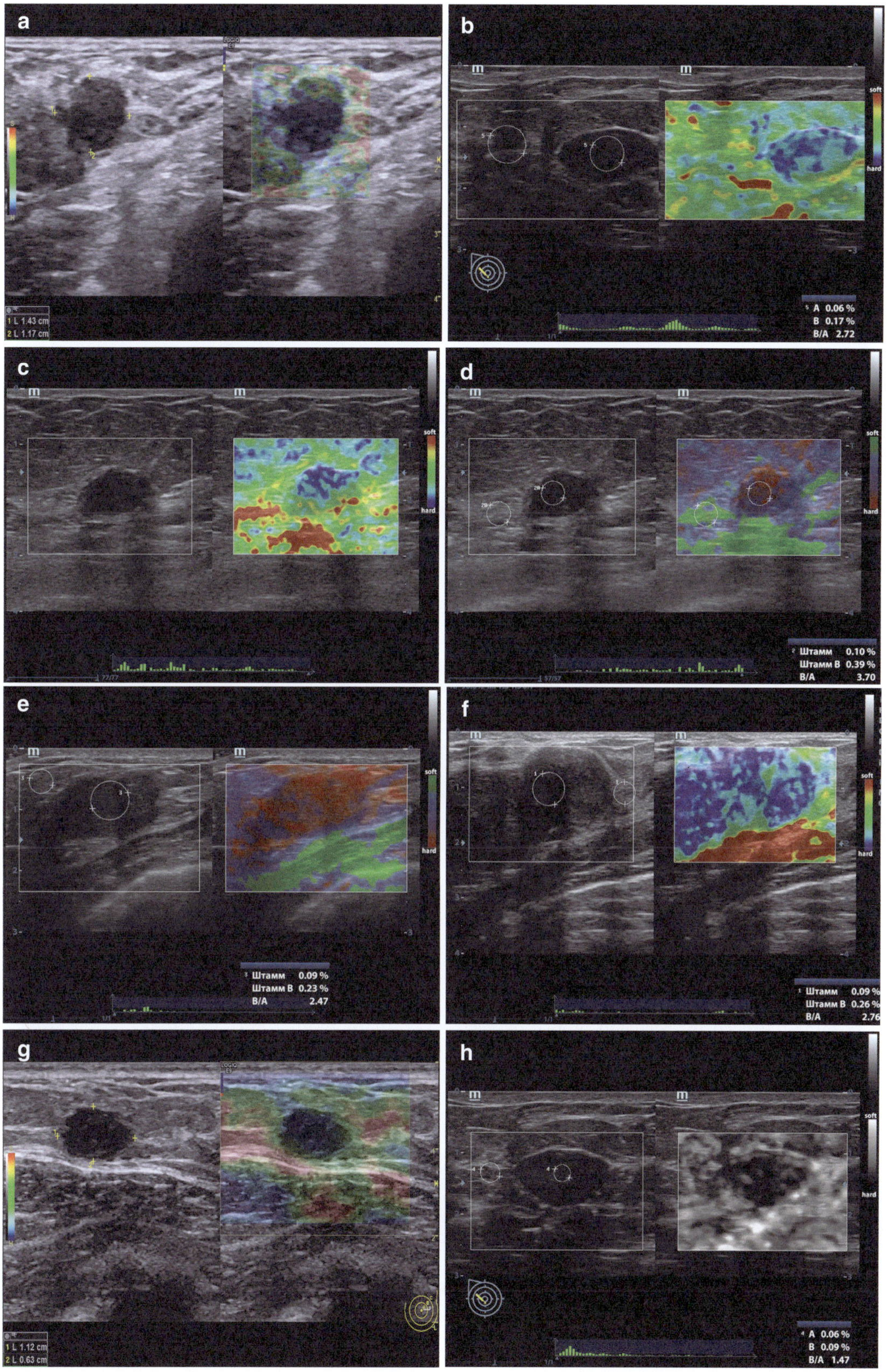

Fig. 5.3 Breast fibroadenoma. (**a**–**h**) Compression US elastography. Irregular coloring of the mass

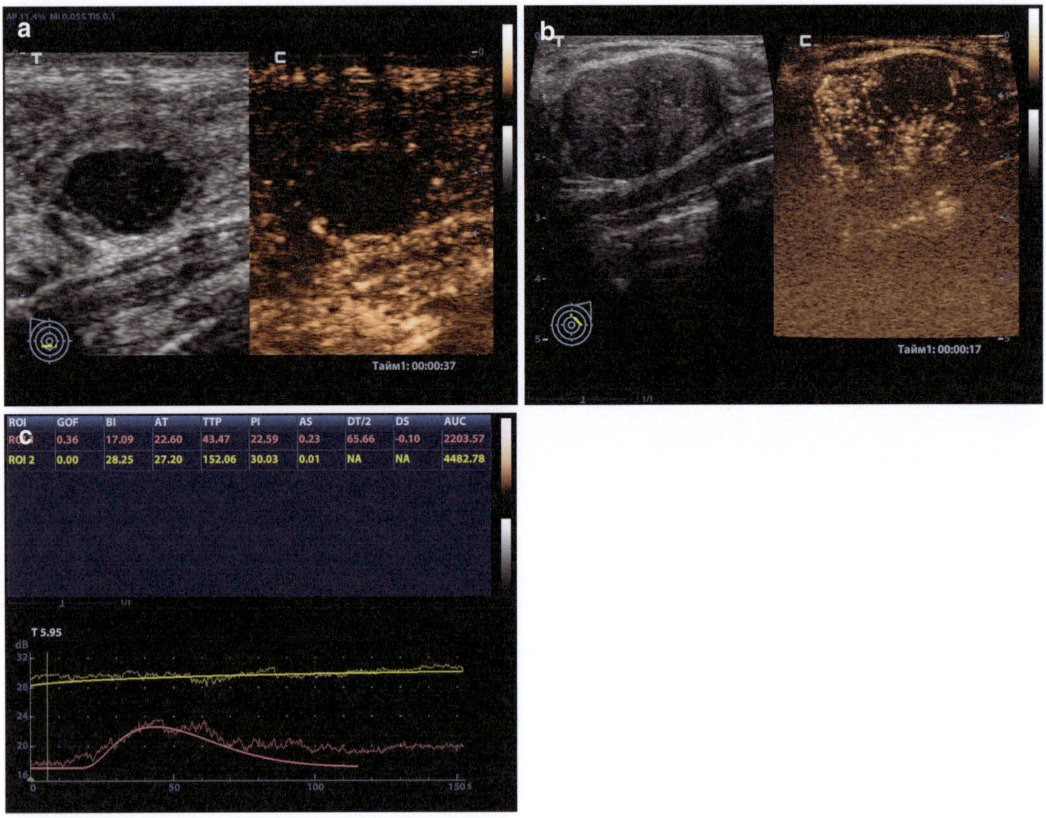

Fig. 5.4 Breast fibroadenoma. (**a–c**) CEUS. SonoVue, 2.4 mL. Asymmetric peripheral enhancement

and a less dramatic washout gradient (70–150 s). Quantitative indices are significantly higher in fibroadenomas compared to breast cancer.

In some cases, fibroadenomas are characterized by intense, irregular contrast enhancement and presence of wide vessels directed toward the center of the lesion (Fig. 5.5).

According to Sencha et al. (2015), CEUS may determine the need for repeated biopsy of verified FA.

The sensitivity of US in the diagnosis of breast fibroadenoma accounts for 89–91.2% with specificity of 78–92.5% and diagnostic accuracy of 91–92.7%.

Once a FA is found, a biopsy with cytological (histological) investigation is performed to determine the type of the tumor and the degree of proliferation of glandular epithelium. Growing FA, the size exceeding 2 cm, and expressed proliferation of glandular epithelium (especially with dysplasia or atypia) are indications for surgical treatment.

Phyllodes tumor (phyllodes fibroadenoma, intracanalicular fibroadenoma with a cell stroma) is a mixed connective tissue and epithelial tumor. It was first described in 1838 by J. Muller as cystosarcoma phyllodes. It demonstrates the incidence not exceeding 0.5–2% of all breast lesions and 2.5–5.4% of all FA (Trufanov et al. 2009). Phyllodes tumor affects women of any age and exhibits two peaks in 16–20 years and 40–50 years. The tumor is, as a rule, represented with a solitary lesion. It may lie dormant for a long period and suddenly start fast growth. Pregnancy can induce its growth. Due to fast increase of phyllodes tumor in size, it is often diagnosed being quite large. It is clinically represented with a well-circumscribed lesion of lobulated structure. Giant tumor can occupy the major part of the breast, induces

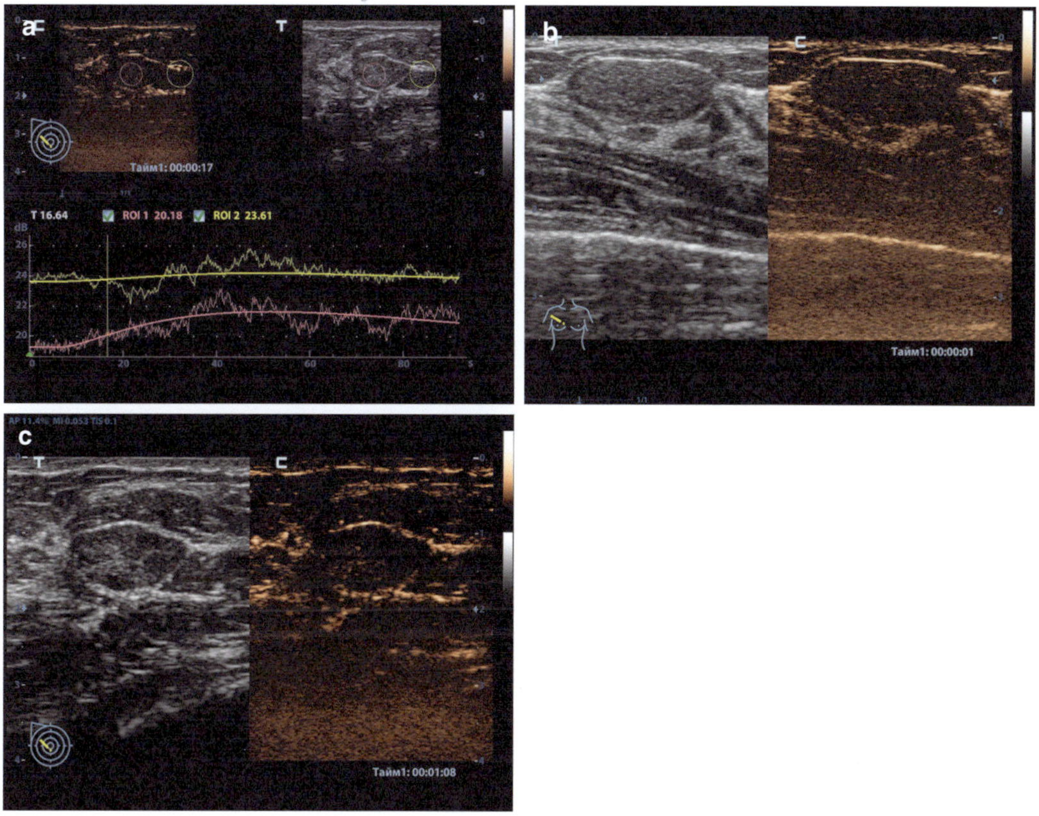

Fig. 5.5 Breast fibroadenoma. (**a**–**c**) CEUS. SonoVue, 2.4 mL. Intranodular centripetal enhancement

skin thinning, and activates subcutaneous venous pattern.

There are three main disease types:

- Simple (benign) phyllodes tumor, 40–80%
- Borderline (intermediate) phyllodes tumor, 10–20%
- Malignant phyllodes tumor, 5–30%

Characteristic US features of phyllodes tumor are listed below (Fig. 5.6):

- Hypo- or isoechoic breast lesion
- Irregular echostructure with multiple anechoic fluid collections and incorporations (especially in large lesions)
- Roundish shape
- Distinct contours, regular borders
- Often with symmetric lateral shadows and posterior acoustic enhancement
- Expressed intranodular hypervascularity with CDI, PDI, and 3DPD
- Irregular mosaic staining with US elastography
- Strain ratio above 2.5

In cases of malignant transformation of connective tissue component, they may develop different sarcomas, such as fibro-, lipo-, hondro-, osteo-, or rhabdomyosarcomas. Malignant transformation of connective tissue and epithelial components results in carcinosarcomas. Early detection of phyllodes tumor assumes its accurate differentiation from fibroadenoma. As compared with fibroadenoma, phyllodes tumor has more cellular stroma with complex architectonics and often with larger degree of nuclear poly-

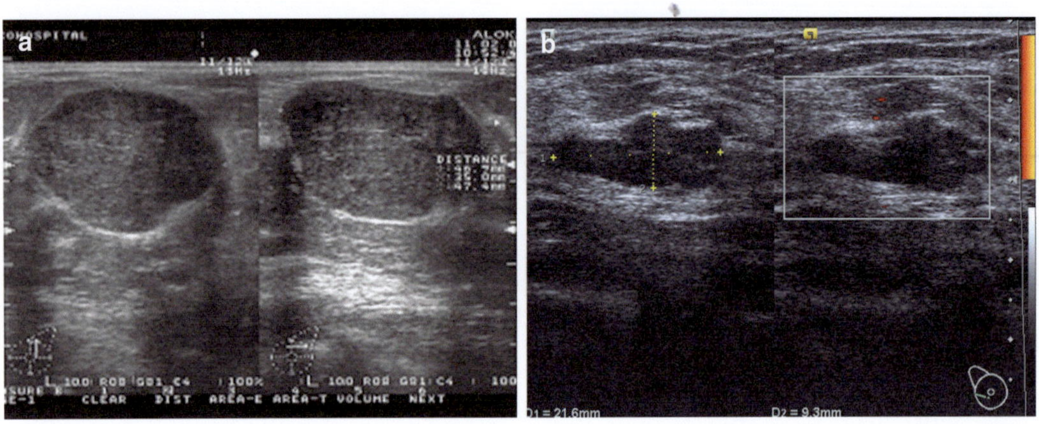

Fig. 5.6 Phyllodes breast tumor. (**a**) Grayscale US. (**b**) PDI

morphism. The type of growth is defined with histological examination of core biopsy samples.

Juvenile (giant, cellular) fibroadenoma is a benign fibroepithelial tumor with enlarged convoluted ducts, usually with papillary-cribose proliferation of the epithelium and stroma, with edema and/or desmoplasia.

Juvenile fibroadenomas are more often bilateral than typical adult fibroadenomas. They are characterized by rapid growth, reaching large sizes in short time. Ultrasound characteristics of juvenile fibroadenomas usually do not differ from the "classical" adenomas of the parenchyma. They look like hypovascular lesions of medium or low echogenicity, oval shape, homogeneous structure, with distinct, even contours, and extremely large size, reaching 10 cm or larger (Fig. 5.7).

Morphologically, juvenile fibroadenoma is a variant of a typical fibroadenoma with a number of specific histological signs. Juvenile fibroadenoma is a benign fibroepithelial tumor with dilated tortous ducts, usually with papillary-cribriform epithelial proliferation. Proliferation of stromal cells with edema and/or desmoplasia is noted. Stromal cells can be moderately polymorphic, but not atypical.

Lipoma is a benign tumor originating from adipose tissue. It accounts for 9% of all breast lesions (Rozhkova 1993). True lipoma consists of mature adipose tissue surrounded with a capsule. It is represented with a mobile soft lesion of roundish or oval shape with palpation, which is often (not always) accurately delimited from the surrounding tissues. US diagnosis of breast lipoma, as a rule, is not difficult.

Characteristic US features of breast lipoma are listed below (Fig. 5.8):

- Lesion of decreased or normal echodensity, comparable to normal adipose breast tissue
- Sometimes irregular structure at the expense of fibrous incorporations
- Easily deformed with compression
- Without posterior enhancement or shadow
- Always avascular with CDI, PDI, and 3DPD
- Regular mosaic staining with compression US elastography
- Strain ratio 1.0–2.0
- No apparent enhancement of vascularization with CEUS
- No regional lymph node enlargement

Differential diagnosis with liposarcoma is always necessary. The latter exhibits fast growth, relatively decreased echodensity, tuberous margins, increased density with elastography and palpation, and pathological vascularization. Tumor biopsy verifies the diagnosis.

Intraductal papilloma is represented with a lesion that grows within the lumen of lactiferous ducts of the breast. Solitary or multiple lesions

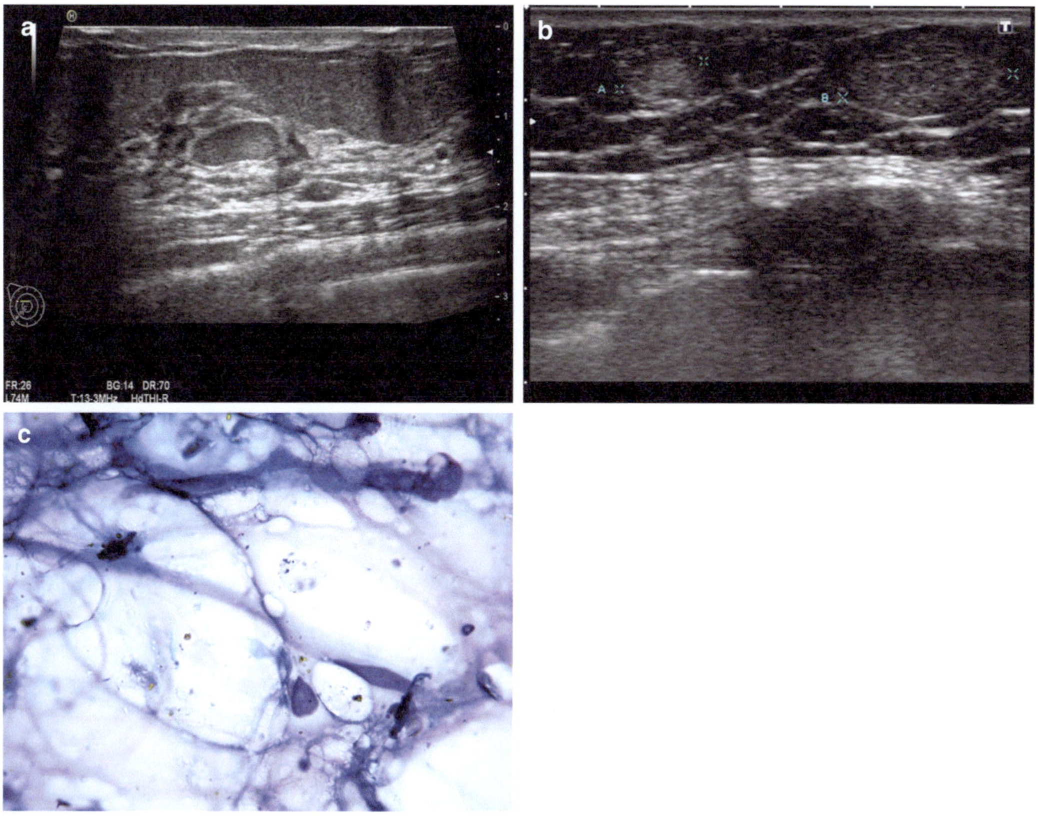

Fig. 5.7 Juvenile fibroadenoma. (**a**, **b**) Grayscale US. (**c**) Pappenheim-stained smears, original magnification, ×100

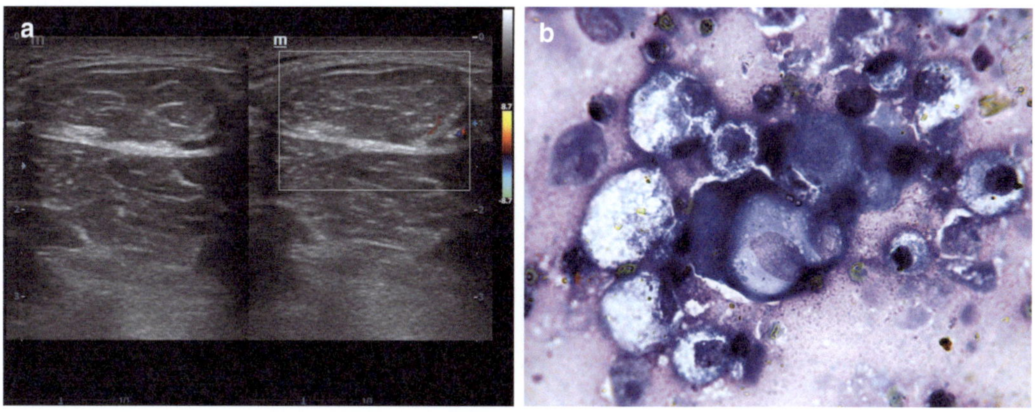

Fig. 5.8 Breast lipoma. (**a**) Grayscale US and CDI. (**b**) Pappenheim-stained smears, original magnification, ×1000

may arise. Intraductal papilloma is associated with abnormal discharge from the nipples. Similar discharge less often occurs at duct ectasia or fibrous mastopathy. However, 13% of cases of bloody nipple discharge and 7% of cases of serous discharge are consequences of ductal breast carcinoma. One basic method of revealing intraductal masses is ductography—the method of artificial contrasting of lactiferous ducts with iodine-containing water-soluble agents while performing X-ray mammography (refer to Sect. 3.1 in Chap. 3). Intraductal lesions are the absolute indication for breast surgery. Ductography usually follows routine mammography and cytology of nipple discharge smears. Triad of cytologic features including macrophages, erythrocytes, and papillary structures or separate glandular epithelial cells is typical for intraductal papilloma. Nevertheless, ductography is contraindicated in patients with inflammatory process in breast ducts or breast carcinoma. That aims to avoid spreading of the infection in the first cases and cancer cells in the second. The value of US in diagnosis of intraductal pathology is limited with such factors as resolution of the equipment (conventional scanner detects lesions greater than 2–3 mm) and the size of an intraductal lesion (tumors are often smaller than 2 mm).

Echographic features of intraductal papilloma are the following (Fig. 5.9):

- Isolated dilatation of the duct (ducts) in the retroareolar area or on the breast periphery
- A solid papillary lesion of ordinary or increased echodensity with lobulated bordering located within a cystic cavity

Ductal papillomatosis of peripheral or terminal ducts (further than 3 cm from the nipple) accompanied with atypical epithelial hyperplasia with cytology is highly suspicious for ductal cancer.

Only large intraductal papillomas with dilatation of lactiferous ducts can be confidently diagnosed with US. Ultrasonographic mistakes at early stages of the disease are not rare.

Atheroma is retention cyst of the sebaceous gland located in the benign skin and subdermal tissues, which occurs by increased sweating of the sebaceous gland, occlusion of its duct, and forming of a capsule around the fatty content. It accounts for 0.2% of all breast lesions (Rozhkova 1993). Atheroma is clinically represented with a dense formation with clear contours, painless, welded to the skin. Atheromas quite often inflame and abscess. Local edema, hyperemia, morbidity, and fluctuation can be revealed in these cases.

Atheroma exhibits the following US features (Fig. 5.10):

- Hypoechoic or anechoic lesion
- Closely adjacent to the skin with scission of skin layers
- Accurately boarded
- Avascular with CDI, PDI, and 3DPD
- Without color pattern with compression US elastography
- Normal elastometry indices

Various combinations of breast lesions are possible (Fig. 5.11). For example, FA may be detected in combination with cysts (often with FBD), lipomas, fibrolipomas, oleogranulomas, cancer, etc.

All breast diseases may also appear in an accessory mammary gland.

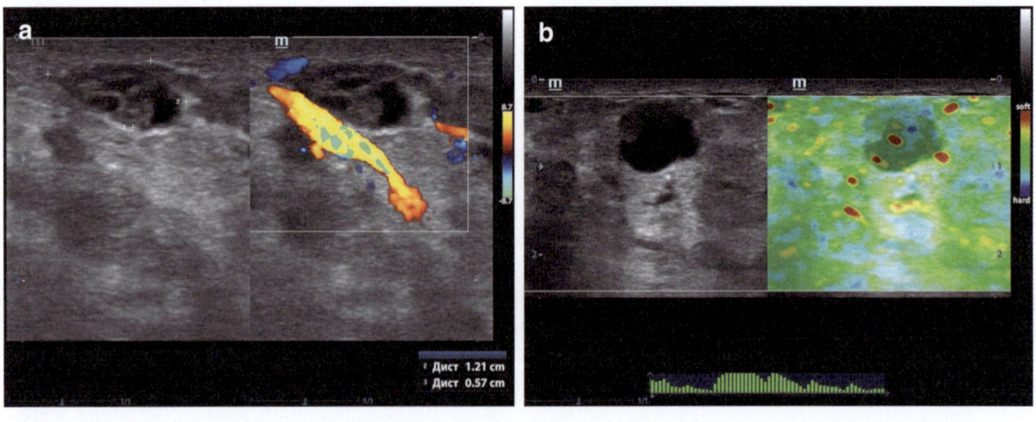

Fig. 5.9 Intraductal papilloma of the breast. (**a**) Grayscale US and CDI. (**b**) Compression US elastography

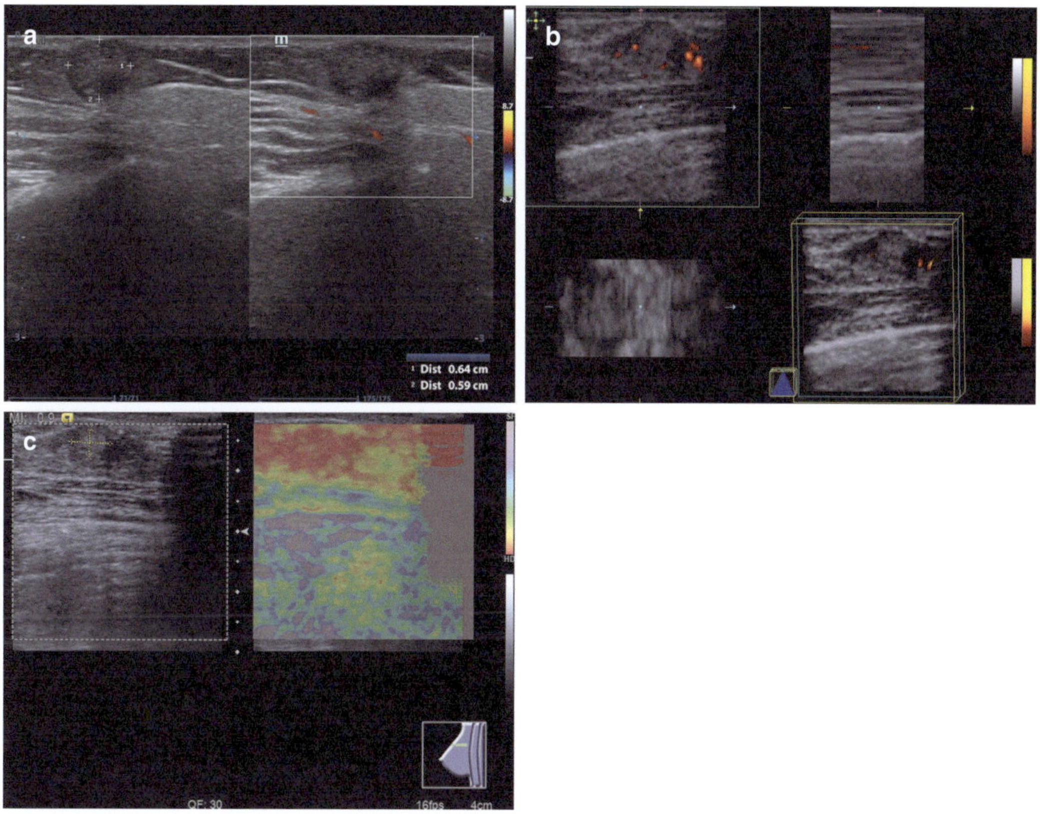

Fig. 5.10 Atheroma. (**a**) Grayscale and CDI. (**b**) 3DPD. (**c**) Compression US elastography

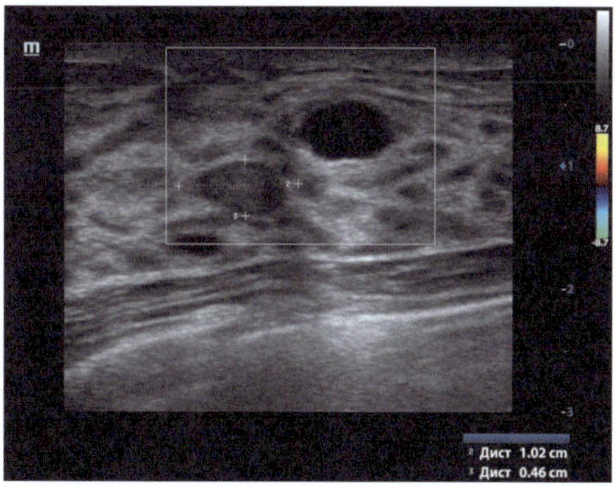

Fig. 5.11 Fibroadenoma and a cyst. Grayscale US and CDI

6 Multiparametric Examination: Basic and Innovative Methods of Ultrasound in Diagnosis of Breast Cancer

Alexander N. Sencha, Yury Patrunov, Ekaterina Sencha, Ella Penyaeva, and Valeriy Rodionov

Abstract

Grayscale ultrasound (US) is the principal ultrasound imaging modality to diagnose breast diseases and breast cancer in particular. Nodular type of breast cancer (up to 80% of breast carcinoma) is characterized by the presence of a lesion within breast structure that can be revealed in grayscale mode or other US regimens. Infiltrative (diffuse) types of breast cancer usually exhibit clinically evident local signs. Ultrasound is highly sensitive (85–93%) in detection of a tumor in any clinically doubtful situation and can provide guidance for biopsy with morphological verification. Paget's cancer is an intraductal epidermotropic eczema-like breast cancer, which originates from the ostia of large milk ducts of the nipple and involves the nipple and the areola and spreads to other parts of the breast. Assessment of the elasticity (stiffness) of tissues for early diagnosis and differentiation of malignant breast conditions is undoubtedly promising and prospective. Contrast-enhanced ultrasound (CEUS) is an informative technology for visualization of the blood flow in breast tumors and identification of neoangiogenesis, which is a characteristic for malignancy. The sensitivity of CEUS in the detection of breast cancer in women is 88%, specificity 90%, and accuracy 89%. Different classifications of breast cancer, including breast imaging-reporting and data system (BI-RADS), morphological types of tumors, and ultrasound correlations are also provided.

A. N. Sencha (✉)
Division of Visual Diagnostics, National Medical Research Center for Obstetrics, Gynecology and Perinatology named after Academician V.I. Kulakov of Ministry of Healthcare of Russian Federation, Moscow, Russia

Y. Patrunov · E. Penyaeva
Department of Ultrasound Diagnostics of Radiology Center, Yaroslavl Railway Clinic, Yaroslavl, Russia

E. Sencha
Department of Ultrasound Diagnostics, Federal State Budget Hospital "9 Treatment and Diagnostic Center" of the Ministry of Defense of the Russian Federation, Moscow, Russia

V. Rodionov
Department of Breast Diseases, National Medical Research Center for Obstetrics, Gynecology and Perinatology named after Academician V.I.Kulakov of Ministry of Healthcare of Russian Federation, Moscow, Russia

The first publications devoted to differential diagnosis of breast pathology with US technologies in A-mode belong to J.J. Wild and D. Neil (1951) and in B-mode to J.J. Wild and J.M. Reid (1952). Before the middle of the 1970s of the twentieth century, breast lesion larger than 1 cm could be successfully detected only in 8% of cases. In the 1980s, echography was considered an additional diagnostic procedure to clinical survey and

G. T. Sukhikh, A. N. Sencha (eds.), *Multiparametric Ultrasound Diagnosis of Breast Diseases*,
https://doi.org/10.1007/978-3-319-75034-7_6

mammography. US today is a highly effective (Chap. 1, Table 1.1) and mandatory method of examination, which is utilized along with mammography, clinical survey, and palpation in diagnosis of breast pathology, including early and differential diagnosis of malignancies (Zabolotskaya and Zabolotsky 1997; Trofimova 2000; Korzhenkova 2004; Komarova 2006; Sencha et al. 2013).

Diagnostic potential of US is based on the ability of tissues with different acoustic resistance to reflect US (cyclic sound pressure waves with a frequency greater than 20,000 Hz). Modern US scanners work in real time, giving the opportunity to observe the locomotion of organs in natural time course. The development of new diagnostic equipment, introduction of digital US scanners, modern high-frequency probes of 7.5–15 MHz, and complex utilization of modern options and technologies significantly increased the diagnostic possibilities of sonography.

The complex of modern US technologies for diagnosis of breast diagnostics confers the following options:

1. Grayscale regimen
2. Tissue harmonics
3. Adaptive coloring
4. Color Doppler imaging
5. Power Doppler mapping
6. Three-dimensional reconstruction of grayscale images and real-time 3D
7. Three-dimensional reconstruction of the image in vascular regimen
8. Panoramic scan
9. Spectral pulse Doppler
10. US elastography (compression and shear wave)
11. Contrast-enhanced ultrasound (CEUS)
12. Other options (multi-slice view, volume CT view, etc.)

Wide range of frequencies and options of US scanning facilitates daily work of US specialists providing detailed image of breast and surrounding tissue for a short time period. Modern algorithms of automatic optimization based on signal preprocessing optimize the influence of tissue irregularity and minimize noises and artifacts.

According to Sencha et al. (2011), the average age of breast cancer patients is 58 years.

Some US signs suspicious for breast malignancy according to our data are listed below:

1. Irregular shape of the breast lesion
2. Rough borders
3. Indistinct contours
4. Decreased echodensity
5. Heterogeneous structure
6. Hyperechoic incorporations and microcalcifications
7. Posterior acoustic shadow
8. Absence of halo

CDI, PDI, and 3DPD reveal the following features:

Lesions that are smaller than 2 cm in size demonstrate avascular structure. Larger lesions (more than 2 cm in size) are hypovascular or hypervascular.

In 3DPD mode irregular distribution of vessels, disorganized vascular pattern, and pathological transformation of vessels are characteristics.

Compression elastography demonstrates hard structure of the lesion with irregular stiffness.

Strain elastography reveals that strain ratio in 76% of breast carcinoma is above 5.1 (22.9 ± 2.14) and ranges from 5.1 to 28.9 depending on histological structure of the lesion. Strain ratio in noninvasive cancer is lower (8.42 ± 3.41) than in infiltrating types (22.64 ± 2.61). In the regimen of virtual touch tissue quantification (ARFI technology), the average velocity of shear wave within malignant breast lesions was 4.1 m/s while 2.9 m/s in the surrounding normal breast tissue.

Enlargement of regional lymph nodes.

According to Sencha et al. (2011), the characteristic ultrasound signs of breast cancer are as follows: irregular shape (98.8%), heterogeneity (84.5–96.0%), uneven contours (86.7–87.6%), hypoechogenicity (88.4–96.6%), dorsal attenuation of the ultrasound signal (77.9%), dorsal amplification (11.1–19.0%), absence of peripheral halo (73.9%), rough borders (67.0%), and microcalcifications (24%). CDI, PDI, and 3DPD in the lesions of smaller than 2 cm in size usually reveal no vascularity (94.4%). In larger lesions (more than 2 cm in size), hypovascularity (56%) or hypervascularity (32.0%) is often observed. 3DPD facilitates to determine irregular distribution of blood vessels within the tumor with pathological tortuosity (32%) and chaotic vascular pattern. Enlarged regional lymph nodes can be detected in 37.5%.

6.1 Grayscale Mode

Grayscale (2D, B-mode) US is the principal ultrasound imaging modality to diagnose breast diseases and breast cancer in particular (Figs. 6.1 and 6.2).

Grayscale imaging supplies basic information on the character of pathological process, thus decreasing the number of unspecified diagnoses.

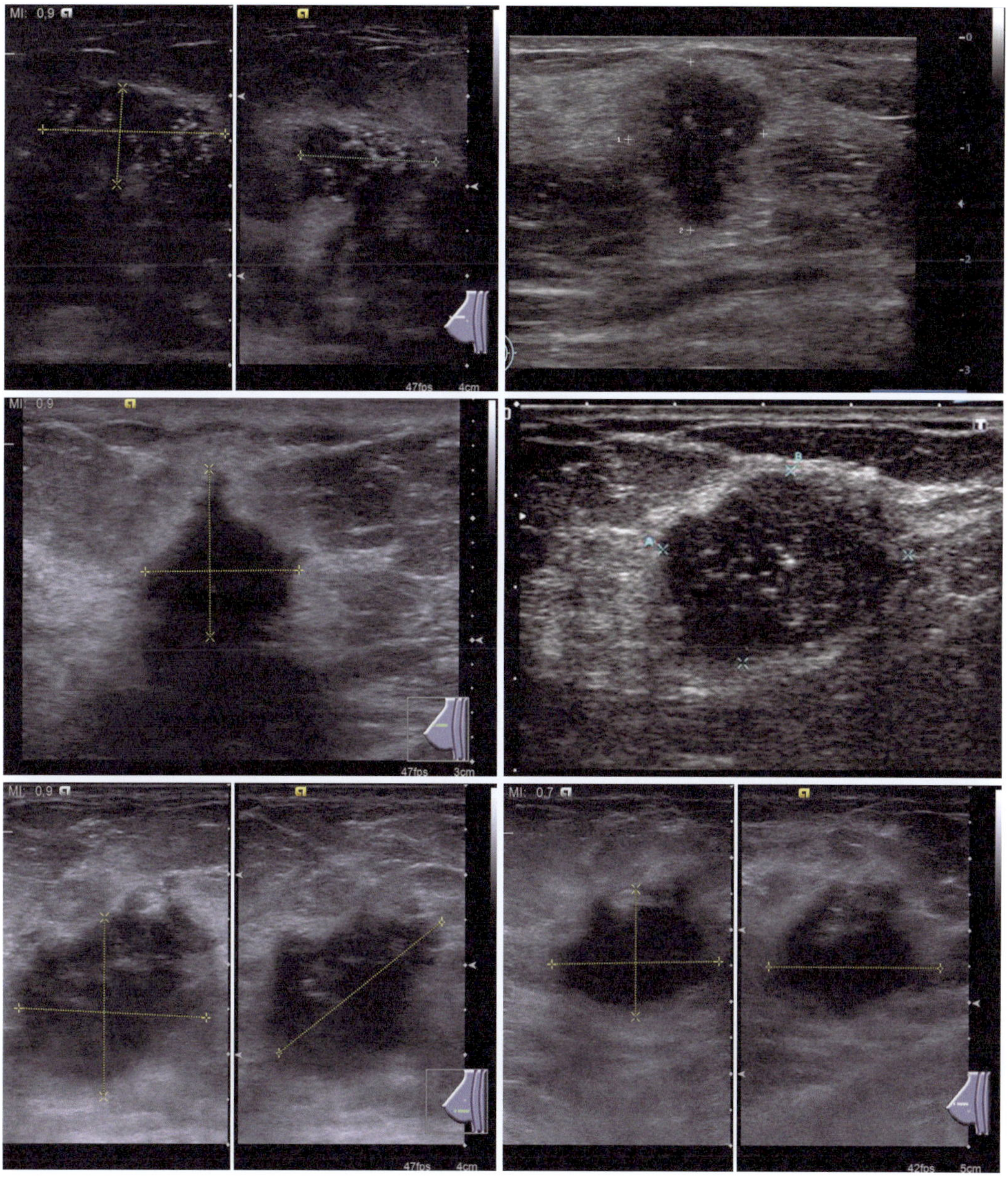

Fig. 6.1 Breast carcinoma. Nodular type. Grayscale US

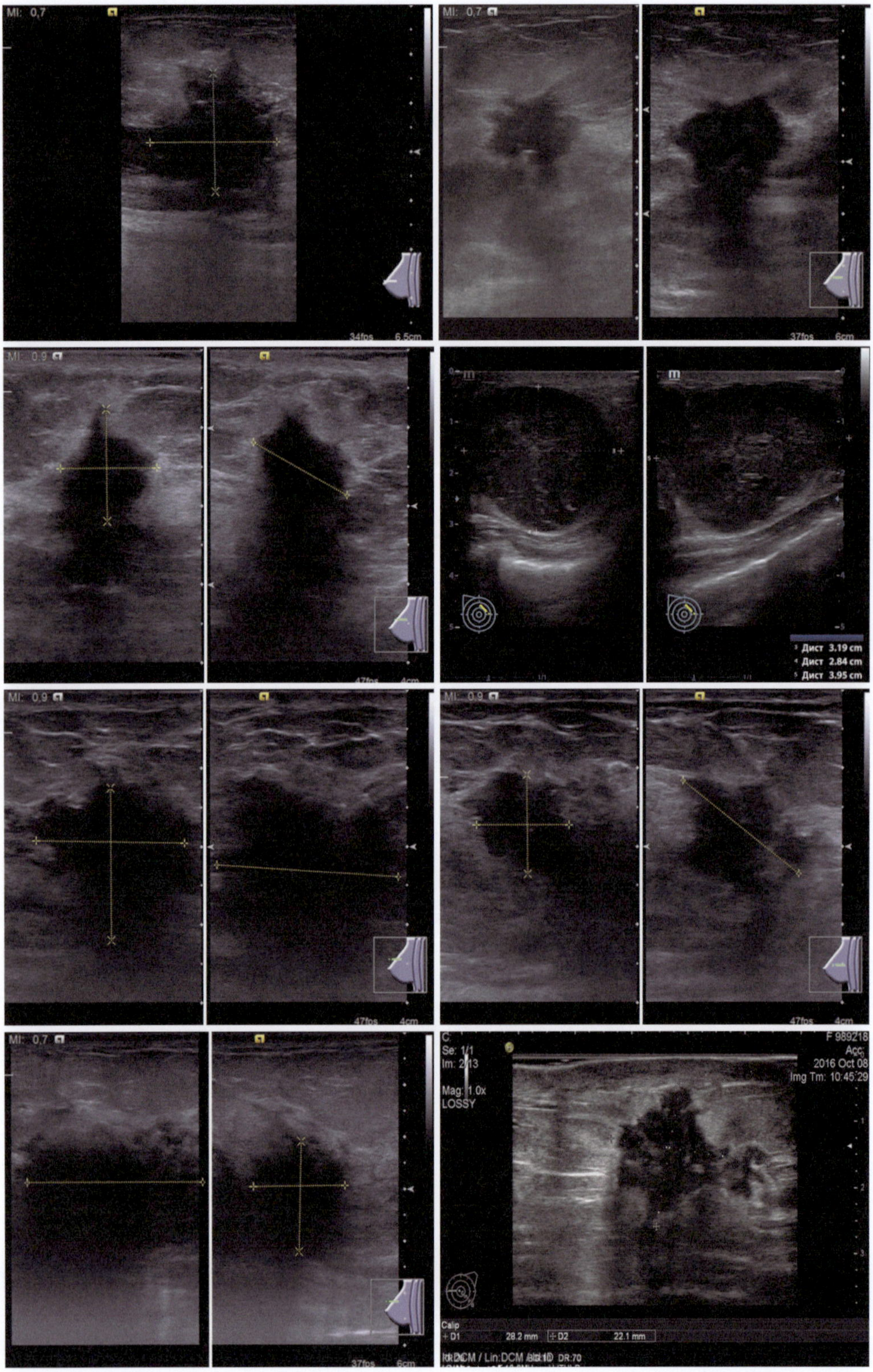

Fig. 6.1 (continued)

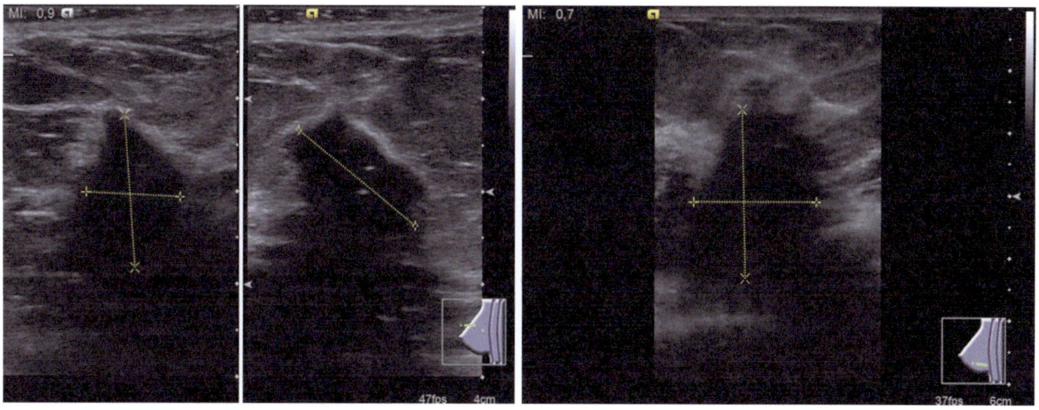

Fig. 6.1 (continued)

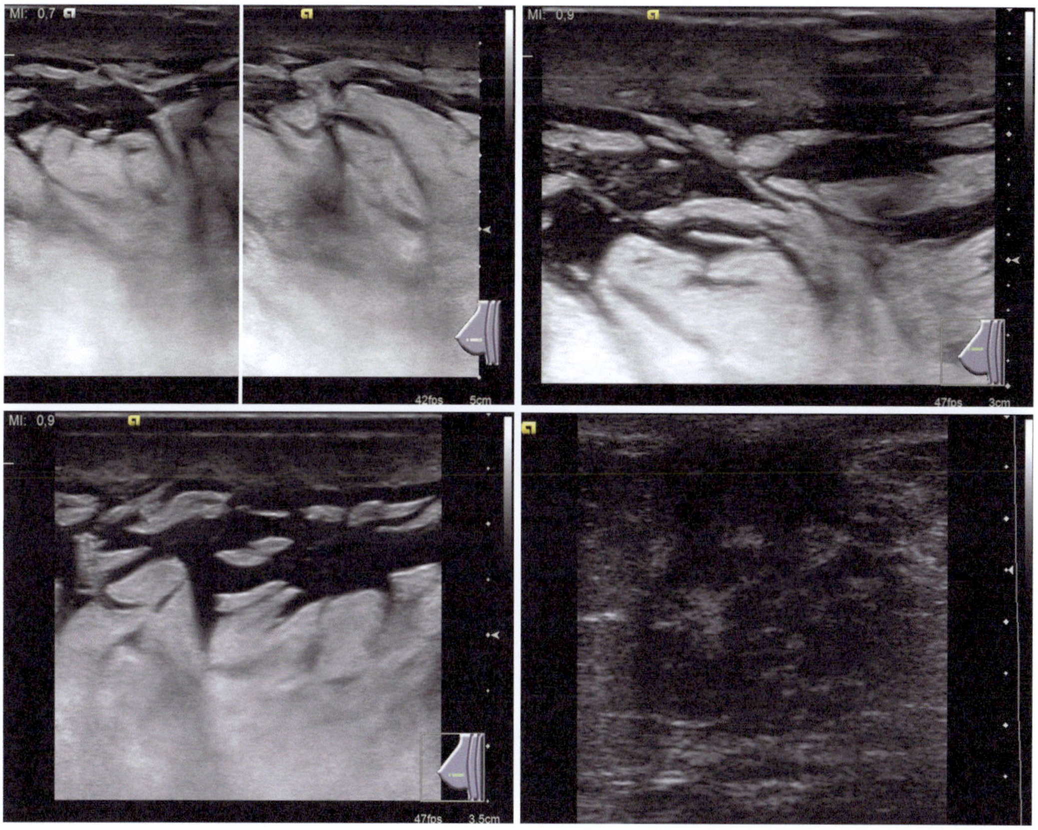

Fig. 6.2 Breast cancer. Edematous-infiltrative type. Grayscale US

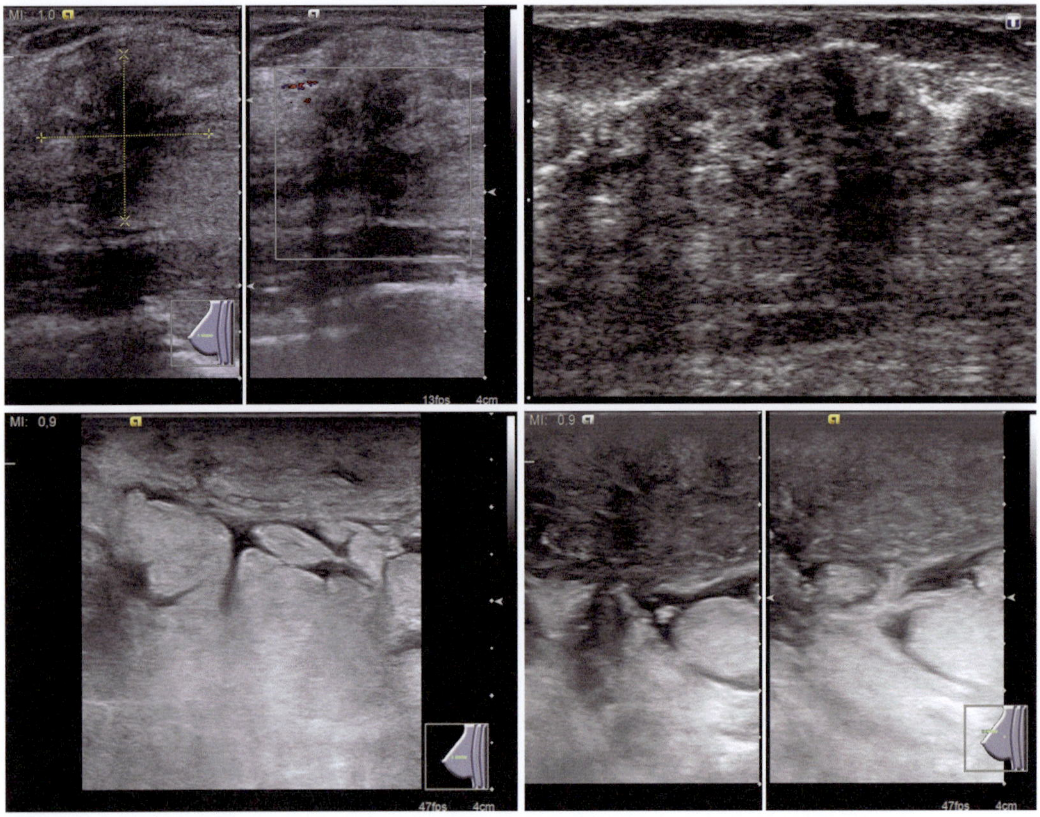

Fig. 6.2 (continued)

A wide range of histological types of tumoral growth invoke the interest to search for correlations between morphological and ultrasound structures.

Breast carcinoma exhibits nodular or diffuse (infiltrative) types of growth.

Nodular type of breast cancer (up to 80% of breast carcinoma) exhibits a lesion within the breast that can be detected in grayscale mode or other US regimens (Fig. 6.1). According to Zabolotskaya and Zabolotsky (1997), up to 50% of all cancers originate from the upper-outer quadrant of the breast; 15% are located in the upper-inner quadrant, 10% in the lower-outer, 5% in the lower-inner, and up to 17% in the central area. The lesion can demonstrate infiltrating or expansive growth. Nodular type of breast carcinoma can be accompanied with the change in breast shape, nipple inversion, pain and discomfort in the breast independent of the phase of menstrual cycle, abnormal discharge from the nipple, and palpable dense breast lesion.

Breast tumors have the following size with US by the time of their detection: 0.5–1.0 cm, 25%; 1.1–3.0 cm, 69%; and larger than 3.0 cm, 68% (Sencha et al. 2011). US image of the lesion depends on tumor size.

According to Ciatto et al. (1994), Marquet et al. (1995), Vetshev et al. (1997), and Trofimova (2002), US picture of breast carcinoma is quite variable. The basic criteria of breast cancer with grayscale US are the following: irregular shape of the lesion, heterogeneity of echostructure, rough uneven contours, and posterior acoustic shadow of various intensities often emerging from posterior or lateral aspects of the tumor.

Sometimes the mass can have a posterior acoustic shadow (Haylenko et al. 2005).

Haylenko et al. (2005) and Sinyukova et al. (2007) noted microcalcifications within tumor in 33% of cases and consider this fact an important diagnostic sign of cancer. According to Zabolotskaya and Zabolotsky (1997), microcalcifications are found in 65% of intraductal breast cancer.

Breast carcinoma can be unilateral or bilateral (in 3–15% of cases). The cancer within the second breast can arise simultaneously with the tumor of the first breast or appear 10 or more years later (Rozhkova 1993). Multicentric cancer is observed in 18% of women, and synchronous affection of the second breast is detected in 43% of cases. The number of "daughter tumors" of multicentric carcinoma may vary. They are most often located near the primary tumor and rarely affect other breast quadrants. According to Sinyukova et al. (2007), the sensitivity of grayscale US in revealing multicentric breast carcinoma is 83.6% with specificity of 86.9% and diagnostic accuracy of 79.9%.

The incidence of cancer in the accessory breast is 0.2–0.3% of overall breast cancer incidence. Most publications report axillary localization (55–65%) of affected accessory breasts. Infiltrative ductal cancer accounts for up to 79%, while medullary and lobular types account for 9.5% of cases.

The most common infiltrative (diffuse) types of breast cancer are the following:

- Edematous-infiltrative
- Inflammatory
- Mastitis-like
- Erysipeloid
- Testaceous

Edematous-infiltrative type is the most common. It usually exhibits clinically evident local signs: edema of the breast, skin hyperemia, and hyperthermia. Ultrasound is highly sensitive (85–93%) in detection of a tumor in any clinically doubtful situation and can provide guidance for biopsy with morphological verification (Kolesnik et al. 2014). Breast X-ray remains the least sensitive method for this type of cancer, since the tumor is often difficult to detect on the background of tissue edema (in 16–80% of cases depending on the mammographic method), but this diagnostic tool remains mandatory.

The following signs (Fig. 6.2) often characterize infiltrative type of breast carcinoma in grayscale regimen:

- Thickening of the skin
- Increase in the echodensity of subcutaneous fat and parenchyma
- Loss of structural differentiation
- Dilation of lactiferous ducts and lymph vessels
- Enlargement of regional lymph nodes

Primary infiltrative type of breast carcinoma does not exhibit any lesion against local swelling of the breast. Secondary infiltrative type is characterized by a combination of swelling and a lesion. US diagnosis of primary infiltrative breast carcinoma is difficult. Skin thickening, local swelling of the breast tissue, dilatation of lymph vessels, and abnormal regional lymph nodes may serve as US signs.

MRI and CT/PET for edematous-infiltrative cancer are supplementary tools to assess the extent of the tumor and detect lesions of adjacent organs and regional lymph nodes.

Paget's cancer is an intraductal epidermotropic eczema-like breast cancer, which originates from the ostia of large milk ducts of the nipple and involves the nipple and the areola and spreads to other parts of the breast. It accounts for 0.5–5% of all breast neoplasms. J. Paget was the first to describe it in 1874 as the cancer of the areola and nipple, which manifests as a chronic eczema.

Paget's disease course is variable. Common signs confer palpable mass of the nipple and areola, itching, burning, nodular induration and erosion in the nipple area, and nipple discharge. Rarely, a mass is found near the nipple, while the changes in the nipple area are secondary. Echography usually detects a subareolar mass (Fig. 6.3).

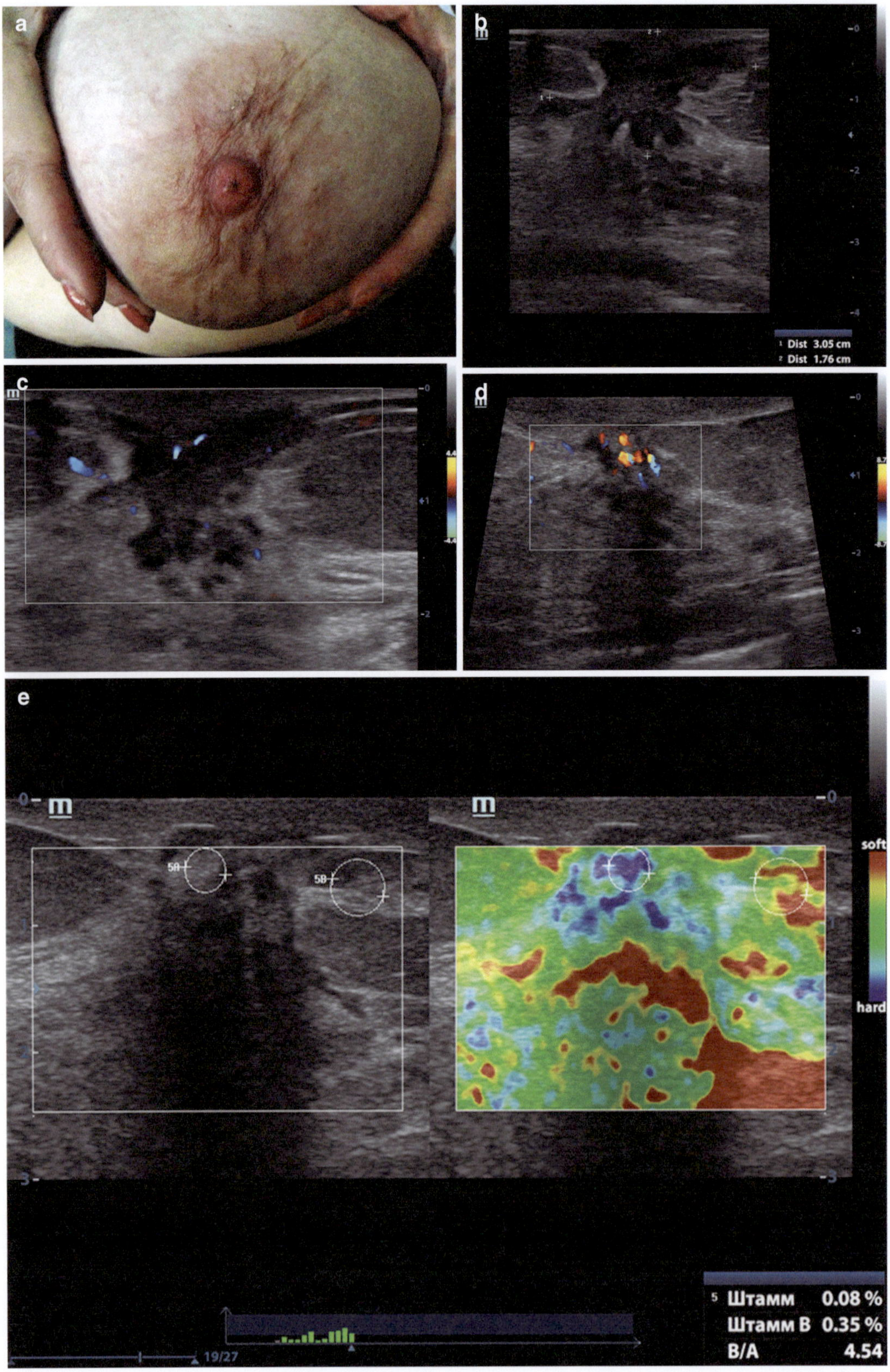

Fig. 6.3 Paget's cancer. (**a**) View of the breast. (**b**) Grayscale. (**c**, **d**) CDI. (**e**) Compression US elastography

Paget's cancer is finally verified by cytology of the nipple discharge or with open biopsy.

Breast US has certain disadvantages in the detection of lesions against adipose involution and in assessment of ductal extension of the tumor. The tumors that are located in retromammary space in large breasts and small lesions (smaller than 0.5 cm in size) may be left undetected. One significant disadvantage of US is operator dependency (Zabolotskaya and Zabolotsky 2005).

6.2 Color-Coded Modes: Duplex Study

Color Doppler mapping (color Doppler imaging, CDI; color flow imaging, CFI; color flow mapping, CFM) is an US technology of blood flow imaging based on registration of velocities of blood flow with further coding with different colors and superimposing on 2D grayscale image (Fig. 6.4).

CDI normally detects poor vascular pattern in the breast tissue. Color pattern, as a rule, is presented by solitary color points, which are distributed in a relatively regular way in all quadrants of the breast (Fisenko 1999; Harchenko et al. 1993; Sandrikov and Fisenko 1998). A technique of measurement of the number of color (vascular) patches in 1 cm^2 and calculation of color pixel density has been suggested (Sohn et al. 1997). Cosgrove et al. (1990, 1993) consider 0.11 of the vessel per 1 cm^2 (1.76% of the field of view) to be a sign of cancer. According to Folkman (1995), one significant feature of the breast cancer is vascular asymmetry.

Vascular pattern in the tumor and surrounding tissue with CDI depends on the size of the mass. Thus, tumors up to 2 cm in size exhibit vascularity in 37.4% of cases with enhanced vascular pattern around the lesion in 51.4% of cases.

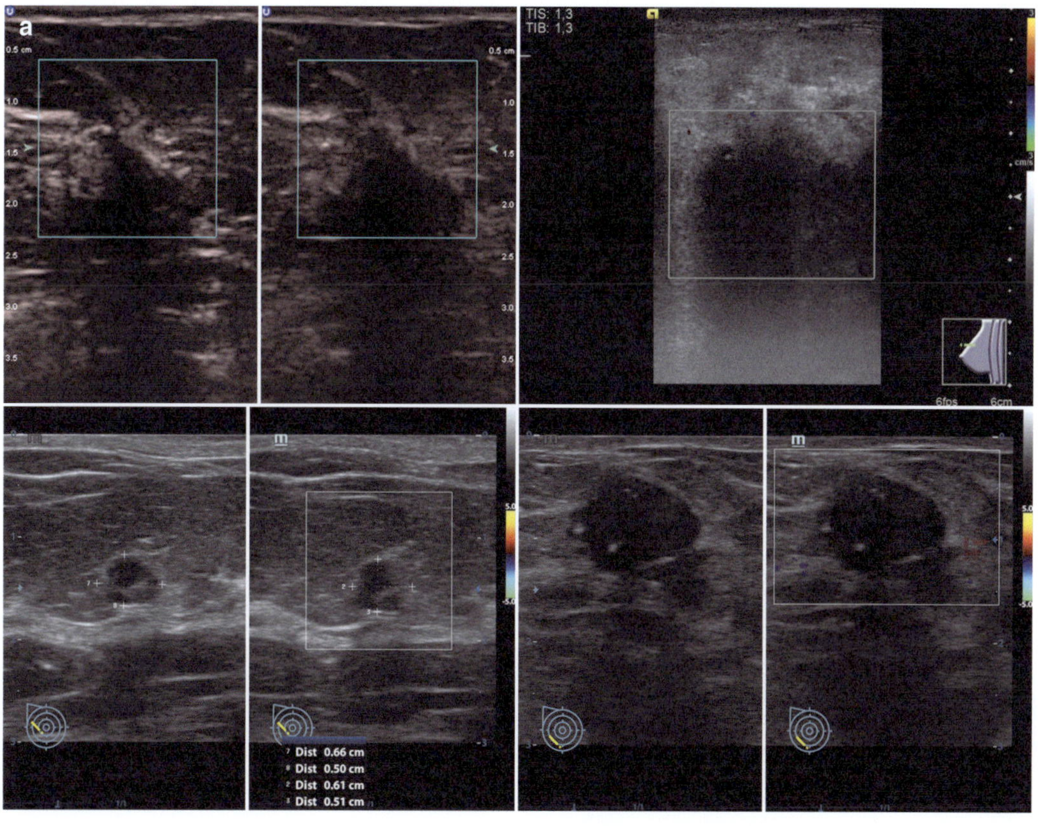

Fig. 6.4 Breast cancer. CDI. (**a**) 1–4. Avascular malignant tumor. (**b**) 1–7. Vascularized mass

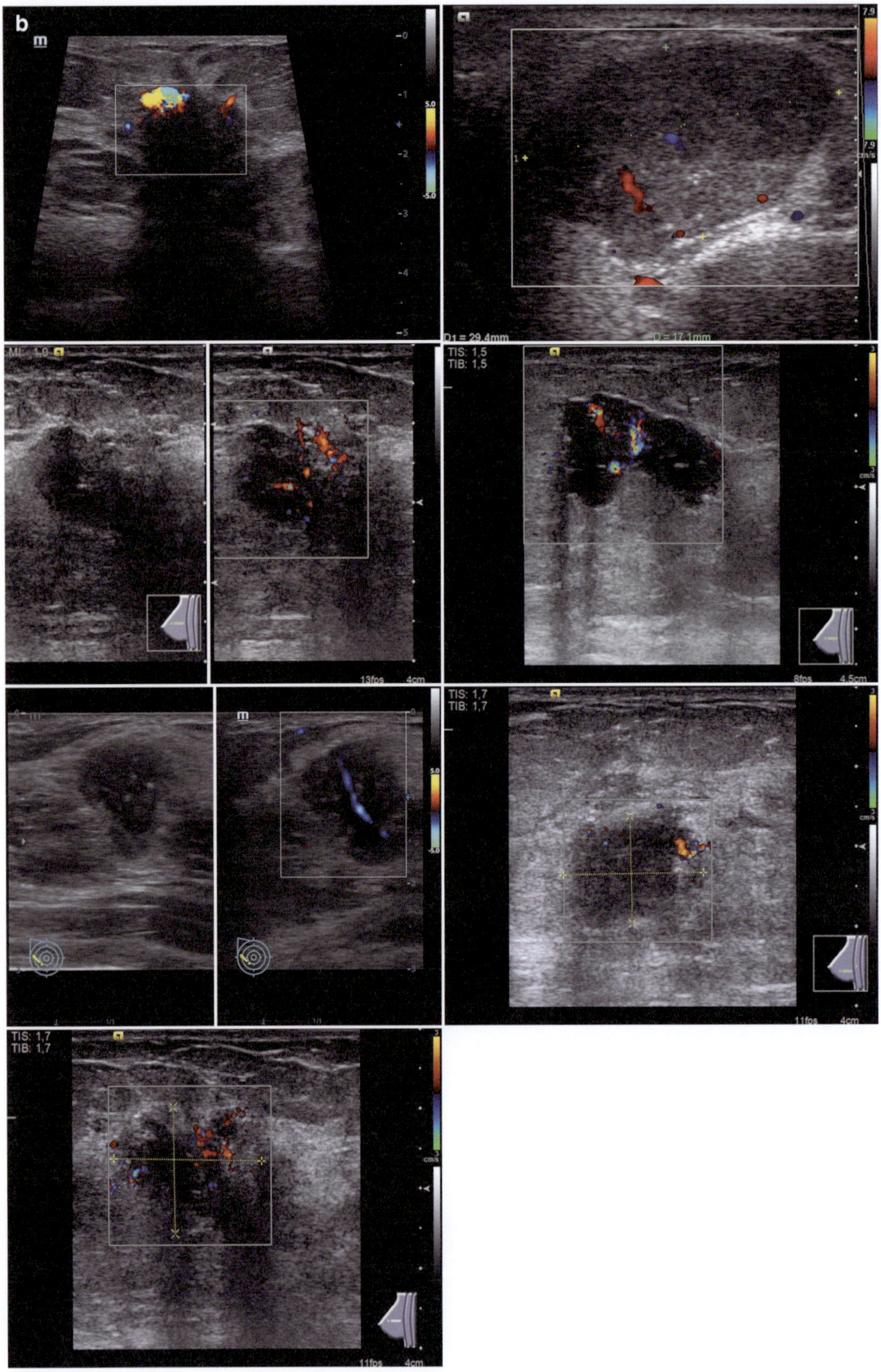

Fig. 6.4 (continued)

Tumors of 2–5 cm exhibited vascularity in 97% and 92.6% of cases, respectively, and in all cases for both indices in tumors over 5 cm.

Tumor growth is often associated with neovascularization and development of own pathological vascular rete. Neoangiogenesis of a malignant tumor results in vascular architectonics, which differs from the same of a benign lesion and physiological breast changes. According to Holcombe et al. (1995), the large number of vessels within a malignant breast lesion suggests its higher stage and possible metastases in axillary lymph nodes.

According to Madjar et al. (1995), the vessels in a malignant breast neoplasm can be detected in 43–100% of instances with 5–14 arteries (8–11 on the average) identified within the tumor. The authors report that the presence of two and more vessels within a tumor is a typical sign of cancer. Infiltrative cancer is reported vascularized in 100% of cases. It has specific characteristics with pulse wave Doppler, such as absence of diastolic component and arteriovenous shunts. Trufanov et al. (2009) report that the majority of malignant breast tumors are well vascularized and exhibit intranodular (72.6%) or mixed (13.8%) type of vascular pattern.

Madjar et al. (1995) suggested counting all vessels detected within the nodule for quantitative assessment of the vascularity of breast lesions. According to their data, benign lesions demonstrated 2 arteries on the average, while malignant up to 11. Sohn et al. (1997) report correlation between vascularization and size of the tumor. Fiedler et al. (1996) consider that CDI is effective only in tumors larger than 1–2 cm in size as blood flow was identified in 90% of cases, whereas in tumors smaller than 1 cm, blood flow was identified in 41.7%. Sohn et al. (1997) consider that the mentioned methods of scoring are too labor-consuming and are not reliable in practice due to high operator and scanner dependency.

Cosgrove et al. (1993) differentiate three types of blood flow within a lesion: perinodular, intranodular, and mixed. Lesions are often divided into hypervascular (with multiple arterial and venous vessels), hypovascular (with 2–3 color pixels), and avascular (without color pixels within) (Harchenko et al. 1999). Sinyukova et al. (2007) differentiate three patterns of blood flow within breast masses, as follows: with an individual vessel, with local increase in blood flow, and with diffuse vascularization.

Nadareishvili et al. (2002) suggested to divide Doppler signals in lesion structure in four types according to their shape: individual, linear, chaotic, and branching. Depending on localization the intratumoral blood flow is divided into three groups: central (up to 6.4%), peripheral (25.9%), and mixed (67.7%).

The vessels within malignant breast lesions are often located chaotically with multiple anastomoses and arteriovenous shunts. They often have irregular caliber (narrow and wide parts) and looped or spiral shape (Madjar et al. 1995). Dilation of vessels within breast carcinoma results from several factors, such as local increase in the temperature and the influence of an oxide of nitrogen due to malignant process. These aspects explain the increase in local vascularity of breast carcinoma with CDI and PDI (Cosgrove et al. 1990; Fisenko 1999).

According to Madjar et al. (1995), breast carcinoma is often surrounded with a hypervascular area. Lee et al. (1995) and Fisenko and Sandrikov (1998) report that the presence of vascular structures within the nodule or around it is suspicious for breast carcinoma.

Trofimova (2000) reports that vascularization can be detected in 90.5% of malignant lesions (in 100% of tumors larger than 4 cm in size and in 76% of tumors smaller than 2 cm). The vessels in malignant neoplasms were characterized with irregular caliber (narrow and dilated segments), collaterals, and branching. Smirnova (1995) and Trofimova (2000) observed absence of vascularity in 85–95% of lesions and consider that blood vessels can be detected only within the tumors of the size larger than 2 cm and are associated with expressed cellular proliferation.

According to Shevchenko (1999), absence of neovascularization in a solid breast lesion, which is highly suspicious for cancer, does not permit to exclude its malignant nature. Almost 31% of cancers appear avascular. Alternatively, CDI can detect vessels in normal breast.

Some authors report a "twinkling" artifact with CDI due to microcalcifications within cancer structure (Gromov and Kubova 2004; Trufanov et al. 2009).

The sensitivity of CDI in the diagnosis of breast cancer is 60–82% with specificity of 39–76%.

CDI has some disadvantages, such as aliasing in cases of high velocities, background noise, and dependence on the angle between the US beam and blood flow.

Power Doppler imaging (PDI) allows to obtain angle-independent images of smaller vessels with more accurate contours (Fig. 6.5). According to Zabolotskaya and Zabolotsky (2000), PDI is capable to define larger number of vessels (as compared with CDI) in all breast malignancies, especially in infiltrative carcinoma.

Sensitivity of PDI in the diagnosis of breast cancer is 67–95% with specificity of 45–80%.

PDI disadvantages are high dependence on motion of surrounding structures with movement artifacts and coloring of perivascular areas.

Pulsed-wave Doppler allows to measure the quantitative indices of the following blood flow (Fig. 6.6):

- In the medial and lateral branches of the afferent thoracic artery on both sides (interpectoral blood flow)
- In blood vessels of the parenchyma (intraparenchymal blood flow)
- In the vessels of the lesion (intranodular blood flow)

Trofimova (2002) considers that assessment of blood flow only within breast lesion is enough. Nevertheless, in cases of infiltrative cancer, there appears the necessity to compare vascular pattern with contralateral area in the other breast.

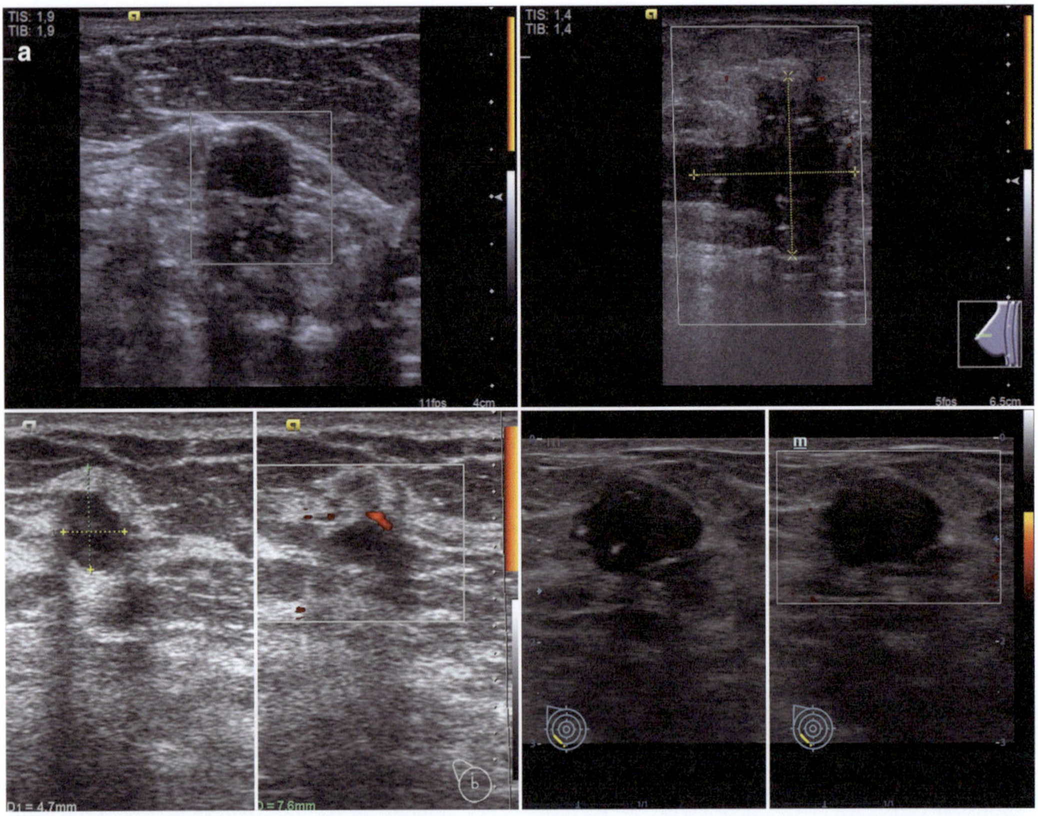

Fig. 6.5 Breast cancer. Power Doppler imaging. (**a**) 1–4. Avascular malignant tumor. (**b**) 1–8. Vascularized tumor

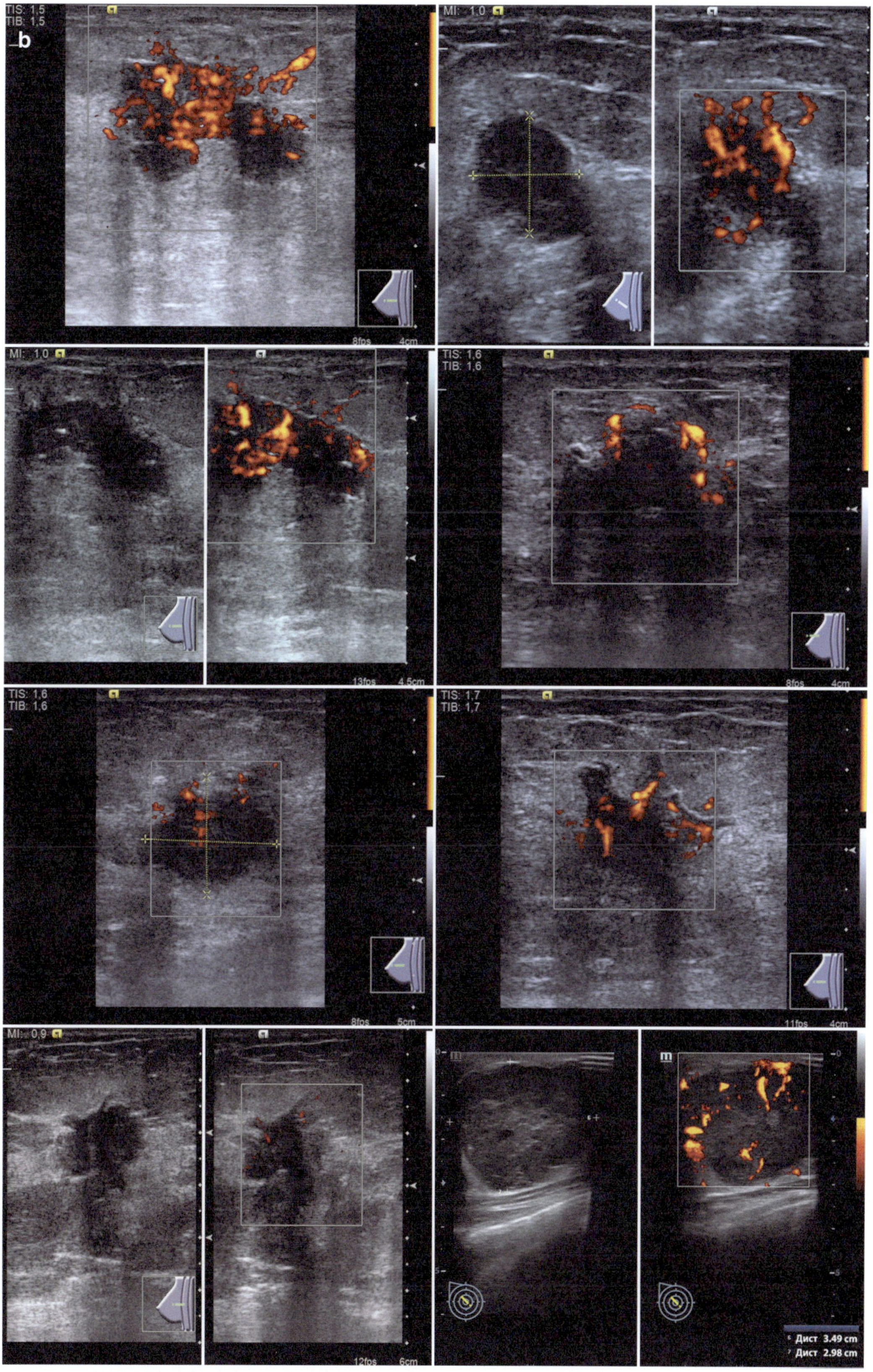

Fig. 6.5 (continued)

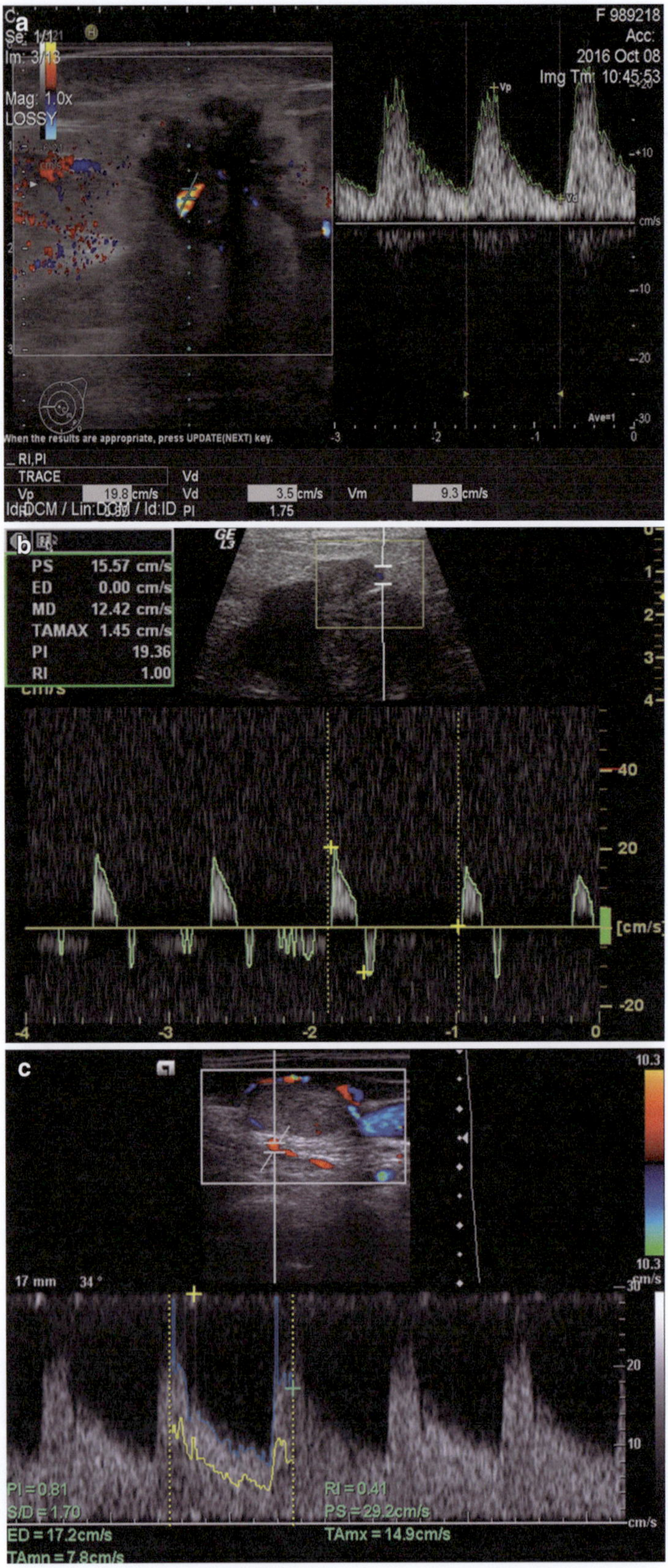

Fig. 6.6 Breast cancer. Pulsed-wave Doppler. (**a**, **b**) Measurement of intranodular blood flow. (**c**, **d**) Measurement of intraparenchymal blood flow

Fig. 6.6 (continued)

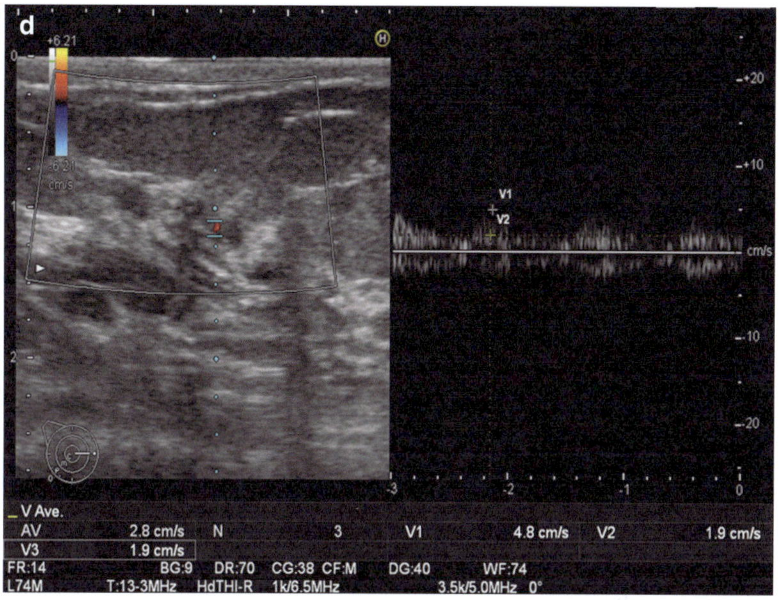

Sohn et al. (1997) report the value of pulsed Doppler data of blood flow in branches of lateral thoracic artery, pectoral branch of the thoracoacromial trunk, and medial mammary branches of the internal thoracic (internal mammary) artery of affected and normal breast.

Some authors advise to measure PSV in the tumor, while others insist on the PSV and EDV measurement with calculation of RI and PI. Pulsed Doppler can confirm blood flow enhancement within a lesion in comparison with that in normal parenchyma; in rare cases vascularization is identical. The intensity of blood flow of the lesion is often related not so much with its morphological structure but with its size (Lelyuk and Lelyuk 2007). According to Svensson (1997), the indexes of blood flow in the vessels of a malignant tumor directly depend on its volume, and enlargement in size results in the increase of spectral characteristics. Haylenko et al. (2005) reported that the indicators of blood flow in malignancies with CDI and PDI also exhibit direct correlation with lesion's volume.

Many researchers analyzed different parameters of vascularization and suggest the following Doppler criteria of malignancy: high EDV of intranodular blood flow, high RI, and high PI. In the opinion of De Albertis et al. (1995), breast carcinoma is characterized with presence of several (more than two) vascular areas, high PSV, and high PI.

According to Harchenko et al. (1993), PSV in the vessels of normal breast tissue is 0.06 ± 0.02 m/s, while the average PSV within cancer is 0.3 m/s. Pulsed Doppler in breast carcinoma is thought to exhibit the following figures: PSV, 0.05–0.47 m/s; EDV, 0.07–0.09 m/s; RI, 0.67–0.81; and PI, 1.47–1.76 (Trofimova 2000; Fisenko and Sandrikov 1998; Madjar et al. 1995; Youssefzadeh et al. 1996). According to Lee et al. (1995), PSV in 67% of breast carcinomas exceeds 0.15 m/s.

According to Shevchenko (1999), the velocities of arterial blood flow in malignant tumors are as follows: PSV, 4.6–56.6 cm/s (average value 18.98 cm/s); EDV, 0.3–9.8 cm/s (average value 2.99 cm/s); and RI, 0.56–1.34 (average value 0.82). The larger the number of vessels in a tumor, the higher blood velocities and RI are registered.

Trofimova (2000) reported the following blood flow parameters within breast carcinoma: PSV, 0.27 (0.06–0.91) m/s; EDV, 0.07 (0.01–0.33) m/s; RI, 0.76 (0.31–1.42); and PI, 1.71 (0.46–8.09). She noticed that blood flow parameters in the vessels around the tumor are close to the data obtained in the areas of mastopathy. Lee et al. (1995) did not reveal any difference between the vascular pattern around benign breast tumor and healthy tissue of contralateral breast.

According to Trufanov et al. (2009), the increase in RI, PSV, and EDV is a characteristic for malignant breast lesions. The authors also noticed that the same parameters are often observed in women with only diffuse breast changes.

Spectral characteristics of blood flow in the vessels of infiltrative breast carcinoma are very variable, starting from almost normal curve with pulsed Doppler ending with shunts to low resistive pathological vessels, irregular dilatations, disorganization of vascular pattern, and different caliber of detected vessels (Zabolotskaya and Zabolotsky 2000).

Sinyukova et al. (2007) noticed that pulsed wave Doppler for breast carcinoma is the most subjective US modality among all diagnostic techniques.

According to Sohn et al. (1997), the methods of quantitative assessment of imaged vessels are labor-consuming and unreliable. Most often, no regularity in the change of velocities and indexes is detected. Wide distribution of indicators of pulsed Doppler does not supply any significant diagnostic information, often fails to serve a criterion for differential diagnosis of breast lesions, and can be only considered an accessory sign.

The combination of grayscale US with spectral and color Doppler permits to obtain additional information and increases the sensitivity of US in diagnosis of cancer from 82–97% to 93–99% and specificity from 59% to 83–97% (Possover et al. 1994; Sohn et al. 1997). The majority of authors note the following criteria for differential diagnosis of breast carcinoma: arteriovenous shunts, change in PSV and EDV, absence of end-diastolic component, increased RI, detection of more than three vessels, and irregular course and calibers of vessels within the lesion (Yang et al. 1996; Trofimova 2000).

The sensitivity Doppler imaging in diagnosis of breast carcinoma is 81–99%; specificity, 71–98%; and diagnostic accuracy, 82–93% (Fisenko and Sandrikov 1998; Trofimova 2000).

6.3 3D Image Reconstruction and Multiplanar Scan

3D image reconstruction is advantageous over other imaging methods, which provide only plane images. 3D US in breast cancer allows to assess not only the number and structure of lesions within the breast structure but also their margins, presence of calcifications, and the growth and spread in detail and to assume the volume of affected and intact breast tissue (Fig. 6.7). 3D provides additional information on the relationship of normal and abnormal structures and allows objective assessment of the lesion in dynamics, such as the change in shape and inner structure, especially against fibrous changes in recurrent tumors. The possibility of rotation and obtaining multi-slice images facilitates perception of depth and topographic relationship of normal and abnormal structures. Sometimes it enables to reduce diagnostic terms and to improve early diagnosis of breast malignancies.

The advantages of 4D (real-time 3D) ultrasound in the diagnosis of breast cancer are faster and more accurate spatial visualization of blood flow in the lesion with better differentiation of artifacts in real time, which makes it possible to conduct detailed differential diagnosis of mixed or incomplete types of vascularization in a breast tumor.

3D reconstruction in vascular regimen (3D power Doppler imaging, 3DPD) often allows more accurate assessment of the pathological transformation of the vessels of the lesion, their distribution, and chaotic course.

Spatial reconstruction is mostly used to assess visual characteristics of vascular structures: spatial symmetry of vessels and their branching and presence of asymmetric protrusions, narrowings, and lacunar dilatations. Analysis of the 3D construction in 3DPD mode shows the details of perinodular and intranodular vascularization and disorganization of the vascular pattern in the tumor (Fig. 6.8). Intranodular and perinodular vessels in breast cancer are often twisted and asymmetric and have fragmented spatial arrangement.

Panoramic scan enables to reconstruct extended images that include several adjacent fields of view and are larger than a conventional scan. This facilitates precise measurements of long objects (Fig. 6.9). The way of presentation of obtained data in panoramic scan often helps to characterize pathological foci in cases of

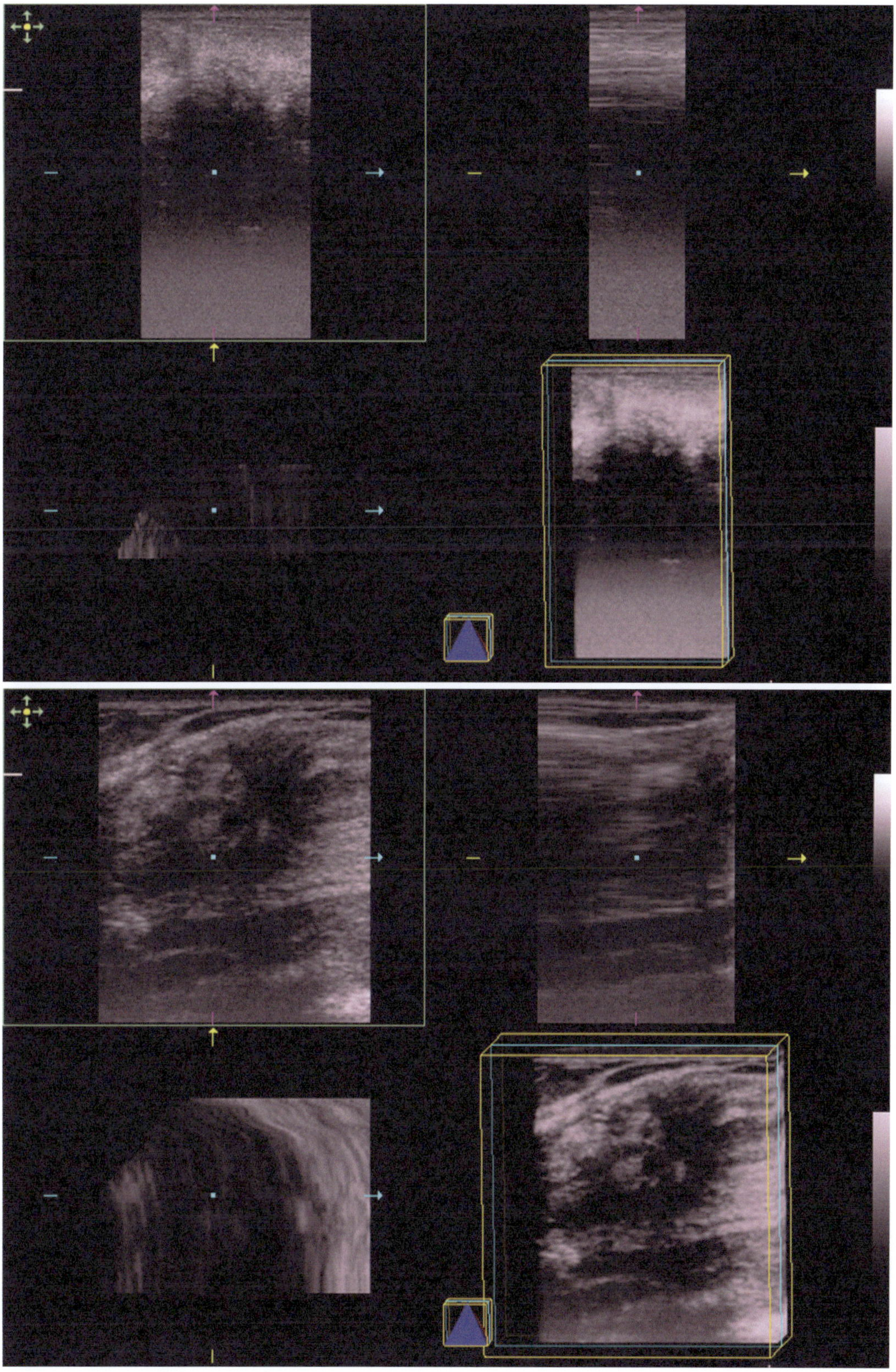

Fig. 6.7 1–4. Breast cancer. 3D ultrasound

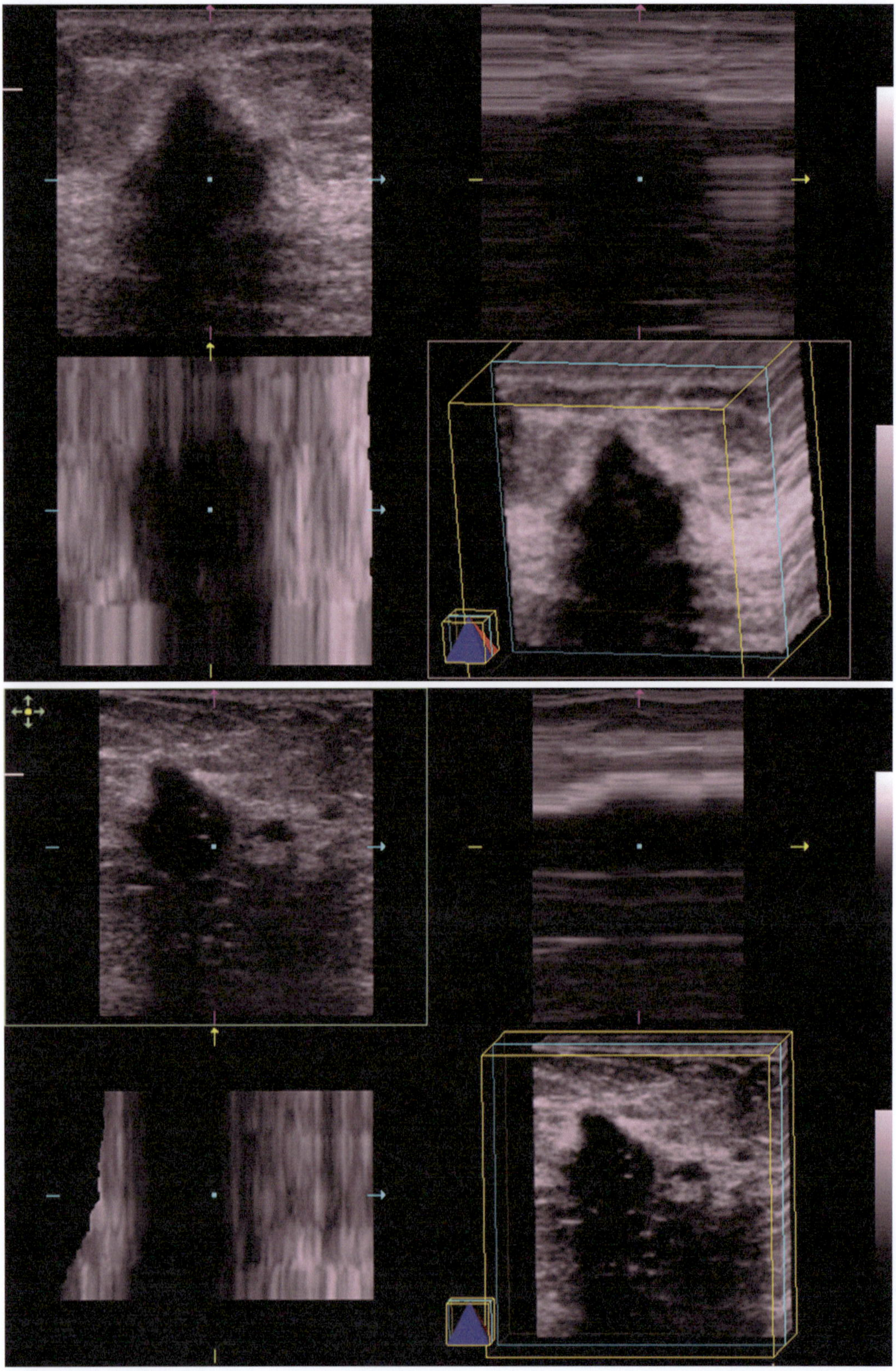

Fig. 6.7 (continued)

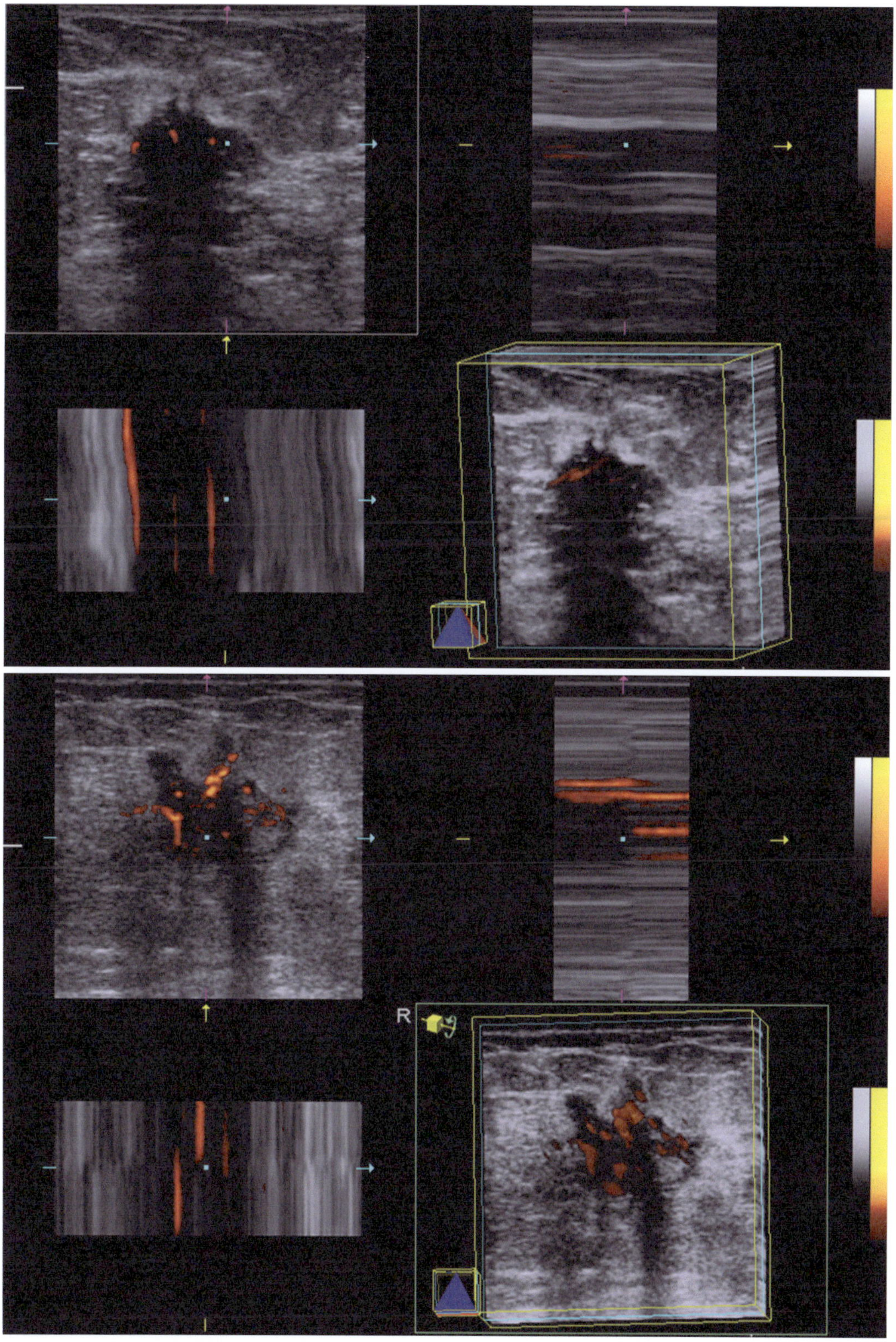

Fig. 6.8 Breast cancer. 3DPD. 1–8. Echograms

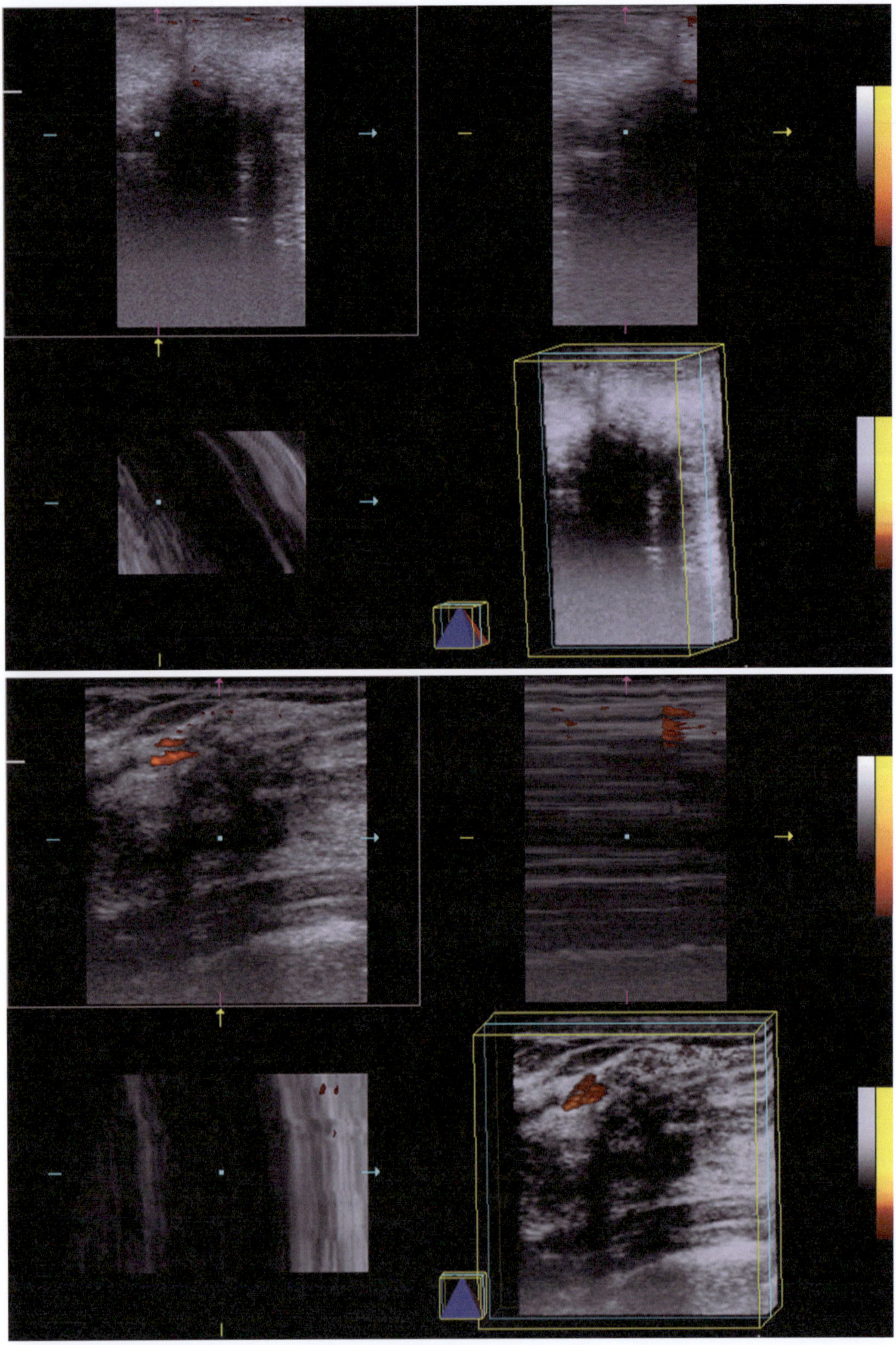

Fig. 6.8 (continued)

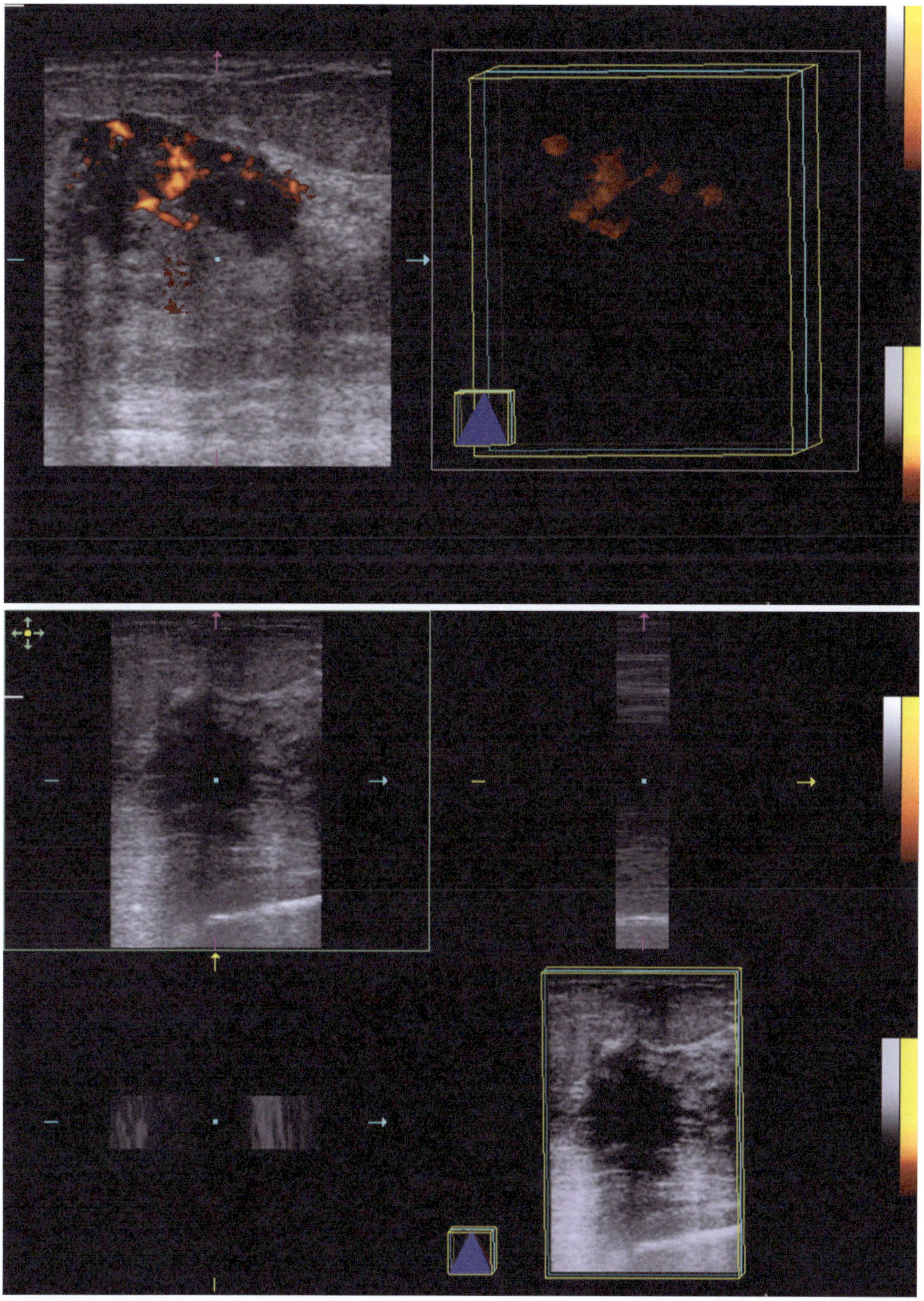

Fig. 6.8 (continued)

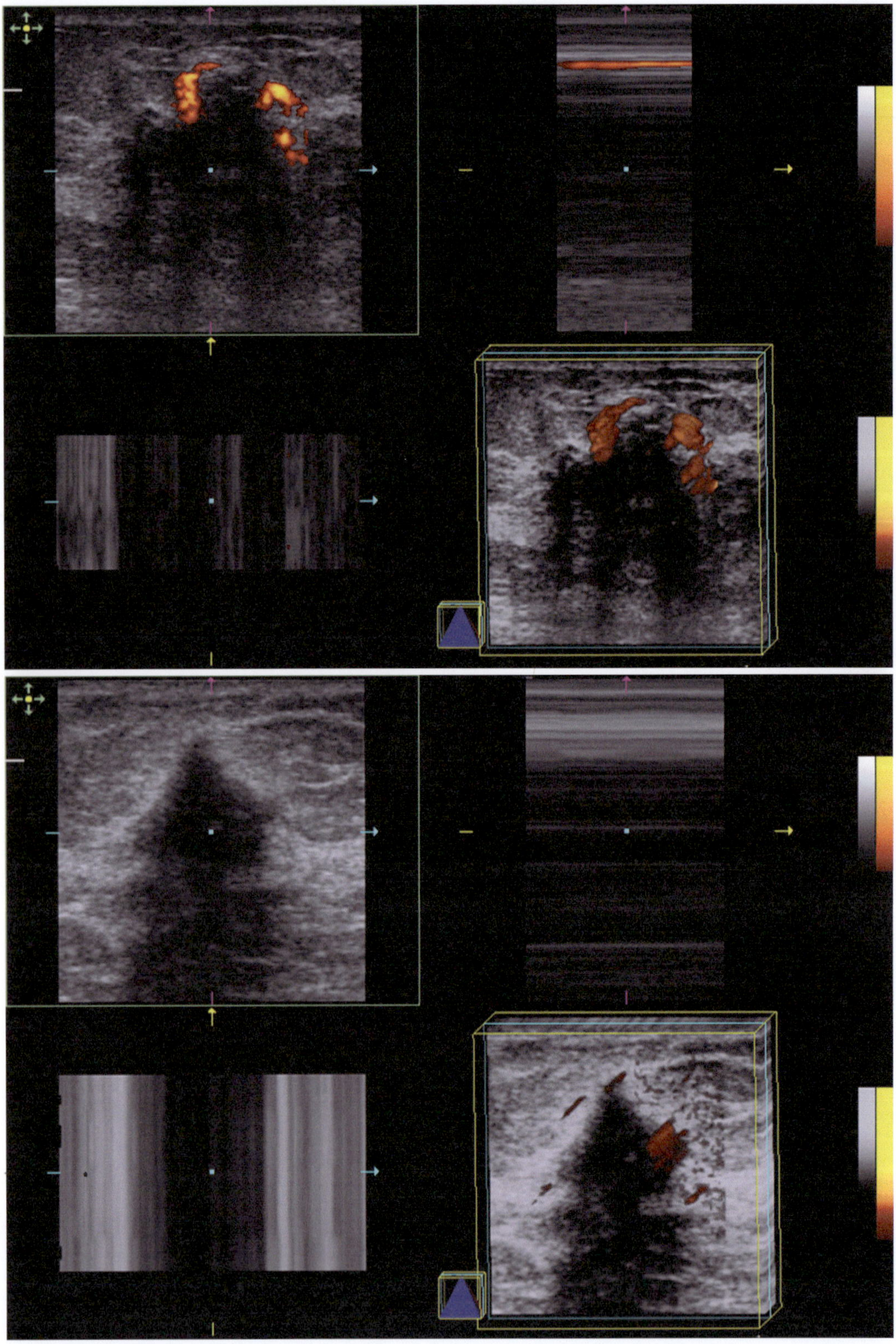

Fig. 6.8 (continued)

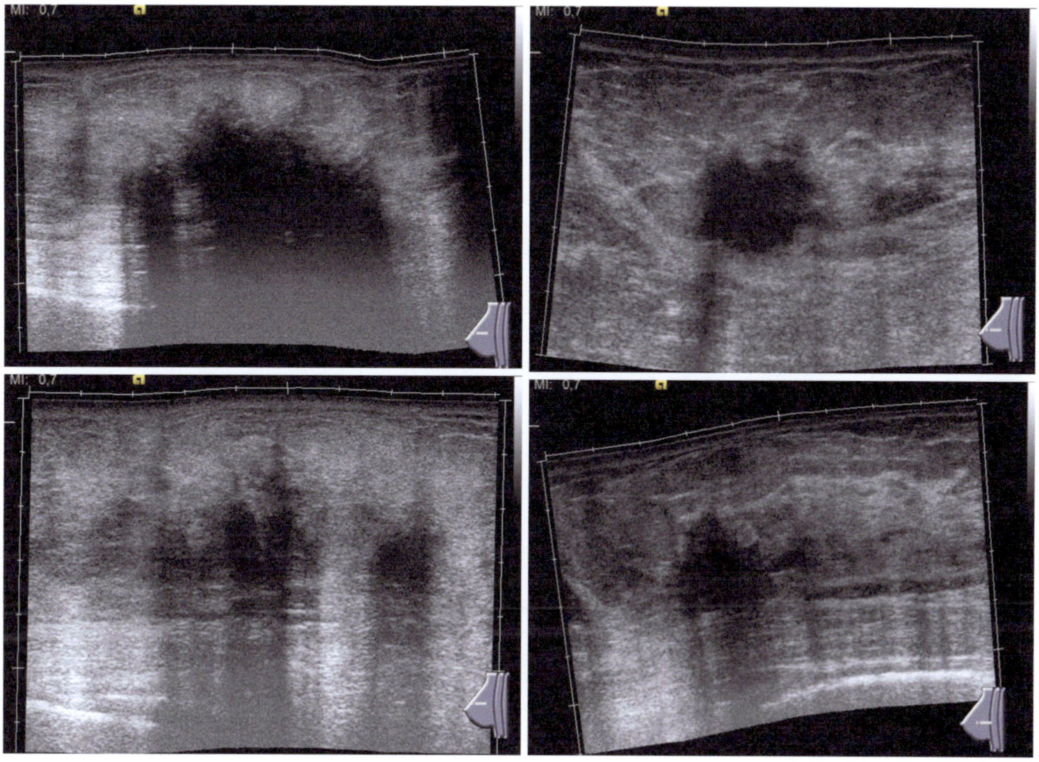

Fig. 6.9 Breast cancer. Panoramic scan. 1–4. Echograms

multicenter growth, assess invasion, and plan surgical intervention.

The multi-slicing technique is a software algorithm, which transforms 3D US image in a series of consecutive sections of 0.5–5 mm in any plane similar to CT. It permits a more objective and reliable way of analysis of the breast image associated with better accuracy (Fig. 6.10). Currently this technique is seldom used in the diagnosis of breast pathology.

Constant improvement of traditional methods and creation of new technologies is a continuous process, which results in perfection of diagnostics and healthcare in general.

Introduction in clinical practice of "hybrid" technologies assuming joint or simultaneous use of various hi-tech diagnostic procedures and technologies of US and other imaging methods is very promising.

Diagnostic accuracy of ultrasound in the detection of breast cancer is 78–94%, sensitivity, 58–100%; and specificity, 65–97% (refer to Chap. 1, Table 1.1). Its diagnostic accuracy increases with the size of the lesion: 87.3% for nodes up to 10 mm, 87.2% for 1–2 cm, 88.0% for 2–5 cm, and 100% for lesions over 5 cm.

Numerous modes of ultrasound image optimization in grayscale, color mapping, 3D, and enhanced filtration technology depending on the zone of interest significantly improve the quality of visualization and reduce the number of artifacts and noise. A wide range of post-processing options significantly reduces the examination time.

6.4 Ultrasound Elastography

Ultrasound elastography is a special technique for visualizing tissues and organs based on the difference in the elastic properties (elasticity) of normal and pathological tissues, determining their deformation under compression or vibration.

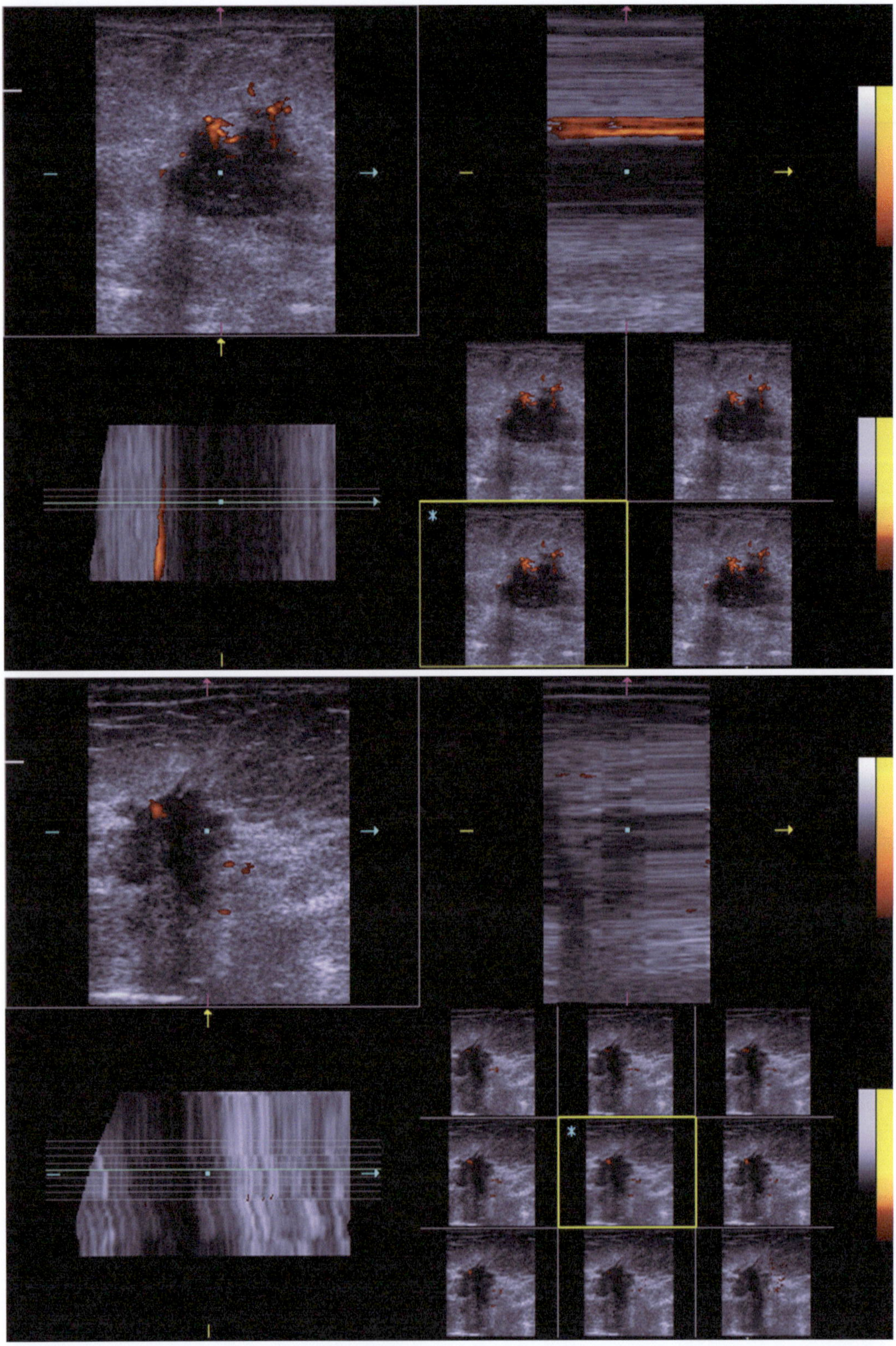

Fig. 6.10 Breast cancer. Multi-slice. 1–4. Echograms

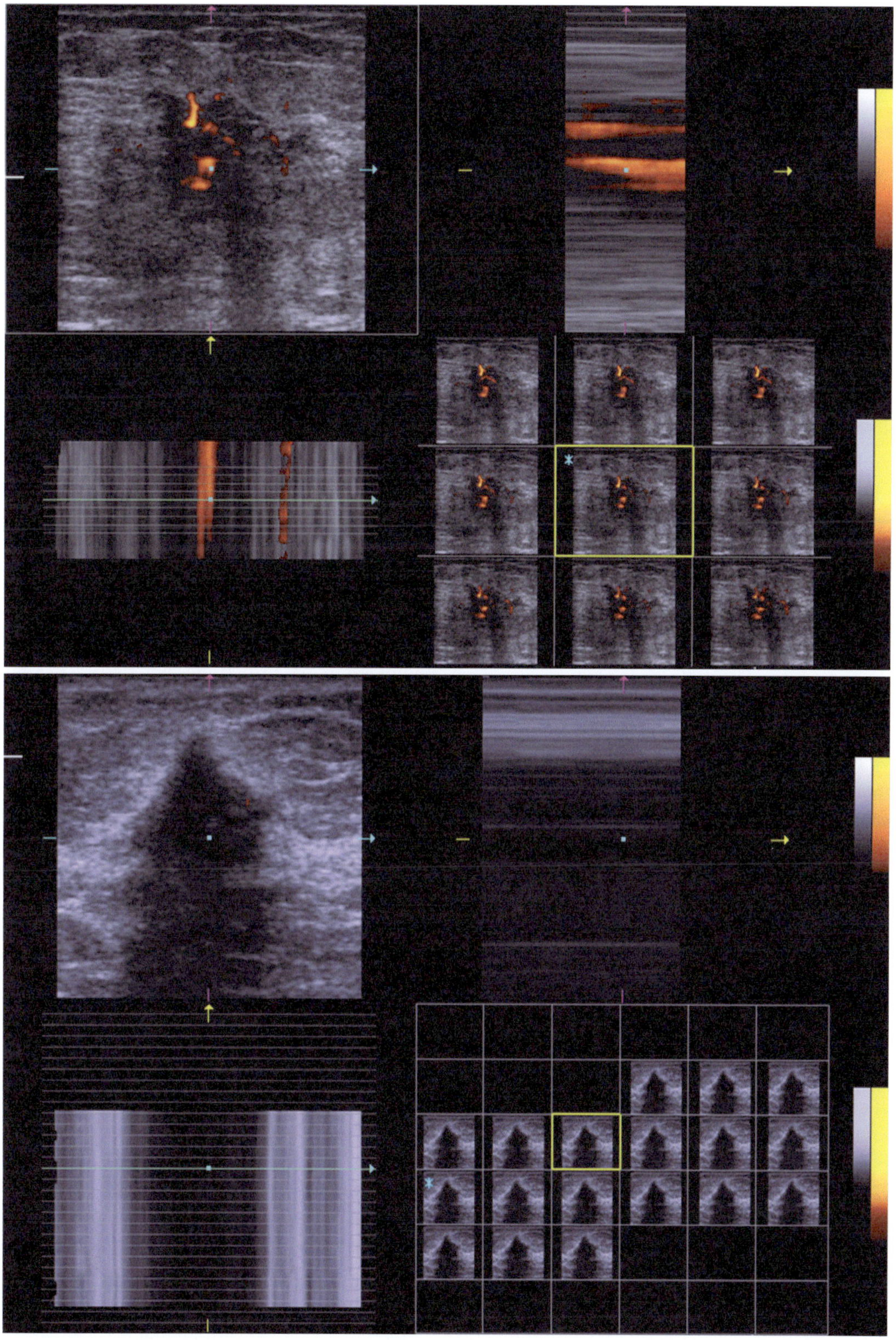

Fig. 6.10 (continued)

The methods of elastography are classified according to the methods of deformation and evaluation:

1. Quasistatic (static) elastography, or compression elastography, with the evaluation of tissue deformation (*strain elastography*—SE) and the possibility of estimation the strain ratio at the different examination sites (SR)
2. Dynamic elastography, using:
   - Mechanical impulse or vibrational pressure, using the arising shear waves (transient elastography) (*transient elastography*—TE)
   - Acoustic radiation pressure created by a long ultrasound signal, with assessment of the resulting longitudinal deformations
   - Acoustic radial force impulse (ARFI) generated by ultrasound signals focused at different depths, with the assessment of shear wave velocity (*shear wave elastography—SWE*)

Compression elastography is most common in daily practice. The method of compression was initially the most widespread due to high resolution and feasibility.

Compression elastography (ultrasound elastography, RTE, CEUS, strain imaging, static strain imaging) is a technology for visualization of tissue irregularities by their shear characteristics. It displays the difference in elasticity (stiffness) of normal and pathological tissues based on the evaluation of local deformation under dosed compression or vibration.

Compression can be applied from the outside (e.g., by the hand of the examiner); by the pulsating vibrations of the walls of the major blood vessels, heart, and chest; by a special vibrator; and statically or dynamically, once or several times with certain intervals. Compression US elastography is based on the expanded combined autocorrelation method, which analyzes standard echographic images of deformed tissues. It uses special mathematical algorithms that are precisely configured to detect any lateral displacement of the lesion. Due to various elasticity, heterogeneous elements of tissues contract differently under external compression. This allows to detect hard zones and diagnose cancer at early stages.

Compression US elastography requires the following certain rules to obtain reliable data: US probe is positioned perpendicularly to the skin over the lesion. Compression time varies from 2 to 5 s. Periodic compression is performed to obtain several images with minor artifacts. The analyzed area should necessarily contain some normal breast tissue for correct comparison with the stiffness of the lesion. Time expense to the examination is usually 1–5 min. The overall time for breast US with elastography does not exceed routine time of 10–20 min.

An elastogram is an image, which results from overlaying of the "compressive" image onto the grayscale image. Tissue elasticity image is coded with shades of gray or color palettes. Hard structures are usually colored with dark or blue. Soft areas are usually marked with light or red. Intermediate colors are applied, respectively. Scanners usually offer several color maps, such as "blue-green-red," shades of gray, or customized maps with shades of red or other colors.

Tissues under the US probe are deformed with compression (strain). Abnormal tissues exhibit unique features—malignant tumors are "hard" as compared with surrounding normal tissues.

Uniform compression of the whole breast is impossible due to comparatively small size of US probe. Normal breast parenchyma with moderate compression exhibits relatively regular, homogeneous, and symmetric fine-grained pattern (refer to Chap. 3). Compression of individual breast segments or lesions is performed more effectively.

The advantage of compression US elastography is that this technique is relatively simple (though not always easily reproducible).

Disadvantages of manual compression with compression US elastography are as follows:

- Inability to obtain quantitative data about tissue stiffness with Young's modulus, because the distribution of pressure in the examined area is unknown. However, it is possible to carry out quantitative comparison of the difference in relative deformations in the site of interest and in the surrounding tissues.
- Correlation of the deformation and the compression force is nonlinear and depends on

time. This is associated with viscosity and uneven elasticity of the tissues.

- Elasticity of the tissue in different planes is not similar. In addition, the investigated areas comprise various liquid inclusions, borders of adjacent organs, scars, etc.
- Echo signal may be distorted during tissue deformation.
- Sensitivity of the method decreases with depth. This is due to the fact that biological tissues, in addition to elasticity, possess viscosity. This leads to the decrease of static pressure with depth and, consequently, to a decreased deformation of deeper tissues.
- Dependence of the result on the force and direction of compression and thus on the experience and skills of an examiner.
- Difficulties in performing compression in certain cases.
- Possible patient's discomfort or pain.
- Significant "noise" and ultrasound artifacts due to the characteristics of the examined structures, arterial pulsation, movements, etc.

The requirements for obtaining elastograms with minimal distortion are listed below:

- Location of the examined structures not deeper than 3–4 cm
- Homogeneity of nearby tissues
- Absence of flat anatomical structures, which make sliding movements
- Some distance between the lesion and the probe
- Absence of damping structures, for example, large veins
- The area of applied pressure should be larger than the examined site
- Limited number of target lesions

Quantitative and qualitative diagnostic criteria for the assessment of US elastography are developed. Qualitative criterion is the analysis of distribution of breast tissue elasticity, quantitative-strain ratio - characterizes the ratio of the degree of deformation of breast lesion and normal surrounding tissues (Rozhkova et al. 2010; Sencha et al. 2013).

Zubarev (2009) reports five types of stiffness of lesions depending on color pattern with US elastography. Dark-blue (stiff) staining that corresponds to the fifth type of color pattern is a characteristic for breast carcinoma. The data obtained with US elastography facilitate differential diagnosis of breast lesions of tumoral nature in complex and doubtful cases.

Rozhkova et al. (2011) add two more types of pattern: three-leveled, which is a characteristic for fluid-containing lesions, and mosaic. Malignant breast lesions, according to the authors, are characterized by the fourth and fifth types according to Ueno classification in 78.6%. The fourth type was identified in 62.5% of breast carcinoma and was characterized by homogeneous blue staining of the tumor with normal elasticity of surrounding tissues. The fifth type of sonoelastogram, which is a characteristic only for cancer, reflected typical features of dense lesions with infiltrating growth. Benign breast lesions, according to the authors, are characterized by the first, second, sixth, and seventh types of elastogram depending on the contents in 85.2% of cases.

Sencha et al. 2011, in a series of 88 cases of compression US elastography, demonstrated that breast carcinoma is more often (in 76.1%) characterized by intense, well-circumscribed hard (stiff) staining (Fig. 6.11). Mixed (blue-green-red) pattern was observed in 12.5% (Fig. 6.12). Additionally, 81.8% of breast lesions exhibited irregular color pattern (Fig. 6.13).

Sencha et al. (2011) report that 22.7% of the malignant lesions are measured 0.5–10 mm different size on grayscale and elastographic images. The malignant lesions with elastography were larger than on grayscale image in 85% and smaller in 15% of cases (Fig. 6.14).

According to Sencha et al. (2011), compression US elastography fails to specify breast disease in 11.4% of patients. This appears as the absence of any color pattern within the lesion, similar color of the lesion and the surrounding structures, or significant artifacts (Fig. 6.15).

Complex use of B-mode and compression US elastography significantly improves the diagnostic accuracy of US: the sensitivity reaches 73.7–96%, specificity 74.7–99%, accuracy 82.5–86.9%, positive predictive value 51.1–97%, and negative predictive value 60.7–99% (Rozhkova et al. 2010; Sencha et al. 2011).

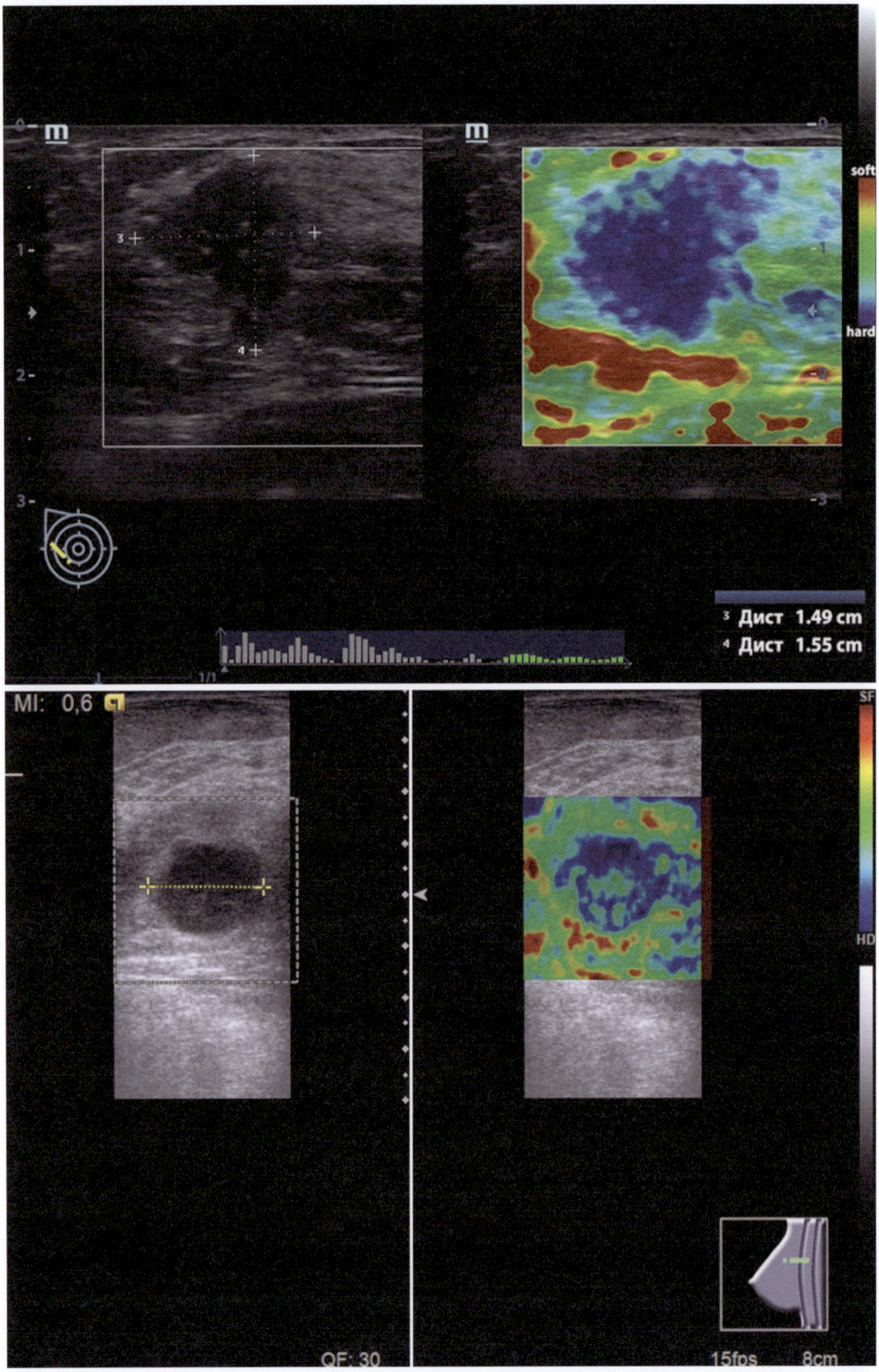

Fig. 6.11 Breast cancer. Compression US elastography. 1–8. Intensive stiff color of the tumor that is different from surrounding parenchyma

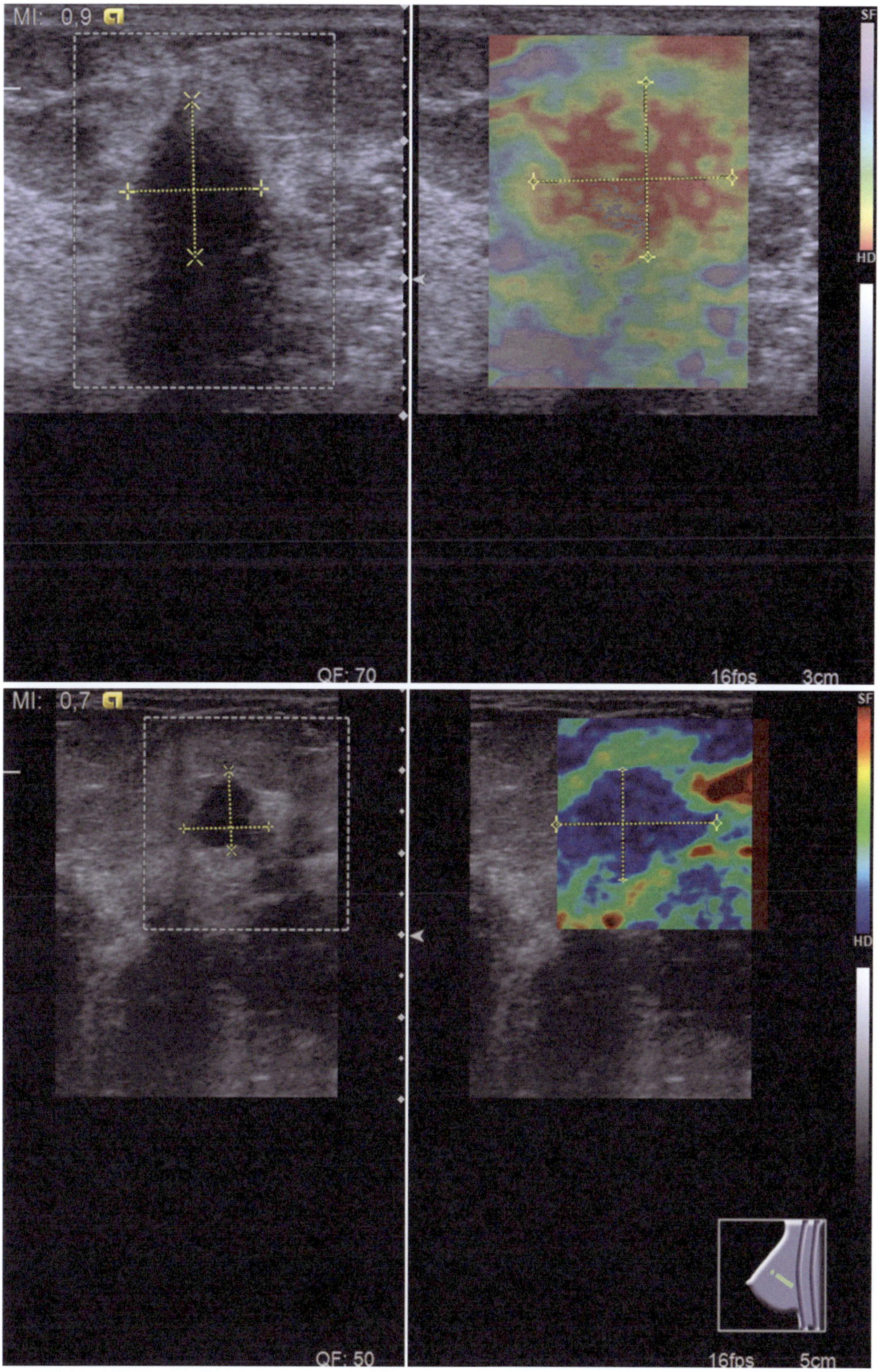

Fig. 6.11 (continued)

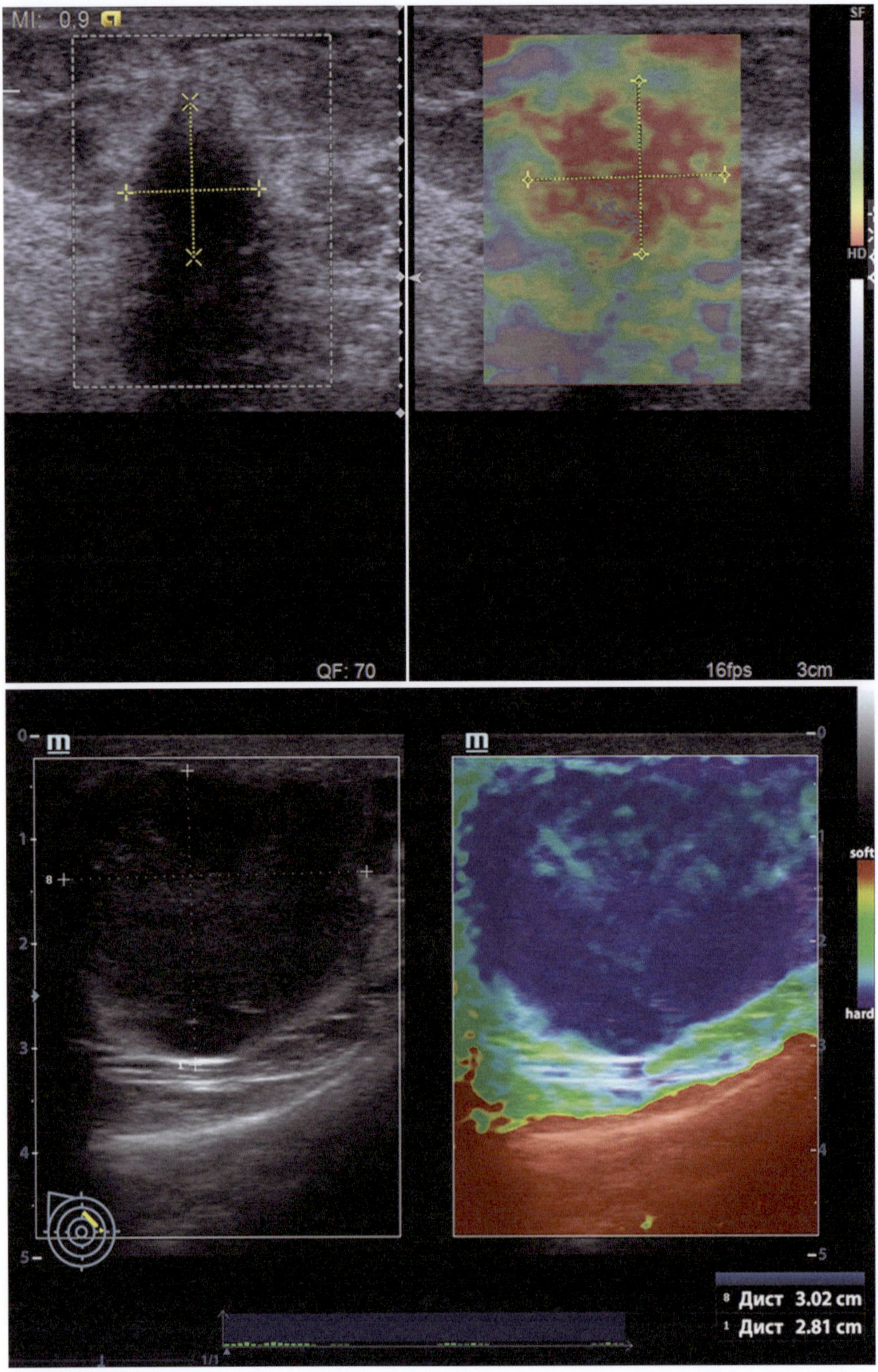

Fig. 6.11 (continued)

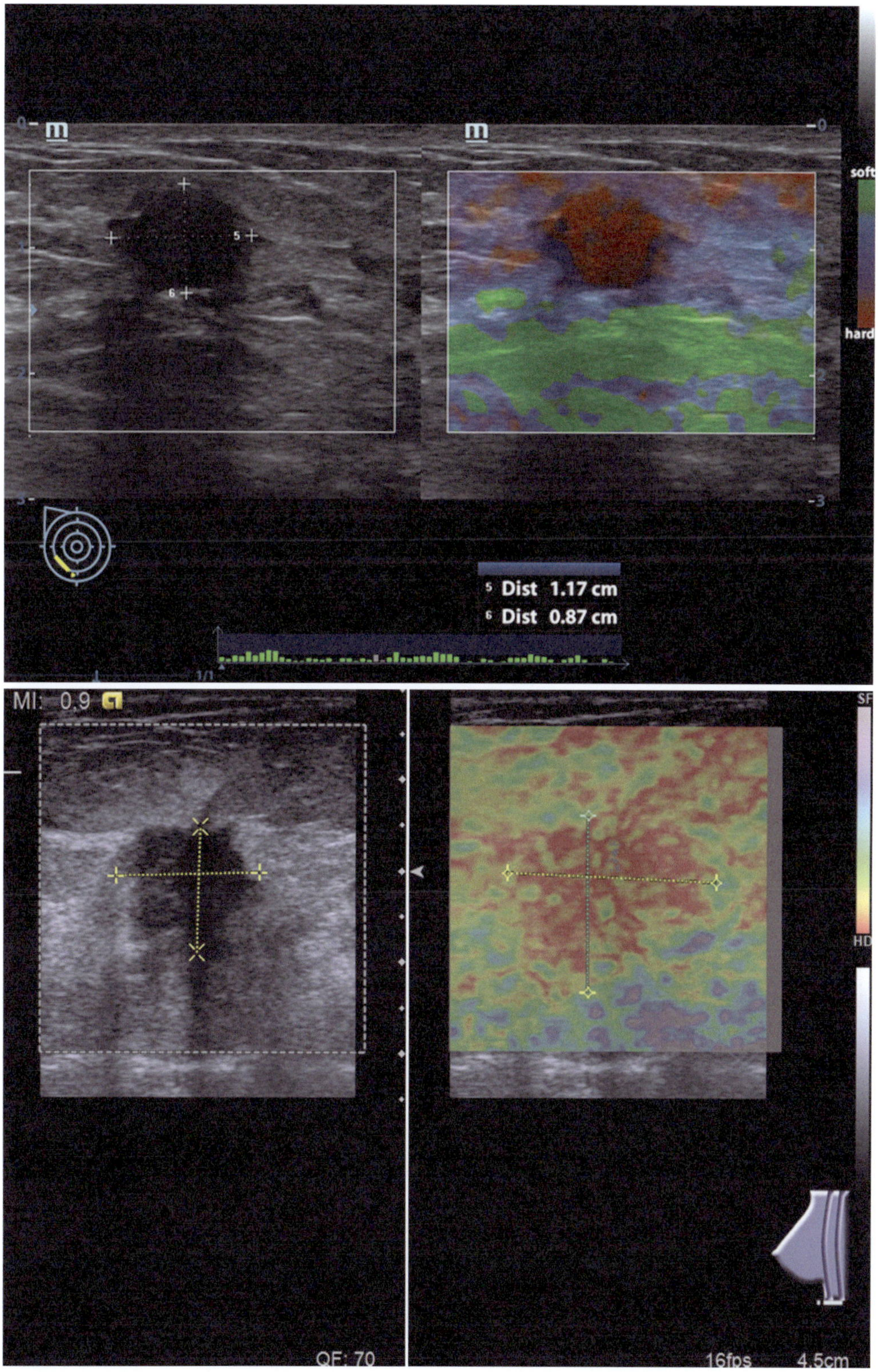

Fig. 6.11 (continued)

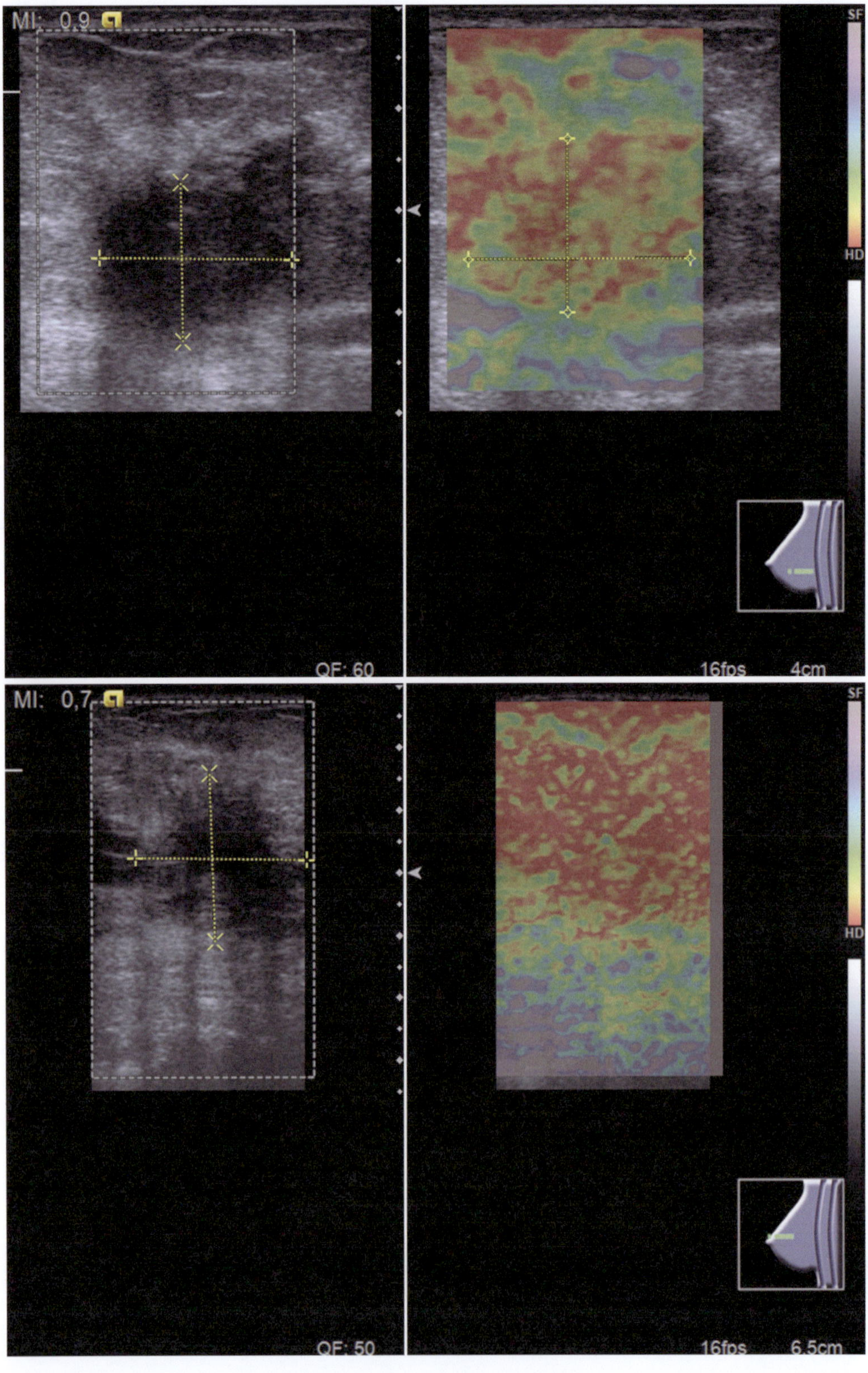

Fig. 6.12 Breast cancer. Compression US elastography. 1–8. Mixed coloring

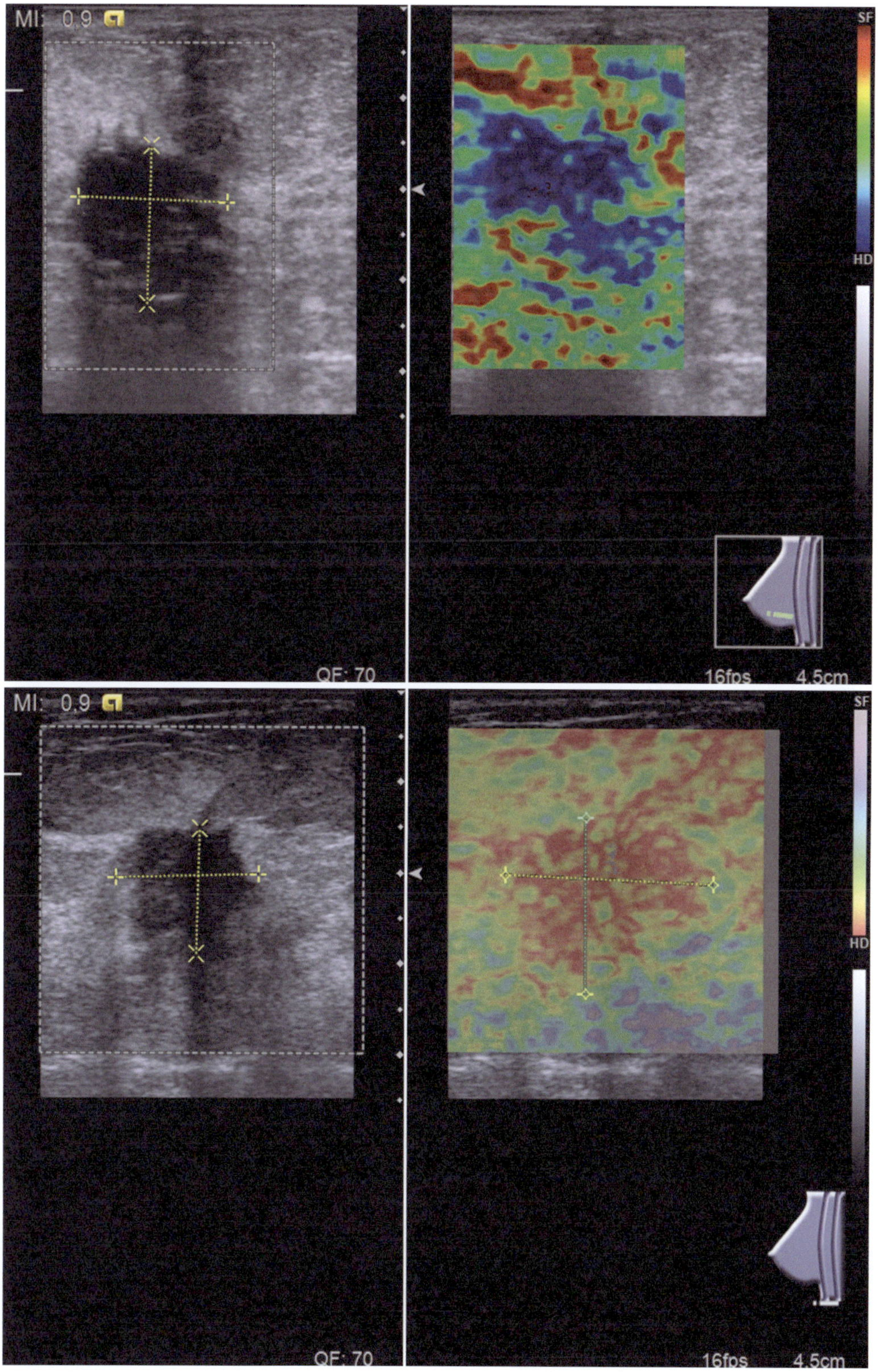

Fig. 6.12 (continued)

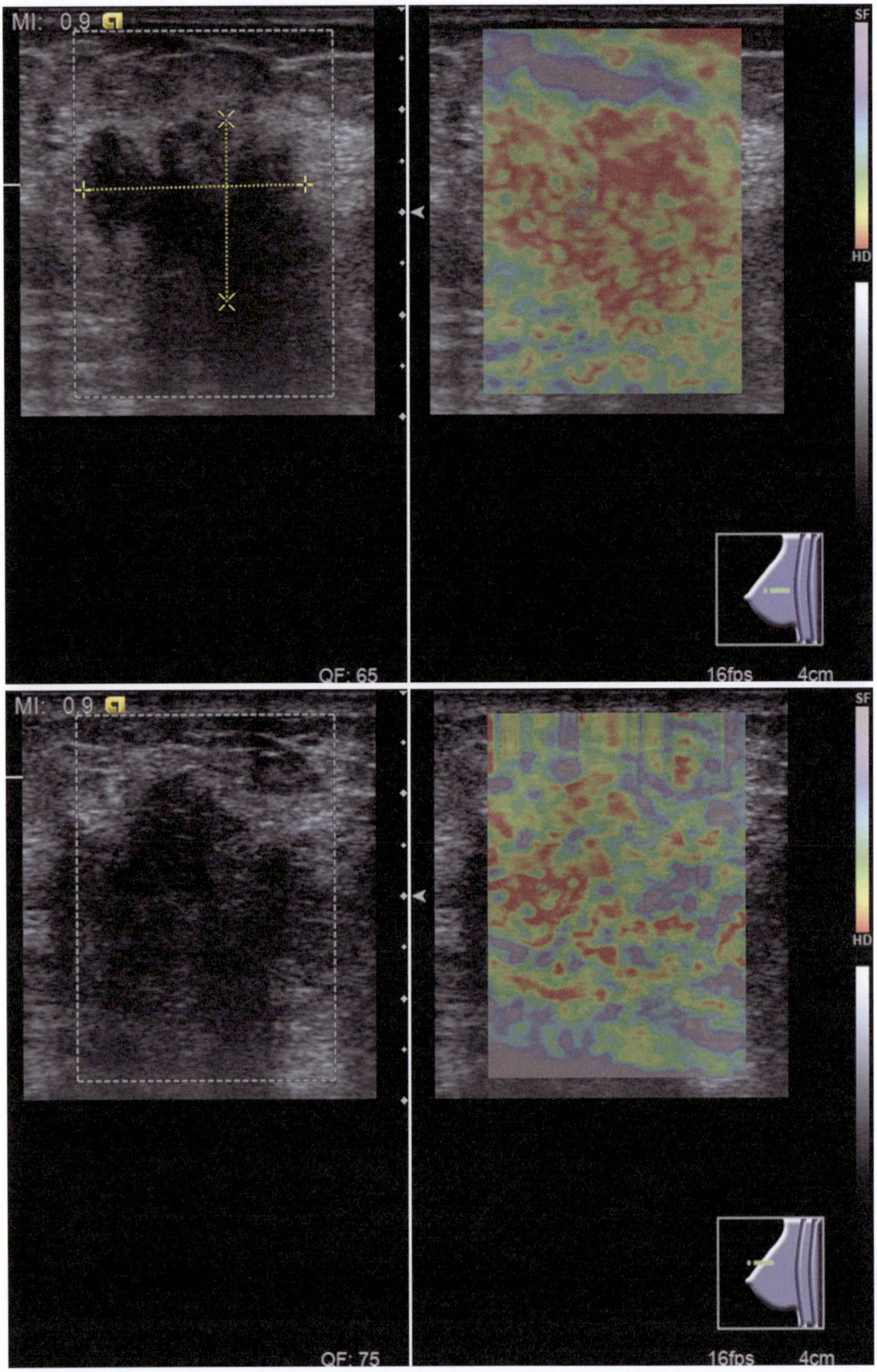

Fig. 6.12 (continued)

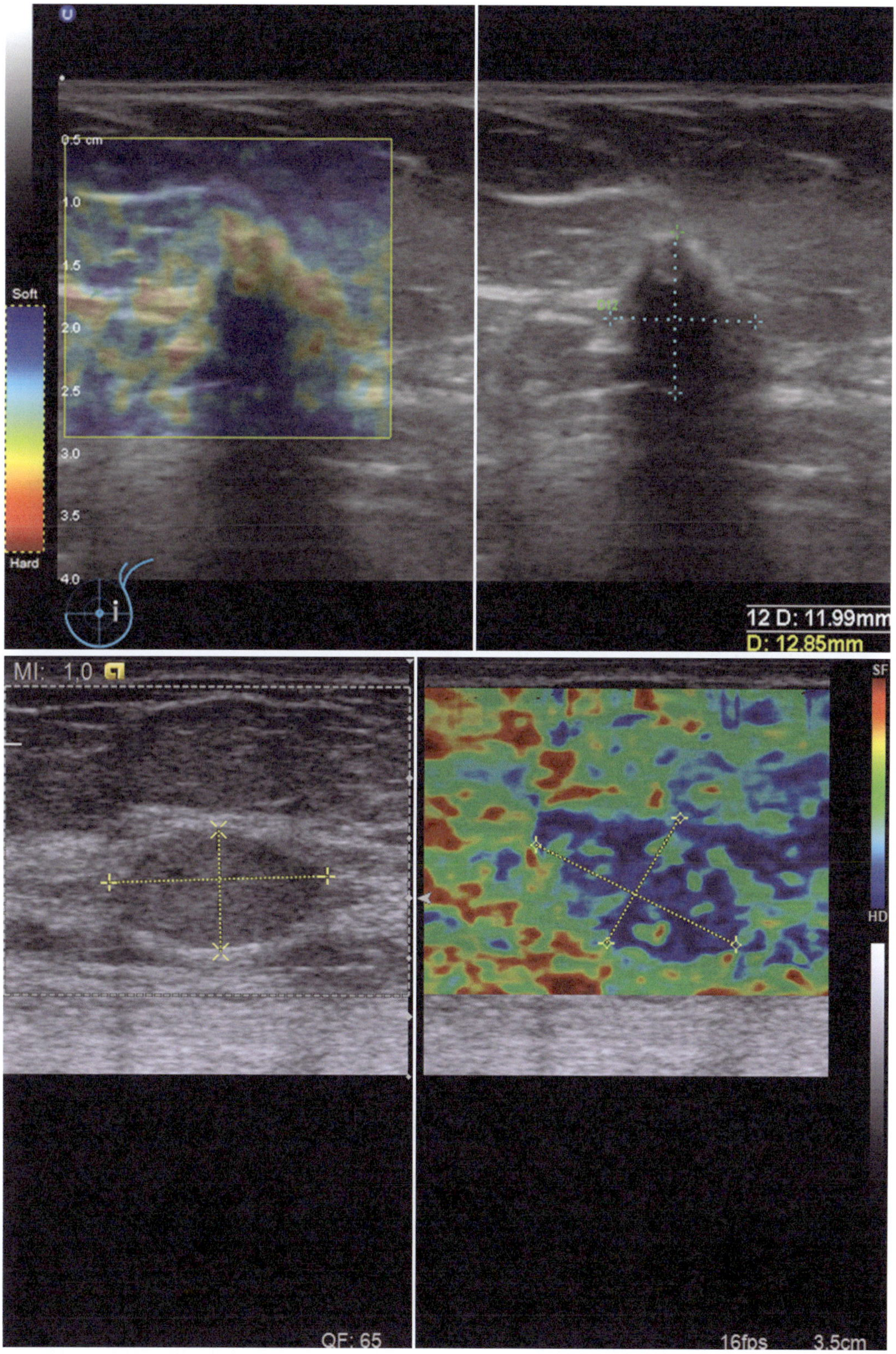

Fig. 6.12 (continued)

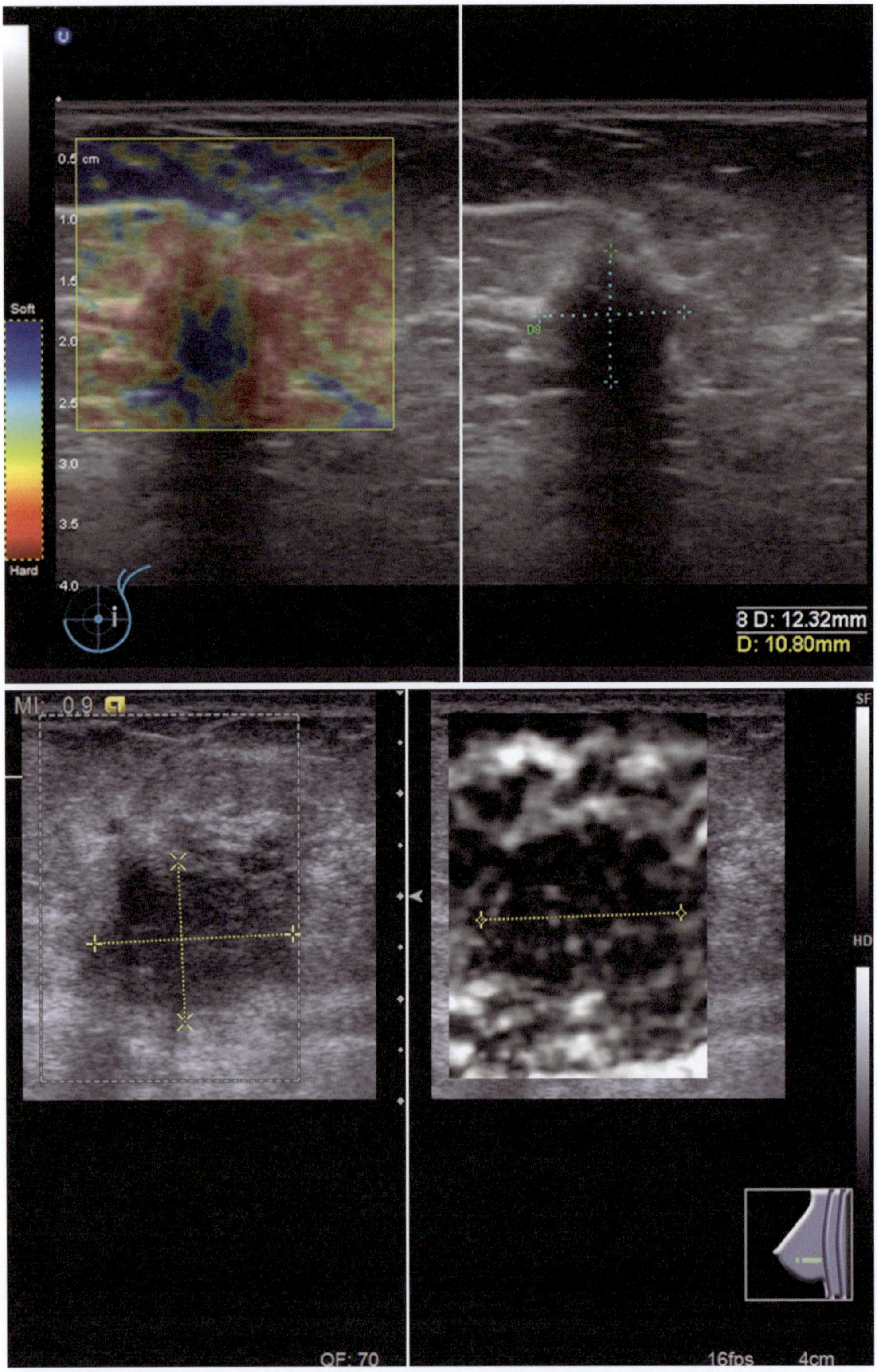

Fig. 6.13 Breast cancer. Compression US elastography. 1–4. Irregular tumor coloring

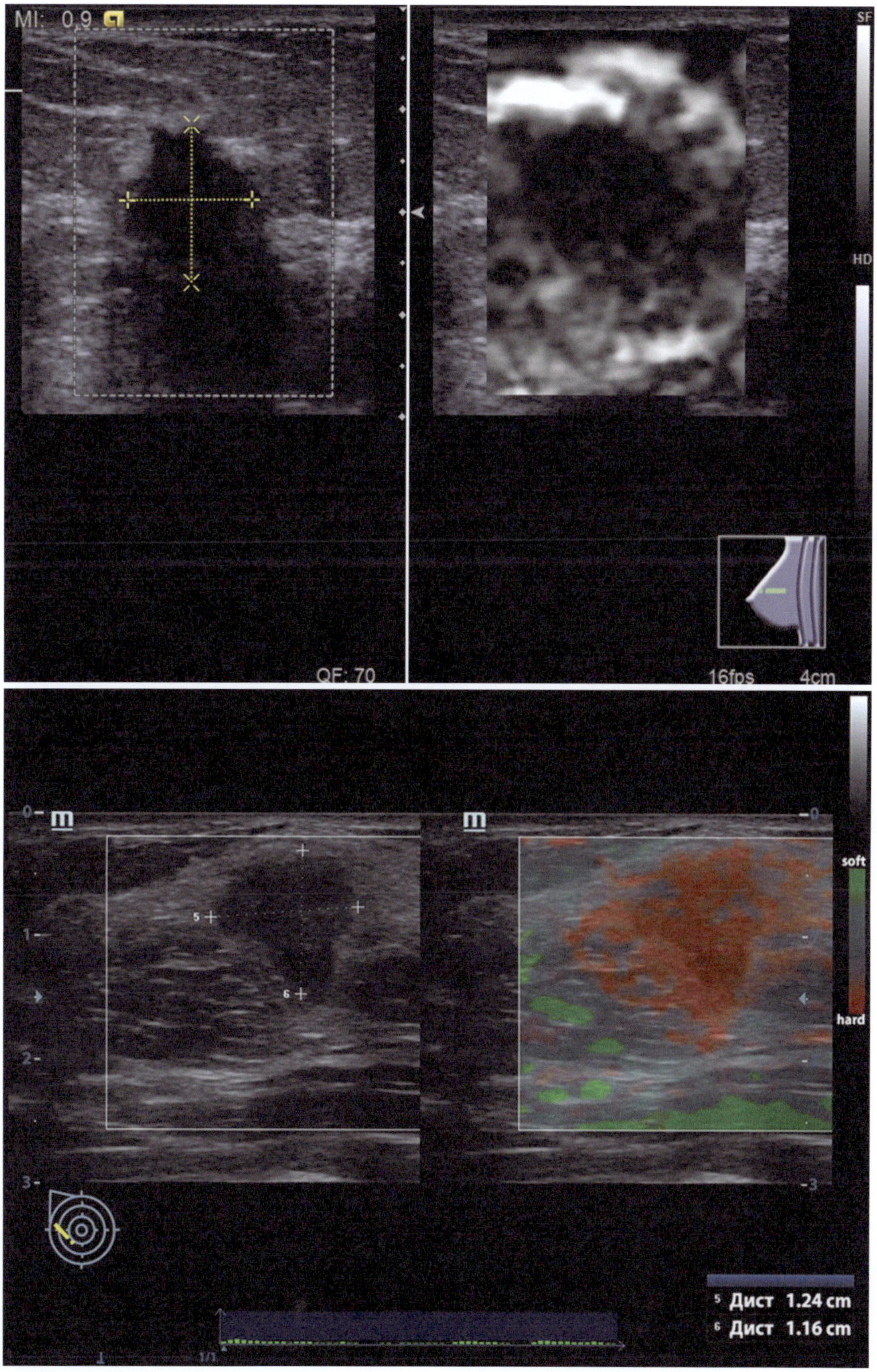

Fig. 6.13 (continued)

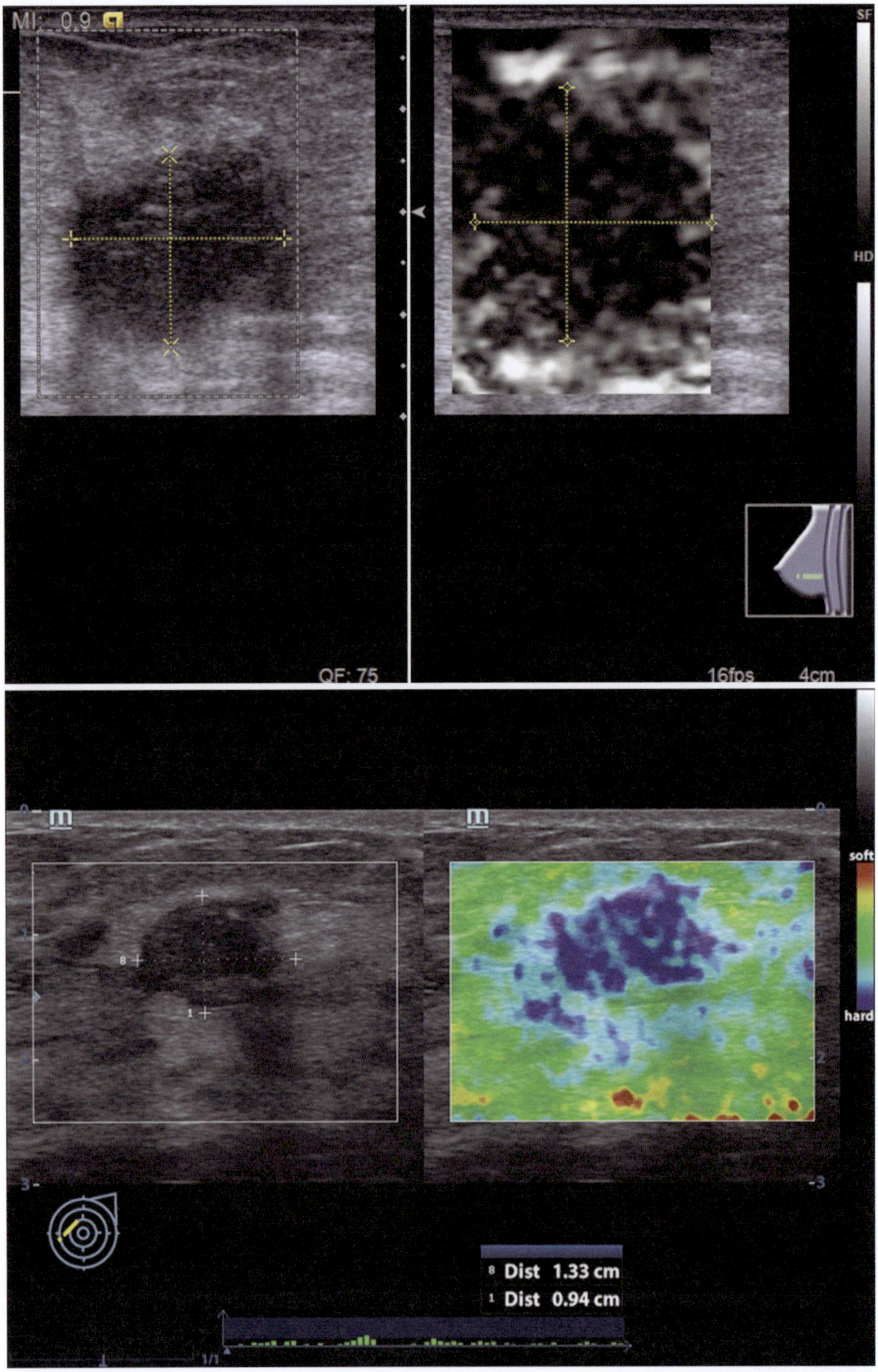

Fig. 6.14 Breast cancer. Compression US elastography. 1–6. Different tumor sizes on grayscale and elastographic images

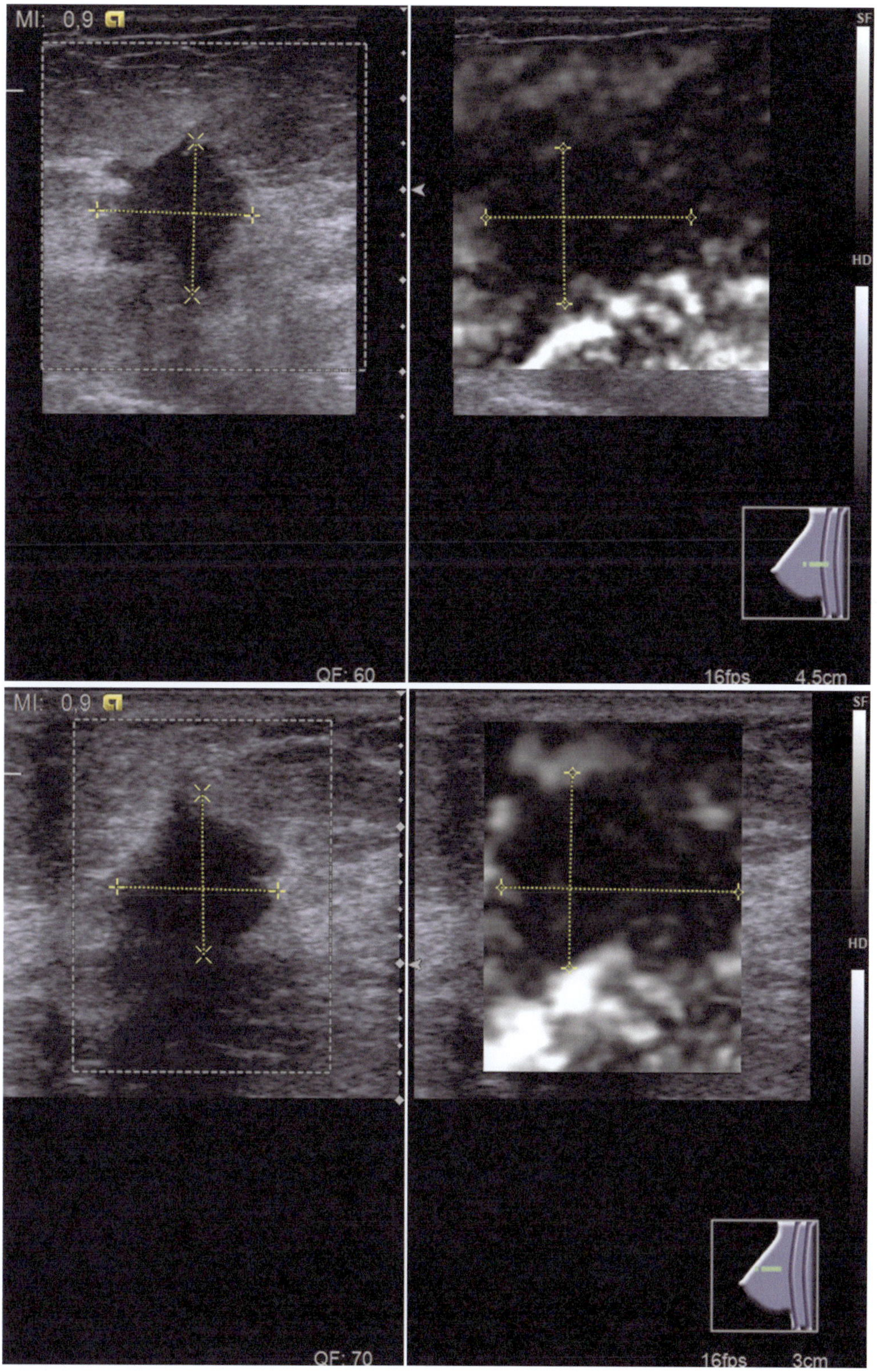

Fig. 6.14 (continued)

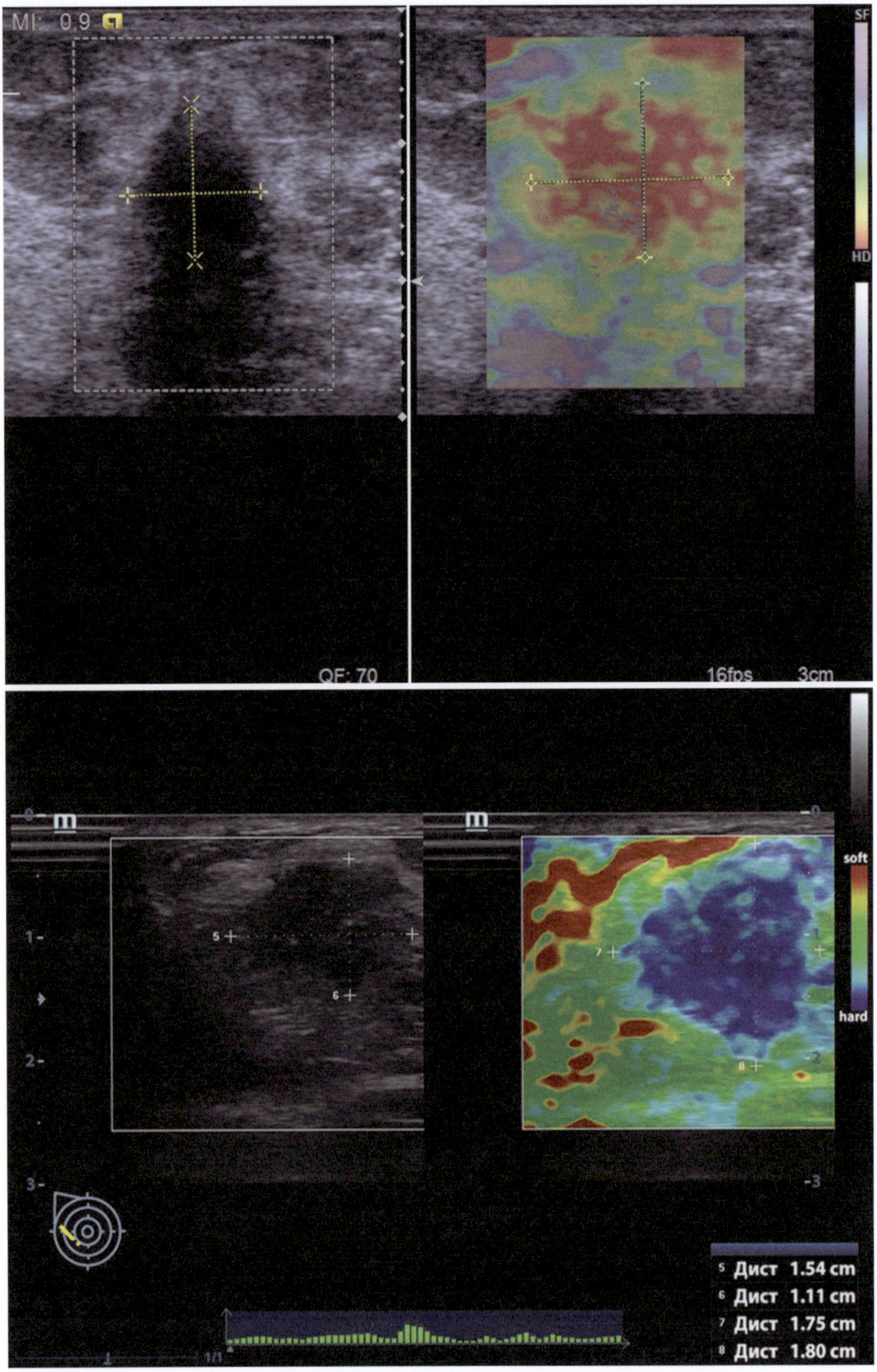

Fig. 6.14 (continued)

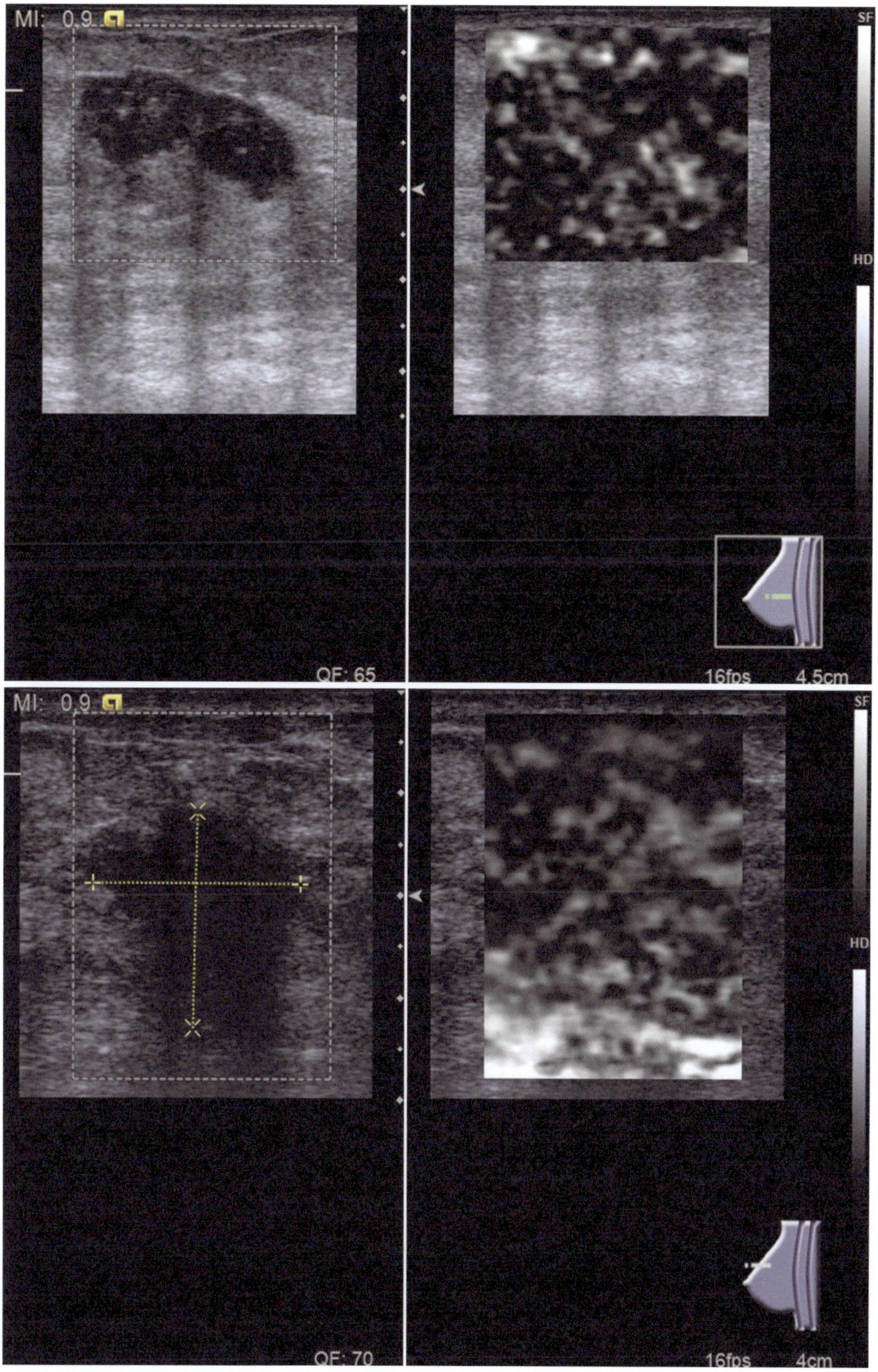

Fig. 6.15 Breast cancer. Compression US elastography. 1–4. Tumor cannot be differentiated with compression US elastography from the surrounding tissues

However, compression US elastography is often subjective. Thus the method fails to reveal agglomerations of microcalcifications in an area <1.5 cm and the majority of intraductal neoplasms. Therefore, it cannot be used as a screening method. US elastography is valuable for masses smaller than 3 cm in diameter and located at depth of 1–3 cm. It is compromised by the lesions smaller than 0.5 cm (Rozhkova et al. 2010).

The higher the tissue density (typical malignant tumors), the higher the shear wave velocity (Piscaglia et al. 2011). Thus, the shear wave velocity is an indicator and a reliable feature of tissue density. The higher the index, the stiffer the tissue. Shear waves in heterogeneous tissues spread in a more complex way and may be distorted due to reflections from the borders of structures with different acoustic impedances. The technology of assessment of shear wave velocity helps to obtain reliable results and allows to assess the stiffness of deeply located lesions, which are impossible to assess with compression elastography.

Shear wave elastography permits objective definition of the velocity of shear waves in tissues and calculation of Young's modulus of elasticity in kPa. It enables quantitative elastographic assessment of the status of the breast tissue (Postnova et al. 2011; Mitkov et al. 2011). Elastometry works in real time and is completely quantitative and in many aspects operator independent.

Quantitative indicators of ultrasound elasticity of tissues are Young's modulus, shear wave velocity, elasticity indices, strain ratio, SWE-ratio, etc. Young's modulus for the normal breast is 18–24 kPa, for fibrous tissue 96–244 kPa, and for breast cancer 22–560 kPa (Fig. 6.16).

One example of the technology of shear wave elastography is acoustic radiation force impulse (ARFI). ARFI (virtual touch) is a method of radiologic imaging with an amplified acoustic pulse, assessing elasticity with the use of a remotely generated, focused acoustic beam with a short (longer than 100 μs) acoustic compression pulse directed toward the examined site to excite the tissue and to monitor its response (an offset). The method is based on Young's law, stating that the tissue elasticity is inversely related to the velocity of shear wave. The amplitude of the resulting displacement indicates the relative stiffness of structures (e.g., pathological foci) within a soft tissue; quantitative measurements of tissue stiffness are possible by determination of the shear wave velocity (Zubarev 2009) (Fig. 6.17).

US probe during ARFI measurements is positioned over the lesion with sample volume gate in its center. The time of measurement that passes in automatic regimen after pressing of a certain key of the scanner as a rule does not exceed 2–5 s. After the calculation of the average shear wave velocity within the tumor (3–5 measurements), the same is carried out in 2–3 areas of normal breast parenchyma on the distance of more than 1–1.5 cm from its border. The comparison of results and analysis usually does not take more than 1–5 min. The general time of breast US with the use of complex US options, including ARFI, does not exceed 10–20 min.

Shear wave velocity threshold for differentiation of breast cancer with ARFI mode is 3.23 m/s, the reproducibility of SWE measurements is 40.3–44.4%, and the sensitivity and specificity are 82.4% and 80.4%, respectively (Mitkov et al. 2013, 2014, 2015).

The other method of quantitative analysis is *strain ratio* (elasticity modulus, stiffness coefficient, elasticity coefficient, SWE-ratio index, etc.), which is calculated as a ratio of strain index of the lesion to the same of normal tissue (Fig. 6.18).

The higher the tissue density (that is common for malignant tumors), the higher the shear wave velocity (Piscaglia et al. 2011). Thus, the wave velocity measured with this technique is a reliable indicator of tissue density. According to Zubarev (2009), intraductal breast carcinoma in situ is characterized with the strain ratio of 5.2, infiltrative lobular cancer 16.58, fibroadenoma 1.02 ± 0.21, and benign intraductal papilloma 1.37. He reported the sensitivity of this method in the diagnosis of breast lesions is 78.9%, specificity 95.2%, and diagnostic accuracy 90.1%.

Rozhkova et al. (2011) reported that strain ratio in 83.2% of breast carcinomas was higher

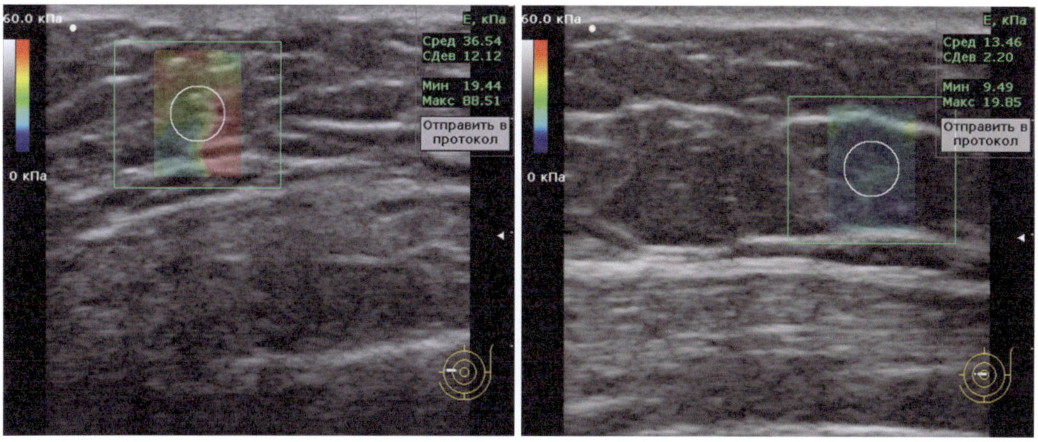

Fig. 6.16 Measurement of Young's modulus of breast parenchyma

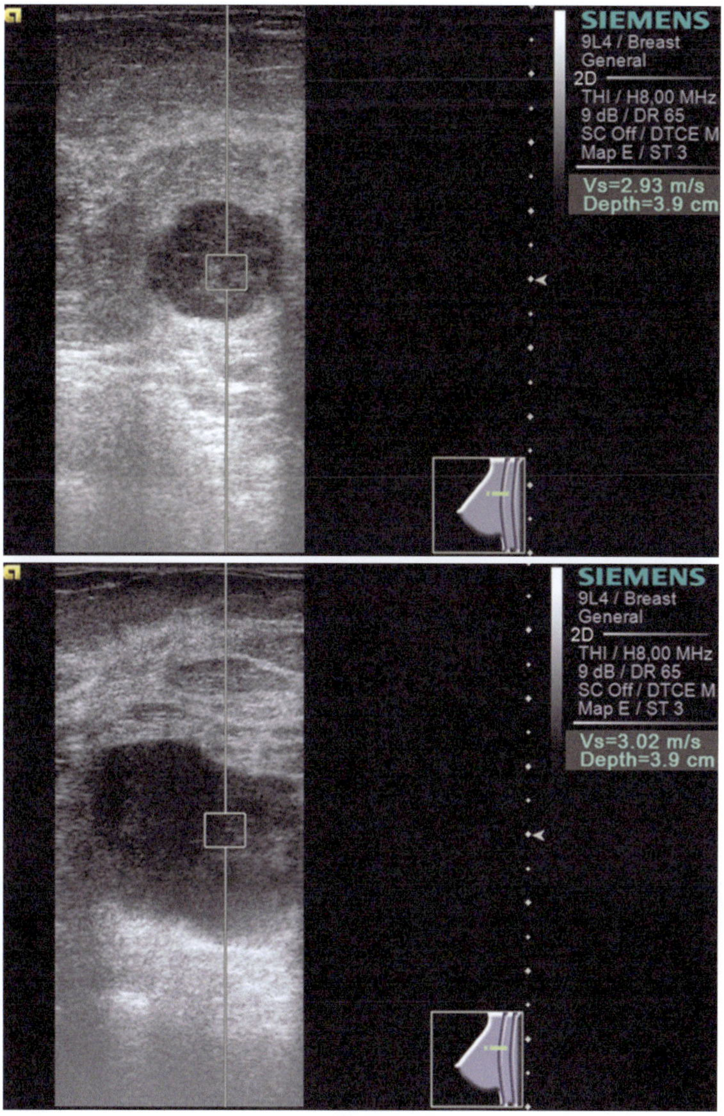

Fig. 6.17 Breast cancer. ARFI. Shear wave velocity measurement in the tumor

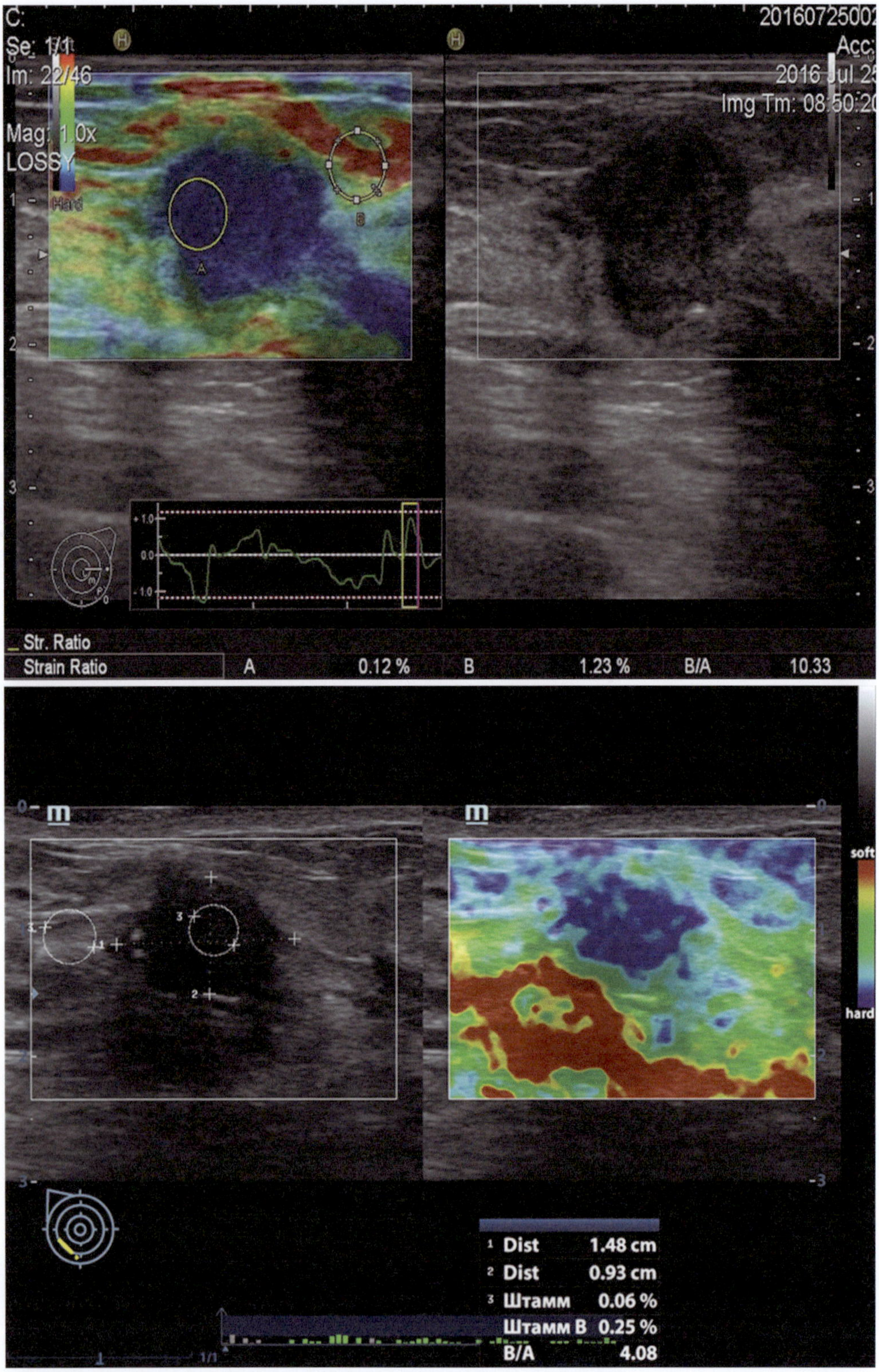

Fig. 6.18 Breast cancer. Sonogram. Strain ratio measurement. High stiffness coefficient

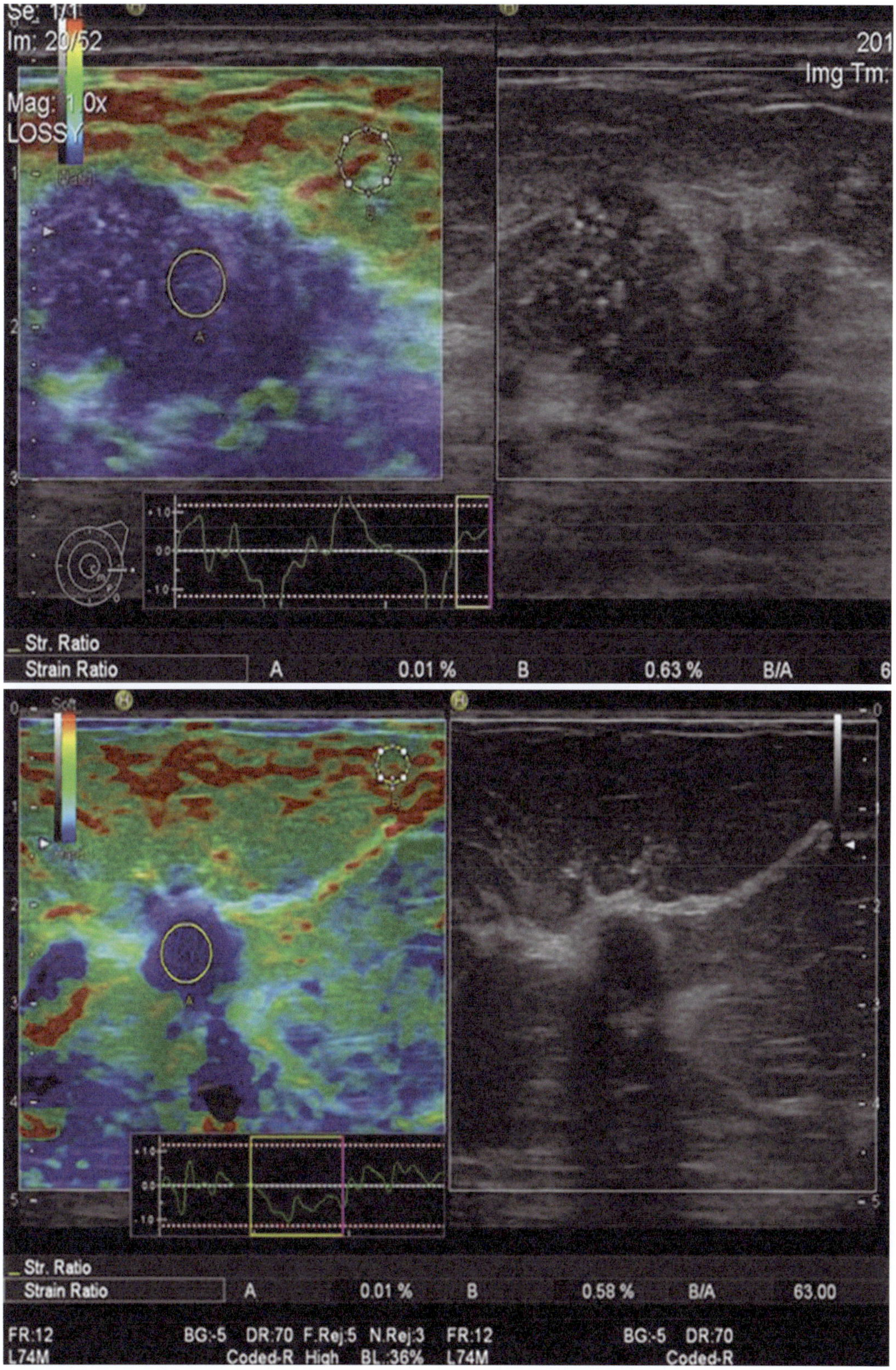

Fig. 6.18 (continued)

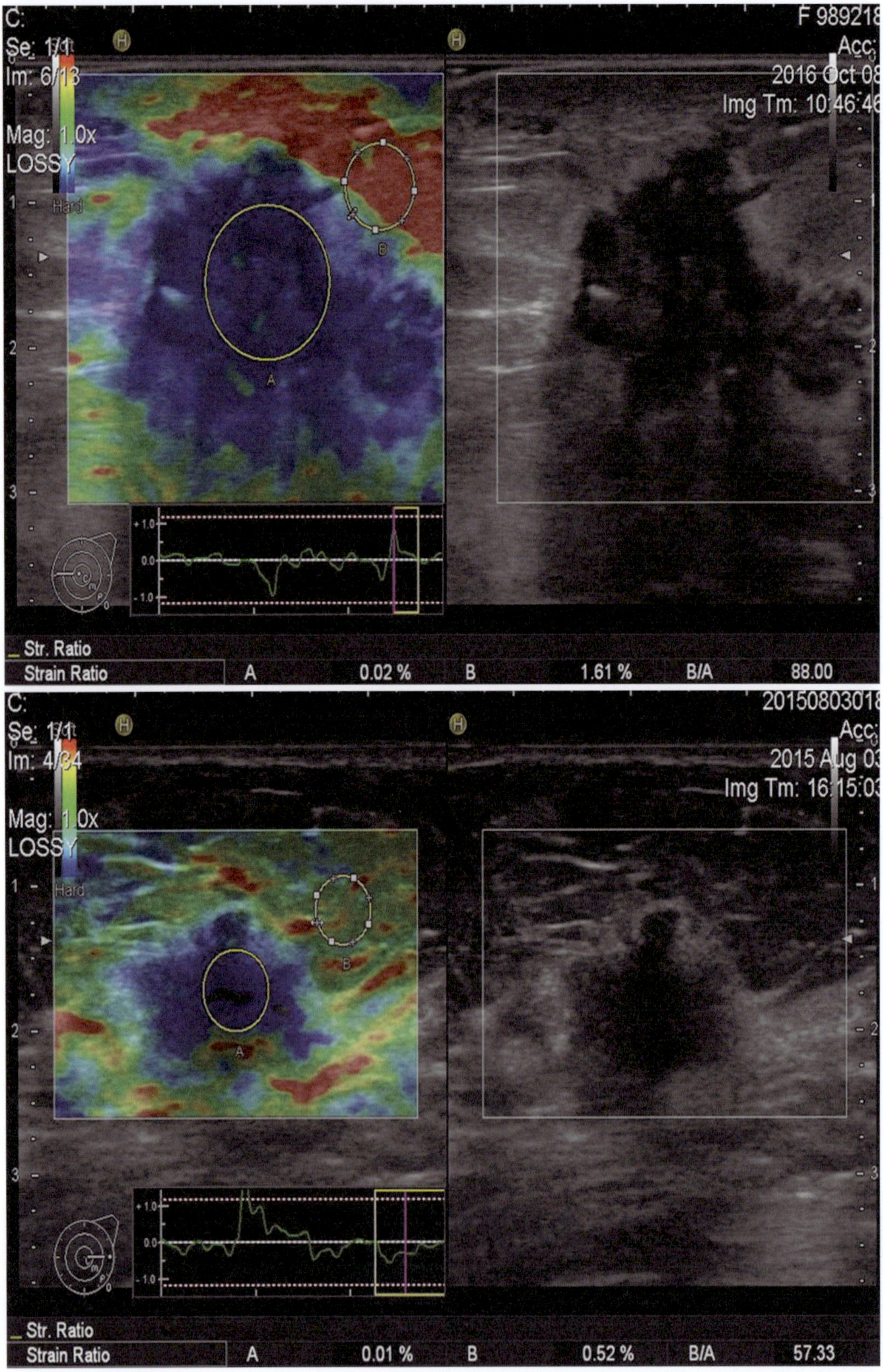

Fig. 6.18 (continued)

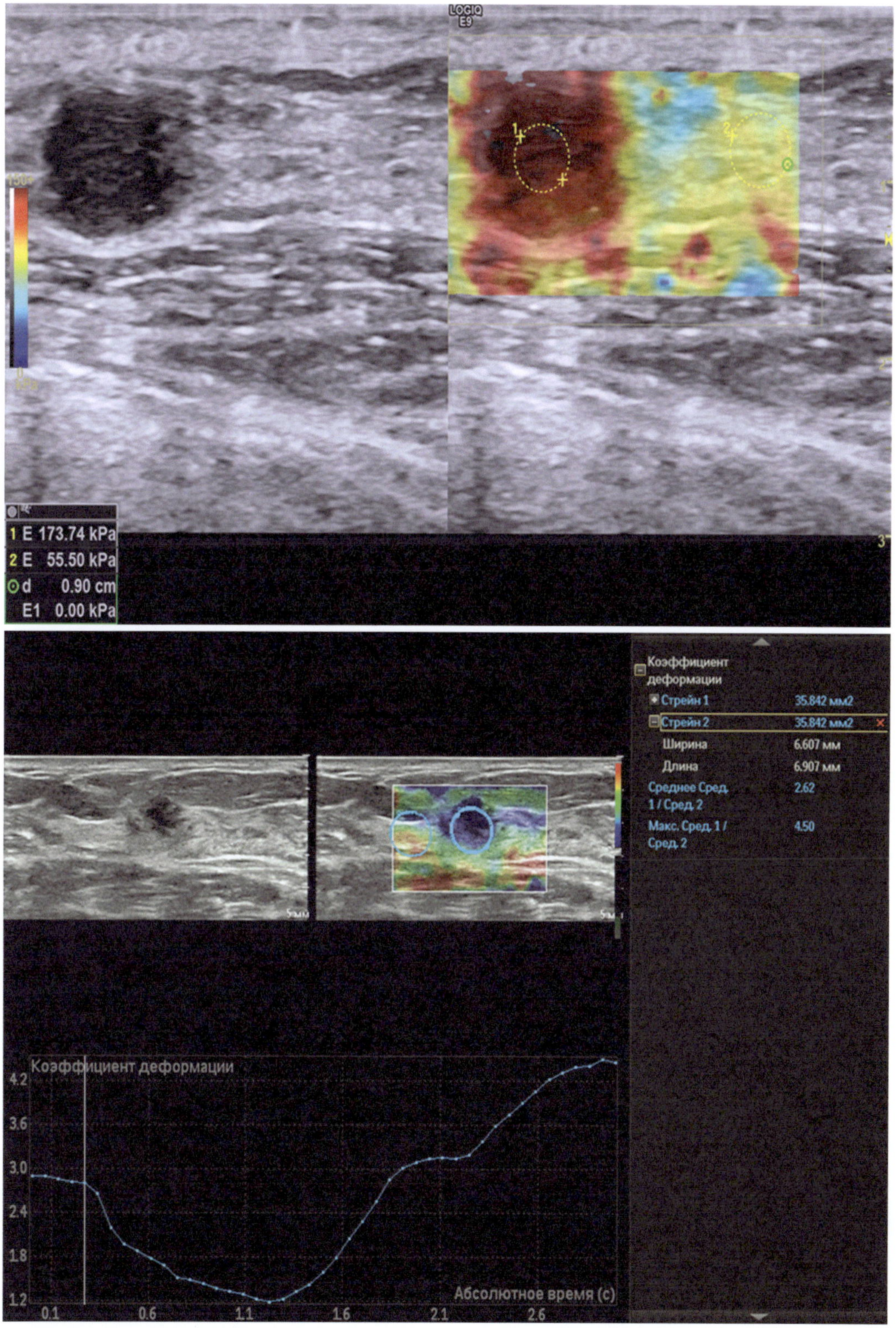

Fig. 6.18 (continued)

than 4.3 (22.9 ± 2.14 on the average) and ranged from 4.3 to 102.1 depending on histological structure of the lesion. Strain ratio was lower in noninvasive tumors (11.33 ± 4.51) than in infiltrative types of cancer (25.51 ± 2.58). Benign breast lesions in 94% demonstrated strain ratio below 4.3.

According to Postnova et al. (2011), stiffness of fat lobules is 4–20 kPa, of cysts 1.7–10, of FA 9–30, and of breast cancer 41–297 kPa.

According to Rozhkova et al. (2011), US elastography has a number of limitations. First of all, it permits assessment of the breast changes, which can be imaged with routine US. US in combination with US elastography cannot be used as a screening method. Second, elastography is of low value in cases of diffuse changes and significant increase in its density involving the whole breast (e.g., infiltrative type of breast carcinoma without any dominant lesion, diffuse mastitis, and early postradiation changes). Third, it is thought that the quality of elastogram depends on the size of a lesion. Elastography is of better value in lesions smaller than 2 cm. Severe heterogeneity of the lesion, presence of fluid collections, large calcifications, and small (subcentimetric) and large lesions are also associated with certain difficulties in correct measurements of shear wave velocities with ARFI (Sencha et al. 2011).

Quantitative US elastography exhibits good reproducibility and does not implicate significant additional time expenses (Evans et al. 2010; Mitkov et al. 2011). Some authors report very high interobserver variability of free-hand compression US elastography. To achieve better reproducibility of compression US elastography, the manufacturers of US scanners introduced quality factors, which reflect the quality of obtained image in real time and the possibility of its interpretation. The higher the quality factor, the more reliable the data is. Some data, which lie below 60%, cannot be interpreted at all owing to major artifacts. Such approach allows not only to introduce the quality standards for interpreting of elastograms but also to develop the skills of effective work with US elastography in US specialists.

Incorporation of US elastography in the diagnostic complex increases the specificity of traditional US in diagnosis of breast carcinoma from 76 to 94.5% and the sensitivity in impalpable tumors in particular from 66.7 to 87.5% (Rozhkova et al. 2011).

Some studies, on the contrary, have found a decrease in the sensitivity of the combination of ultrasound in B-mode with elastography, if compared to ultrasonography in B-mode.

US elastography is an innovative ultrasound technology for the early diagnosis and dynamic follow-up of patients with various breast diseases, which is practically applicable (including screening) and prospective (Sencha et al. 2013; Rozhkova et al. 2011).

Perspective trends of the development of elastographic technique are three-dimensional and real-time triplex elastography. Unification of ways of shear wave velocity and elastic modulus measurement, as well as of other criteria of compression in different manufacturers' equipment, requires special attention.

The place of ultrasound elastography in diagnostic flow charts for breast tumors has not been definitely determined yet. Assessment of the elasticity (stiffness) of tissues in early diagnosis and differentiation of malignant and benign breast conditions is undoubtedly promising and prospective. Recent European guidelines and recommendations for clinical elastography, as well as certain recommendations on the standardized technique of compression elastography of the breast, thyroid gland, and regional lymph nodes (Borsukov et al. 2016), will promote the unification and increase the level of its reproducibility.

6.5 Contrast Ultrasound

Modern imaging methods often utilize contrast agents. Contrasts are used in classical X-ray diagnostics and computed tomography and paramagnetics in MRI. A contrast agent migrating with the blood to the examined organs facilitates their visualization either due to the increase of tissue density (X-ray contrast preparations) or due to the change of the magnetic properties of tissues by amplification of the tissue signal with paramagnetic substances. The sensitivity of US in detecting blood vessels in the breast or its tumors can be significantly increased by the use of intravenously injected contrast agents.

Contrast-enhanced ultrasonography (CEUS) is an ultrasound examination with contrast enhancement after intravenous administration of a contrast agent.

The first works on the use of echocontrasts in the A- and M-modes of ultrasound scanning were published in 1968–1969. Contrast-enhanced echography in the diagnosis of breast tumors has been applied since 1990. Introduction of new generation of ultrasound contrast agents significantly increased the interest for CEUS in evaluation of tumor perfusion and differential diagnosis of breast pathology.

One advantage of CEUS as compared with contrast-enhanced CT and MRI is that it allows continuous real-time study. It is based on the resonance effect of small circulating particles with special acoustic properties. The most important of these acoustic effects are listed below:

- Amplification of the reflected echo signal
- Reduction of echo attenuation
- Circulation of contrast agents within vascular system or their selective capture by certain tissues

Ultrasound contrast agents are able to modify one of the three interactions between the ultrasound and tissues—absorption, reflection, and refraction. Contrast agents for ultrasound are microbubbles (2–6 nm) of air (or other gases) in various capsules. The difference in the acoustic impedance between microbubbles and the surrounding tissues in vivo provides amplification of the acoustic signal reflected by the bubbles.

To visualize small blood vessels, it is necessary that ultrasound contrast agents amplify the echoes of the blood to a level much higher than the echoes of the surrounding tissues or be used in a mode providing simultaneous suppression of the echoes from the contrast-free tissues. Contrast agents increase the number of reflecting surfaces, which significantly increase the amount of reflected US registered by an ultrasound probe. Hence, echo signal in the contrast-containing area appears much higher than the signal from the surrounding tissues. Since US contrasts are intravascular, the ability of the blood to backscatter the echo increases, the blood becomes hyperechoic, and the signal-noise ratio improves. The increase in acoustic backscattering leads to the increase in echo signal intensity from the blood flow and the echodensity of the image of vascularized tissues in grayscale mode. This is especially important when the details of the examined structure are not sufficiently distinguishable.

The main indications for breast CEUS are listed below:

- Solid lesions of medium to low echogenicity, suspicious for malignancy (BI-RADS 4) prior to FNAB
- Solid lesions of medium to low echogenicity, suspicious for malignancy (BI-RADS 4) with no signs of atypia at cytology
- Complex cysts (BI-RADS 3, BI-RADS 4), with solid component
- A mass with unclear or confusing characteristics with different diagnostic tests (BI-RADS 3)
- A mass, which has changed its ultrasound appearance (echogenicity, uniformity, vascularization, elasticity) within a short period of time (BI-RADS 3)
- A breast mass after endoprosthetics or gel injection
- Recurrent breast tumor
- A mass in the accessory lobe
- A mass, which is not suspicious for malignancy with US but is accompanied by metastatic lesions in axillary lymph nodes

Breast CEUS is based on the detection and specification of microcirculation in the organ in general and in a pathologic mass in particular and on the detection of neoangiogenesis within the tumor, which is a well-known feature of malignant neoplasms. The use of contrast agents significantly improves visualization of vascular architectonics. The number of detected vessels increases from 36 to 95%.

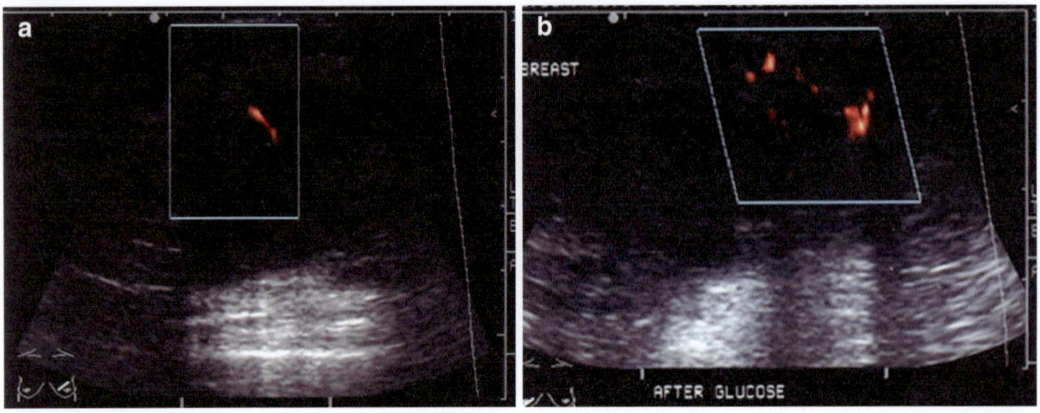

Fig. 6.19 Breast cancer. Echograms. PDI. (**a**) Before administration of 40% glucose. (**b**) 15 min after glucose administration. Enhanced tumor vascularity

An advanced technology of contrast echography with 40% glucose has been introduced to improve the visualization of vessels and differentiation of tumors. Some authors report that intravenous administration of glucose provides better visualization of the tumor borders, its heterogeneity, and additional atypical, adjacent and smaller vessels in grayscale and color-coded modes (Fig. 6.19).

Blood flow velocity in the arteries of breast carcinoma is higher than in normal tissue and is confidently registered with contrast echography. The detectability of the vascular pattern increases in small tumors up to 77.4–89.7%; enlargement of the diameter of the vessels is observed in 84.9% of cases.

Using the presence of blood vessels as a criterion for malignant neoplasm of mammary gland, some authors noted an increase in sensitivity (from 36 to 95%) and of positive and negative prognostic value, but a decrease in specificity (from 86 to 79%) due to hypervascularity of some benign tumors. There is some difference between carcinoma and fibroadenoma in the distribution of microvessels. It is supposed that the higher the differentiation of the tumor, the more uniform is the vascular pattern. This may explain the absence of difference in vascularization of low-grade malignant tumors and benign masses.

Preparation, methodology, and technique of contrast agent administration (in particular SonoVue) in ultrasound imaging for differential diagnosis of focal breast pathology are in many ways similar to those for other organs. The patient is placed in a standard supine position. Introduction of a contrast agent, recording of a video loop, and the visual analysis of contrast-enhanced image occur simultaneously in real time, while the quantitative analysis needs post-processing of ultrasound images (Fig. 6.20).

For breast examination, as a rule, 2.4–5.0 mL of SonoVue is introduced intravenously as a bolus injection. The best results are achieved with bolus intravenous administration of 4.8 mL of SonoVue followed with 5 mL saline flash.

Qualitative criteria for assessing temporal and spatial characteristics of echo contrasting of breast masses (as well as of other organs) are the following:

- Detection of vascularity (vessels filled with contrast) within the examined area
- Intensity of vascularization as compared with normal parenchyma
- Type of vascular architectonics (e.g., “steps,” “wheels,” “basket,” peripheral-nodular type, etc.)
- Dynamics of contrast enhancement with time (fast/slow, early/late)
- Dynamics of contrast washout

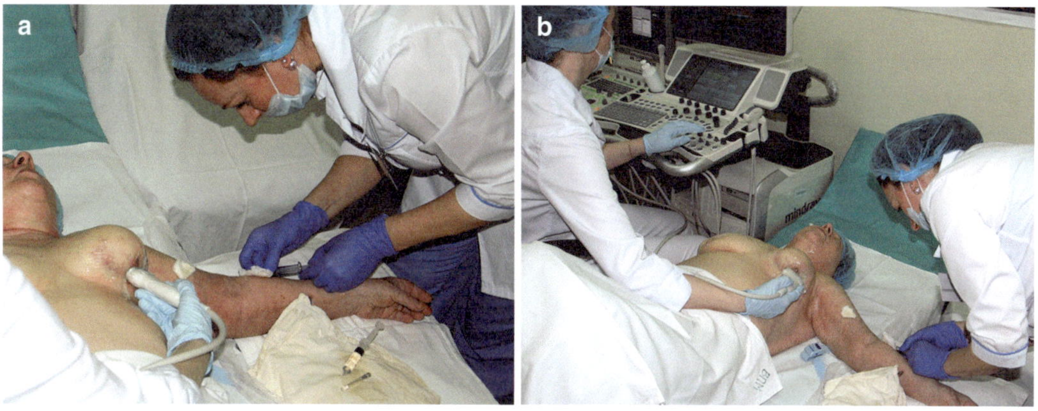

Fig. 6.20 Breast CEUS. Position of the patient and of medical personnel

The quantitative characteristics of echo contrasting of breast masses are as follows:

- Time to peak (TTPs)—the time interval from the start of contrast injection to the time of maximum contrast accumulation
- Peak intensity (PI, dB)—maximum intensity of the enhanced lesion
- Descending time (DT/2, c)—the time of half-life of the contrast within the lesion

Breast CEUS can reduce the number of biopsies. CEUS was as an alternative to MRI, especially for the first 18 postoperative months, when postoperative scars and granulomas may have an intensive capillary network, which decreases with time.

Unfortunately, most published data on the use of ultrasound with contrast enhancement do not correlate with the density of microvessels determined histologically, and so far this technique failed to provide higher diagnostic accuracy. Since the breast is a superficial organ, a diagnostic biopsy is safe and considered the "gold standard" of breast examination. Nevertheless, noninvasive differential diagnosis of malignant and benign tumors remains in demand.

US contrast microbubbles (SonoVue) always remain within vessel lumen, as opposed to contrast-enhanced MRI, when the contrast agent migrates from microvessels into extravascular space. Thus, the area of US enhancement and the curves of contrast accumulation strictly comply with vascularity and neoangiogenesis and are not associated with tumor extravascular space.

CEUS is the only imaging technique that allows long-term real-time monitoring of all phases of contrast enhancement. This ensures accurate identification of tumor microcirculation. Breast lesions are thoroughly evaluated with CEUS against hypovascular background that is advantageous to other parenchymatous organs.

It is a sensitive imaging technique, which supplements other methods of assessment of local breast vascularity. High accuracy of contrast echography is noted in the study of neoangiogenesis while monitoring the residual or recurrent tumor.

There is a problem with examination of small-sized lesions, which are often invisible in B-mode. Limited field of the view does not allow to apply this technique for examination of the entire breast. In fact, the contrast imaging technology is not yet mature enough to replace conventional ultrasonography or ultrasound-guided biopsy. Nevertheless, breast CEUS gives some interesting results and looks quite promising.

Although malignant breast masses are generally considered highly vascular, the ability to visualize the circulatory network within the tumor with conventional CDI and PDI is limited, as these methods have low sensitivity to slow blood flow and deep blood vessels. Heterogeneous intense contrast enhancement with CEUS is characteristic for malignant breast pathology (Fig. 6.21).

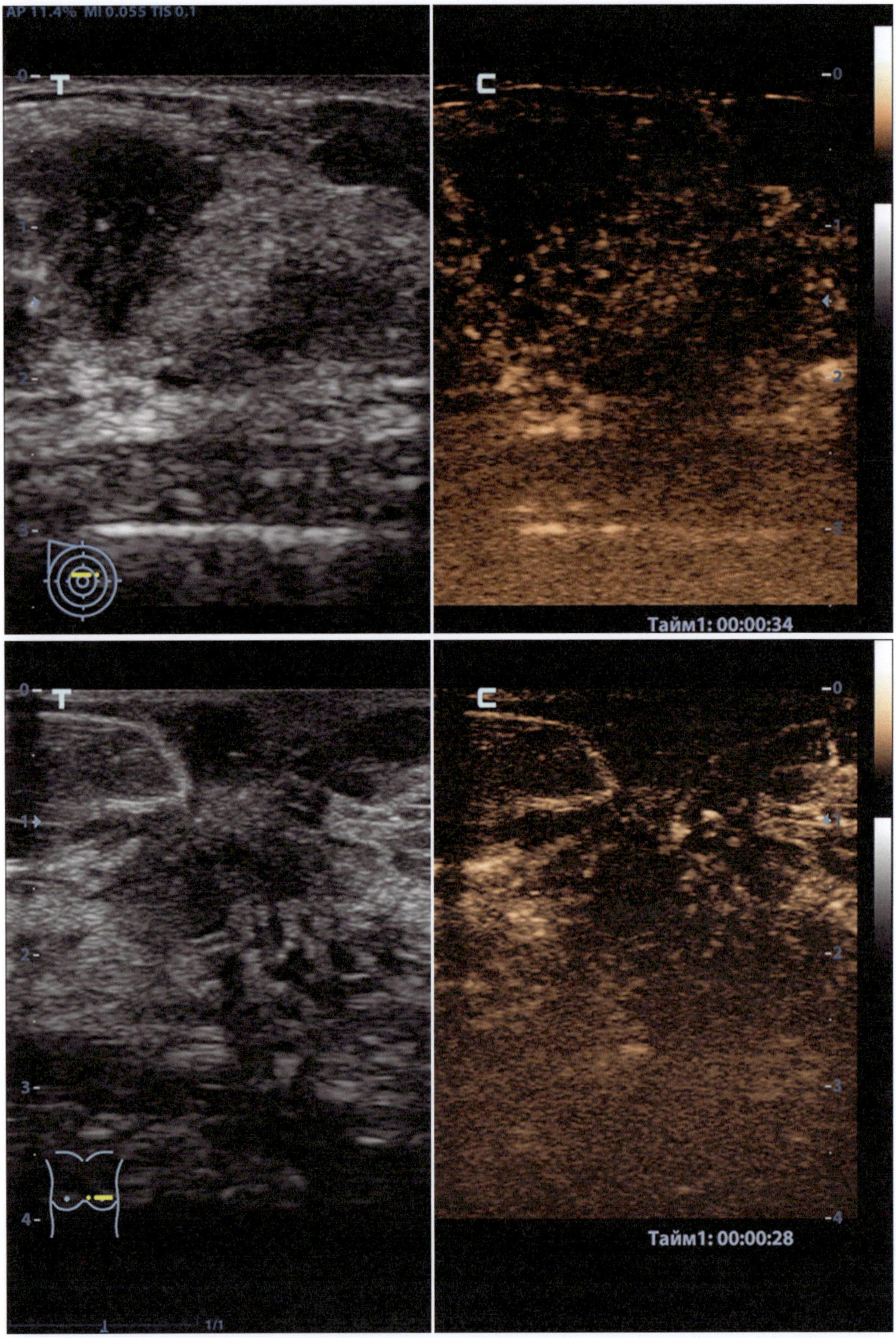

Fig. 6.21 (1–4) Breast cancer. CEUS. SonoVue, 2.4 mL. Asymmetric enhancement

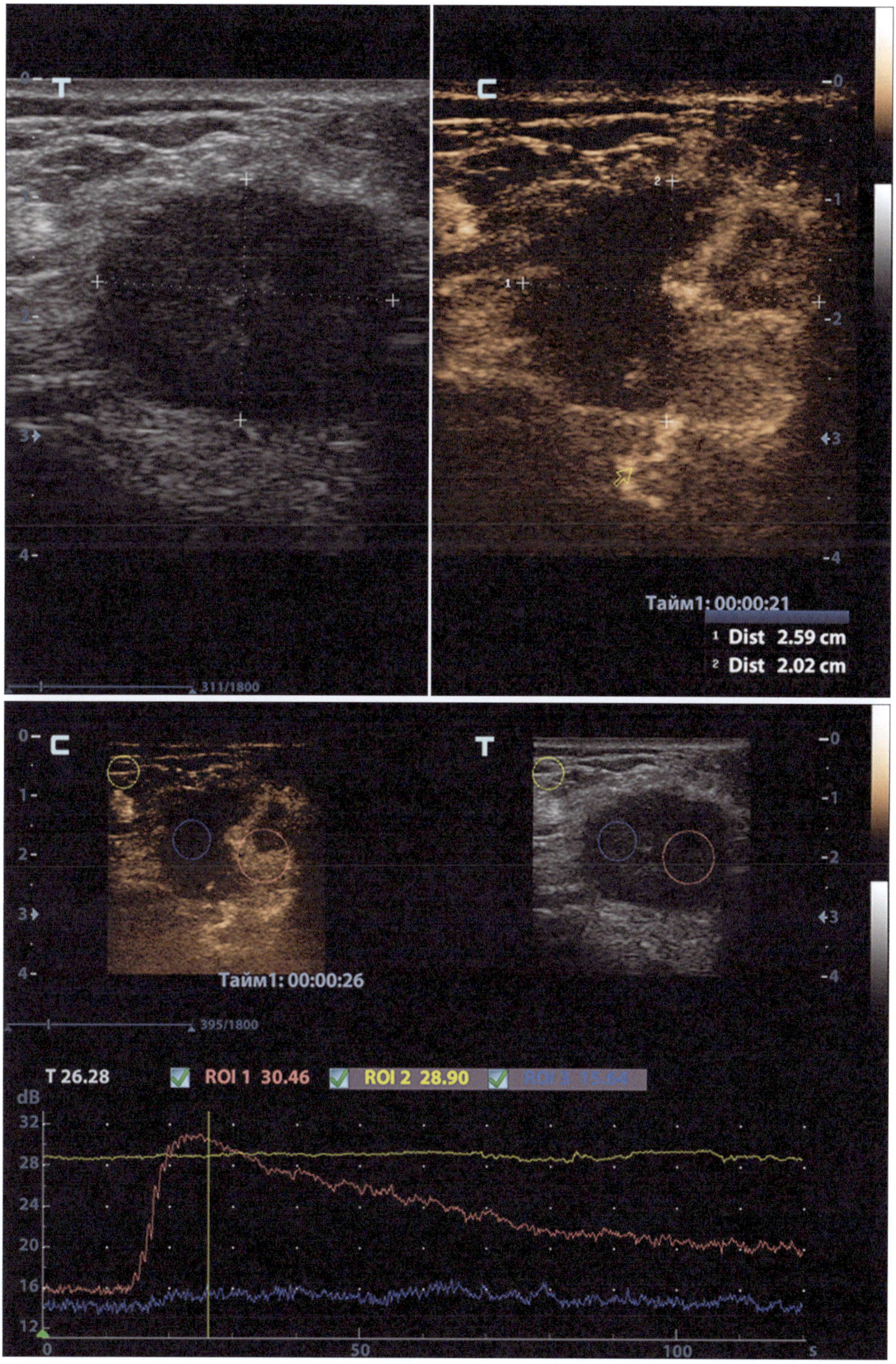

Fig. 6.21 (continued)

Heterogeneous and intense contrast enhancement in carcinoma reflects the rete of branching vessels, chaotically and atypically located in the arterioles and venules, arteriovenous shunts, which provide rapid washout of contrast agent from the tumor. In some cases (in 15%) of breast cancer, marginal accumulation of contrast is observed, and contrast enhancement occurs in a certain area of the tumor. Perhaps, this is due to perfusion deficiency inside the tumor, which depends on the degree of fibrosis and degeneration. In any case, the area of contrast enhancement should be suspicious for malignancy, and targeted biopsy of this site under ultrasound guidance will be most valuable (Sencha et al. 2015). There were cases when a malignant tumor exhibited only peripheral contrast enhancement.

Chaotic vascular pattern and irregular caliber of vessels with abnormal blood flow velocities are typical for most breast tumors (Fig. 6.22). The following changes are specific for fast-growing tumors: uneven decrease of the vessels caliber, elongated and spiral vessels, arteriovenous shunts, dichotomous branching, and roughness of the vascular wall. Correlation between vascular disorganization and the degree of tumor anaplasia is very high (Sencha et al. 2015). Automatic multiplanar color mapping of contrast enhancement and its graphical analysis facilitate examination (Fig. 6.23).

Relative risk of malignancy is significantly increased, when vessels with irregular course and flow velocities are identified with US. In contrast, fibroadenoma, the most common benign breast tumor, generally has a poor vascular network with vascular distribution predominantly around the mass, with a uniform and minor branching of the vessels. However, about 10% of all breast diseases, including inflammatory processes, immature fibroadenomas, and phyllodes tumors, may have expressed blood supply with mosaic blood flow. On the other hand, in some cases of intraductal carcinoma, according to pathology data, blood perfusion through capillaries can be significantly hampered by intense fibrosis and narrowing of the vessels caliber.

According to Sencha et al. (2015), a quantitative analysis of contrast enhancement in focal breast cancer in women revealed the following data: mean time to peak 21.89 ± 1.6 s, peak intensity 21.8 ± 0.8 dB, and descending time 53.67 ± 5.04 s. To compare with FA, the corresponding figures are as follows: mean time to peak 32.08 ± 1.2 s, peak intensity 27.04 ± 0.7 dB, and descending time 79.13 ± 3.1 s. In men, these indices were approximately in the same range. In breast cancer, the mean time to peak was 22.27 ± 1.3 s, peak intensity 34.25 ± 1.4 dB, and descending time 49.87 ± 6.0 s. In gynecomastia time to peak was 32.08 ± 1.2 s, peak intensity 25.6 ± 1.1 dB, and descending time 78.56 ± 2.2 s.

According to Zhang et al. (2013), a quantitative analysis of contrast enhancement showed that peak intensity in benign pathology was higher (16.52 ± 4.15 dB) than in the group with malignant lesions (13.86 ± 3.36 dB) ($p = 0.007$). Time to peak (TTP) was longer for benign masses (19.86 ± 4.87 s) than for malignant ones (16.52 ± 4.85 s) ($p = 0.009$). Descending time (DT/2) was 80.55 ± 18.65 s in benign masses versus 65.16 ± 20.28 s in malignant tumors ($p = 0.006$).

Interpretation of the CEUS findings is difficult for masses, where vascularity is reduced or minimal, for example, with adenosis, fibrotic changes, scars, and some types of fibroadenomas. Quantitative characteristics of contrast enhancement may depend on the method of administration of the contrast agent (bolus, cannula, Infusomat, etc.), the patient's age (tumor perfusion is lower in patients older than 60 years), size, histological type (time to peak, as a rule, is higher in carcinoma in situ and low-grade invasive carcinomas), and tumor homogeneity (contrast washout in invasive tumors is very fast due to arteriovenous shunts).

Nevertheless, biopsy with pathological examination is still the principal verification method.

Thus, CEUS is an informative technology for visualization of the blood flow in breast tumors and identification of neoangiogenesis, which is characteristic for malignancy. The use of ultrasound contrast agents for evaluation of vascular perfusion creates certain prospects for differential diagnosis of detectable focal breast masses.

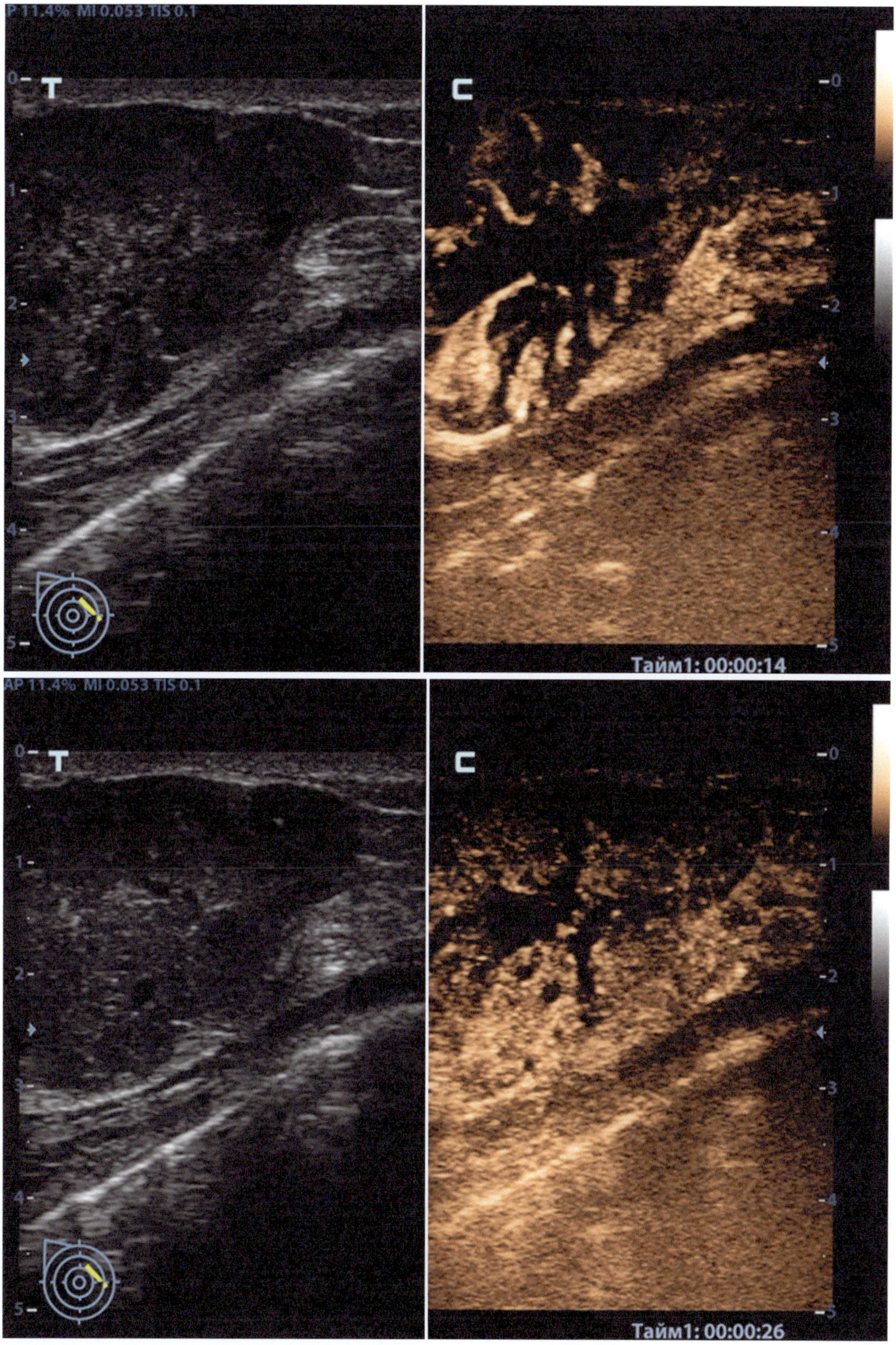

Fig. 6.22 Breast cancer. CEUS, SonoVue, 2.4 mL. Chaotic intranodular enhancement, disorganized vascular pattern, and abnormal vessels

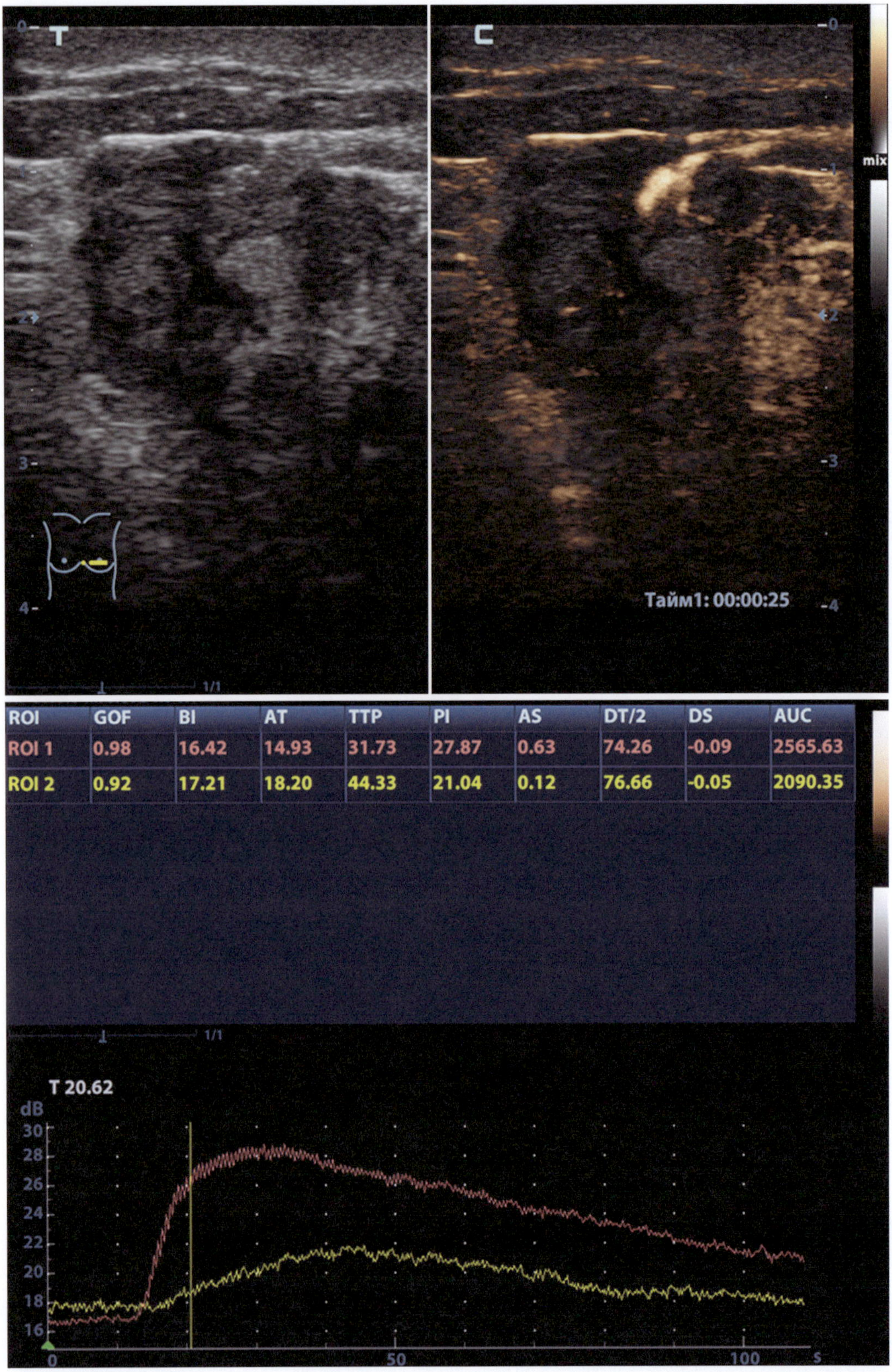

Fig. 6.22 (continued)

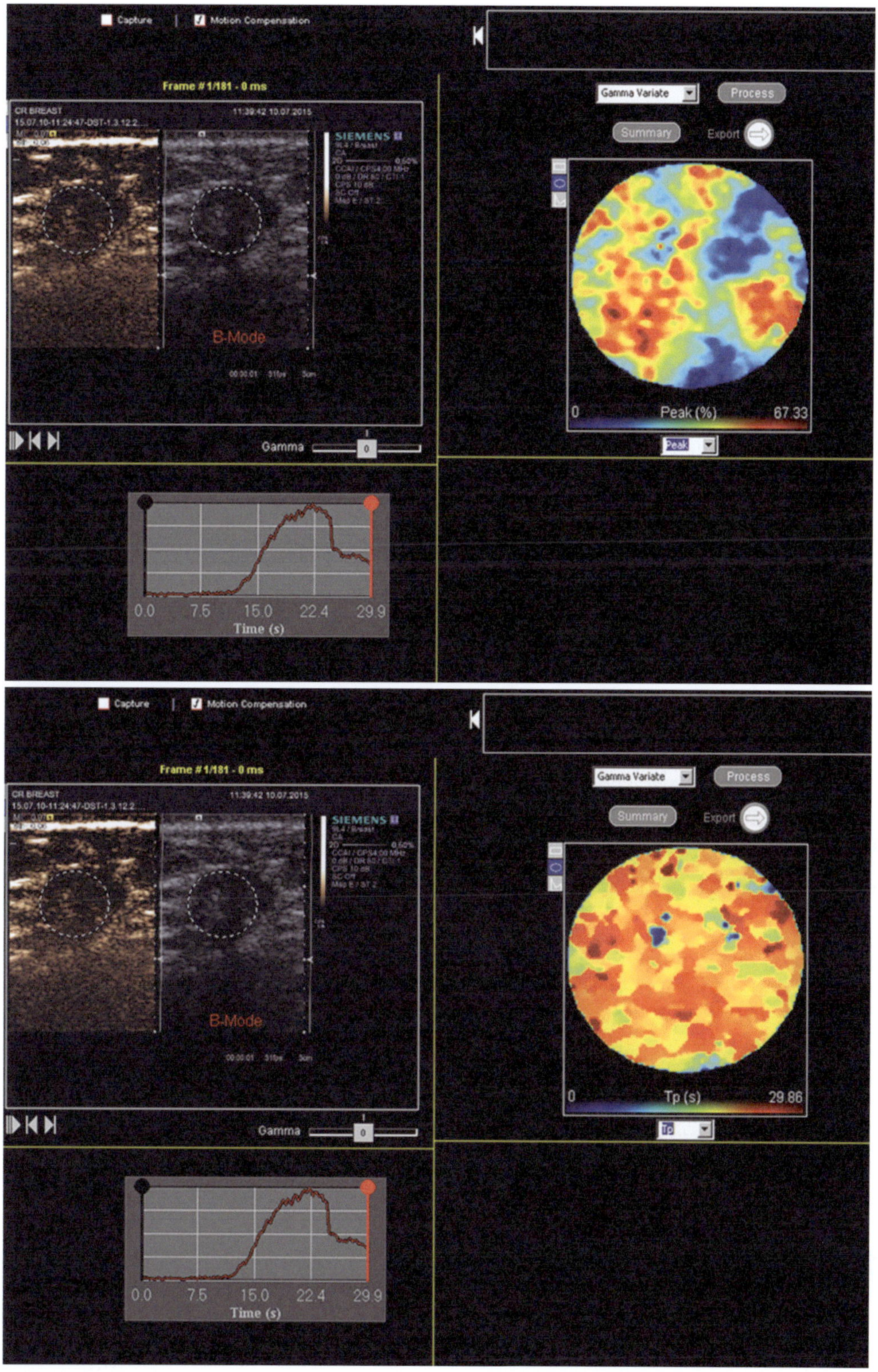

Fig. 6.23 Breast cancer. CEUS, SonoVue, 2.4 mL. Multiparametric color mapping of contrast enhancement

Sensitivity of CEUS in the detection of breast cancer in women is 87.5%, specificity 90%, and accuracy 88.5% (Sencha et al. 2015). For breast cancer in men, these indices are 83.3%, 80%, and 81.25%, respectively.

CEUS can be effectively used for assessment of early response to chemotherapy in aggressive breast cancer and for prediction and monitoring of tumor growth, invasion, and extent.

To date, ultrasound with contrast enhancement is an additional diagnostic technology, which increases the value of complex US in breast cancer. Methodological issues and analysis of the results of CEUS require further data accumulation, standardization of the method, and further promotion of this technology in practical healthcare.

6.6 Classification of Breast Cancer: Morphological Types of Tumors and Ultrasound Correlations

Division of breast tumors into groups, differentiation by stages, is important for determination of tactics, choice of treatment, duration of therapy, volume of surgical intervention, further rehabilitation, follow-up terms, and prognosis.

There are several classifications of breast cancer based on clinical, etiological, histological, ultrasonographic and other criteria that characterize the status of the primary breast tumor, its extent, and local and distant metastases (Table 6.1).

The international classification is carried out according to the TNM system (Sobin 2010). There are several clinical and pathomorphological classifications of breast cancer. Clinical staging is based on the results of clinical examination. Pathomorphological staging is based on the conclusion of a pathologist after surgery.

TNM Classification of Carcinomas of the Breast

TNM Clinical Classification

T: Primary Tumor

- *TX.* Primary tumor cannot be assessed
- *T0.* No evidence of primary tumor

Table 6.1 Breast cancer by stages

Stage 0	Tis	N0	M0
Stage IA	T1*	N0	M0
Stage IB	T0, T1*	N1mi	M0
Stage IIA	T0 T1* T2	N1 N1 N0	M0 M0 M0
Stage IIB	T2 T3	N1 N0	M0 M0
Stage IIIA	T0 T1* T2 T3	N2 N2 N2 N1, N2	M0 M0 M0 M0
Stage IIIB	T4	N0, N1, N2	M0
Stage IIIC	Any T	N3	M0
Stage IV	Any T	Any N	M1

*T1 includes T1mi

- *Tis.* Carcinoma in situ
  - *Tis (DCIS).* Ductal carcinoma in situ
  - *Tis (LCIS).* Lobular carcinoma in situ
  - *Tis (Paget).* Paget's disease of the nipple with no tumor

    Note: Paget's disease associated with a tumor is classified according to the size of the tumor.
- *T1.* Tumor 2 cm or less in greatest dimension
  - *T1mic.* Microinvasion 0.1 cm or less in greatest dimension

    Note: Microinvasion is the extension of cancer cells beyond the basement membrane into the adjacent tissues with no focus more than 0.1 cm in greatest dimension. When there are multiple foci of microinvasion, the size of only the largest focus is used to classify the microinvasion. (Do not use the sum of all individual foci.) The presence of multiple foci of microinvasion should be noted, as it is with multiple larger invasive carcinomas.
  - *T1a.* More than 0.1 cm but not more than 0.5 cm in greatest dimension
  - *T1b.* More than 0.5 cm but not more than 1 cm in greatest dimension
  - *T1c.* More than 1 cm but not more than 2 cm in greatest dimension
- *T2.* Tumor more than 2 cm but not more than 5 cm in greatest dimension
- *T3.* Tumor more than 5 cm in greatest dimension

- *T4.* Tumor of any size with direct extension to the chest wall or skin only as described in T4a to T4d
- Note: The chest wall includes the ribs, intercostal muscles, and serratus anterior muscle but not the pectoral muscle.
  - *T4a.* Extension to the chest wall
  - *T4b.* Edema (including peau d'orange) or ulceration of the skin of the breast or satellite skin nodules confined to the same breast
  - *T4c.* Both 4a and 4b, above
  - *T4d.* Inflammatory carcinoma

    Note: Inflammatory carcinoma of the breast is characterized by diffuse, brawny induration of the skin with an erysipeloid edge, usually with no underlying mass. If the skin biopsy is negative and there is no localized measurable primary cancer, the T category is pTX when pathologically staging a clinical inflammatory carcinoma (T4d). Dimpling of the skin, nipple retraction, or other skin changes, except those in T4b and T4d, may occur in T1, T2, or T3 without affecting the classification.

N: Regional Lymph Nodes

- *NX.* Regional lymph nodes cannot be assessed (e.g., previously removed).
- *N0.* No regional lymph node metastasis.
- *N1.* Metastasis in movable ipsilateral axillary lymph node(s).
- *N2.* Metastasis in fixed ipsilateral axillary lymph node(s) or in clinically apparent* ipsilateral internal mammary lymph node(s) in the absence of clinically evident axillary lymph node metastasis.
  - *N2a.* Metastasis in axillary lymph node(s) fixed to one another or to other structures
  - *N2b.* Metastasis only in clinically apparent* internal mammary lymph node(s) and in the absence of clinically evident axillary lymph node metastasis
- *N3.* Metastasis in ipsilateral infraclavicular lymph node(s) with or without axillary lymph node involvement or in clinically apparent* ipsilateral internal mammary lymph node(s) in the presence of clinically evident axillary lymph node metastasis or metastasis in ipsilateral supraclavicular lymph node(s) with or without axillary or internal mammary lymph node involvement.
  - *N3a.* Metastasis in infraclavicular lymph node(s)
  - *N3b.* Metastasis in internal mammary and axillary lymph nodes
  - *N3c.* Metastasis in supraclavicular lymph node(s)

    * *[Note: Clinically apparent is defined as detected by imaging studies (excluding lymphoscintigraphy) or by clinical examination or grossly visible pathologically.]*

M: Distant Metastasis

- *MX.* Distant metastasis cannot be assessed.
- *M0.* No distant metastasis.
- *M1.* Distant metastasis.

pTNM Pathological Classification

pT: Primary Tumor

The pathological classification requires the examination of the primary carcinoma with no gross tumor at the margins of resection. A case can be classified pT if there is only microscopic tumor in a margin. The pT categories correspond to the T categories.

Note: When classifying pT, the tumor size is a measurement of the invasive component. If there is a large in situ component (e.g., 4 cm) and a small invasive component (e.g., 0.5 cm), the tumor is coded pT1a.

pN: Regional Lymph Nodes

pNX. Regional lymph nodes cannot be assessed (not removed for study or previously removed).

pN0. No regional lymph node metastasis.*

pN1mi. Micrometastasis (larger than 0.2 mm but not larger than 2 mm in greatest dimension).

pN1. Metastasis in one to three ipsilateral axillary lymph node(s) and/or in internal mammary nodes with microscopic metastasis detected by sentinel lymph node dissection but not clinically apparent.**

pN1a. Metastasis in one to three axillary lymph node(s), including at least one larger than 2 mm in greatest dimension.

pN1b. Internal mammary lymph nodes with microscopic metastasis detected by sentinel lymph node dissection but not clinically apparent.

pN1c. Metastasis in one to three axillary lymph nodes and internal mammary lymph nodes with microscopic metastasis detected by sentinel lymph node dissection but not clinically apparent.

pN2. Metastasis in four to nine ipsilateral axillary lymph nodes or in clinically apparent*** ipsilateral internal mammary lymph node(s) in the absence of axillary lymph node metastasis.

pN2a. Metastasis in four to nine axillary lymph nodes, including at least one that is larger than 2 mm.

pN2b. Metastasis in clinically apparent internal mammary lymph node(s), in the absence of axillary lymph node metastasis.

pN3. Metastasis in ten or more ipsilateral axillary lymph nodes; or in infraclavicular lymph nodes; or in clinically apparent ipsilateral internal mammary lymph nodes in the presence of one or more positive axillary lymph nodes; or in more than three axillary lymph nodes with clinically negative, microscopic metastasis in internal mammary lymph nodes; or in ipsilateral supraclavicular lymph nodes.

pN3a. Metastasis in ten or more axillary lymph nodes (at least one larger than 2 mm) or metastasis in infraclavicular lymph nodes

pN3b. Metastasis in clinically apparent internal mammary lymph node(s) in the presence of one or more positive axillary lymph node(s) or metastasis in more than three axillary lymph nodes and in internal mammary lymph nodes with microscopic metastasis detected by sentinel lymph node dissection but not clinically apparent.

pN3c. Metastasis in supraclavicular lymph node(s).

Note: * Cases with only isolated tumor cells (ITC) in regional lymph nodes are classified as pN0. ITC are single tumor cells or small clusters of cells, not more than 0.2 mm in greatest dimension, which are usually detected by immunohistochemistry or molecular methods but which may be verified on H&E stains. ITCs do not typically show evidence of metastatic activity (e.g., proliferation or stromal reaction).

** Not clinically apparent = not detected by clinical examination or by imaging studies (excluding lymphoscintigraphy)

*** Clinically apparent = detected by clinical examination or by imaging studies (excluding lymphoscintigraphy) or grossly visible pathologically

pM: Distant Metastasis

The pM categories correspond to the M categories.

Clinical groups: operable breast cancer (Stages 0, I, IIA, IIB, IIIA), locally advanced (inoperable) breast cancer (Stages IIIB, IIIC), metastatic breast cancer, or recurrence of the disease

Breast Cancer in the International Classification of Diseases (ICD-10, 2010)

C50.0 Nipple and areola
C50.1 Central portion of the breast
C50.2 Upper-inner quadrant of the breast
C50.3 Lower-inner quadrant of the breast
C50.4 Upper-outer quadrant of the breast
C50.5 Lower-outer quadrant of the breast
C50.6 Axillary tail of the breast
C50.8 Overlapping lesion of the breast
C50.9 Breast, unspecified

WHO Histological Classification of Tumors of the Breast (Tavassoéli and Devilee 2003)

Epithelial Tumors

- Invasive ductal carcinoma, not otherwise specified (NOS)—8500/3
  - Mixed type carcinoma
  - Pleomorphic carcinoma—8022/3
  - Carcinoma with osteoclastic giant cells—8035/3
  - Carcinoma with choriocarcinomatous features
  - Carcinoma with melanotic features
- Invasive lobular carcinoma—8520/3

- Tubular carcinoma—8211/3
- Invasive cribriform carcinoma—8201/3
- Medullary carcinoma—8510/3
- Mucinous carcinoma and other tumors with abundant mucin
  - Mucinous carcinoma—8480/3
  - Cystadenocarcinoma and columnar cell mucinous carcinoma—8480/3
  - Signet ring cell carcinoma—8490/3
- Neuroendocrine tumors
  - Solid neuroendocrine carcinoma
  - Atypical carcinoid tumor—8249/3
  - Small cell/oat cell carcinoma—8041/
  - Large cell neuroendocrine carcinoma—8013/
- Invasive papillary carcinoma—8503/
- Invasive micropapillary carcinoma—8507/
- Apocrine carcinoma—8401/
- Metaplastic carcinomas—8575/3
  - Pure epithelial metaplastic carcinomas—8575/3
  - Squamous cell carcinoma—8070/3
  - Adenocarcinoma with spindle cell metaplasia—8572/3
  - Adenosquamous carcinoma—8560/3
  - Mucoepidermoid carcinoma—8430/3
  - Mixed epithelial/mesenchymal metaplastic carcinomas—8575/3
- Lipid-rich carcinoma—8314/3
- Secretory carcinoma—8502/3
- Oncocytic carcinoma—8290/3
- Adenoid cystic carcinoma—8200/3
- Acinic cell carcinoma—8550/3
- Glycogen-rich clear cell carcinoma—8315/3
- Sebaceous carcinoma—8410/3
- Inflammatory carcinoma—8530/3
- Lobular neoplasia
  - Lobular carcinoma in situ—8520/2
- Intraductal proliferative lesions
  - Usual ductal hyperplasia
  - Flat epithelial atypia
  - Atypical ductal hyperplasia
  - Ductal carcinoma in situ—8500/2
- Microinvasive carcinoma
- Intraductal papillary neoplasms
  - Central papilloma—8503/0
  - Peripheral papilloma—8503/0
  - Atypical papilloma
  - Intraductal papillary carcinoma—8503/2
  - Intracystic papillary carcinoma—8504/2
- Benign epithelial proliferations
  - Adenosis including variants: sclerosing adenosis, apocrine adenosis, blunt duct adenosis, microglandular adenosis, and adenomyoepithelial adenosis
  - Radial scar/complex sclerosing lesion
  - Adenomas
    Tubular adenoma—8211/0
    Lactating adenoma—8204/0
    Apocrine adenoma—8401/0
    Pleomorphic adenoma—8940/0
    Ductal adenoma—8503/0

Myoepithelial Lesions

- Myoepitheliosis
- Adenomyoepithelial adenosis
- Adenomyoepithelioma—8983/0
- Malignant myoepithelioma—8982/3

Mesenchymal Tumors

- Hemangioma—9120/0
- Angiomatosis
- Hemangiopericytoma—9150/1
- Pseudoangiomatous stromal hyperplasia
- Myofibroblastoma—8825/0
- Fibromatosis (aggressive)—8821/1
- Inflammatory myofibroblastic tumor—8825/1
- Lipoma—8850/0
  - Angiolipoma—8861/0
- Granular cell tumor—9580/0
- Neurofibroma—9540/0
- Schwannoma—9560/0
- Angiosarcoma—9120/3
- Liposarcoma—8850/3
- Rhabdomyosarcoma—8900/3
- Osteosarcoma—9180/3
- Leiomyoma—8890/0
- Leiomyosarcoma—8890/3

Fibroepithelial Tumors

- Fibroadenoma—9010/0
- Phyllodes tumor—9020/1

  - Benign—9020/0
  - Borderline—9020/1
  - Malignant—9020/3
- Periductal stromal sarcoma, low grade—9020/3
- Mammary hamartoma

Tumors of the Nipple

- Nipple adenoma—8506/0
- Syringomatous adenoma—8407/0
- Paget's disease of the nipple—8540/3

Malignant Lymphoma

- Diffuse large B-cell lymphoma—9680/3
- Burkitt lymphoma—9687/3
- Extranodal marginal zone B-cell lymphoma or MALT type—9699/3
- Follicular lymphoma—9690/3

Metastatic Tumors: *Tumors of the Male Breast*

- Gynecomastia
- Carcinoma
  - Invasive—8500/3
  - In situ—8500/2

6.6.1 Ultrasound BI-RADS Classification of Breast Masses

Lack of continuity of primary care and communication between health workers responsible for diagnosis of breast pathology (mammologist, oncologist, ultrasound specialist, radiologist, surgeon), variety of algorithms, and sequence of application of various diagnostic (ultrasound, mammography, MRI) and invasive (core and fine needle biopsy) techniques often lead to misinterpretation of the obtained results, significant increase of the time of additional examination, erroneous referrals of patient data, and detection of already advanced, often metastatic, disease.

In the 1990s, the American Society of Radiologists, in collaboration with the National Cancer Institute, the Centers for Disease Control and Prevention, the Food and Drug Administration, the American Medical Association, the American Society of Surgeons, and the Society of American Pathologists, has developed a classification (scale) aimed to standardize the assessment of results of mammography according to the risk of malignancy (BI-RADS). The main goal of the developed system was to develop a unified language and terms for interpreting the results of visualization of the breast and adequate recommendations for further clinical tactics.

BI-RADS (breast imaging-reporting and data system) is a system for interpreting and recording of breast visualization and classification of certain radiological signs according to the risk of malignancy detected with breast mammography/US/MRI, which allows planning the management of patients depending on the assigned category.

BI-RADS scale in the evaluation of imaging methods (mammography, ultrasound, CT, MRI) is a mandatory step for reports in the leading clinics in the United States, EU countries, Australia, and Kazakhstan. The scale allowed to significantly improve the interpretation of the findings and standardize therapeutic and diagnostic algorithms.

Introduction of this scale into practice is important for assessment of ultrasound findings. Since the ultrasound and mammographic images of various pathological processes are different, direct application of BI-RADS scale for assessment of US images is impossible. At the same time, the general principles of classifying the images into categories are similar (Table 6.2).

The protocols of radiologic studies, as a rule, along with BI-RADS implement the principle of nosological diagnosis. The absolute majority of findings with mammography and ultrasound are classified as BI-RADS 1 (Table 6.3).

The BI-RADS terminology for ultrasound (US BI-RADS) differs from that for mammography (see Chap. 1).

Conclusion on the ultrasound findings should have the following structures:

- Indication for the examination
- Statement of scope and technique of breast US examination

Table 6.2 US BI-RADS classification system

BI-RADS category	Radiologic examination findings	Recommended approach
0	Incomplete	Further investigation with other methods
BI-RADS 1	Negative	Repeat examination in 12 months
BI-RADS 2	Benign	Repeat examination in 12 months
BI-RADS 3	Probably benign (malignancy risk is less than 2%). This specific case includes grouped, point, isodense microcalcifications; a homogeneous, well-defined mass; and an impalpable local asymmetry which resembles a fused fibrous-glandular tissue	Repeat examination in 6 months
BI-RADS 4	Suspicious (2–95% risk of malignancy)	Further investigation with other methods, including biopsy
BI-RADS 5	Highly suggestive of malignancy (risk of malignancy >95%)	Further investigation with other methods, including biopsy
BI-RADS 6	Known biopsy—proven malignancy	Individual plan of neoadjuvant treatment

Table 6.3 Correspondence of BI-RADS categories and diagnosis (ICD-10)

BI-RADS category	Incidence (n = 11,595)	%	Characteristics	Nosologic diagnosis
BI-RADS 1	9822	84.7	No pathologic structures	Fibrous-fatty involution, diffuse fibrous-glandular mastopathy
BI-RADS 2	886	7.6	A mass with distinct borders, even or uneven contours, weak or moderate degree of intensity of shadows, and absence of pathological changes in surrounding structures	Fibroadenoma, lipoma, cyst, oleogranuloma, galactocele, intramammary lymph node
BI-RADS 3	197	1.7	Calcifications (of doubtful nature) and masses with distinct or indistinct contours and increased radiological density	Multiple cysts, fatty necrosis, fibroadenomas with atypical manifestations
BI-RADS 4	54	0.47	Diffuse changes or masses of various sizes, with indistinct borders, even or uneven contours, calcifications of doubtful nature	Atypical cysts (cystadenoma papilloma, cystadenocarcinoma), phyllodes tumors, sclerosing adenosis, local fibrosis, fat necrosis, malignant tumors
BI-RADS 5	277	2.3	Masses with high radiological density and indistinct, uneven contours (fescue, tautness, radiance); reorganization of surrounding tissues	Breast cancer (invasive, noninvasive), metastatic tumors, sarcoma, malignant phyllodes tumors
BI-RADS 6	246	89	Histologically confirmed diagnosis of breast cancer	Breast cancer, metastatic tumors, sarcoma, malignant phyllodes tumors

- Succinct description of the overall breast composition (screening only)
- Clear description of any important findings
- Comparison to previous examination(s), including correlation with physical, mammography, or MRI findings
- Composite reports
- Assessment
- Management

Assessment of ultrasound images according to US BI-RADS assumes allocation of certain categories.

Category 0: Assessment is incomplete. Needs additional imaging evaluation

In many instances, the US examination completes the evaluation of the patient. If US is the initial study, other examinations may be indicated. An example would be the need for mammography if US were the initial study for a patient in her late 20s evaluated with US for a palpable mass that had suspicious sonographic features. Another example might be where mammography and US are nonspecific, such as differentiating between scarring and recurrence in a patient with breast cancer treated with lumpectomy and radiation therapy. Here, MRI might be the recommendation. A need for previous studies to determine appropriate management might also defer a final assessment.

Category 1: Negative. There is nothing to comment on

Various variants of normal breast. The volume and structure of breast correspond to the age, constitution, and physiological state of the patient (Fig. 6.24). There are no direct or indirect signs of pathological processes. This category is for sonograms with no abnormality, such as a mass, architectural distortion, and thickening of the skin or microcalcifications. For greater confidence in rendering a negative interpretation, an attempt should be made to correlate the ultrasound and mammographic patterns of the breast tissue in the area of concern.

Recommendations: routine examination according to age (usually one time per year).

Category 2: Benign finding(s)

This includes benign breast conditions (Fig. 6.25):

- Simple cysts
- Lipoma
- Atheroma
- Intramammary lymph nodes
- Breast implants
- Typical fibroadenoma
- Oleogranuloma
- Local fibrosis
- Duct ectasia
- State after endoprosthesis replacement
- Postoperative changes

Recommendations: examination every 6–12 months; biopsy is not recommended. Indications for FNB should be determined individually: in cysts, for therapeutic and diagnostic purposes and in soft breast masses, to make decision on surgical treatment.

Category 3: Probably benign—short-interval follow-up suggested

This includes benign breast conditions with cancer probability less than 2% (Fig. 6.26):

- Growing fibroadenoma
- Areas of fat necrosis
- Nodular hyperplasia of the parenchyma
- Abscess
- Atypical or complex cysts and fluid-containing masses with signs of inflammation

Recommendations: preference is given to examination every 6–12 months. According to the indications or at the patient's request, ultrasound-guided FNB with antibacterial preventive treatment (in inflammatory conditions) and subsequent ultrasonographic control may be

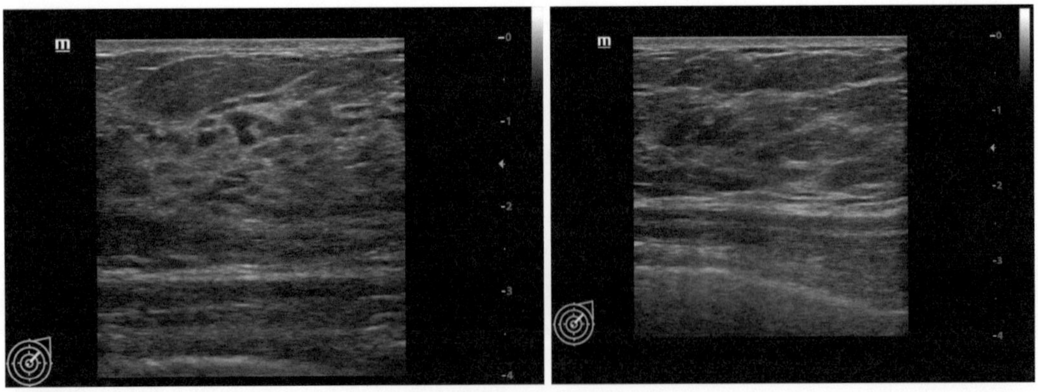

Fig. 6.24 US BI-RADS 1. Normal breast. Grayscale US

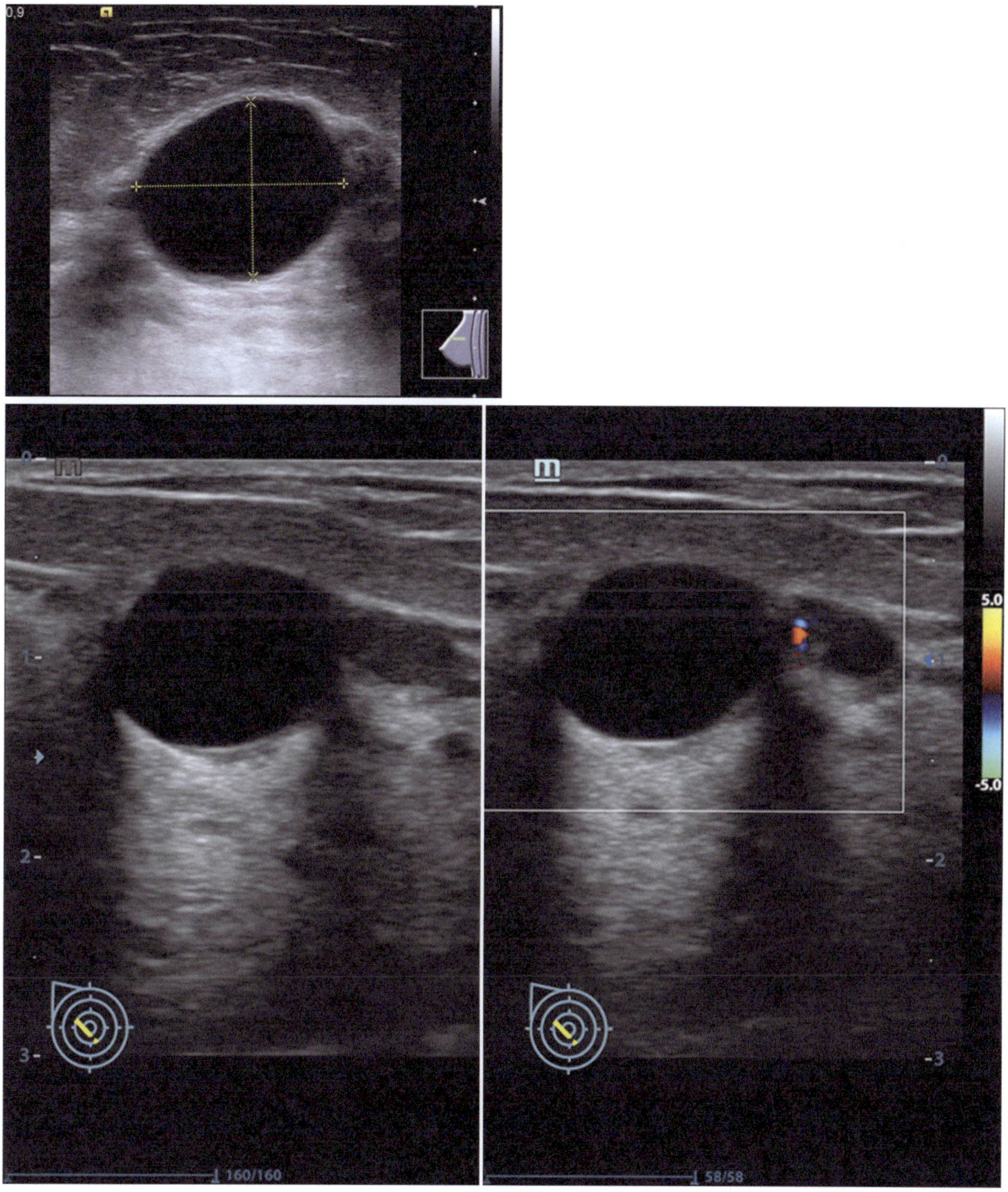

Fig. 6.25 US BI-RADS 2. Simple cyst. Grayscale, CDI

applicable. If dynamic ultrasonography proves signs suspicious for malignancy, the case is converted into Category 4. At favorable dynamics or stability, the case is converted to Category 2.

Category 4: Suspicious abnormality—biopsy should be considered

The observed changes are suspicious for malignancy with a probability of 2–94%. A low, moderate, and high cancer probabilities are distinguished (Categories 4a, 4b, and 4c, respectively). These include the following positions (Figs. 6.27, 6.28, and 6.29):

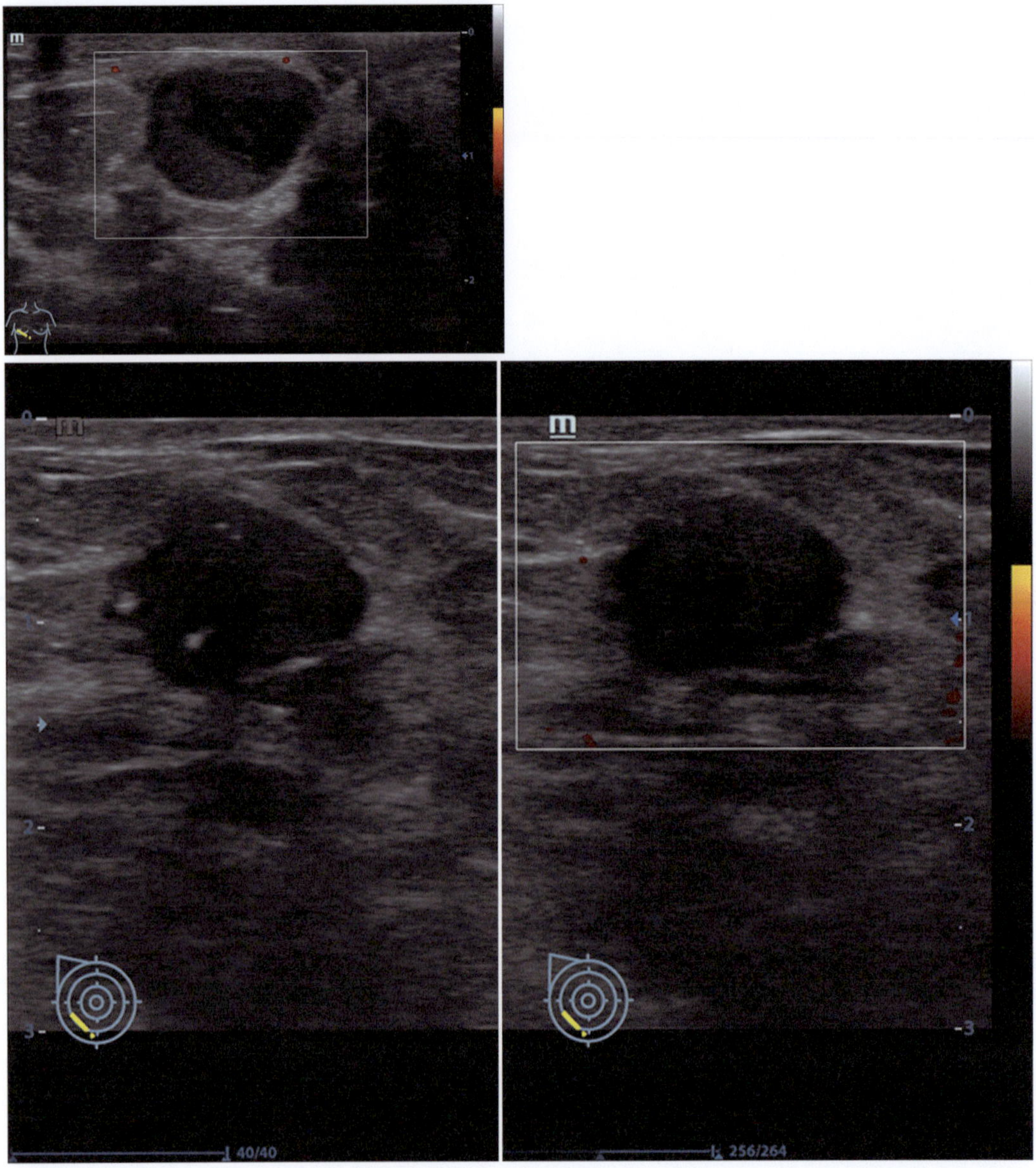

Fig. 6.26 US BI-RADS 3. Complex cysts. Grayscale, PDI

- A mass that does not demonstrate reliable signs of FA and has no complete certainty about its benign nature.
- A FA over 3 cm (suspicious for a phyllodes tumor) or fibroadenomas with uneven contours, attenuation of echo, and indistinct contours.
- Atypical cysts with intracystic masses
- Ductal tumors
- Lesions with uncertain echographic pattern
- Signs of mastitis without positive dynamics after anti-inflammatory and antibacterial treatment
- Zones of nodular parenchymal hyperplasia with or without positive dynamics after conservative treatment
- Local asymmetric hyperplasia and dilatation of peripheral milk ducts

Recommendations: Morphological verification of the diagnosis should be carried out with

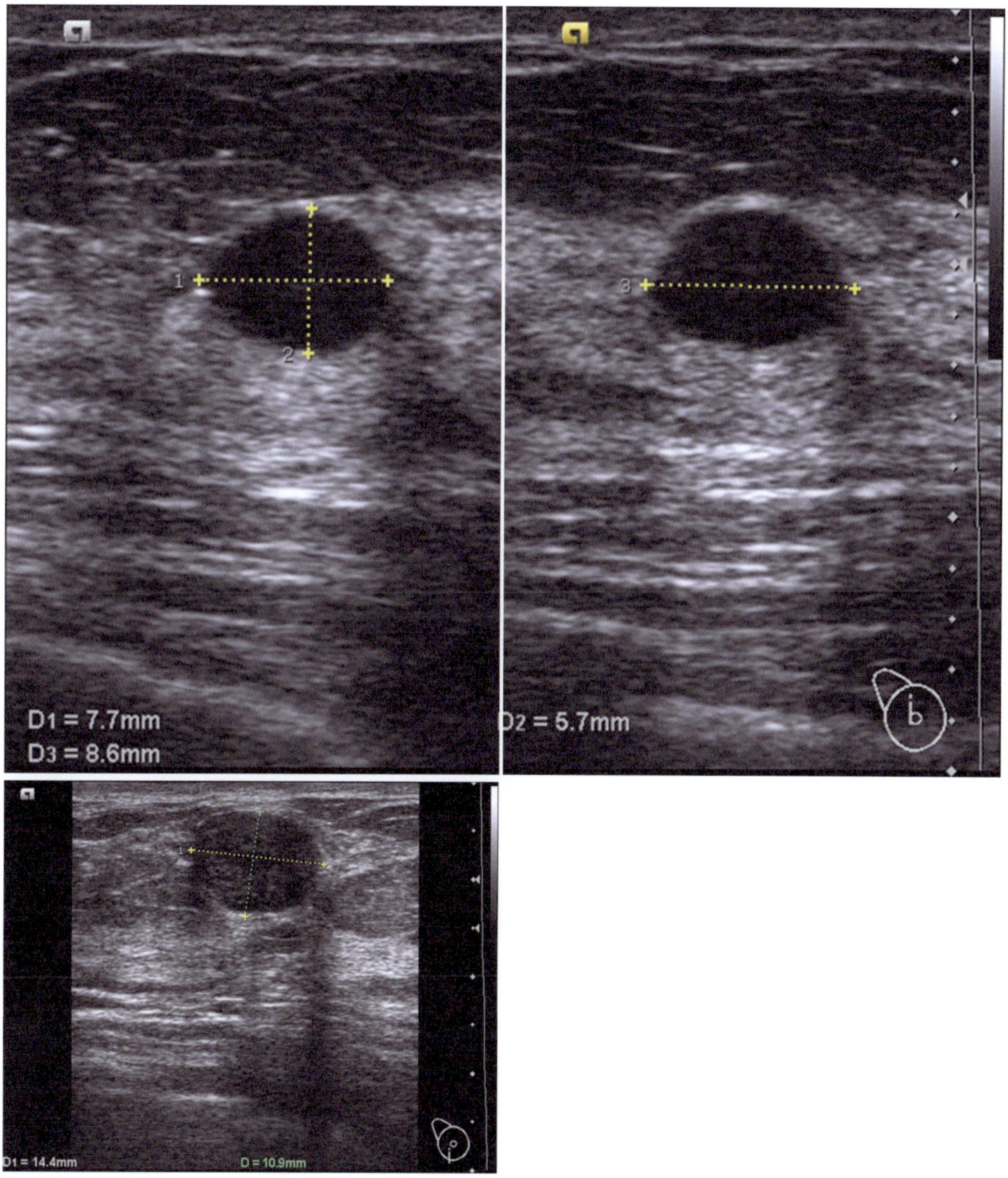

Fig. 6.27 US BI-RADS 4a. Fibradenomas. Grayscale US

targeted core biopsy or FNAB with morphological verification of the diagnosis. To assess the nodular structures, a core needle biopsy with a histological examination of tissue samples is recommended. In the case of benign tumor, ultrasound checkup is recommended in 6 months.

Category 5: Highly suggestive of malignancy—appropriate action should be taken

Signs of breast cancer with a probability of 95% and higher (Fig. 6.30). Morphological verification with pathology and immunohistochemical study is indicated. An ultrasound assessment of the extent of breast cancer is necessary. If the puncture and verification are suggestive of benign disease or uncertain, the mass is classified as US BI-RADS 4, implying thorough ultrasound checkup in 6 months.

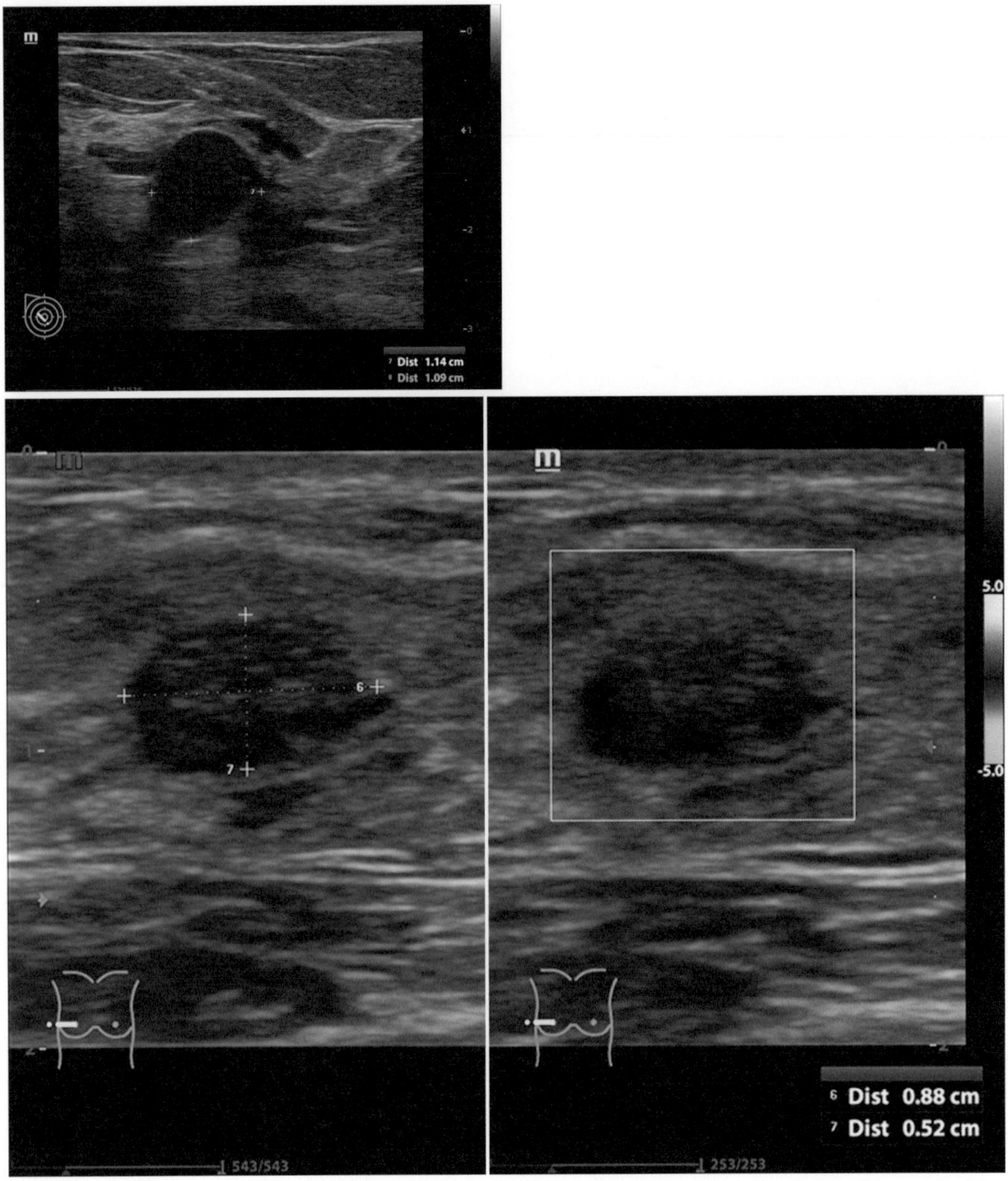

Fig. 6.28 US BI-RADS 4b. Fibradenoma with increase of the greatest dimension by 6 mm for the last 6 months. Grayscale US, CDI

Category 6: Known biopsy-proven malignancy—appropriate action should be taken

A morphologically confirmed breast cancer before specific treatment initiation (Fig. 6.31).

Compliance with the BI-RADS scale is usually determined throughout the examination and is included into the report.

BI-RADS is a constantly evolving system. Discussions are still going on division of Category 4 to subcategories. Introduction of new ultrasound technologies (elastography, CEUS, etc.) forces to evaluate their compatibility with BI-RADS scale.

Ultrasound elastography is an important supplement for differentiation of breast pathol-

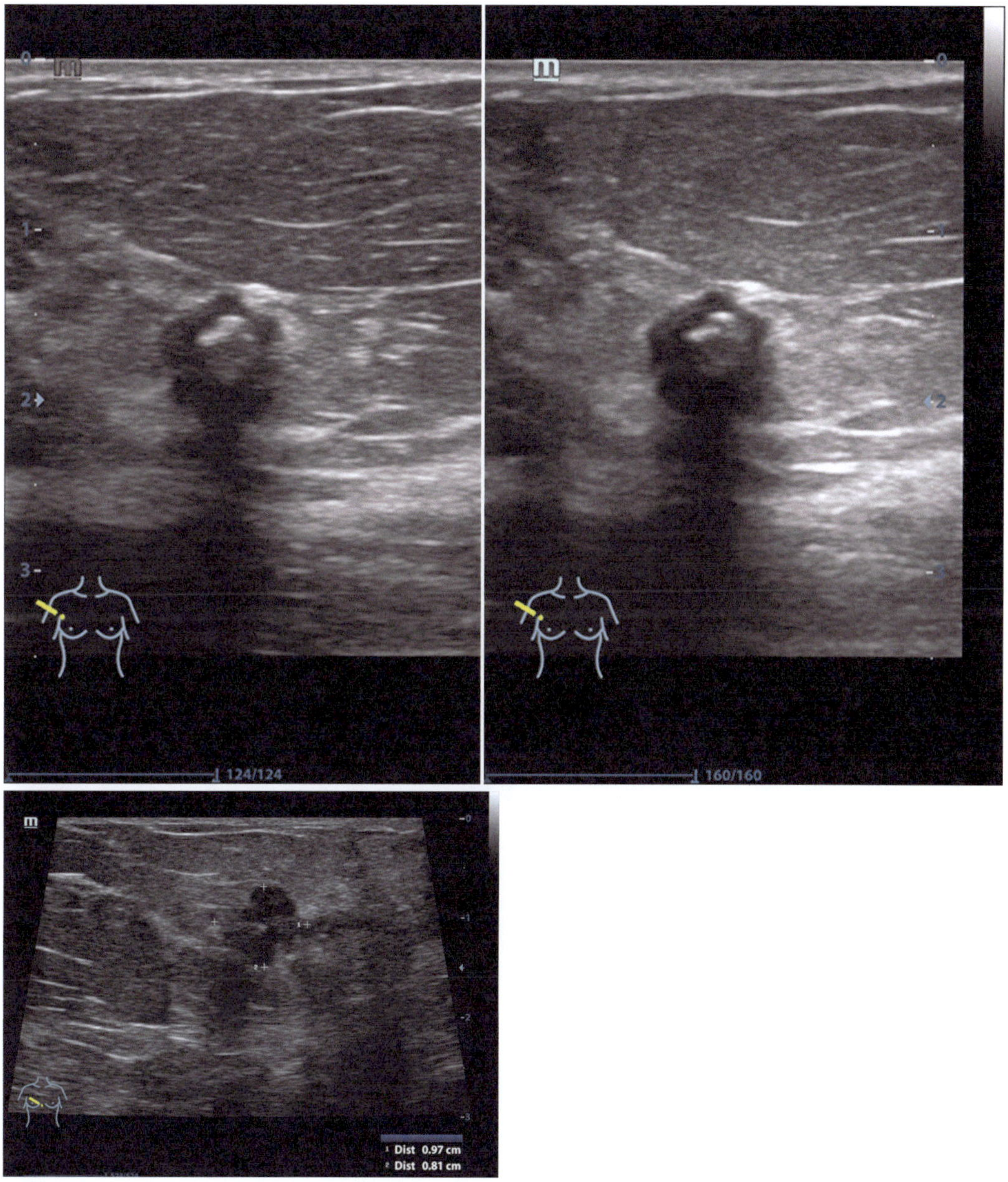

Fig. 6.29 US BI-RADS 4c. Minor breast cancer. Suspicious US signs of malignancy. Grayscale US

ogy to BI-RADS system (Sencha et al. 2015). It allows accurate characterization of stiffness of suspicious masses, detailization of the extent of malignant lesions, analysis of changes after treatment, and prediction of the course of the disease.

Ultrasonography is often used to assess breast abnormalities that were previously detected with mammography or clinically. When allocating a BI-RADS category basing on mammographic and US data, the diagnostic capabilities of these methods in each specific case should be considered. Standardization of lexicon for description of findings and development of a unified examination protocol are expected to facilitate the communication with physicians.

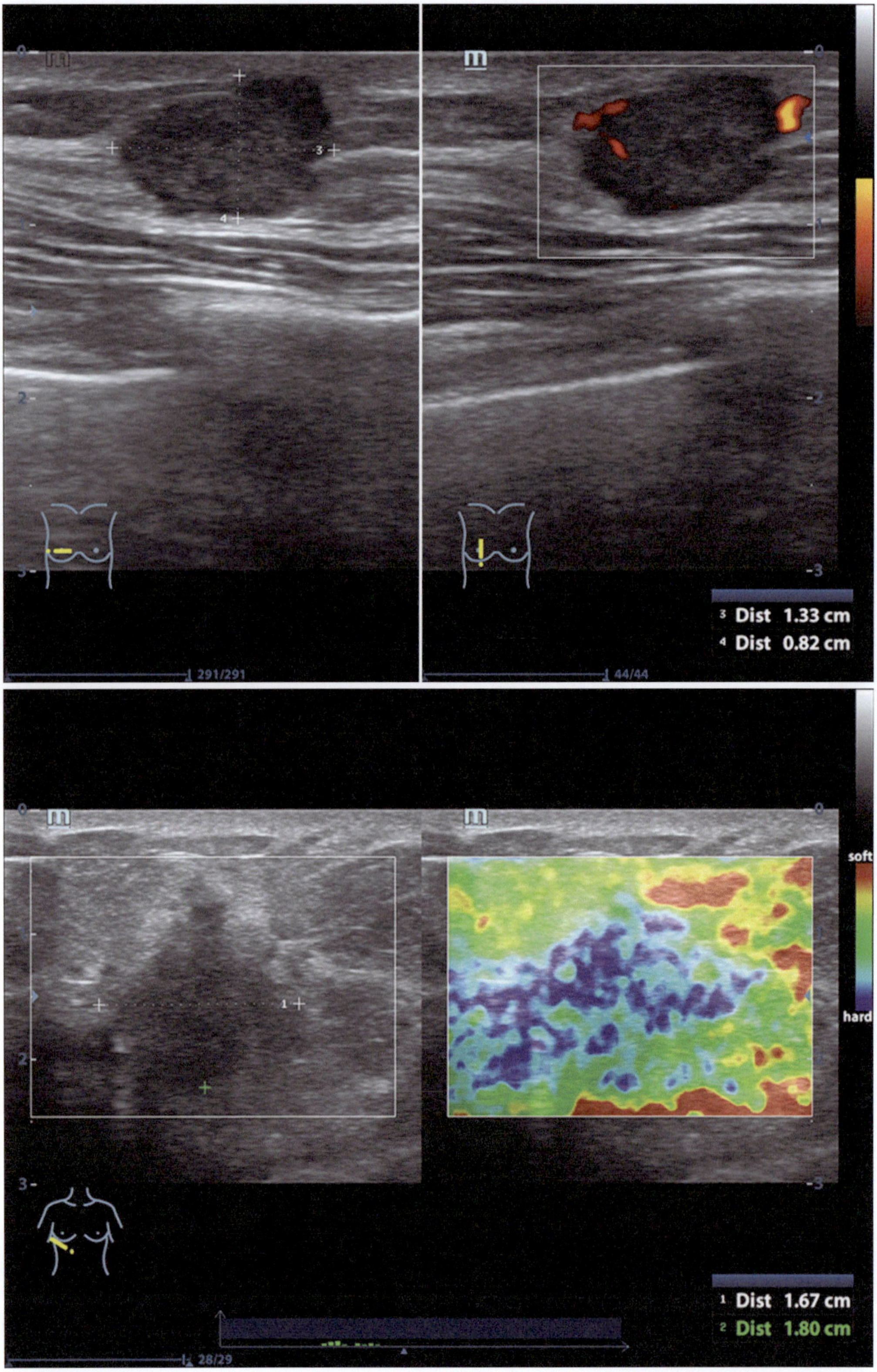

Fig. 6.30 US BI-RADS 5. Breast cancer. Typical ultrasonographic signs of malignancy. Grayscale US, PDI, US elastography

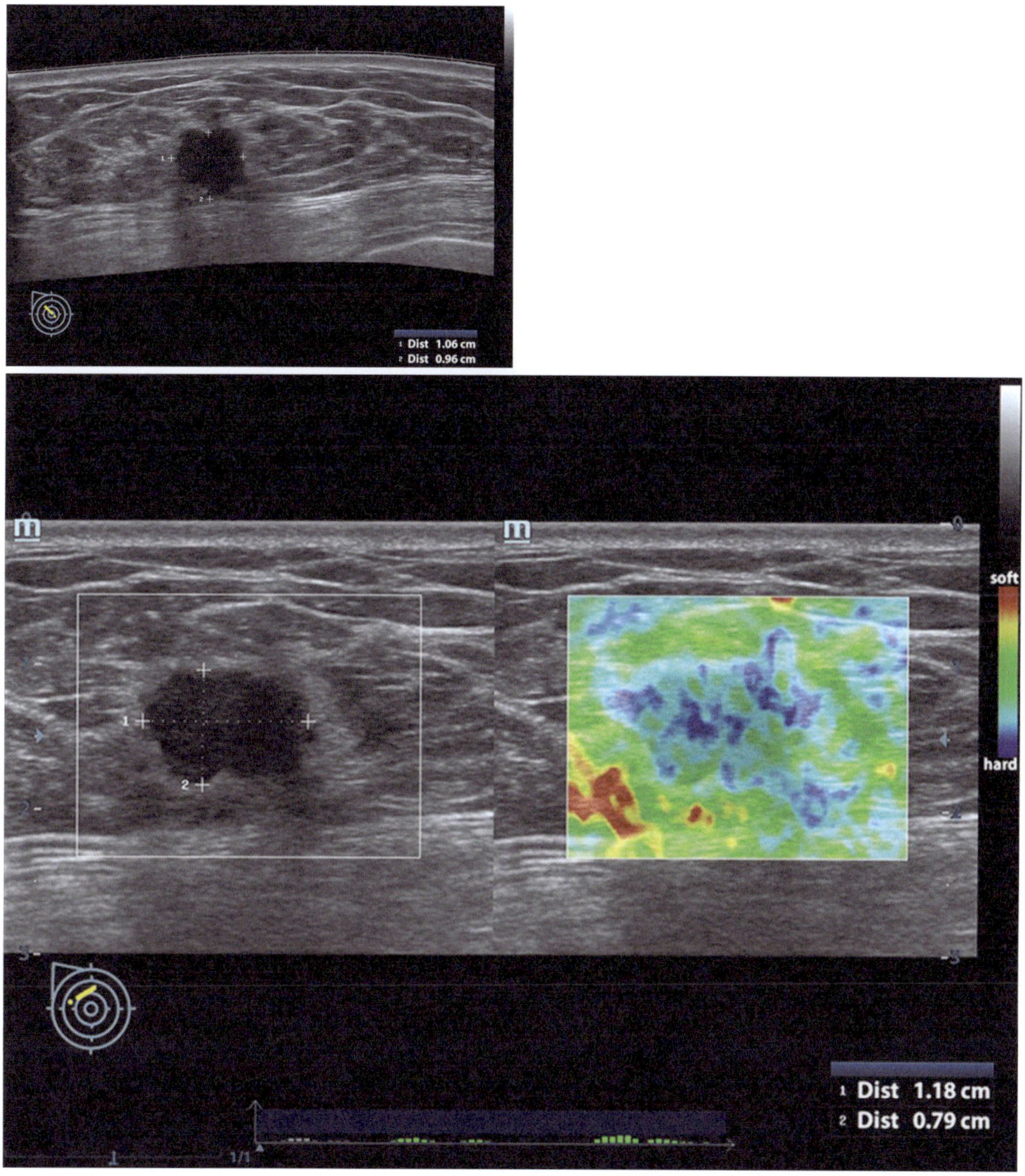

Fig. 6.31 US BI-RADS 6. Breast cancer. Grayscale US, panoramic scan, US elastography

The use of US BI-RADS system is different from traditional image assessment. The main goal is, along with clear specification of the nature of the detected changes (fibroadenoma, cyst, cancer, etc.), the planning of further follow-up in specific time intervals and providing key information for invasive procedures and treatment. BI-RADS scale ensures the continuity of the appropriate interventions by different specialists, in different health facilities, or in different regions and helps to reduce the operator dependency of US. BI-RADS specification takes little time, but it has significant impact on patients' management.

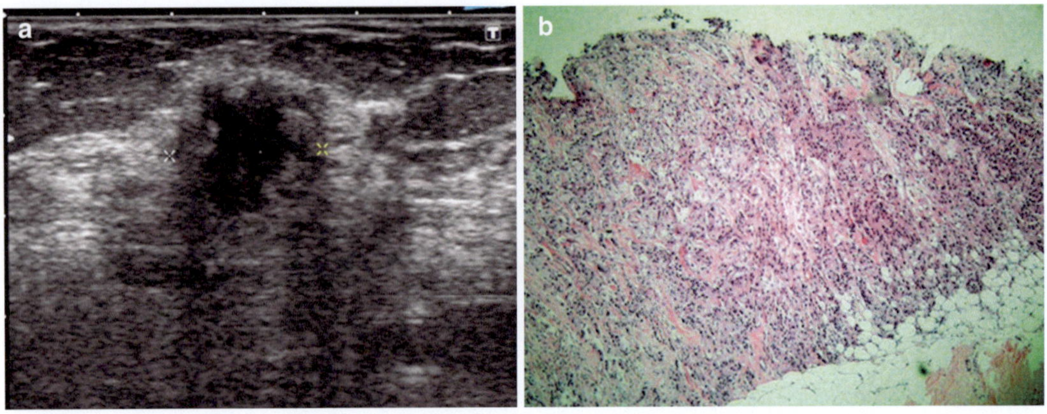

Fig. 6.32 Invasive ductal carcinoma. (**a**) Grayscale US. (**b**) H&E stained section, original magnification, ×100

6.6.2 Ultrasound Image of Various Types of Breast Cancer

Invasive ductal cancer (59%) dominates among all types of breast cancer. There are also several other cancer types with a smaller incidence: invasive lobular (8%), tubular (7%), cancer in a cyst (5%), mucous (4%), medullary (4%), and others (13%) (Sencha et al. 2011). The prevalence of TNM cancer stages is as follows: T in situ, 7%; T1N0M, 20%; T1N1M0, 7%; T1N2M0, 2%; T1N3M0, 1%; T2N0M0, 30%; T2N1M0, 11%; T2N2M0, 3%; T3N1M0, 1%; T3N1M1, 1%; and T4NM, 10%. In 7% of cases, the stage of breast cancer remains unspecified (Sencha et al. 2011).

Attempts have been made to assume morphological structure of a tumor basing on US image. However, US with CDI, PDI, 3D, and other options in the majority of cases does not allow differentiation of morphological type of breast carcinoma. The difficulties in distinguishing morphological structure of lesions are also a consequence of the fact that one third of cancers (31.5%) are combined tumors.

The main task of an ultrasound specialist is to detect breast cancer, while its type specification is a task of a pathologist.

Invasive ductal carcinoma exhibits a set of features for reliable differential diagnosis with benign lesions and other malignancies. Infiltrating duct cancer accounts for more than 70% of all invasive breast cancer types (Haylenko et al. 2005).

US features of ductal breast carcinoma are the following (Fig. 6.32a):

- Hypoechoic
- Homogeneous echostructure
- Indistinct rough contours
- Increased echodensity of the surrounding tissues
- Posterior acoustic shadow
- A- or hypovascularity in CDI, PDI, and 3DPD
- High PI and RI of blood flow within the lesion
- Intensive coloring with US elastography

Macroscopically, invasive ductal cancer is a solid dense lesion of oval or stellar shape. Histologically it corresponds to adenocarcinoma with prevalence of stromal fibrosis (Fig. 6.32b).

Lobular cancer in situ (alveolar cancer, acinar cancer, non-infiltrative lobular cancer) is the type of breast cancer, which is initially a pool of malignant cells surrounded by epithelium, not involving the basal membrane, but potentially invasive. It is most prevalent at the age of 45–50 years. As a rule, it exhibits no clinical symptoms, mammographic, or US features. It is an occasional finding at breast biopsy for nodular mastopathy (Fig. 6.33).

Invasive lobular cancer accounts for 5–15% of all invasive breast carcinomas. It shows as dense nodules with indistinct borders. It demonstrates scirrhous growth and intraorganic spread and is often bilateral (13%, according to Haylenko et al. 2005).

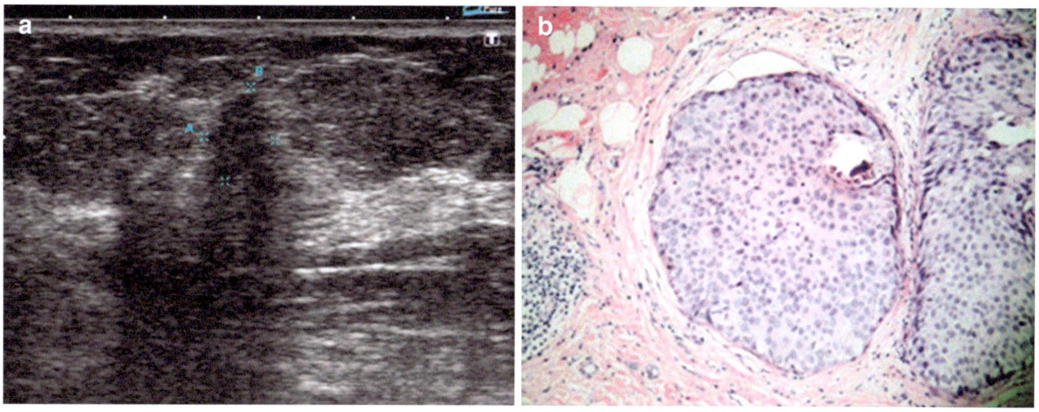

Fig. 6.33 Lobular carcinoma in situ. (**a**) Grayscale US. (**b**) H&E stained section, original magnification, ×100

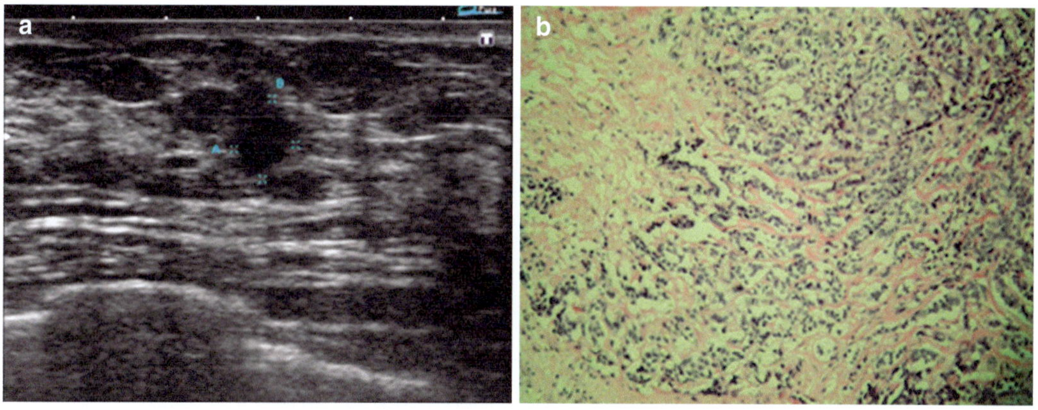

Fig. 6.34 Invasive lobular carcinoma. (**a**) Grayscale US. (**b**) H&E stained section, original magnification, ×400

It exhibits the following US features (Fig. 6.34):

- Focal (sometimes multicentric) lesion
- Irregular shape
- Hypoechoic pattern
- Heterogeneous structure
- Lumpy
- Indistinct contours and irregular borders
- A- or hypovascular at CDI, PDI, and 3DPD
- Intensive coloring with US elastography

Breast cancer with scirrhous growth exhibits the prevalence of stroma fibrosis and is characterized with the following US features (Fig. 6.35):

- Hypoechoic lesion
- Heterogeneous echostructure
- Irregular shape
- Lumpy, rough borders
- Uneven contours
- A- or hypovascular at CDI, PDI, and 3DPD
- Intense hard coloring with US elastography

It is macroscopically presented with dense nodules without clear boundaries and often bilateral and exhibits scirrhous growth with intraorganic diffusion. This type of cancer dominates in the group of X-ray-negative tumors; therefore US is advantageous in its diagnosis.

According to Marquet et al. (1995), scirrhous breast lesion is more often imaged as a lesion with indistinct contours. It is a consequence of invasive growth and star-like speculated shape results from connective tissue. According to Ueno (1996) and Mihaylov and Skrynnik (1997),

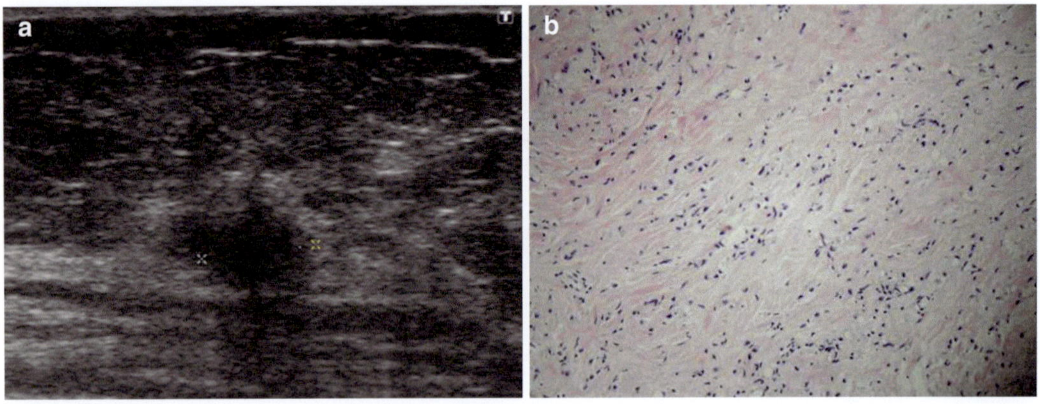

Fig. 6.35 Scirrhous breast carcinoma. (**a**) Grayscale US. (**b**) H&E-stained image of a section, original magnification, ×100

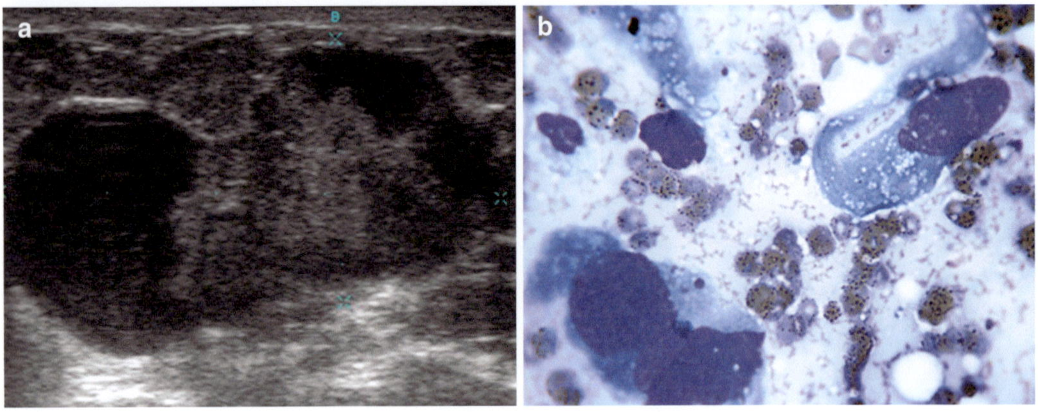

Fig. 6.36 Breast sarcoma. (**a**) Grayscale US. (**b**) Pappenheim-stained image of a section, original magnification, ×1000

posterior shadowing assumes significant connective tissue component within tumor structure.

Breast sarcomas account for 0.2–4.0% (in 3% in women, in 0.5% in men) (Trufanov et al. 2009) of all malignant breast lesions (Rozhkova 1993; Korzhenkova 2004) and occur at any age.

Characteristic US features of breast sarcoma (Fig. 6.36) are listed below:

- Hypoechoic lesion
- Heterogeneous echostructure with anechoic inclusions
- Even indistinct borders
- Large size (often)
- Hyper- or hypovascularity at CDI, PDI, and 3DPD
- Intense, irregular (more often "mosaic") coloring at CEUS elastography
- Rare metastases in axillary lymph nodes

Mucinous cancer (colloid, gelatinous, mucous, cricoid) is a rare cancer with relatively good prognosis. Macroscopically it shows as well defined breast lesion with gray wet gelatinous surface at section. Microscopy reveals solid or mucinous complexes of monomorphic cells containing mucous in their cytoplasm, among massive mucus agglomerations.

US features mucinous breast carcinoma (Fig. 6.37) are listed below:

- Hypoechoic lesion
- Heterogeneous echostructure

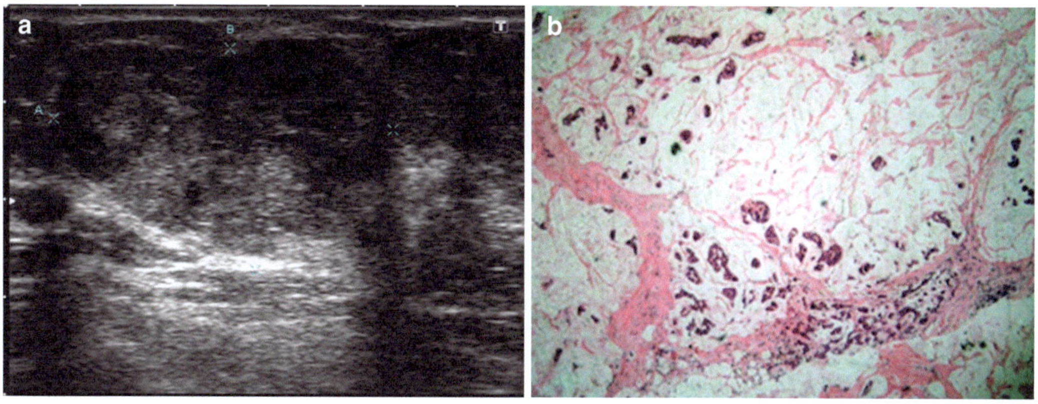

Fig. 6.37 Mucinous breast cancer. (**a**) Grayscale US. (**b**) H&E-stained image of a section, original magnification, ×400

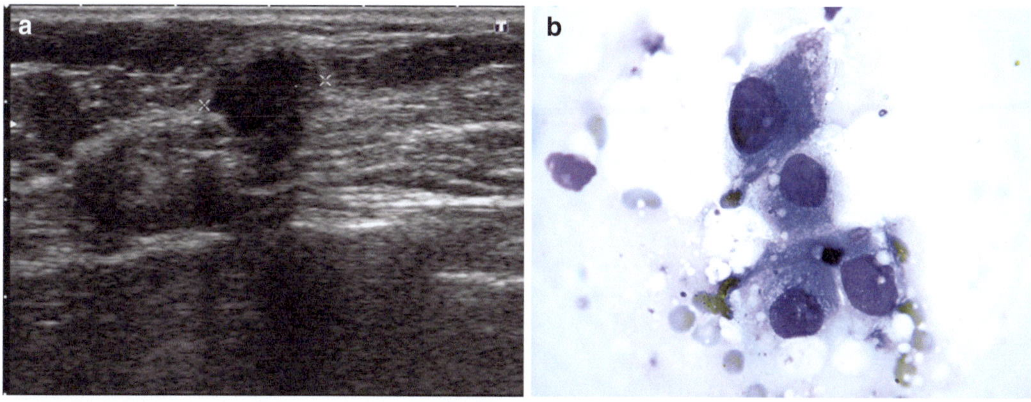

Fig. 6.38 Medullary carcinoma. (**a**) Grayscale US. (**b**) Pappenheim-stained image of a section, original magnification, ×1000

- Polycyclic rough borders
- Distinct or indistinct contours
- Sometimes posterior amplification, more rarely acoustic shadow
- A- or hypovascular at CDI, PDI, and 3DPD
- Intense, irregular "mosaic" coloring at US elastography
- Rare metastasis in axillary lymph nodes

Medullary breast carcinoma is most often represented as an accurately circumscribed nodule of grayish color, soft consistence, and impure structure, which exhibits the following US features (Fig. 6.38):

- Roundish shape
- Decreased echodensity
- Heterogeneous echostructure, often with anechoic incorporations
- Accurate contours
- Irregular borders
- A- or hypovascular pattern in CDI, PDI, and 3DPD
- Decreased, irregular "mosaic" staining with US elastography

Tubular breast carcinoma (Fig. 6.39) is a rare type of cancer, belonging to the group of infiltrative ductal cancer, but with a favorable clinical course and prognosis. It is often met at senior age and rarely metastasizes. Microscopy shows unilaminate tubules of slightly angular, extended shape. Stroma is characterized by expressed fibrosis and hyalinosis. The foci of

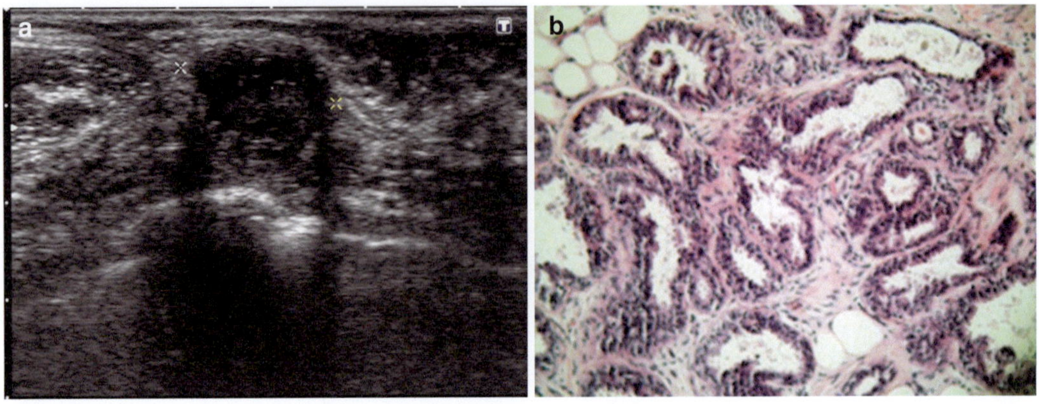

Fig. 6.39 Tubular breast carcinoma. (**a**) Grayscale US. (**b**) H&E-stained image of a section, original magnification, ×100

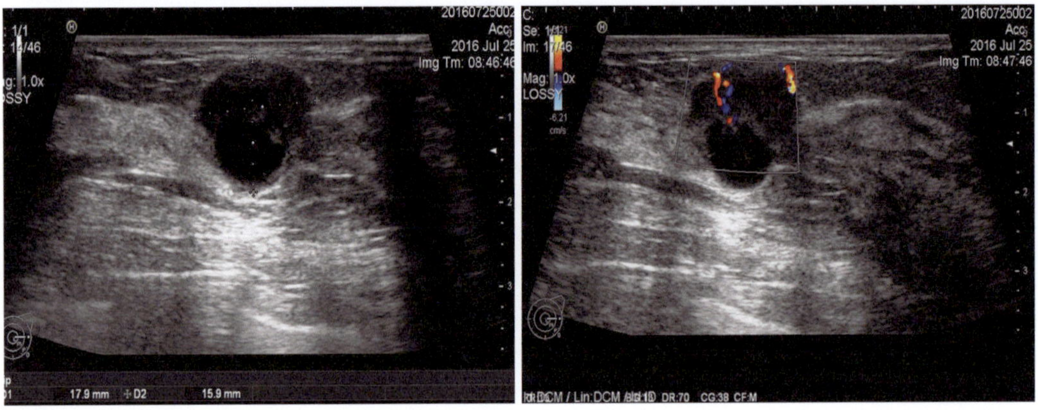

Fig. 6.40 Papillary breast cancer. Grayscale US and CDI

periductal and perivascular elastosis are often observed.

Tubular breast carcinoma sonographically is usually defined as a lesion <2 cm of mixed echogenicity, with heterogeneous structure, even or rough borders, and indistinct contours and often with distal acoustic shadow, and is avascular with CDI, PDI, and 3DPD and intensively irregularly colored with US elastography.

Papillary cancer is a rare type of breast cancer, affecting mostly elderly women. Microscopically, it is represented by numerous papillae of polymorphic, less often monomorphic epithelial cells. Ultrasound often defines it as a cancer in the cyst, with proliferation of hypervascularized solid component. It may reach 2–4 cm in size (Fig. 6.40).

Intraductal breast cancer accounts for 2% of all cancers of the breast. Microscopically, the tumor is usually represented by dilated lactiferous ducts filled with solid proliferates of polymorphic cells. Ultrasonographic features of the intraductal cancer are as follows (Fig. 6.41):

- Low or mixed echodensity
- Heterogeneous echostructure
- Multiple microcalcifications
- Often necrotic areas
- Dilatation of lactiferous ducts
- Extensive process (often with invasive growth and involvement of adjacent lobules)
- Different degrees of vascularization in color-coded modes
- Various stiffness with compression US elastography and elastometry

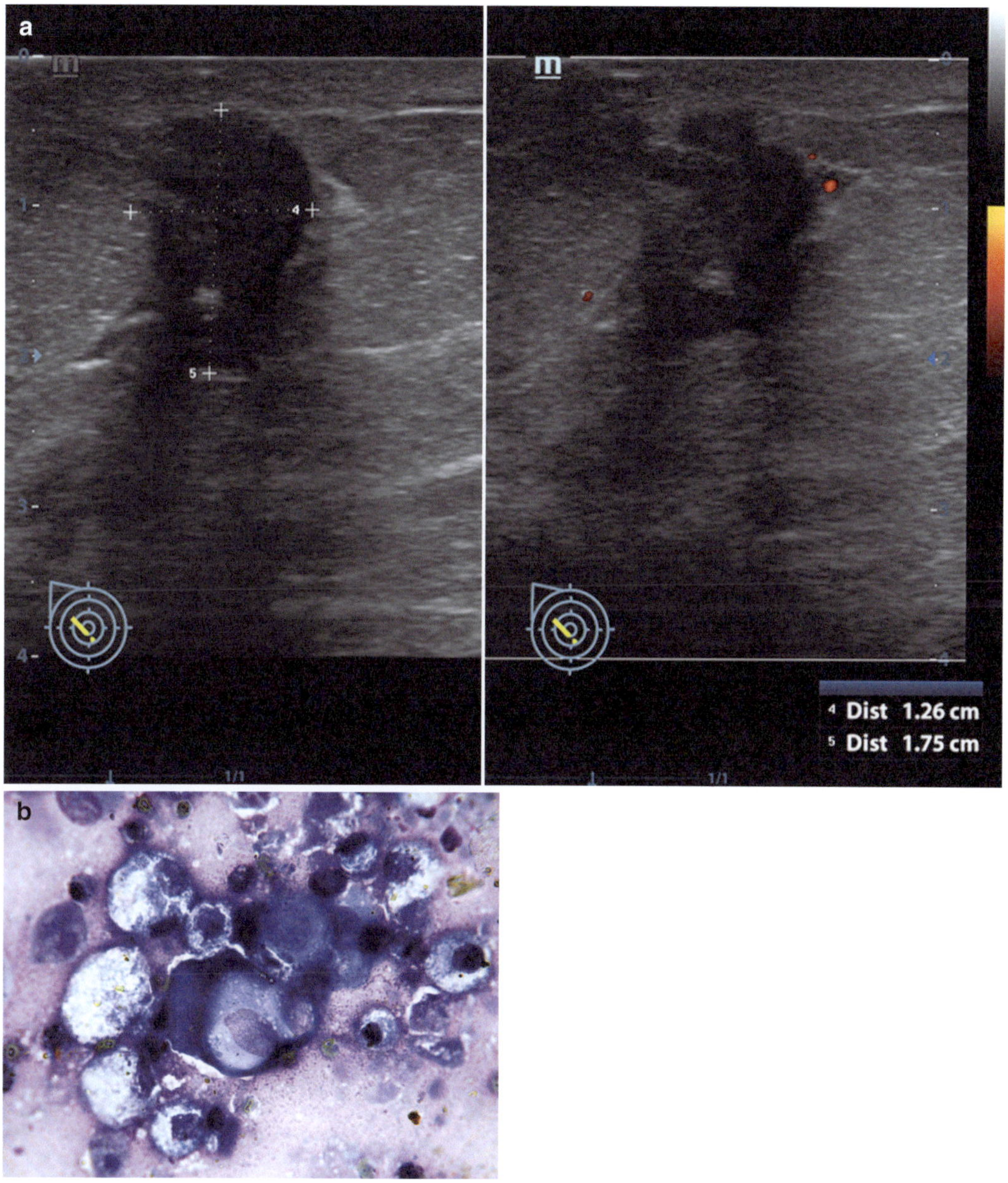

Fig. 6.41 Intraductal breast cancer. (**a**) Grayscale US and PDI. (**b**) Pappenheim-stained image of a section, original magnification, ×1000

None of US features of breast carcinoma is absolutely reliable. The majority of signs should be considered only in a complex with other criteria and the data of other methods (Sencha et al. 2009). Routine and new US technologies permit to sort out the features of lesions, which are characteristic for malignancies, to facilitate differential diagnosis in the majority of complex diagnostic cases.

A set of US techniques available at every particular scanner should be used by an ultrasonographist to classify the patients into the following groups:

- Patients with normal breast, who do not require further thorough examination or follow-up. They are recommended to undergo breast examination once in 1–2 years.

- Patients with breast lesions that do not require surgical treatment. They are subject to follow-up with breast examination once in 6–12 months.
- Patients with breast masses suspicious for malignancy. Further examination (breast biopsy with morphologic verification) is necessary. Subsequent surgery may apply.

High qualification of US specialists and cooperation of doctors of different specialties, following the principles of continuity of diagnostic process, and utilization of all available technologies, enable early detection of malignant breast tumors and optimal patient management.

An example of US report of a patient with breast cancer

Name, surname. __S__ Age__41__

Outpatient examination. Date____

Patient's record____

US scanner____

First day of last menses____

Breasts are mainly presented by adipose tissue. Glandular tissue is up to 11 mm thick. Fibrous tissue is expressed moderately in all quadrants. Lactiferous ducts within the right breast are moderately dilated up to 0.4 cm, mainly in outer quadrants. A homogeneous hypoechoic lesion of 2.3 × 3.1 cm in size of irregular star-like shape with indistinct, rough boundaries is located in upper-outer quadrant (10 o'clock position) of the right breast. The lesion is hypovascular with CDI, PDI, and 3DPD (three color pixels in the central area). It demonstrates intense irregular hard (blue) staining with sonoelastography.

Enlarged axillary lymph nodes are detected on the right side up to 1.0–2.2 cm in size, hypoechoic with irregular structure, and disorganized blood flow pattern. The lymph nodes of over groups are not enlarged.

Conclusion: Right breast lesion suspicious for carcinoma. US BI-RADS 5. Sonographic signs of metastasis in the right axillary lymph nodes.

Biopsy of the lesion and right axillary lymph nodes is recommended.

7 Breast Diseases in Pregnant Women: Possibilities of Ultrasound Diagnostics

Alexander N. Sencha and Ella Penyaeva

Abstract

Mammary glands undergo significant physiologic changes during pregnancy and lactation in response to the increase in circulating hormone levels. Ultrasound is the first-line test for palpable breast masses in pregnant or breastfeeding patients. US images of normal breasts may vary depending on terms of pregnancy and duration of lactation. In the first trimester, the breast structure in a pregnant woman may be similar to the nonpregnant state: glandular tissue prevails, with clear granularity and narrow lactiferous ducts. In the second trimester, glandular tissue becomes more thick achieving 25–30 mm, the structure of parenchyma becomes more granular and diffusely hypoechoic due to increase of fat-free fibroglandular component, lactiferous ducts are about 3 mm wide, and vascularization of the parenchyma may be enhanced. At term, a diffuse duct ectasia of various degrees can be noted. During the entire lactation period, parenchyma is hyperechoic with significantly dilated (>3 mm) lactiferous ducts in grayscale images. Hypervascularized parenchyma shows in color imaging. During pregnancy and lactation, the mammary gland is subject to a number of specific changes, which can lead to the appearance of certain disorders, including benign changes that are associated with physiological changes in the body during pregnancy/lactation: inflammatory and infectious changes, juvenile papillomatosis, benign tumors, and malignant tumors. Specific features of breast cancer associated with pregnancy are usually aggressive in course, late diagnosis, and poor prognosis. The primary diagnosis, clinical stage, and extent of breast cancer in pregnant women in 85% are based on US findings.

A. N. Sencha
Division of Visual Diagnostics, National Medical Research Center for Obstetrics, Gynecology and Perinatology named after Academician V.I. Kulakov of Ministry of Healthcare of Russian Federation, Moscow, Russia

E. Penyaeva (✉)
Department of Ultrasound Diagnostics of Radiology Center, Yaroslavl Railway Clinic, Yaroslavl, Russia

7.1 Possibilities and Efficacy of Imaging Modalities for Diagnosis of Breast Pathology in Pregnant Women

Breast examination in a pregnant or breastfeeding woman, with specification of palpable masses, detection of impalpable masses, differential diagnosis, and making decision on further management is a common task for a radiologist.

Mammary glands undergo significant physiologic changes during pregnancy and lactation in

G. T. Sukhikh, A. N. Sencha (eds.), *Multiparametric Ultrasound Diagnosis of Breast Diseases*,
https://doi.org/10.1007/978-3-319-75034-7_7

response to the increase in circulating hormone levels (estrogen, progesterone, and prolactin). These changes usually start from the eighth week of gestation. This initial period is characterized by significant development of lactiferous ducts and enlargement of the glandular lobules. At the same time, stromal component of the breast parenchyma is subject to involution, along with the enhanced vascularization and infiltration of the lobules with mononuclear cells. Proliferation and differentiation of the lobules, alveoli, and lactiferous ducts occur in the first and second trimesters; alveolar epithelium becomes secretory. The lobular structures intensively grow due to epithelial proliferation, especially in the parenchyma, in the second and third trimesters. Under the increase of prolactin level during the third trimester, the epithelium continues to differentiate, and finally colostrum fills alveoli and ducts. After childbirth, lactogenic effect of prolactin results in significant milk production. These physiologic changes may strongly affect the possibility and quality of visualization of the mammary gland and make examination of pregnant and breastfeeding patients really complex. A clinician, when inspecting breast of a pregnant woman, may consider a mass as a physiologic sign of pregnancy. Moreover, physiologic alterations may mask a developing tumor.

On the one side, highly informative imaging tests (mammography, US, MDCT) are necessary for correct diagnosis; on the other, concerns about the fetus' safety limit the means for diagnostic, sometimes leading to false-negative results. Contrast agents and radioisotopes are not safe for a fetus. A puncture biopsy (necessary to obtain material for pathologic study) during pregnancy may result in a persistent lactiferous duct fistula and complicate neoadjuvant treatment.

Ultrasonography, mammography, and MRI are used for detection and differential diagnosis of breast pathology in pregnant women. Application of imaging modalities during pregnancy is now well defined.

Mammography during pregnancy is usually safe. Nevertheless, both pregnant patients and their doctors may be concerned about high risk of ionization. This test is recommended during pregnancy only if a malignancy is suspected or already proved by core needle biopsy. Sensitivity of breast X-ray during pregnancy is lower than of US: 78–90% (Yang et al. 1996). Mammography may be useful for detection of microcalcifications (undetectable with US) and for evaluation of the severity of the disease, including multifocal, multicentric, and contralateral lesions. Therefore, bilateral breast X-Ray is recommended for any patient with a suspicious breast mass detected at physical examination or US and in any patient diagnosed with pregnancy-associated breast cancer.

Routine annual screening with mammography is not performed during pregnancy. Women over 40 years of age are recommended to undergo screening not earlier than 3 months after cessation of lactation and complete involution of breast parenchyma and return to normal function and baseline density.

MRI with contrast enhancement is usually not recommended during pregnancy, because gadolinium-based contrasts are classified by the US FDA as Category C for pregnancy. Despite the absence of evidence of teratogenic effect of gadolinium-based contrasts in humans, no prospective controlled trials evaluating such effects have been performed. The European Society for Urogenital Radiology has issued a guideline stating that gadolinium-based contrasts can be safely introduced during pregnancy, as there is no evidence on teratogenicity. However, these agents are known to pass placental barrier in detectable amounts, and therefore, residual minor amounts of gadolinium in amniotic fluid may dissociate to toxic-free ions of gadolinium.

Contrast-enhanced MRI may be safely performed in lactating patients with breast cancer for assessment of the disease extent and evaluation of the surrounding structures.

Taking into account diagnostic challenges of contrast-enhanced MRI in lactating women, use of MRI for screening in high-risk patients is also limited. Postponing of screening until lactation cessation may be reasonable.

Radioisotope scan of the skeleton for detection of metastases of breast cancer is rarely used in pregnant women, because this test provides

0.00194 Gy radiation to the fetus. PET-CT with isotope fluor-18-fluorodeoxyglucose (18-FDG) is necessary for search of metastases, a primary lesion, and a so-called CUP (cancer unknown primary) syndrome or for monitoring of the cancer treatment.

US-guided core needle biopsy, being radiation-free and feasible, is the procedure of choice in cases where histologic verification of suspicious breast cancer is needed in pregnant women. Stereotactic biopsy is safe and can be applied in early pregnancy and also for verification of suspicious lesions undetectable by US. MRI-guided procedures may also be performed in breastfeeding women.

When performing interventions under imaging control, a patient should be fully informed and instructed. They should be assured that local anesthesia with lidocaine does not adversely affect the fetus. Breastfeeding patients should be informed on the possible presence of some blood and lidocaine in the breast milk after the biopsy due to dilatation of lactiferous ducts and enhanced vascularization of the parenchyma during pregnancy and lactation.

The technique of diagnostic procedures in pregnant patients does not differ from that applied in nonpregnant women. Prior to mammography, MRI, or US, a woman is advised to breastfeed her baby or to squeeze the milk, in order to reduce the density of the breast parenchyma. A test can be performed without any preparation as well.

7.2 Mammary Glands During Pregnancy and Lactation: Ultrasound Features

US is the first-line test for palpable breast masses in pregnant or breastfeeding patients. Outstanding advantages of US include safety due to absence of the ionizing radiation, accessibility, no need for preparation, high diagnostic value, and sensitivity for pregnancy-associated tumors. Efficacy of US in diagnosis of breast cancer in pregnant women was confirmed in many studies.

The US images of normal breasts may vary depending on terms of pregnancy and duration of lactation.

In the first trimester, the breast structure in a pregnant woman may be similar to the nonpregnant state: glandular tissue prevails, with clear granularity and narrow lactiferous ducts (Fig. 7.1).

In the second trimester, glandular tissue becomes more thick achieving 25–30 mm, the structure of parenchyma becomes more granular and diffusely hypoechoic due to increase of fat-free fibroglandular component, lactiferous ducts are about 3 mm wide, and vascularization of the parenchyma may be enhanced (Fig. 7.2)

At term, a diffuse duct ectasia of various degrees can be noted (Fig. 7.3)

During the entire lactation period, parenchyma is hyperechoic with significantly dilated (>3 mm) lactiferous ducts in grayscale images. Hypervascularized parenchyma shows in color imaging (Fig. 7.4).

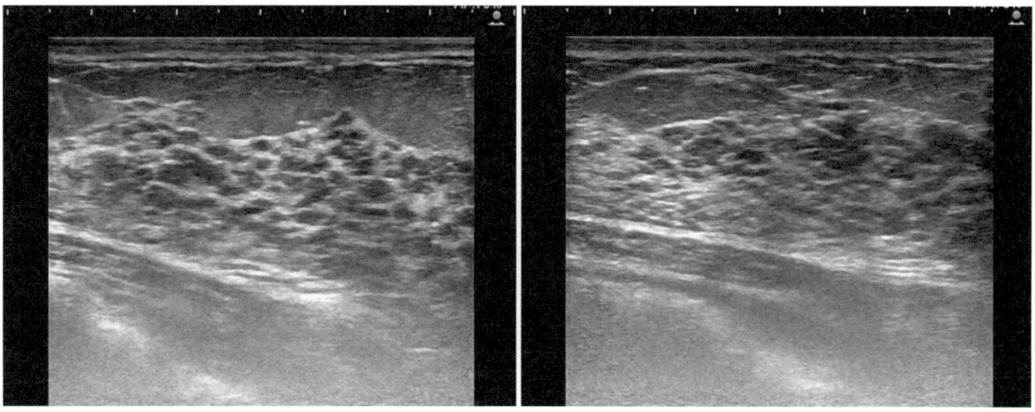

Fig. 7.1 US structure of the mammary gland during pregnancy, 10 weeks of gestation. Grayscale US

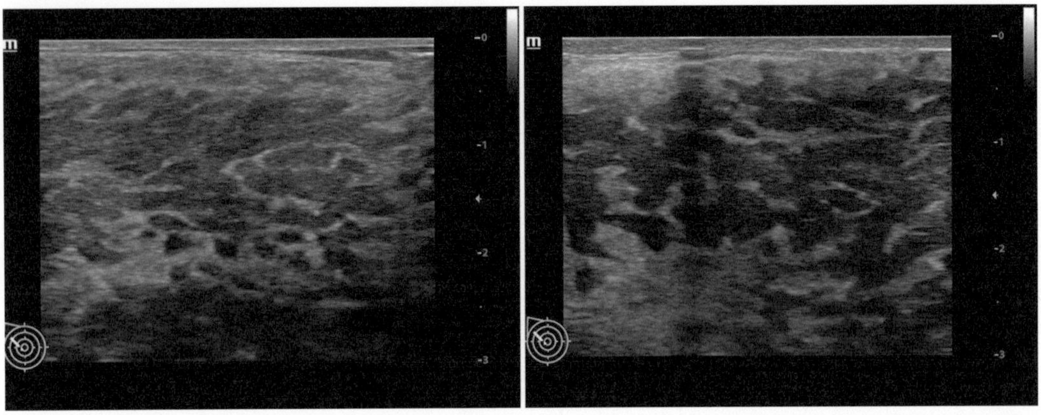

Fig. 7.2 US structure of the mammary gland during pregnancy, 23 weeks of gestation. Grayscale US

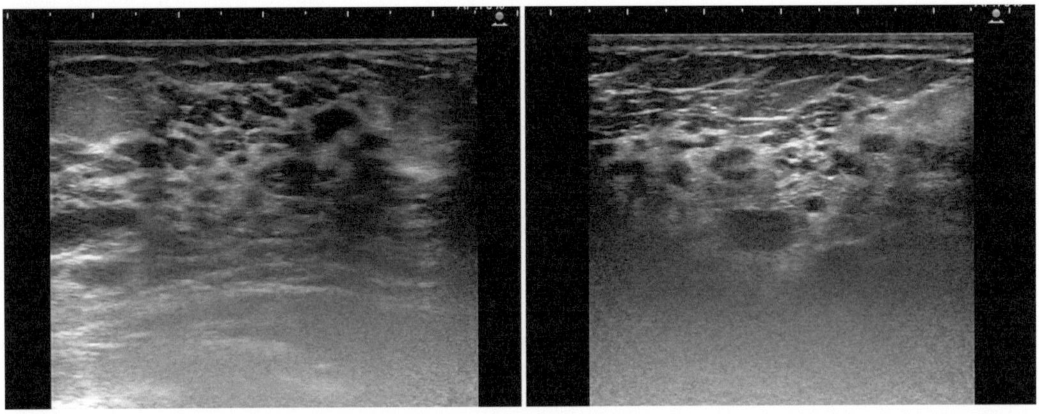

Fig. 7.3 US structure of the mammary gland during pregnancy, 39 weeks of gestation. Grayscale US. Dilated lactiferous ducts

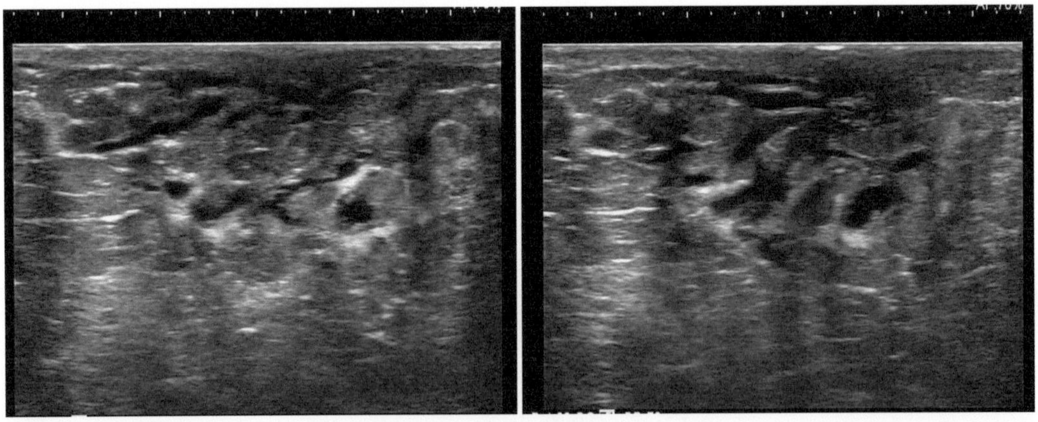

Fig. 7.4 US structure of the mammary gland during lactation. Grayscale. Dilated lactiferous ducts

As soon as lactation is accomplished, the glandular compartments of the mammary gland gradually reduce in volume, alveolar cells become atrophic, fibrotic layers become rough and dense, and lactiferous ducts narrow. The structure of the mammary gland returns to pre-pregnant state.

7.3 Pathologic Breast Conditions During Pregnancy

During pregnancy and lactation, the mammary gland is subject to a number of specific changes, which can lead to the appearance of certain disorders, including benign changes that are associated with physiological changes in the body during pregnancy/lactation: inflammatory and infectious changes, juvenile papillomatosis, benign tumors, and malignant tumors.

Any palpable formation of the breast in a pregnant or breastfeeding patient requires a fast assessment with an appropriate imaging technique and targeted intervention.

Types of pathologic breast conditions associated with pregnancy and lactation

1. Benign pathology associated with physiological breast changes
   - Gestational and secretory hyperplasia
   - Spontaneous bleeding from the nipple
   - Galactocele
   - Gigantomastia
2. Inflammatory and infectious breast diseases
   - Postpartum lactation mastitis
   - Granulomatous mastitis
3. Diseases associated with fibrocystic mastopathy
   - Juvenile papillomatosis
4. Benign breast tumors
   - Tumors associated with pregnancy/lactation
     – Lactating adenoma
   - Morphological and physiological changes in fibroadenoma related to pregnancy/lactation
     – Fast-growing fibroadenoma
     – Fibroadenoma with infarction (foci of necrosis)
     – Fibroadenoma with secretory hyperplasia or lactational changes
5. Malignant tumors
   - Breast cancer
   - Sarcoma
   - Burkitt's lymphoma

Multiparametric ultrasound can effectively detect and differentiate the majority of benign breast masses in pregnant patients. Any suspicious lesion detected with ultrasound can be quickly verified, if necessary, with US-guided core needle biopsy. Identification of suspicious axillary lymph nodes or clinically undetectable multifocal (in the same quadrant), multicenter (in another quadrant), or contralateral lesion can facilitate rapid and effective preoperative diagnosis.

FA is the most common benign breast tumor in young women. These tumors are sensitive to hormones. As a result, **FA during pregnancy and lactation** often enlarges in response to increased hormone levels.

Typical US image of a FA in a pregnant woman does not significantly differ from the one of non-pregnant woman. Specific features of gestational FA are round or oval shape, decreased echogenicity, heterogeneity of echostructure, internal hyperechoes, clear even contours and borders, pseudocapsule, and absence of posterior acoustic shadow, often hypovascularization (Fig. 7.5).

However, ultrasound picture of FA during pregnancy can often be atypical, due to the presence of heterogeneity of the structure, appearance of cystic inclusions, increased vascularization, and dilated milk ducts. In the presence of atypical features such as small lobular structure, uneven edges, heterogeneous echostructure, distal acoustic shadow, and pronounced hypoechogenicity, transcutaneous core needle biopsy is indicated to confirm the diagnosis and exclude breast cancer. If a FA during pregnancy outgrows its blood supply, an infarction can occur. In this case a patient may feel a painful mass, and the structure of the tumor becomes more heterogeneous.

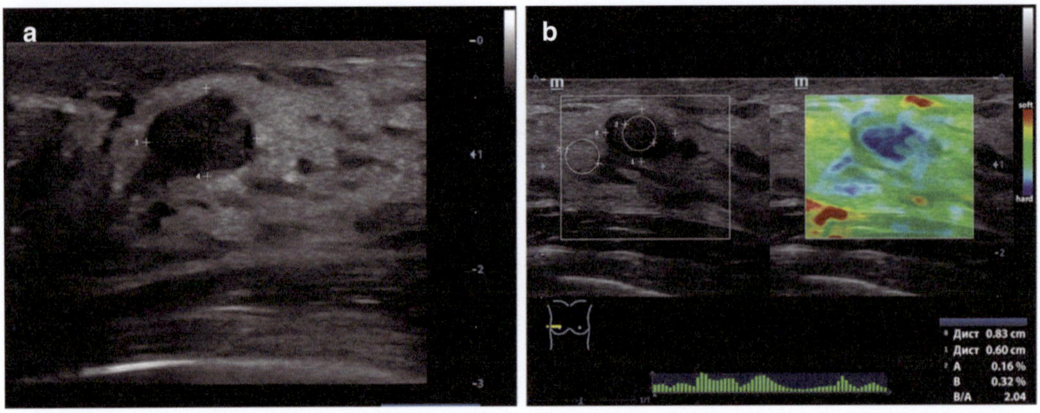

Fig. 7.5 Breast FA during pregnancy. (**a**) Grayscale US. (**b**) Compression elastography

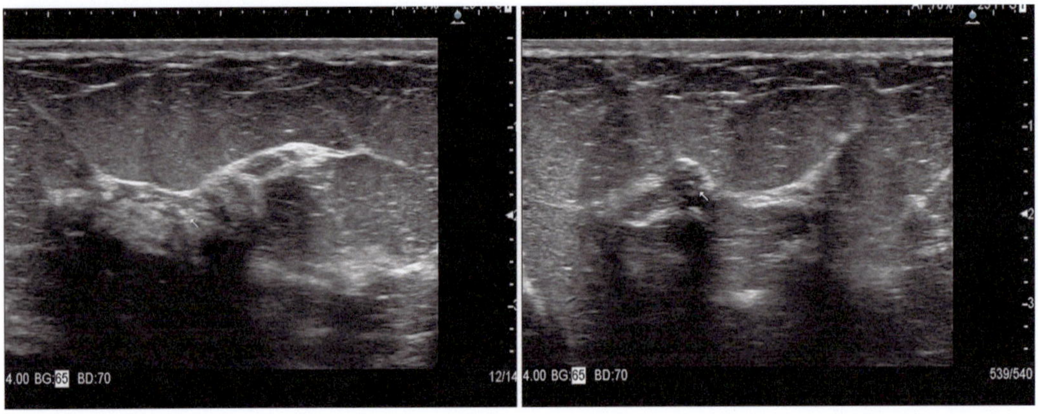

Fig. 7.6 Microcalcifications in gestational hyperplasia. Grayscale US

Microcalcifications in gestational hyperplasia can be detected with mammography or ultrasonography. Microcalcifications often have no acoustic shadow and are usually visualized as diffuse or focal round hyperechogenic inclusions. Linear structures or lesions with uneven borders are rare (Fig. 7.6). To confirm the diagnosis, a fine needle biopsy with subsequent cytology is often performed.

Spontaneous spotting from a nipple is a rare condition during pregnancy and lactation. It usually occurs in the third trimester of pregnancy, when microcirculation and blood flow significantly increase along with significant changes of the epithelium. It leads to bleeding even with minimal injuries. Cytological examination of the nipple discharge should be carried out with greater caution. When bloody discharge occurs from one duct, galactography and ultrasound scan are usually performed to exclude breast cancer and other masses of breast parenchyma.

Cysts, fibroadenomas, and other benign masses are also often detected in the breast during pregnancy. As a rule, these are pre-existing conditions, which have been already noted before pregnancy. They require dynamic monitoring after pregnancy. Ultrasound characteristics of the benign masses during pregnancy are usually similar to those in nonpregnant women (see Sect. 4.5 in Chap. 4, Fig. 7.7).

After pregnancy, benign masses may change in size, structure, vascularity, and stiffness, often with positive dynamics.

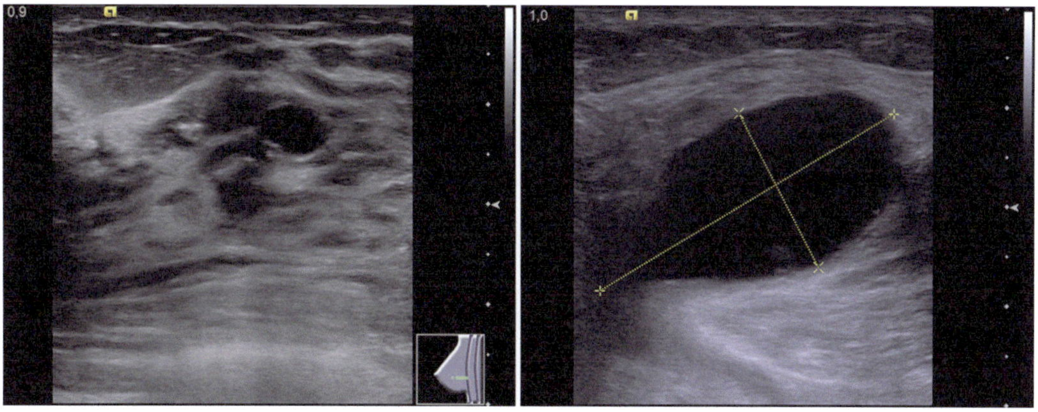

Fig. 7.7 A simple breast cyst during pregnancy (24 weeks of gestation). Grayscale US

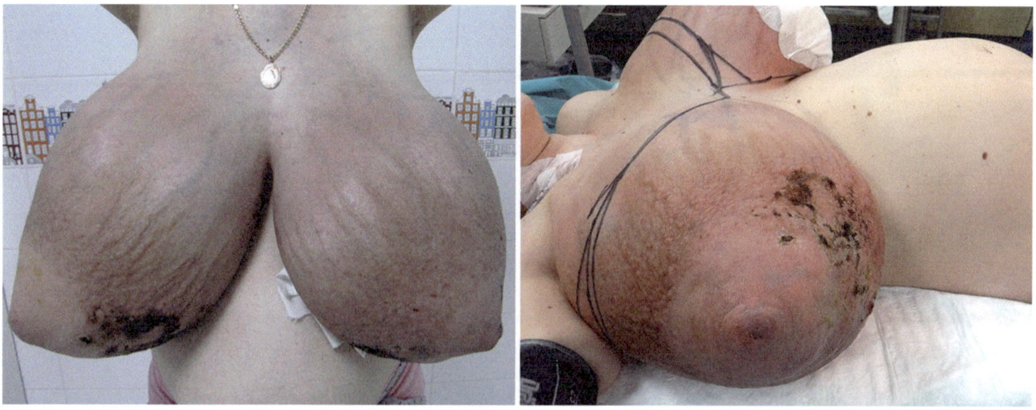

Fig. 7.8 True gestational gigantomastia. View of mammary glands

Gigantomastia (macromastia, megalomastia) is a rare benign breast pathology, manifesting with rapid symmetric enlargement of the mammary glands. The disease can occur both in puberty (see Chap. 4), and during pregnancy (Fig. 7.8).

Gestational gigantomastia is more often observed in women with repeated pregnancies (without or with a previous history of breast enlargement during previous pregnancies). Palmuth was the first to describe gigantomastia in pregnancy in 1648. Since then, about 100 cases were published. The incidence of gestational gigantomastia in pregnancy in 1935–1960 was 1 per 28,000, and that in 1989–2009 was 1 per 100,000 pregnant women. The exact etiology and pathogenesis of gigantomastia are still not clear.

Gigantomastia quickly leads to physical discomfort and suffering, including psychological disorders. Patients with gigantomastia are often stressed by their appearance and suffer from depression and social desadaptation. Gigantomastia is often associated with severe pain, ulcers, necrosis, and hemorrhages. Without appropriate treatment, infectious complications may follow (mastitis, abscesses, or other).

Ultrasonographic features of gestational gigantomastia (as well as of the juvenile gigantomastia) (see Chap. 4) are as follows (Figs. 7.9 and 7.10):

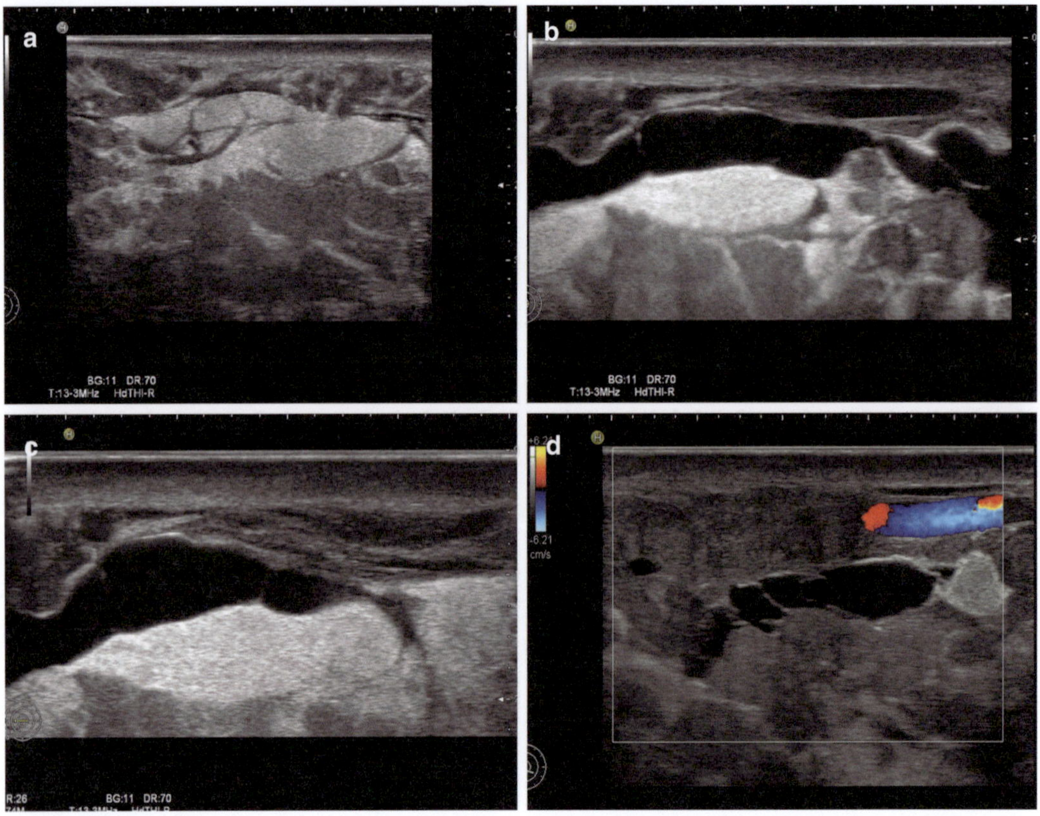

Fig. 7.9 True gestational gigantomastia. Ultrasound image of the breast transformation. Inhomogeneity of the parenchyma structure, lymphatic duct dilatation, and superficial veins. (**a–c**) Grayscale US. (**d**) CDI

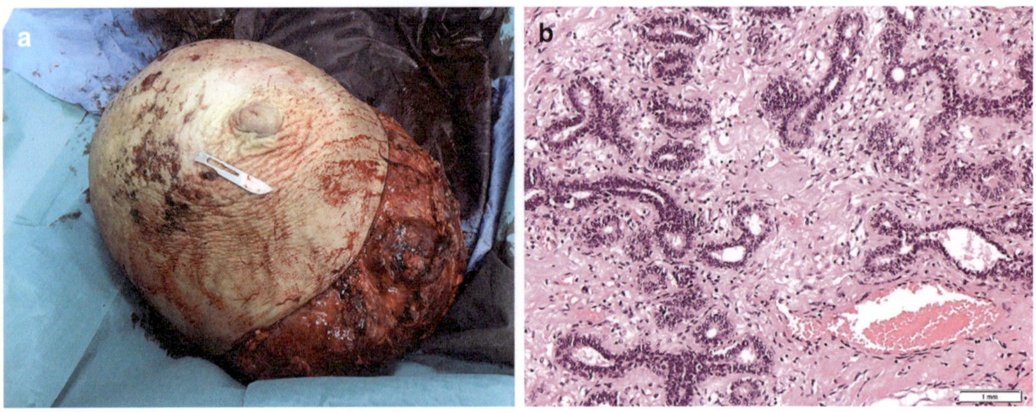

Fig. 7.10 True gestational gigantomastia. (**a**) Gross pathology of the removed breast. (**b**) H&E stained section; original magnification, ×200. Hyperplasia of the lobules and ducts with preservation of their normal histoarchitectonics; in the stroma there are many dilated blood vessels

- Pronounced edema of the skin and subcutaneous fat and decreased echogenicity and heterogeneity of the structure.
- Presence of enlarged lymphatic vessels.
- Heterogeneity of the structure of the parenchyma.
- Unevenly expressed duct ectasia.
- Delated superficial veins and/or varicosities in parenchyma, sometimes with "spontaneous contrasting" of blood flow, colored in color regimens.
- Inhomogeneity of density of various parts of parenchyma in the modes of ultrasound compression elastography; average strain ratio at different sites can reach 1.8–2.1.
- Normal size and echostructure of regional lymph nodes.

Gigantomastia under normal prolactin levels should be distinguished from mastitis, juvenile hypertrophy of the breast, normal glandular changes during pregnancy, benign masses (FBD, fibroadenoma), Hodgkin's lymphoma, and infiltrative breast cancer.

The treatment of gigantomastia is still a debatable issue and may include various options from drug therapy to surgical correction. The reports on the operative treatment of macromastia during pregnancy and subsequent successful childbirth are very few. In most cases, surgery (mastectomy or reduction mammoplasty) provides the best outcomes.

Currently, contrast-enhanced ultrasound during pregnancy and lactation is not recommended. The use of radiopharmaceuticals and dyes can also become a serious barrier for biopsy of the sentinel lymph nodes. The effect of technetium on the fetus is unknown, and the use of blue dye (isosulfan) can cause anaphylactic reaction in a patient and cause miscarriage and fetal abnormality.

7.4 Breast Cancer During Pregnancy

The most common cancers during pregnancy are cervical cancer, breast cancer, lymphomas, and leukemia (Serov and Sukhikh 2014).

According to the WHO definition, breast cancer associated with pregnancy (pregnancy-associated cancer (PA breast cancer), gestational breast cancer) is breast cancer diagnosed during pregnancy or lactation within 1 year after the termination of pregnancy.

PA breast cancer implies three clinical situations:

1. PA breast cancer is diagnosed during pregnancy.
2. PA breast cancer is diagnosed during lactation.
3. PA breast cancer is diagnosed within 1 year after termination of pregnancy.

Gestational cancer is the most common malignancy in pregnancy, with incidence of 1 case per 1000–10,000 pregnancies, and is the most common cause of death from cancer in pregnant and breastfeeding women (Serov and Sukhikh 2014). Breast cancer ranks the first among all cancers in pregnant women, accounting for 5–17%. Studies by the Swedish national health registry showed that the incidence of gestational breast cancer increased between 1963 and 2002 from 16.0 to 37.4 per 100,000 pregnant women. If the women, who had abortions, were also included, the incidence of breast cancer associated with pregnancy would increase by more than 7 times and reach 215.8 per 100,000 pregnancies.

In 25% of cases, PA breast cancer is diagnosed before 45 years of age, during the most active reproductive period. Most vulnerable are women aged 32–38 years; 14% of cases of PA breast cancer occur before 35 years of age, 11% before 40 years, and 7.3–10% at 40–45 years. The average age of pregnant patients with breast cancer is thus 33 years. The reason that a previously rare combination of breast and pregnancy is not that rare currently, is the older age of childbearing, and that the cohort of patients has enlarged due to those women, whose breast cancer was detected within the first year after childbirth. It is expected that the incidence of breast cancer associated with pregnancy will grow as more women delay childbearing. This potential increase of morbidity is due to the higher prevalence of the breast cancer in the older groups and the evidence that women with the first pregnancy older than 30 years are two to three times more likely to have breast cancer than women with the first pregnancy under 25. The situation worsens both with the steady increase of the morbidity, affecting also women of reproductive age (the cancer grows "younger"), and, on the other, with the social challenges of the modern world, which sometimes restrict childbirth at a young age, while more women give birth at 30–40 years; this brings them closer to the breast cancer risk group.

Specific features of breast cancer associated with pregnancy are usually aggressive course, late diagnosis, and poor prognosis. In average, the interval before the first signs and the diagnosis is 2–15 months. This is a factor contributing to the severity and the worse prognosis of the disease.

As already mentioned, aggressive forms of the tumor are more common during pregnancy than in the general population of the breast cancer patients. For example, low tumor differentiation is noted in 74% of cases and lymphatic vessel invasion with tumor emboli in 88%. In pregnant women larger tumors are more prevalent, as well as the higher incidence of lymph nodes metastases (56–89% compared to 38–54% in nonpregnant young women). Ten-year survival in patients with gestational breast cancer is 55%, which is lower than in nonpregnant patients (79%). Some authors reported that breast cancer is more probable in women giving birth to girls (63%) than in those delivering boys (37%).

The lack of data on both the effect of pregnancy on the cancer course and on the impact of the chemotherapy on the newborn's health puts a difficult task of choosing optimal methods of diagnosis and treatment and requires further research and guidelines on the management of a pregnancy complicated by the malignant disease.

Physiological changes in the breast during pregnancy (an increase of the volume of glandular tissue, lactostasis, discharge from the nipple) make it difficult for the patient and the doctor to detect the tumor. Late diagnosis of breast cancer during pregnancy leads to the delay of treatment on average for 2–3.5 months. There is evidence that 1 month of delay increases the risk of metastasis to axillary lymph nodes by 0.9% and the delay for 6 months by 5.1%. For this reason, at the time of establishing the correct diagnosis, the disease is often in an inoperable stage. The physiological processes that take place in breast tissue during pregnancy explain the difficulties of the diagnosis: increase in volume and change in breast density and structure. The tumor is often misdiagnosed as mastitis or galactocele. A common error in clinical practice is the diagnosis of lactational mastitis instead of a malignant breast tumor. In addition to the coincidence of the signs of a true lactational mastitis and breast cancer, the clinical and ultrasound patterns may also coincide. No less important factor is the low oncological awareness of obstetrician-gynecologists and other specialists.

Incorrect management of patients with diffuse breast cancer mimicking acute or chronic mastitis is especially common. The following reasons for late diagnosis often arise:

1. A wrong belief of the health practitioners that breast cancer affects mainly pre- and postmenopausal women and is very seldom in pregnant and lactating women.
2. Physiological hyperplasia of the lobules and enlargement of the breast during pregnancy mask the tumor. The breast of a breastfeeding woman is elastic and tense, and it is not always easy to distinguish between galactostasis, mastitis, and tumor. Mammography and needle biopsy are helpful in these cases.

The algorithm of examination of the breast in a pregnant woman is not much different from that in a nonpregnant woman and is based on the principle of safety for the fetus. If a painless mass is detected, the nipple discharge with some inclusions is observed, and if the baby refuses to take milk, ultrasonography is strongly recommended. This will allow to specify the nature of the mass and to assess regional lymph nodes.

Ultrasonography is the optimal diagnostic tool for breast cancer in pregnant and lactating patients. Its sensitivity is 86.7–100%.

The most typical ultrasound signs of breast cancer associated with pregnancy are the following (Fig. 7.11):

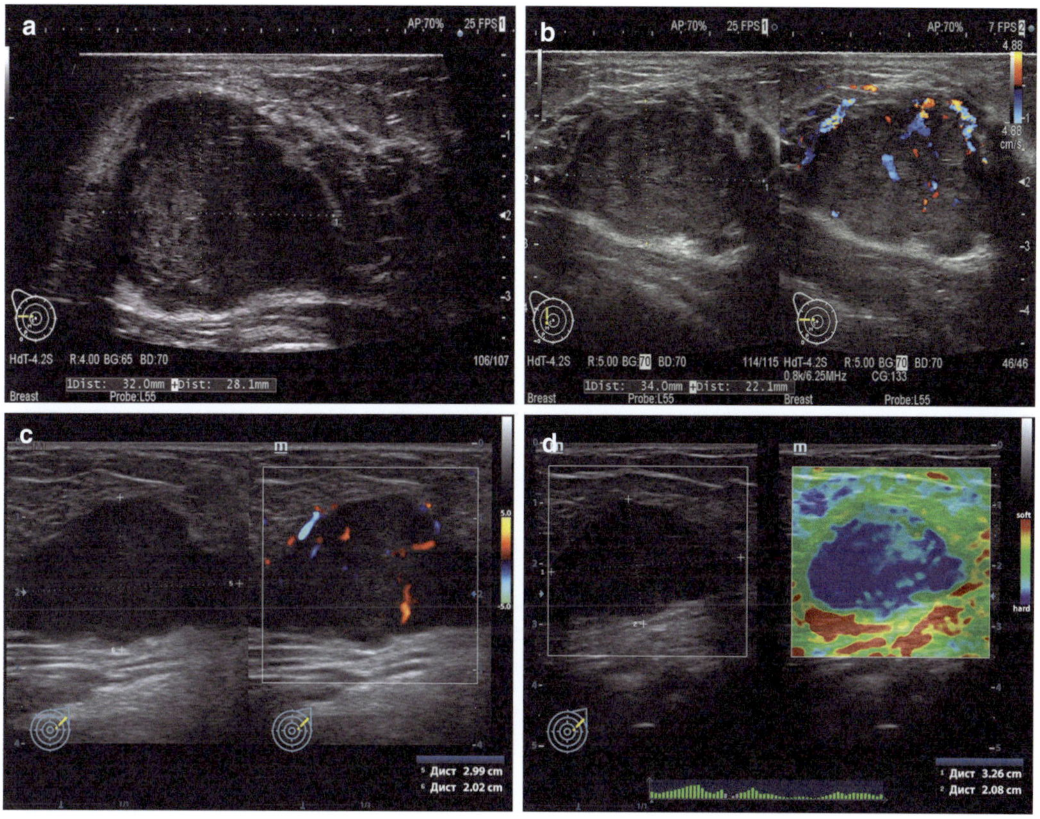

Fig. 7.11 Breast cancer associated with pregnancy. (**a**) Grayscale US. (**b** and **c**) CDI. (**d**) Compression US elastography

- A mass in the parenchyma
- Various, often irregular, shapes
- Often large (more than 2 cm) in size
- Decreased echogenicity
- Heterogeneous structure, often with cystic component
- Sometimes with posterior enhancement
- Thickening of the skin and subcutaneous fat over the mass
- Hypervascularization of the tumor with CDI and PDI
- Good colorability in compression US elastography mode
- The strain ratio > 2.7
- Often metastasis to regional lymph nodes at early stages

A biopsy of any newly detected lesion during pregnancy should be performed as soon as possible to avoid delays in diagnosis.

The primary diagnosis, clinical stage, and extent of breast cancer in pregnant women in 85% are based on US findings. The most common histological and immunohistochemical variants of breast cancer associated with pregnancy are high-intensive invasive ductal carcinoma (estrogen and progesterone receptors-negative) with high incidence of lymphovascular invasion. Despite the similarity of the immunohistochemical profile of pregnancy-associated breast cancers compared to breast cancer in nonpregnant young women, cancer in young women is known to be of a higher class of malignancy and of more low-grade differentiation than breast cancer in elderly women.

The choice of treatment modality for breast cancer during pregnancy is controversial in many aspects. This category of patients has never been included in large multicenter studies. The main challenge is the balance between the safest approach, possible teratogenicity, and assumption of more aggressive course of the disease. The key issue of the treatment strategy is the possibility to keep the pregnancy. Preservation of pregnancy in breast cancer patients is always a difficult decision based on the assessment of the disease extent, the pregnancy term, and the biological characteristics of the tumor in each specific case.

The treatment choice depends, first of all, on the stage of the disease and not on the term of pregnancy. The goal of treating a patient with an oncological disease is not only to achieve the best clinical effect but also to provide better life expectancy and quality. Pregnancy management in the patients with cancer is the task of a multidisciplinary team including specialists in oncology, oncohematology, obstetrics, reproductive and perinatal medicine, genetics, and psychology.

If a patient refuses to undergo any specific cancer therapy, since the priority for her and her family is the safety of the fetus, the treatment is postponed until childbirth. As a rule, the prognosis in patients who chose this option is extremely unfavorable. Another option assumes immediate termination of pregnancy and appropriate treatment of the breast cancer, which will not differ from that in nonpregnant patients. The third option, which for the last decades has become widely used, is prolongation of pregnancy with simultaneous cancer treatment including both surgery and medical therapy.

As a rule, abortion is nearly inevitable in the first trimester, since even with small tumors a comprehensive examination and treatment may cause teratogenic effects, while in the advanced disease the risk of progression is significantly increased. In the second and third trimesters, a choice is possible, taking into account the patient's expectations. At term, in less aggressive and advanced breast cancer, the treatment tactics should take into account the potential teratogenicity of any therapy. Operative treatment is indicated irrespective of the pregnancy term, since modern anesthesia operates techniques, which are safe for a fetus. The volume of surgery is determined only by the extent of the disease.

Treatment of breast cancer implies a comprehensive approach, including surgical intervention, drug treatment, and radiation therapy. Despite the fact that radiation therapy is often used in conventional oncological practice, it is contraindicated for pregnant women. Teratogenic effects of radiation therapy, the threat of development of an oncological disease in child, make it non-applicable throughout the entire pregnancy.

According to the recommendations of the European Society of Oncologists, 2010, surgical treatment can be undertaken in any period of pregnancy (under appropriate anesthesia, proper mother oxygenation, and the fetal heart rate monitoring after 24 weeks of pregnancy). Pregnancy itself does not affect the surgical volume (mastectomy or radical resection of the mammary gland). The life expectancy of patients is similar in both methods of treatment. The approaches of the North American cancer school are somewhat different (recommendations of the National Comprehensive Cancer Network, 2016): radiation therapy is not recommended at any term of pregnancy; therefore, organ-preserving surgical treatment is possible only after childbirth. Mastectomy is possible at any term, while chemotherapy is possible starting from the second trimester. Pregnancy termination is considered only if breast cancer has been diagnosed in the first trimester.

The safety and possible side effects of antitumor drugs during pregnancy are controversial issues. The greatest risk (10–20%) of fetal malformations is due to the chemotherapy in the first trimester of pregnancy; also, the risk of spontaneous abortions increases. Chemotherapy, carried out in the II and III trimesters of pregnancy, can also lead to premature birth and complications, such as myelosuppression in mother and fetus, bleeding and infectious diseases, growth restriction, low fetal body weight, and stillbirth. The impact of chemotherapy on the health of the fetus depends on the type, duration, and dose of the applied drugs, as well as on gestational age.

Long-term effects of chemotherapy during pregnancy are unknown.

Long-term health outcomes for children born by women who had underwent a specific drug treatment for breast cancer during pregnancy have not been reported. According to Serov and Sukhikh 2014, the risk of congenital anomalies in children, whose mothers had received treatment for malignant tumors, is not higher than in general population.

Since patients with gestational breast cancer more often have a locally advanced disease than nonpregnant women, neoadjuvant chemotherapy may be required. The therapeutic effect of neoadjuvant chemotherapy is assessed by comparison of the size of the tumor before and after treatment and by presence of edema and hyperemia. If the disease is monitored during pregnancy, it is necessary to select diagnostic techniques that are safe for the fetus. Dynamic ultrasonography is indicated to evaluate the therapeutic response to neoadjuvant chemotherapy during pregnancy. A control examination including mammography, lung X-ray, abdominal ultrasound, and radioisotope examination of bones is performed after the treatment and in 6–12 months.

The survival rates of nonpregnant and pregnant women with gestational breast cancer of the same age and the disease stage are similar. Nevertheless, breast cancer associated with pregnancy has a worse prognosis than the overall breast cancer. This is attributed to the greater extent of the gestational disease at the time of diagnosis.

7.5 Breast Diseases During Lactation

Multiparametric ultrasound is fundamental in the early and differential diagnosis of various pathologic conditions of the breast during lactation.

Benign lactation calcifications are sometimes observed in lactating patients, who are examined for some breast complaints or for screening. Generally, calcification is not a common mammographic feature of the lactation or postlactation breast. Microcalcifications in secretory hyperplasia can be detected with mammography or ultrasonography; these are usually diffuse or regional spots and can be bilateral or unilateral. Microcalcifications are usually round and diffuse or focal and sometimes have irregular borders or linear shape (Fig. 7.12). To confirm the diagnosis, FNA with cytological examination is often performed.

Ductal and lobular proliferation in the breast tissue during pregnancy leads to lactational changes, which are seen at histologic examination.

Lactating adenoma is a benign pathology of the breast that occurs in response to physiological changes during pregnancy and lactation and is the most common breast mass in pregnancy. Until now, its causes remain unknown

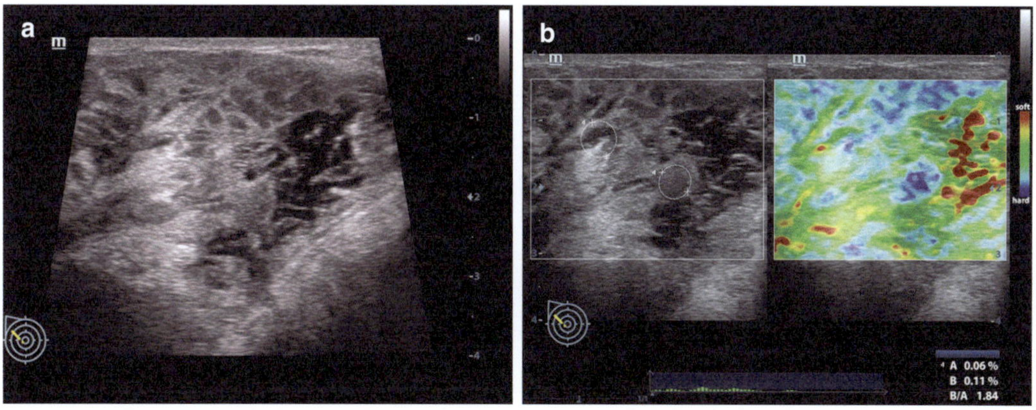

Fig. 7.12 Benign lactation calcification. (**a**) Grayscale US. (**b**) Compression US elastography

and controversial. Some authors believe that lactating adenoma is an ordinary variant of fibroadenoma, tubular adenoma, or lobular hyperplasia, undergoing histologic alterations under the effects of hormones during pregnancy and lactation. Usually, during the third trimester, lactational adenomas decrease in size or regress spontaneously after birth. Sometimes they relapse during next pregnancy. Lactational adenomas may mimic other benign breast tumors, such as fibroadenomas, phyllodes tumors, and non-advanced malignant tumors. Hemorrhages and infarctions are detected in about 5% of cases. Fibroadenomas and lactating adenomas are susceptible to focal necrosis (infarctions).

At echography, lactating adenoma mostly appears as a benign mass similar to the "classical" fibroadenoma of the breast, characterized by moderate or low echogenicity; homogeneity of the structure; round or oval shape; clear, even contours; and hypovascularity (Fig. 7.13).

In the structure of a lactating adenoma, hyperechoic zones (zones of accumulation of the milk fat) are often visualized. Development of necrosis in fibroadenomas is related to the third trimester of pregnancy and lactation. The patients often complain of a sudden pain in the breast, where fibroadenoma is located. At ultrasonography, lobular borders are seen, the echostructure of the mass is usually heterogeneous, and lateral acoustic shadows are noted. With massive necrosis, the mass looks extremely suspicious of cancer. In this case, the diagnosis is easily confirmed by a core needle biopsy.

Hyperplasia of accessory mammary tissue in the axillary region is also benign. The embryonic mammary ridge (milky line) extends from

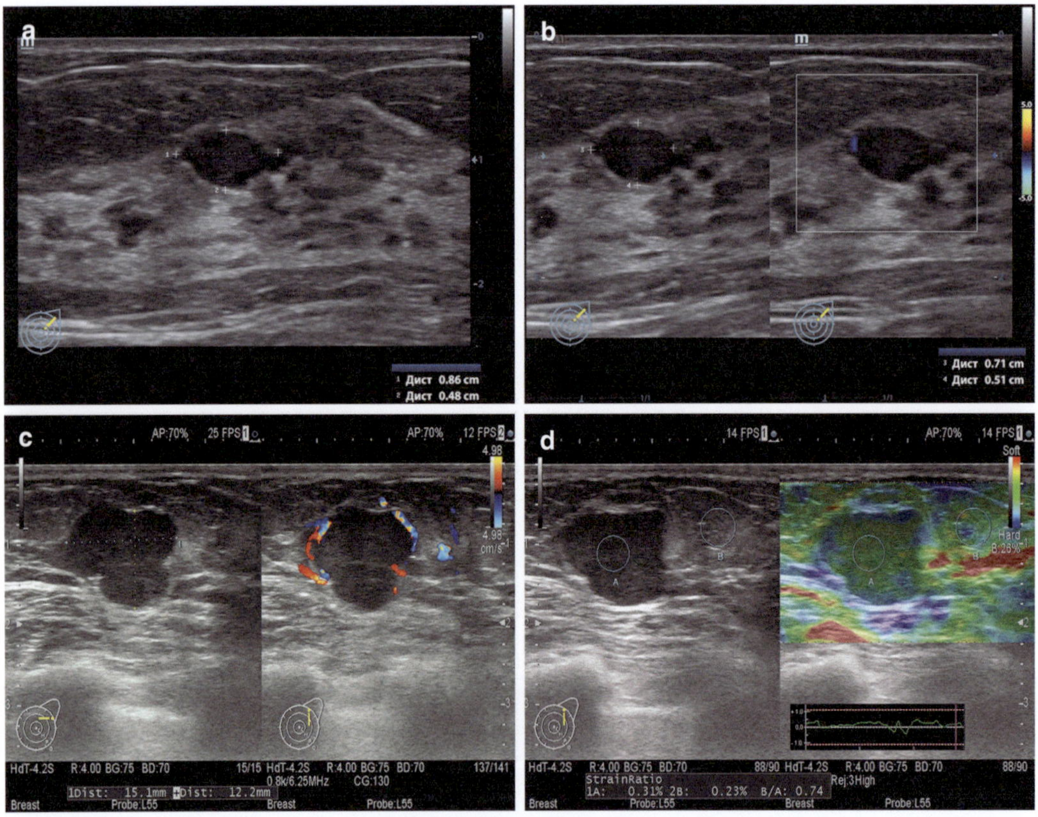

Fig. 7.13 Lactating adenoma. (**a**) Grayscale US. (**b** and **c**) CDI. (**d**) Compression US elastography

the axilla to the groin. Incomplete regression of this ridge during embryo development leads to ectopia of the mammary tissue.

Accessory mammary tissue is found in 0.2–6% of the general population. Ectopic mammary tissue is susceptible to the same hormonal effects and risks of a disease as the eutopic tissue. During menstruation or pregnancy, hormonal stimulation can cause breast induration and discomfort. These patients usually complain of induration and discomfort in the axilla. Ectopic mammary tissue can undergo lactational changes during pregnancy, and, if the areolar-nipple complex is in place, the lactation may occur. The axillary cavity is the most common location of the accessory mammary tissue. At ultrasonography, the accessory mammary tissue has a picture of the ectopic normal (unchanged) fatty lobule of the breast (Fig. 7.14).

All pathological processes in the mammary gland, including those during lactation, may occur in the accessory mammary tissue. Mastitis, abscesses, fibrocystic disease, fibroadenoma and adenoma, a phyllodes tumor, and various forms of breast cancer in the accessory lobule have been reported.

Obstruction of milk ducts occurs frequently during lactation and is caused either by mechanical obstruction on the background of lactational changes or scarring after surgery or infection. Usually, a soft mass is palpated behind the areola or in any other part of the breast.

The ultrasound image varies from a single incompressible formation or duct to a diffuse echoic zone with a hypoechoic halo (Fig. 7.15). In case of recurrent duct obstruction, the obturating neoplasm should be excluded.

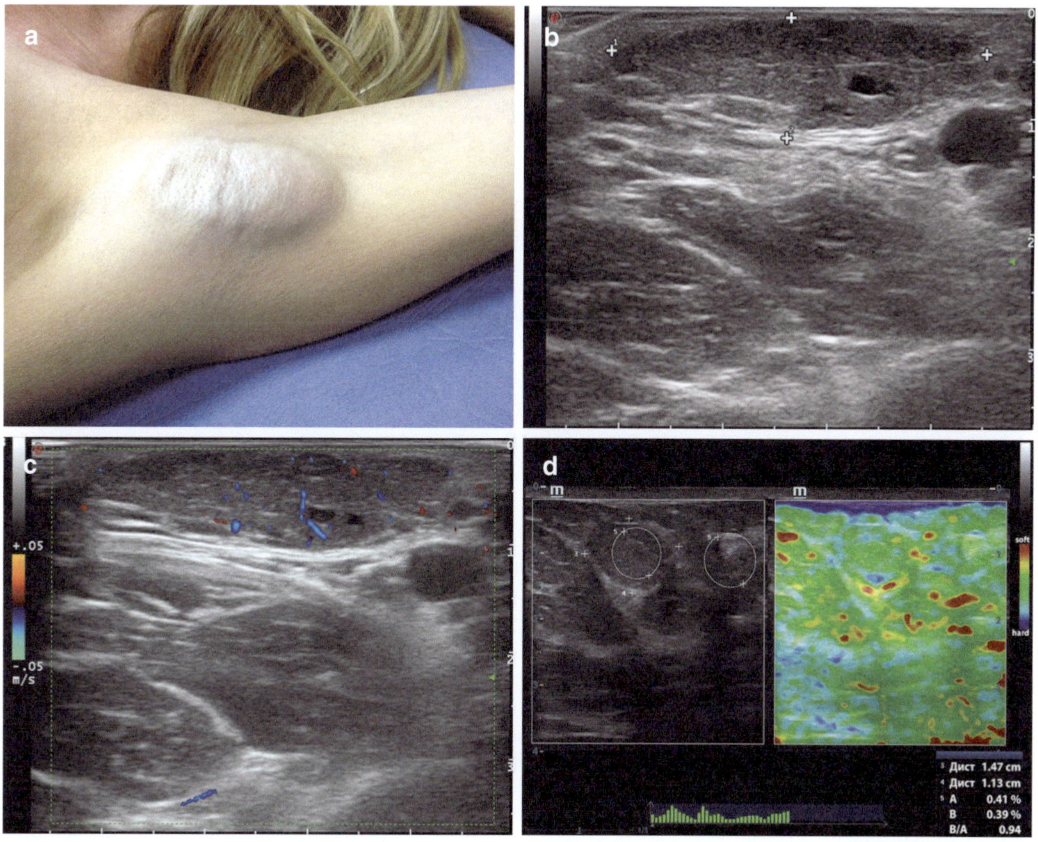

Fig. 7.14 Accessory mammary lobe in the axillary region. (**a**) Photo of a patient. (**b**) Grayscale US. (**c**) CDI. (**d**) Compression US elastography

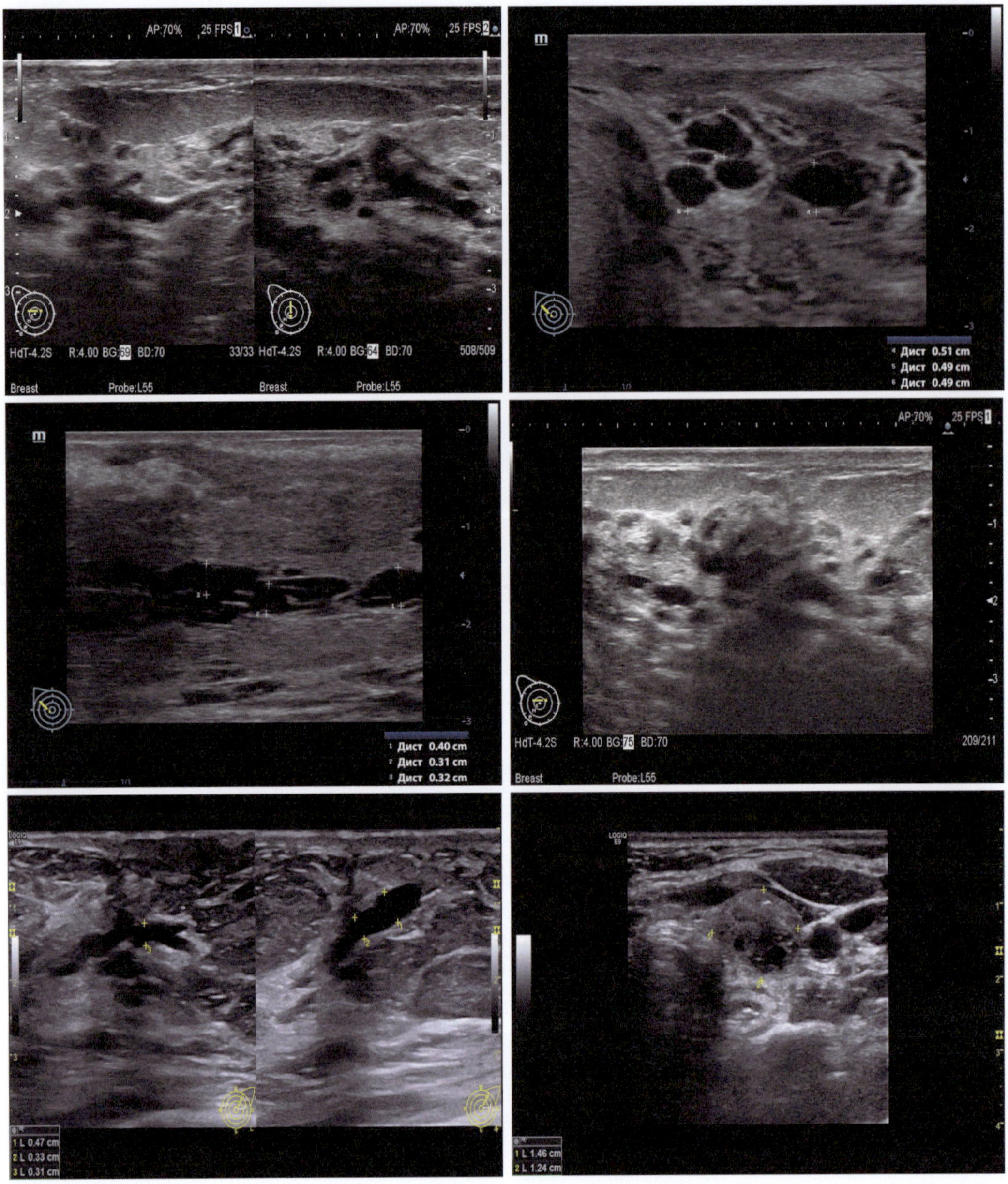

Fig. 7.15 Duct ectasia on the background of lactation mastitis. Grayscale US

Direct aspiration can be performed to relieve the symptoms, prevent abscess, and for diagnostics. The condition is usually treated with warm packs, massage, and frequent milking.

Lactation mastitis is an inflammatory condition of the breast during lactation (with the incidence of 6.6–33% according to WHO), which may be accompanied by an infectious lesion of the parenchyma.

Milk stasis, blocked ducts, induration or physical damage of the breast, and poor attachment of the infant to the breast may cause lactation mastitis. Milk stasis provides an environment for bacterial growth. The most common causative agents of mastitis and abscesses associated with lactation are *Staphylococcus aureus* and *Streptococcus*.

Usually, the patients complain of pain, hyperemia and swelling of the breast (Fig. 7.16a), fever, and chills.

Ultrasonography is the method of choice for the diagnosis of abscesses of the mammary gland.

Ultrasound examination with lactational mastitis can reveal (Fig. 7.16b):

- Thickening of the skin over the affected area
- Heterogeneity of the structure and zones of reduced (or increased) echogenicity in breast parenchyma
- Increased vascularization with CDI and PDI
- Reactive axillary lymph nodes

In recent years, the latent forms of inflammatory breast diseases, characterized by unclear clinical signs or their complete absence, have become very common. A purulent mastitis can be associated with normal or subfebrile temperature, minor proinflammatory blood changes, weak inflammatory reaction, and unchanged structure of the regional lymph nodes.

Treatment usually includes antibiotics, frequent breastfeeding or decanting, and prevention of lactostasis.

Echography can confirm the diagnosis and guide the draining and administration of antibiotics and can be safely used for monitoring of the abscess. Acute bacterial mastitis, as a rule, either resolves under antibacterial therapy or transforms into the abscess of the breast, if the treatment is untimely or inadequate.

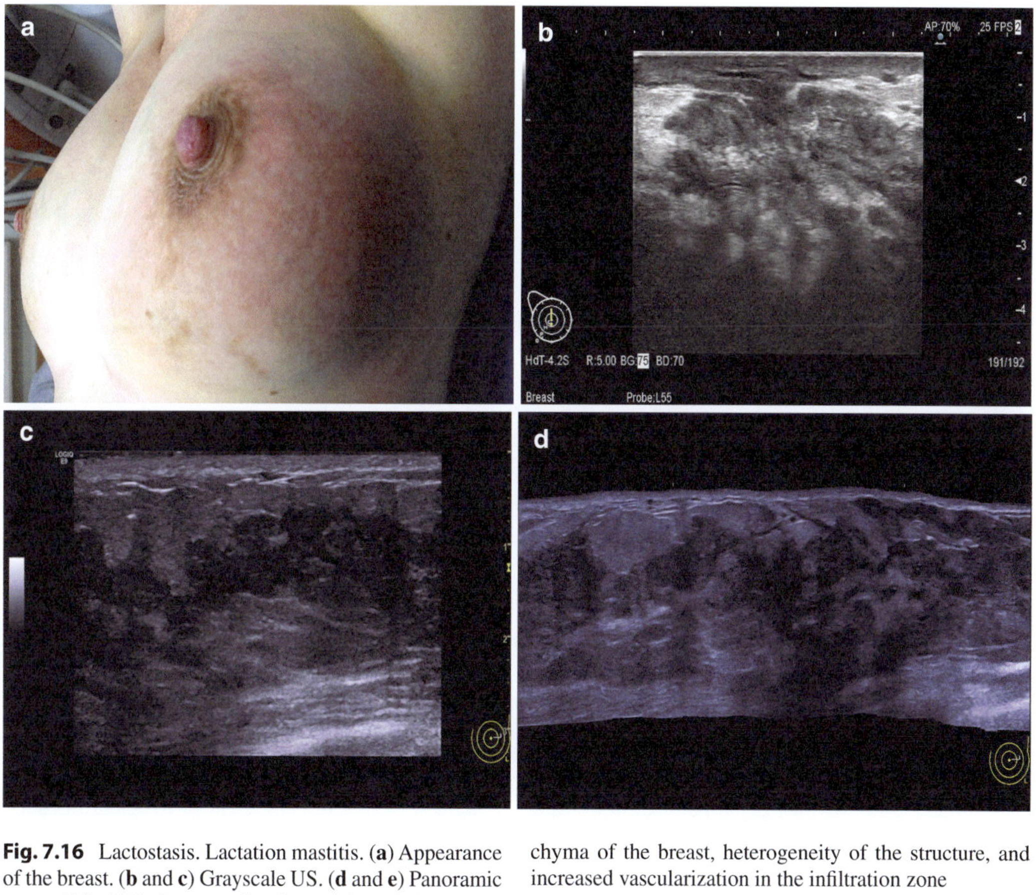

Fig. 7.16 Lactostasis. Lactation mastitis. (**a**) Appearance of the breast. (**b** and **c**) Grayscale US. (**d** and **e**) Panoramic scan. (**f–i**) CDI. Decreased echogenicity of the parenchyma of the breast, heterogeneity of the structure, and increased vascularization in the infiltration zone

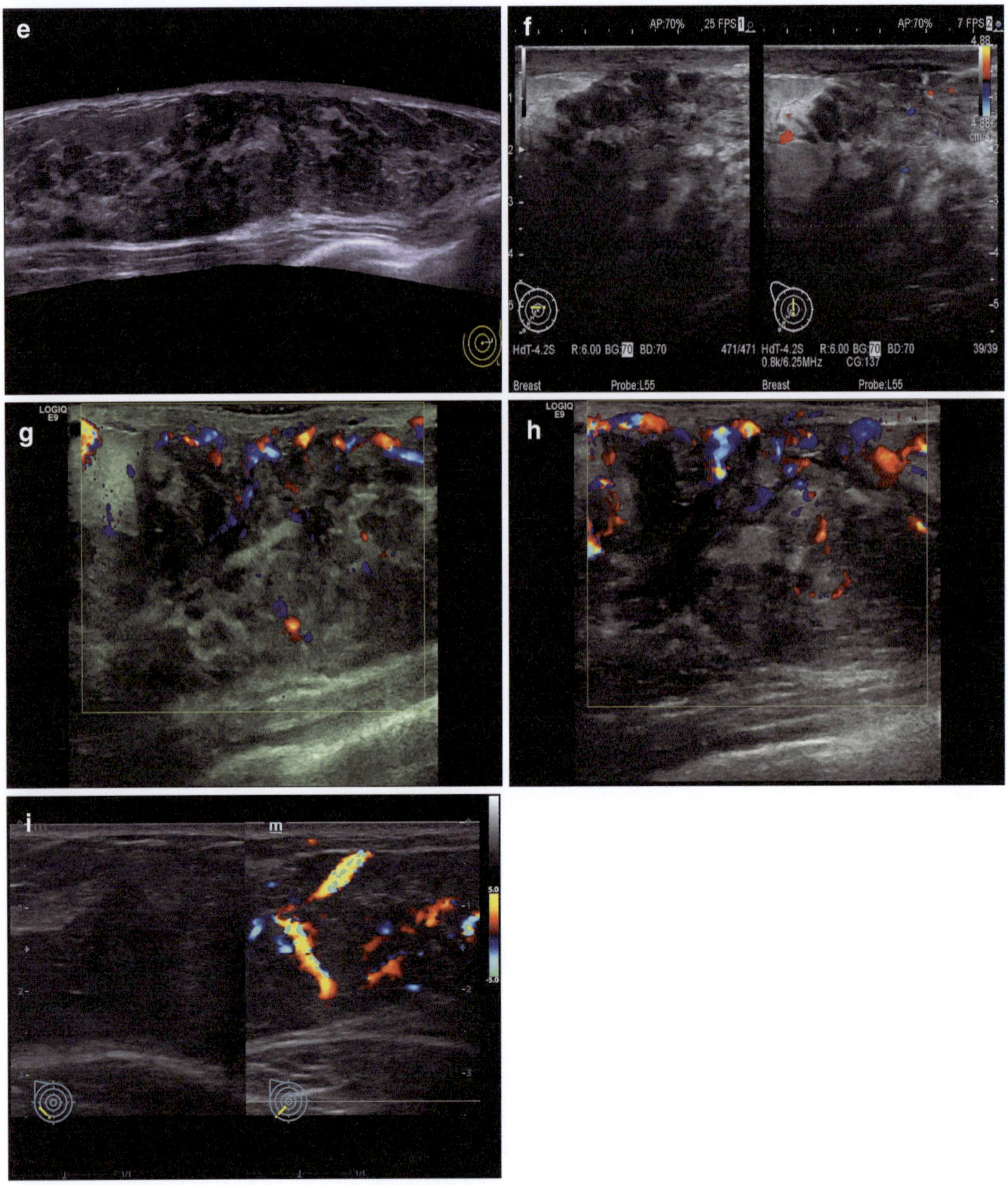

Fig. 7.16 (continued)

About 4.8–11% of mastitis associated with lactation are complicated by breast abscesses. Usually, the patients complain of pain, local hyperemia and swelling, fever, chills, and enlargement of the axillary lymph nodes.

Ultrasonographic features of an abscess are listed below (Fig. 7.17):

- A complex hypo- or anechoic mass
- Various shapes
- Heterogeneous echostructure
- Uneven contours and clear or irregular borders
- Often with distal acoustic echo enhancement
- Avascular, sometimes with peripheral vascularization of surrounding tissues

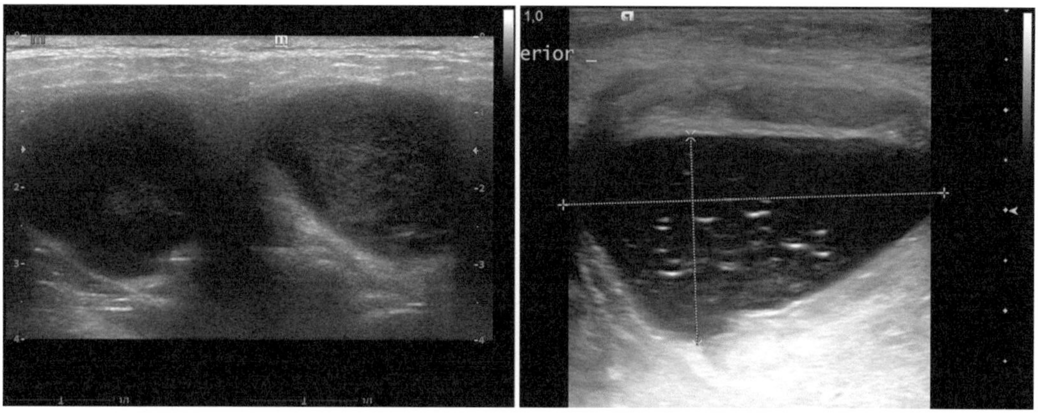

Fig. 7.17 Abscess on the background of lactational mastitis. Grayscale US

Mammography is performed only, if the diagnosis is doubtful and the breast cancer is suspected. Transdermal draining together with antibacterial therapy, as a rule, is effective enough. Warm pads and frequent breastfeeding also help to resolve the symptoms. Mastitis and/or abscess does not affect breastfeeding. Termination of breastfeeding is necessary only under antibacterial therapy with a medication, which may be harmful to a baby, or in case of the surgical draining of the abscess.

Idiopathic granulomatous mastitis is a rare inflammatory disease of the breast of unknown etiology, which often mimics malignant neoplasms. This condition is more common in patients with autoimmune diseases, hyperprolactinemia, and pituitary adenomas, during pregnancy and/or lactation, and in oral contraceptive users.

Ultrasonographic image shows a dense hypovascular mass of decreased echogenicity with uneven contours and heterogeneous structure. It may be accompanied by axillary lymphadenopathy (Fig. 7.18).

Histologic investigation usually reveals a noncaseous granulomatous inflammatory reaction. Tuberculosis, fungal infections, sarcoidosis, Wegener's granulomatosis, and granulomatous reactions associated with carcinomas should be ruled out.

The image is nonspecific and sometimes can mimic malignancy. According to echography, single or multiple heterogeneous hypoechoic inclusions with a tubular configuration are mostly seen, less often a diffuse abscess with fistula formation. MR and X-ray signs are also nonspecific.

Treatment of granulomatous mastitis, especially of resistant or relapsing forms, often comprises a combination of steroid therapy and surgery.

Galactocele is a retention cyst of the mammary gland, single or multicystic, filled with milk, formed during pregnancy and/or lactation. The formation of galactocele is also possible in neonates and children of the younger group (children's galactocele).

Galactocele is the most common benign lesion of the breast in lactating women and can occur in the third trimester of pregnancy, after childbirth or even after the termination of breastfeeding. Galactocele usually occurs as a result of the obstructed outflow through the ducts, leading to the extension of proximal lobular segments. At palpation, one or more soft masses are detected. The image of galactocele varies depending on the amount of fat, protein, and water contents.

Echography shows a hypo- or anechoic mass of oval or round shape, with uneven contours, distinct from the nearby tissues, with a thin capsule (up to 1 mm) of increased echogenicity, in the projection of the areola margin. Its structure

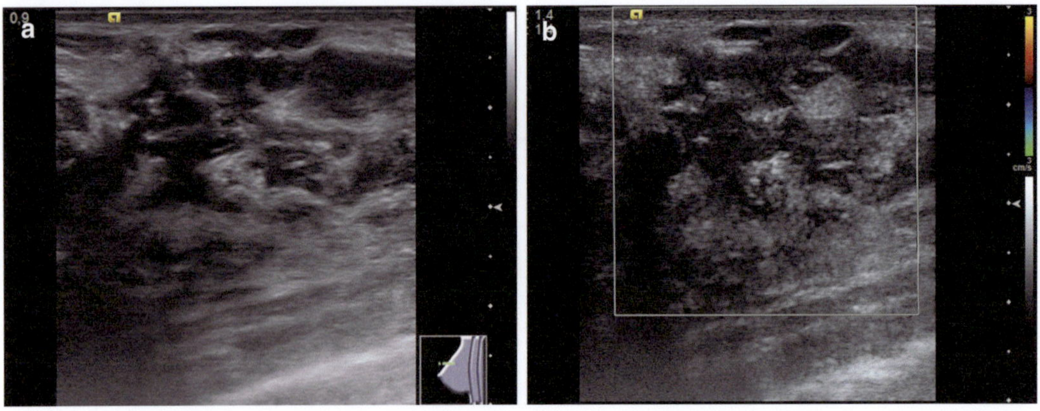

Fig. 7.18 Granulomatous mastitis. (**a**) Grayscale US. (**b**) CDI

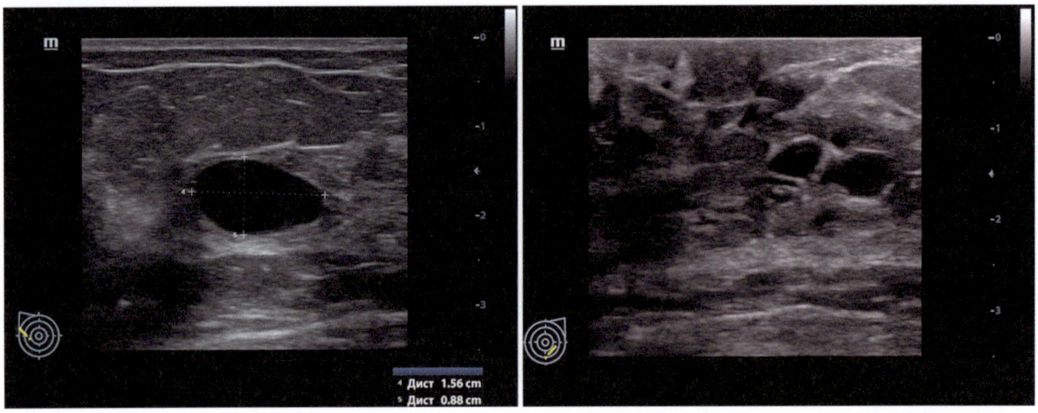

Fig. 7.19 Galactocele of the breast. Grayscale US

is usually heterogeneous due to the presence of dense particles in the cavity ("dairy crumbs") and the liquid (Fig. 7.19). Acoustic effects and echogenicity of galactocele often depend on the size and density of the contents of the dilated duct. Contours range from clear to uneven depending on the degree of surrounding inflammation. In the color-coded regimens, galactocele appears as an avascular structure.

Histologic investigation of the galactocele usually shows cuboidal and flat-lined epithelial cysts, often accompanied by inflammatory and necrotic inclusions. If the galactocele is asymptomatic, or a typical fat-fluid level is found, the condition may be treated conservatively.

Enlarged intramammary and/or axillary lymph nodes. Bilateral, multiple lymph nodes with signs of benign reactive hyperplasia usually accompany regional inflammation, infectious diseases, and rheumatoid arthritis but also may be a sign of the malignant breast cancer and lymphoma (see Chap. 8). These are usually seen in the upper outer quadrant of the breast and in the axillary region (Fig. 7.20).

As a rule, reactive lymph nodes usually demonstrate good differentiation of the hilum and cortex, nonactive hilar blood flow. They are painless when compressed. An important differential feature is the dynamic transformation of the ultrasonographic pattern, changes of the size and

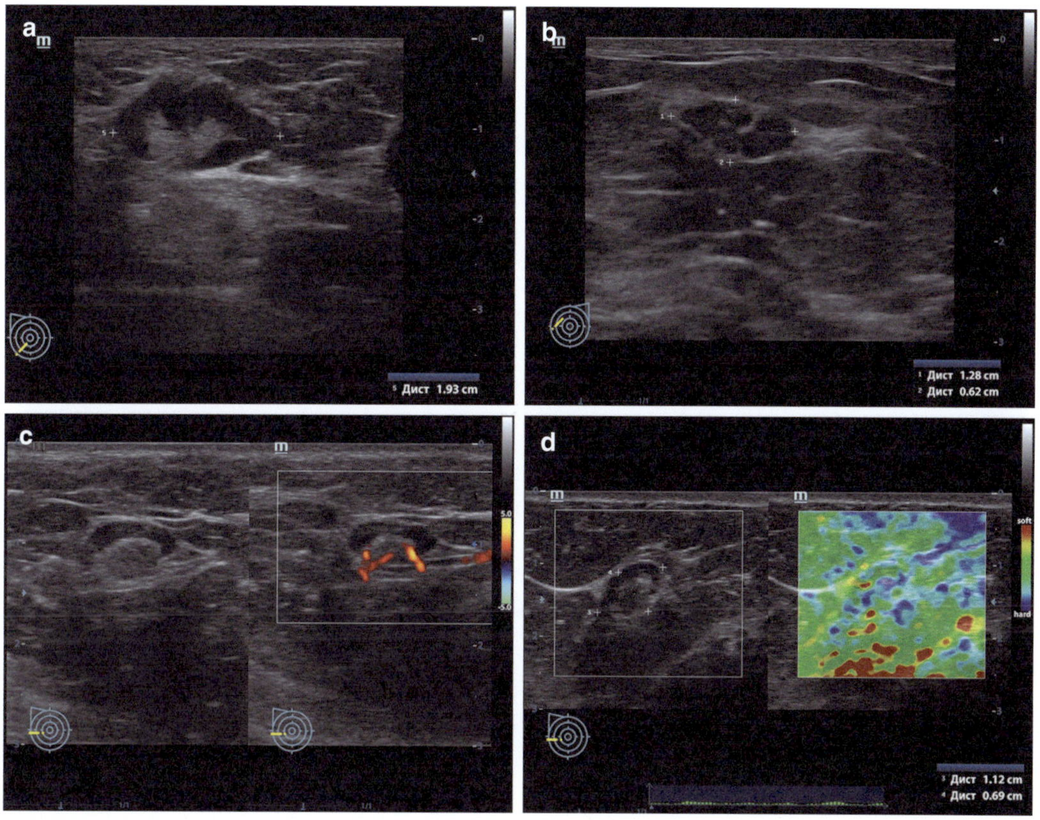

Fig. 7.20 Lactation period. Enlarged reactive lymph nodes. (**a** and **b**) Grayscale mode. (**c**) CDI. (**d**) Ultrasound elastography

structure of the lymph nodes, and vascularization in course of follow-up.

7.6 Pregnancy After Treatment of Breast Cancer

Advances in the treatment of breast cancer over the past 10–20 years have led to an increase in life expectancy after successful treatment of gestational breast cancer in most patients. At an early stage, this disease is almost completely curable. This poses new challenges for medicine: it is necessary to care not only about the effectiveness of treatment but also about the quality of life of patients who have undergone breast cancer. One of the main issues for young women after breast cancer treatment is the chance to have children throughout their later life.

Breastfeeding after breast cancer, even after conservative surgery, is possible and safe. Women should be informed that the tumor cells do not metastasize into the fetal tissues; cessation of lactation is dictated only by the necessity to start the treatment immediately. A belief that a future female child will certainly have breast cancer if the mother has mutations of the BRCA1 and BRCA2 genes is also false. A patient should be aware that the continuation of pregnancy does not worsen the prognosis of early stage breast cancer. The issue of pregnancy after treatment should be addressed with caution. It is necessary to take into account the stage of the disease and the presence or absence of unfavorable prognostic factors. The minimal interval from the completion of treatment to pregnancy should be 2–3 years. After treatment a woman should be followed by an oncologist. The first control examination should be done 6 months after treatment, with repeated examinations annually.

Breastfeeding is not recommended during chemotherapy because the drugs excreted with milk may cause toxic effects to the baby. Before starting treatment, in particular chemotherapy or hormone therapy, the patient should be informed about the possible negative impact of such treatment on her reproductive function. Those who plan a pregnancy after treatment should be offered a consultation of a reproductologist prior to treatment. Accordingly, pregnancy planning should be discussed with the oncologist.

About half of women who had been diagnosed with breast cancer would like to have children after treatment. However, in the past, only 3–5% of such women had successful pregnancy. This was due to the uncertainty of the effect of pregnancy on the further prognosis of cancer and fear that this would increase the risk of relapse. This also led to a high percentage of abortions among this category of women (up to 30% of cases).

Adjuvant chemotherapy reduces the number of fertile patients, but 3–11% of women who had underwent treatment for breast cancer at 35–40 years of age had pregnancy afterward. About 70% of these pregnancies occurred in the first 5 years after treatment for breast cancer.

Pregnancy after treatment of breast cancer is safe irrespective to the presence or absence of hormonal receptors in the tumor. Pregnancy after treatment reduced the risk of death by 41%. Since about 15% of breast cancers occur in women of reproductive age, the medical practitioners should be aware of these new data and not discourage women to have pregnancy after successful treatment of early stage, like it used to be in the past.

It is advisable to test a patient for BRCA-1 and BRCA-2 genes mutation, because of the high risk of inheritance of breast and ovarian cancer by the offspring.

The ideal interval between the end of treatment for breast cancer and the pregnancy is not defined but is assumed to be more than 3–5 years, since the prognosis is not clear until then. Pregnancy is definitely not recommended during the first 6 months due to the possible teratogenic effects of cytostatics. Pregnancy can promote a relapse of the disease and appearance of latent regional and distant metastases.

Thus, a pregnancy is possible after breast cancer treatment. There are no formal international protocols regarding the timing of pregnancy after breast cancer, but most experts agree on no less than 2 years after the diagnosis, no less than 6 months after chemotherapy, and not earlier than 3 months after hormonal or targeted therapy.

The significance of multiparametric ultrasonography for diagnosis of the breast pathology and the detection of malignant tumors associated with pregnancy at all terms, in the postpartum period and during lactation, is extremely important. The method is in demand, accessible, safe, and highly informative.

Concomitant Diseases of Mammary Glands and Other Organs

8

Ella Penyaeva and Alexander N. Sencha

Abstract

Breast diseases are combined with the pathology of other organs in 77% of cases. The primary multiplicity of tumors is now defined as the independent occurrence and development of two or more neoplasms in the body of one patient. In this case, not only different organs of different systems but also paired organs (mammary glands, lungs, etc.) can be affected. Multicentric lesions of one organ can occur as well. Combination of two tumors predominates in the structure of polyneoplasias. The cases of triple localization occur in 5–8% of cases. The risk of developing tumors in patients already having neoplasms is approximately 1.3 times higher than in those who did not previously have neoplasms. The risk of breast cancer depends on the intensity of the proliferation of the lobular and/or ductal epithelium and increases by 3–5 times at preexisting benign breast diseases, especially in combination with diseases of reproductive organs. Metastatic lesions in mammary glands can occur in cases of primary tumors of various localizations. These cases are rare and are often associated with poor prognosis.

E. Penyaeva (✉)
Department of Ultrasound Diagnostics of Radiology Center, Yaroslavl Railway Clinic, Yaroslavl, Russia

A. N. Sencha
Division of Visual Diagnostics, National Medical Research Center for Obstetrics, Gynecology and Perinatology named after Academician V.I. Kulakov of Ministry of Healthcare of Russian Federation, Moscow, Russia

The problem of diagnosis of concomitant conditions of mammary glands and diseases of other organs has been discussed for a long time. Combined pathology is found quite often during examination of women, including imaging techniques (Adamyan et al. 2006; Radzinsky et al. 2016). Breast diseases are combined with the pathology of other organs in 77% of cases. Available published data on concomitant diseases include the associations of the diseases of the breast and the uterus (Adamyan et al. 1989), the thyroid gland, gastrointestinal diseases, and others.

The most common combinations of breast pathology and diseases of other organs are as follows:

1. Fibrocystic mastopathy and uterine myoma
2. Fibrocystic mastopathy and genital endometriosis
3. Mammary gland disease and adnexal masses
4. Mammary gland disease and thyroid pathology
5. Mammary gland disease and pathology of the gastrointestinal tract
6. Primary-multiple breast cancer

Undoubtedly, the most important problem, a difficult task to solve, and an often missed diagnosis

G. T. Sukhikh, A. N. Sencha (eds.), *Multiparametric Ultrasound Diagnosis of Breast Diseases*,
https://doi.org/10.1007/978-3-319-75034-7_8

are different combinations of breast cancer with tumors of other localizations. The incidence of primary combination of breast cancer and malignant tumors of other localizations is 3.8% among all breast cancer patients (38.3% account for endometrial cancer, 26.7% for ovarian cancer, 16.7% for cervical, and 18.3% for colon cancer).

The primary multiplicity of tumors is now defined as the independent occurrence and development of two or more neoplasms in the body of one patient. In this case, not only different organs of different systems can be affected but also paired organs (mammary glands, lungs, etc.). Multicentric lesions of one organ can occur as well. Combination of two tumors predominates in the structure of polyneoplasias. The cases of triple localization occur in 5–8% of cases. Four, five, six, or more tumors in one patient are extremely rare. The prevalence of primary-multiple tumors is estimated to be 0.73–11.7%; the morbidity increases with age.

An important point in the differentiation of multiple tumors is their time of onset. Slinchak (1968) proposed the following classification of combined tumors:

1. Synchronous (arising simultaneously or within a period of up to 6 months) multiple tumors:
   - Multicentric multiple tumors of one organ
   - Systemic tumors and tumors of paired organs
   - Non-systemic multiple tumors of various organs
2. Metachronous (arising at various time intervals exceeding 6 months) tumors:
   - Multicentric metachronous tumors of one organ
   - Systemic metachronous tumors and tumors of the paired organs
   - Non-systemic metachronous tumors

According to the classification proposed by Moertel (1977), primary-multiple tumors are also classified:

1. Multiple primary malignant neoplasms of multicentric origin:
   - The same tissue and organ
   - A common, contiguous tissue shared by different organs
   - The same tissue in bilaterally paired organs
2. Multiple primary malignant neoplasms of different tissues or organs
3. Multiple primary malignant neoplasms of multicentric origin plus a lesion (s) of a different tissue or organ

Development of primary-multiple malignant breast neoplasms within one mammary gland is termed “multicentric tumors” (Fig. 8.1).

Bebyakin (1974) proposed the following classification of concomitant tumors:

1. By combination:
   - Benign
   - Benign and malignant
   - Malignant
2. By the diagnosis sequence:
   - Synchronous
   - Metachronous
   - Synchronous-metachronous
   - Metachronous-synchronous
3. By functional relationship:
   - Functionally dependent
   - Hormonally dependent
   - Unclassified
4. By tissue affiliation:
   - The same tissue
   - Different tissues
5. By the histological structure:
   - The same histological structure
   - Different histological structures
6. Localization:
   - One or paired organs
   - Different organs of the same system
   - Organs of different systems

The risk of developing tumors in patients already having neoplasms is approximately 1.3 times higher than in those who did not previously have neoplasms. The incidence of malignant tumors among relatives of the first degree with primary-multiple malignant neoplasms is seven times higher than the populational incidence of these diseases. Half of patients with

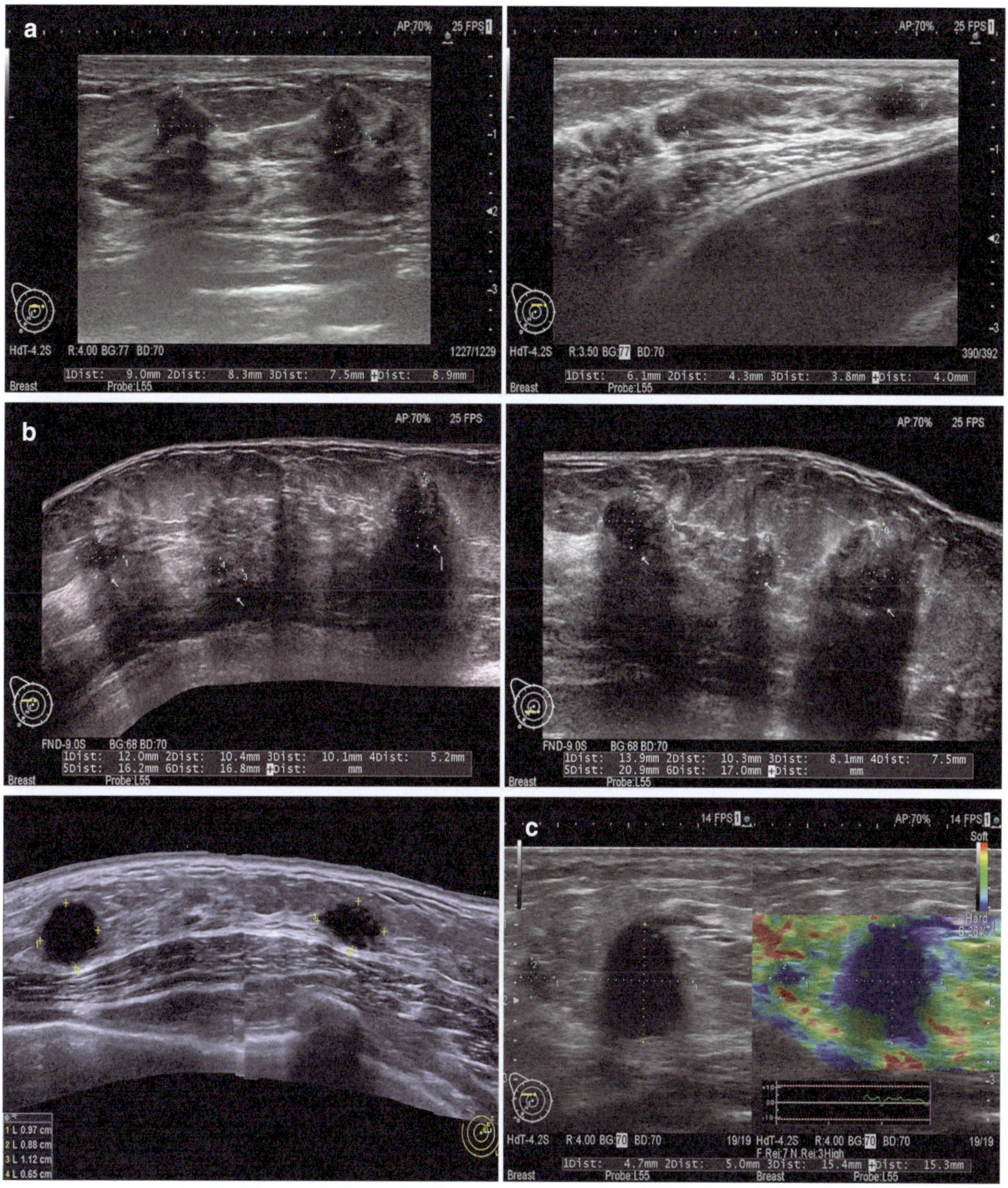

Fig. 8.1 Breast cancer. Multicentric growth of the tumor. (**a**) 1–2 Grayscale US. (**b**) 1–3 Panoramic scan. (**c**) Compression US elastography

primary-multiple malignant tumors have repeated cases of malignant neoplasms in the family, e.g., 43% of patients with stomach and breast cancer.

Primary-multiple breast cancer is a type of cancer associated with malignant tumors of various other localizations. The incidence of primary-multiple breast cancer varies globally from 0.73 to 18.1%. Cancer of multiple localizations (in three or more organs) is observed in 7.2% of patients. Primary-multiple breast cancer is most often combined with neoplasms of female genitalia and colon (Kaprin et al. 2017):

1. Bilateral breast cancer (in 4.6–41.1% of observations)
2. Breast cancer in combination with the tumors:

- Of female genitalia (5.6–41.0%), most often with endometrial cancer (2.0–38.3%), ovarian cancer (26.7%), and cervical cancer (16.7%)
- Of the organs of the digestive system (9.4%), most often with the malignant tumors of the colon (8.6–18.3%) and stomach (5.6%)
- Of the thyroid gland (6.6%)
- Of other organs (the lungs, skin, kidneys, bladder) (2.9–7.2%)

The growth and local metastatic spread of malignant tumors are so diverse and unexpected that it is not always possible to distinguish the second primary-multiple tumor from a recurrence or metastasis.

The detection and registration of primary-multiple neoplasms are carried out in three ways:

- Detection of simultaneously existing tumors
- Detection of a tumor and retrospective definition of the first neoplasm
- Detection of a subsequent tumor occurs in course of the follow-up, which requires a vigorous and detailed medical examination of cancer patients

Breast and ovarian cancer are the diseases of the reproductive system, and therefore they are characterized by a certain similarity of hormonal, metabolic, and behavioral risk factors. These two diseases are the main components of the most frequent hereditary syndrome in humans—so-called breast-ovarian hereditary cancer syndrome. Hereditary carcinomas of breast and ovaries are often caused by mutations in the germline of the BRCA1 and BRCA2 genes (BRCA1/BRCA2 syndromes) and are less associated with other hereditary syndromes, such as Li-Fraumeni and Peutz-Jeghers. The BRCA1/BRCA2 proteins play a special role in DNA repair. Therefore, loss of function due to mutation causes the accumulation of mutations in other genes and the subsequent oncogenesis at an early age. The incidence of detected breast cancer increases from the age of 30 years, ovarian cancer with BRCA1 syndrome from 40 years, and BRCA2 from 50 years. BRCA syndrome is suspected in case of breast cancer in first-degree relatives, especially at a young age (breast and/or ovarian cancer). In the BRCA syndrome, medullary carcinomas predominate, but other types of carcinoma may also be found. Ovarian carcinomas in the syndrome are usually highly differentiated serous, mucinous carcinomas or borderline tumors. There is an increased risk of breast cancer in men with BRCA1/BRCA2 mutations. A family history of breast cancer was a high-risk factor of developing malignant neoplasms of pelvic organs in women.

Ultrasound signs of primary-multiple breast cancer, combined, for example, with ovarian cancer, are usually similar to a typical picture of breast cancer. Nodular types of lesions with pronounced lymphogenous dissemination are more common. They have the following ultrasound characteristics (Fig. 8.2):

- Irregular shape
- Often small (less than 2 cm) in size
- Decreased echogenicity
- Heterogeneous structure
- Thickening of the skin, subcutaneous fat over the mass
- Hypervascularization of the tumor at CDI and PDI
- Good enhancement with CEUS
- Strain ratio more than 2.7
- Frequent metastasis in regional lymph nodes at early stages

Combination of **breast cancer and cervical cancer** is observed in 9.9% of cases; the disease

→

Fig. 8.2 Primary-multiple breast cancer. (**a**) 1–4. Breast tumor. Grayscale US. (**b**) Secondary highly differentiated endometrial adenocarcinoma: (b1) Grayscale US, (b2) CDI, (b3) CEUS

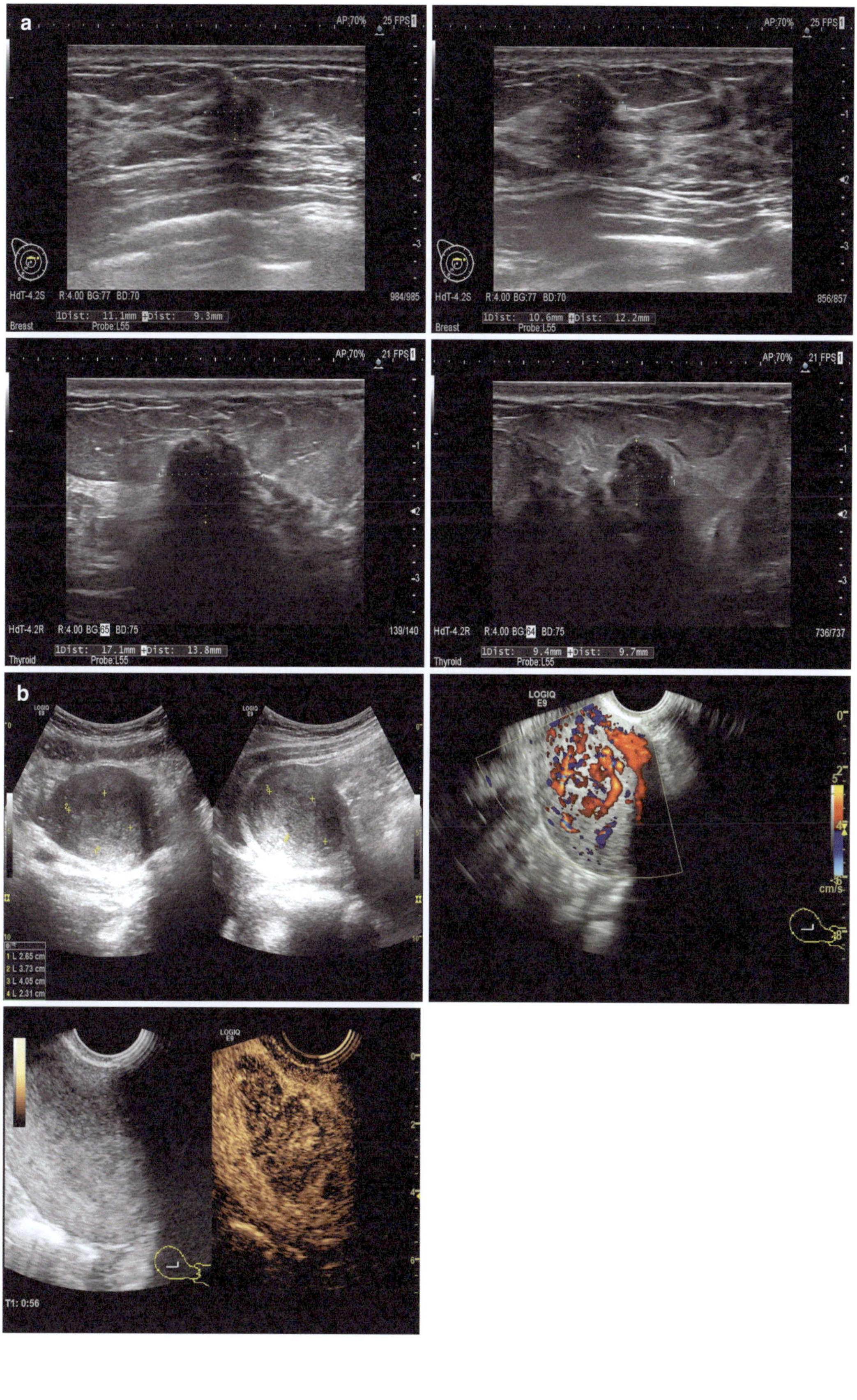
a
AP:70% 25 FPS
HdT-4.2S R:4.00 BG:77 BD:70 984/985
1Dist: 11.1mm 2Dist: 9.3mm
Breast Probe:L55
AP:70% 25 FPS
HdT-4.2S R:4.00 BG:77 BD:70 856/857
1Dist: 10.6mm 2Dist: 12.2mm
Breast Probe:L55
AP:70% 21 FPS
HdT-4.2R R:4.00 BG:65 BD:75 139/140
1Dist: 17.1mm 2Dist: 13.8mm
Thyroid Probe:L55
AP:70% 21 FPS
HdT-4.2R R:4.00 BG:64 BD:75 736/737
1Dist: 9.4mm 2Dist: 9.7mm
Thyroid Probe:L55
b
1 L 2.65 cm
2 L 3.73 cm
3 L 4.05 cm
4 L 2.31 cm
LOGIQ E9
cm/s
T1: 0:56

is metachronous in 90.9% of observations, and in 42.7% of cases, the first tumor was breast cancer (Kaprin et al. 2017).

In patients with **gynecological conditions,** breast diseases are diagnosed in 50–80% of cases. The similarity in mechanisms of the development of genital and breast diseases, mostly associated with various hormonal disorders, is confirmed by numerous studies and indicates an increase in cancer risks in patients with combined pathology (Adamyan et al. 2006; Radzinsky et al. 2016). **Chronic inflammatory pelvic disease** is one of the key factors of breast conditions such as fibrocystic mastopathy. Hyperplastic processes in the uterus (myoma, endometriosis, endometrial hyperplasia, or their combinations) are often accompanied by tumors (including breast cancer), as well as by diffuse mixed or predominantly glandular breast disorders, which are more often referred to as breast proliferative diseases. Risk factors for the development of breast and genital diseases may be untimely menarche, reproductive failures, and intrauterine interventions, which, along with pelvic inflammatory disease, lead to damage to endo- and myometrium and hormonal disorders.

The risk of breast cancer depends on the intensity of the proliferation of the lobular and/or ductal epithelium and increases by 3–5 times at preexisting benign breast diseases, especially in combination with diseases of reproductive organs.

The impact of the **hormonal background** on the development of fibrocystic breast disease was reported. Hyperandrogenism protects against development of fibrocystic breast disease in **polycystic ovary syndrome**. In the groups of patients who have polycystic ovaries, the frequency of fibrocystic breast disease was statistically higher (56.98% and 91%, respectively) than in the group of patients with normal ovaries (6.83%).

In **benign pathology of mammary glands**, the intensity of expression of steroid hormones is parallel to the degree of hyperplasia. The disease progresses from fibrocystic breast disease (35%) to fibrous adenosis (50%) and lobular and ductal hyperplasia (85%). A positive relationship is observed between the presence of the progesterone receptor and fibroblastic or epithelial proliferation. **Fibroadenomas** of the mammary glands always contain progesterone receptors and estrogen receptors in only 25% of cases. Expression of the progesterone receptors is also very high in benign phyllodes tumors, almost as high as in malignant breast tumors.

A lot of research deals with the influence of **oral contraceptives** on the risk of breast cancer. Epidemiological data demonstrate a correlation between levels of endogenous sex hormones and the risk of breast cancer. The Collaborative Group on Hormonal Factors in Breast Cancer, 1996, published a combined analysis of approximately 90% of studies globally, assessing 53,297 cases of breast cancer and 100,239 women without cancer. The group concluded that women taking oral contraceptives are at a higher risk of breast cancer, but the risk decreases with time after the last use of oral contraceptives and is no longer evident 10 years after discontinuation. Some authors suppose that increased risk of breast cancer in oral contraceptives users is associated with the binding affinity of synthetic estrogen to the estrogen receptor being 90% higher than the binding affinity of natural estrogen. Moreover, ethinyl estradiol is a much more potent hormone and dose-dependently increases the proliferation of breast epithelial cells, therefore increasing the risk of breast cancer.

Metastatic lesions of the mammary gland can occur in primary tumors of various localizations. These cases are rare and are often associated with poor prognosis (see Chapter 10). Metastases of melanoma, lymphoma, ovarian cancer, mild neuroendocrine tumors, and sarcoma are most common in the breast. It is necessary to differentiate such lesions from other benign and malignant mammary gland masses. Outlined lesions often represent hematologically disseminated metastases, whereas metastases with lymphatic dissemination often show diffuse edema of the breast and thickening of the skin. Unlike primary breast tumors, most metastatic lesions of the mammary gland do not exhibit spiculated margins, reactive skin, or nipple. Although calcification is not often

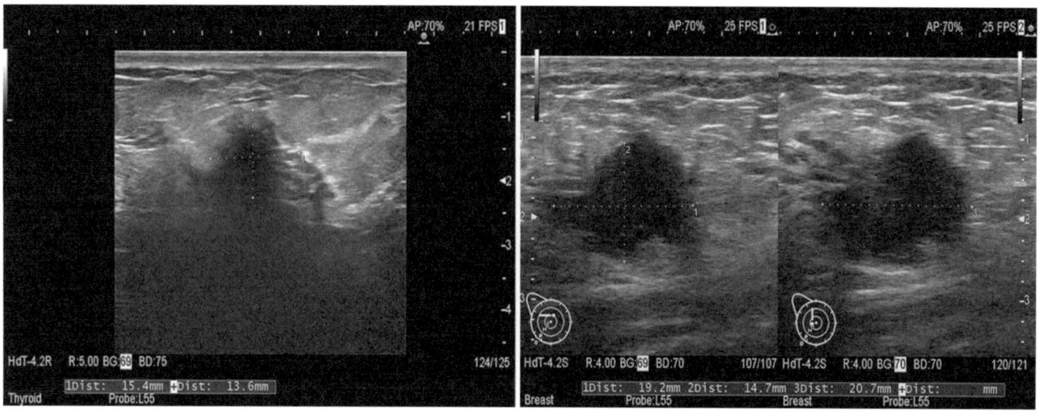

Fig. 8.3 Metastatic lesion of the mammary gland. The primary tumor is ovarian cancer. Grayscale US

present in metastatic lesions, they are more common in patients with primary ovarian cancer (Fig. 8.3).

Publications contain controversial data on possible interrelation of **breast and thyroid diseases**. Many authors report higher incidence of breast cancer in patients with thyroid dysfunction compared with the norm. Thyroid hormones are involved in the regulation of growth and development of the body, cell differentiation, and metabolism. Thyroid pathology is registered in 46% of women with breast cancer, while in the general population, the incidence of thyroid disorders does not exceed 14%.

The risk of breast cancer after thyroid cancer is 1.5–1.89; of thyroid cancer after breast cancer is 1.5–1.68. Possible relationship between breast cancer and thyroid cancer has been described with several publications. According to Kaprin et al. (2017), the incidence of combinations among patients with primary-multiple tumors, one of which was defined as breast cancer, was 6.6%, a synchronous combination was observed in 18.4% and metachronous in 81.6% of cases.

According to Kaprin et al. (2017), breast cancer is combined with **esophageal cancer** in 5.8%, **stomach cancer** in 65.7%, and **colorectal cancer** in 37.8% of cases.

Identification, differential diagnosis, specification of the degree, and extent of comorbid and primary-multiple breast cancer are an important diagnostic issue, which is still far from being solved. Late diagnosis of malignant comorbid and primary-multiple breast tumors is largely due to diagnostic errors at the prehospital stage. Typical preclinical diagnostic errors are incomplete and prolonged examination, irrational diagnostic algorithms, over- or underestimation of the value of certain diagnostic tools, insufficient oncologic alert, and incorrect diagnosis formulation.

In the diagnosis of synchronous primary-multiple breast tumors, the choice of the volume and methods of investigation prior to and during the treatment of neoplasms is important. Great opportunities were also open with introduction of endoscopic and perfection of radiological and ultrasound techniques (Sencha et al. 2015).

A lifelong observation of cancer patients aimed at early detection of multiple tumors is especially important. The probability of second tumor increases at the age interval of 55–70 years, and this should be taken into account when monitoring and planning examination of patients. Some sources recommend lifelong follow-up of patients who have had a malignant tumor of any localization, especially of the breast. Clinical follow-up is recommended at least two times a year, i.e., these patients are automatically included in the group of secondary cancer risk. A significant time interval for the appearance of metachronous tumors necessitates mandatory follow-up throughout the life of the patient.

In case of verified (diagnosed, treated) breast cancer, the examination of patients should include a comprehensive investigation of the below listed organs:

- The second breast
- Uterus
- Ovaries, adnexa
- Stomach
- Skin
- Thyroid gland

The main cause of diagnostic errors is that after detection of one malignant tumor, the possibility of the existence of another seems to be ruled out, and no further examination is carried out, thus neglecting radical effective treatment.

Multiparametric ultrasound, rational algorithms of imaging methods and technologies allow a comprehensive diagnosis of all conditions, including those associated with breast disease such as primary-multiple breast cancer, specification of the nature of the lesion, assessment of the severity and stage of the disease, status of surrounding tissues, and establishment of the treatment tactics and prognosis.

Ultrasound Imaging of Male Breast

9

Alexander N. Sencha and Yury Patrunov

Abstract

The principles of diagnostics and the approaches to breast pathology treatment in men are based on knowledge obtained in the process of diagnosis and treatment of women with similar breast pathology. High efficacy of ultrasound in diagnosis of breast carcinoma in men is the result of high sensitivity (86.9%) and specificity (85.3%). It allows assessing the areas, which are inaccessible to mammography, such as retromammary space, regions of lymph drainage, and the relation of a tumor to the skin and nipple. In the first visit, the correct diagnosis of cancer is established in 20–52% of male patients. The most difficult is the diagnostics of breast cancer comorbid to gynecomastia, which is observed in 12–40% of patients. The image of normal male breast is rather constant and does not depend on age and cyclic physiological features. Gynecomastia is the most common pathologic condition, which accounts for 74% of all processes developing in male breast. A typical feature of gynecomastia is its central location under the nipple. Physiological gynecomastia exhibits three age peaks: in newborn, in puberty, and in senile period. Gynecomastia may periodically accompany diabetes and other diseases. Palpable benign breast masses in men may be represented with tumors (lipoma, fibroadenoma, atheroma, schwannoma, angiolipoma, intraductal papilloma, cyst) or inflammatory lesions (mastitis, subareolar sepsis, abscess, posttraumatic hematoma, adipose necrosis, tuberculosis, syphilis, intramammary lymph nodes, etc.). Breast cancer in men is a rare disease, discussed in the chapter in detail.

A. N. Sencha (✉)
Division of Visual Diagnostics, National Medical Research Center for Obstetrics, Gynecology and Perinatology named after Academician V.I. Kulakov of Ministry of Healthcare of Russian Federation, Moscow, Russia

Y. Patrunov
Department of Ultrasound Diagnostics of Radiology Center, Yaroslavl Railway Clinic, Yaroslavl, Russia

9.1 Imaging Modalities for Male Breast Diseases

Both terms "male breast" and "male mammary gland" are utilized in medical literature. Experimental and clinical studies demonstrate similar origin and development of hyperplastic processes in breast in men and women and common etiology and pathogenetic mechanisms of development of breast carcinoma in male and female organisms. International standard for anatomical terminology (Terminologia Anatomica 1998) omitted the separate term "mamma masculine" because the breast in the male contains no unique elements, but those of the female breast developed to a lesser extent. In the European and

G. T. Sukhikh, A. N. Sencha (eds.), *Multiparametric Ultrasound Diagnosis of Breast Diseases*,
https://doi.org/10.1007/978-3-319-75034-7_9

North American literature, several terms are used for breast carcinoma both in women and in men along with the Latin term "cancer mammae." The common term in English is "breast cancer," but with reference to men, the additional word "male" is applied.

Male breast cancer is often regarded as an exclusively female condition. Patient's visit due to the changes in breast or a tumor is often delayed due to vague symptoms of the disease at early stages. General practitioners' lack of awareness of the early symptoms of breast diseases and low-level knowledge about breast malignancies result in 30–40% of men cancer patients being treated in the initially nonoperable stages of disease. Male breast cancer is a rare disease (<1% of all breast tumors globally). The incidence of the disease has significantly increased for the recent decades.

The principles of diagnostics and the approaches to breast pathology treatment in men are based on knowledge obtained in the process of diagnosis and treatment of women with similar breast pathology. Cases of last stage breast carcinoma in men are most often the consequence of insufficient attention of patients to one's health that results in late medical aid. Sometimes low oncologic awareness of general practitioners may lead to appointment of unreasonable or insufficient medical actions, which often worsen the clinical course. Because of the late address to the doctor, 60% of patients have complications, regional or remote metastases by the time of the diagnosis. Breast carcinoma in 20% of patients remains not diagnosed at all. The mortality among the men with breast carcinoma is up to 0.3% of the mortality from other malignancies.

Until present, there is still no standardized approach to diagnostic assessment and therapy allowing to avoid unnecessary surgical interventions and to provide a specified and effective treatment. Generally, there are no national programs, algorithms, and protocols of medical examination of men. Breast cancer screening in the frames of national programs is targeted only at women. It is considered cost-ineffective to perform screening mammography (ultrasound or X-ray) for all men, as it is being done for all women, taking into account low level of morbidity and rarity of this pathology in the population. Another issue is that men are not focused on this problem and less prone to refer for health care, including screening or testing. Breast disease often falls out of scope during medical examination of men. Only joint efforts of patients and doctors, specific oncologic alertness of clinicians and diagnosticians aimed at early detection of the disease, and appropriate treatment could raise attention to this problem and support early diagnosis and prediction.

The list of technologies for diagnostic assessment is very similar to that used for early and differential diagnostics of breast pathology in women. However, indications, algorithms, and techniques are in some respect specific. Early detection of breast cancer and effective differential diagnostics are of high priority.

In carrying on medical examination of men, the attention should be paid to the size of mammary glands, the shape of the nipples and areola, their symmetry, presence or absence of deformations, lesions, and the state of axillary lymph nodes (Fig. 9.1). It is always necessary to compare the breasts. An oncologically alerted doctor is significantly assured against wrong tactics. This should always be kept in mind during examination of men especially at the age 50–60 years by general practitioners, andrologists, urologists, endocrinologists, and physicians.

During palpation of pathologically changed male breasts, one can detect a mass with uneven borders, which is centrally located behind the nipple or areola or near them. Once an induration is detected, a thorough palpation of this area should be performed to define the size, shape, consistency, mobility of the mass, and the state of skin over it. Thin layer of subcutaneous fat in men, as compared to the same in women, and affinity of the gland to the skin and underlying tissues lead to the fact that the tumor early fixes to the anterior thoracic wall and the skin, the latter becoming wrinkled. However, palpation of a small breast tumor at early stages is often difficult, it's revealing being incidental. The palpation of regional lymph nodes is not always informa-

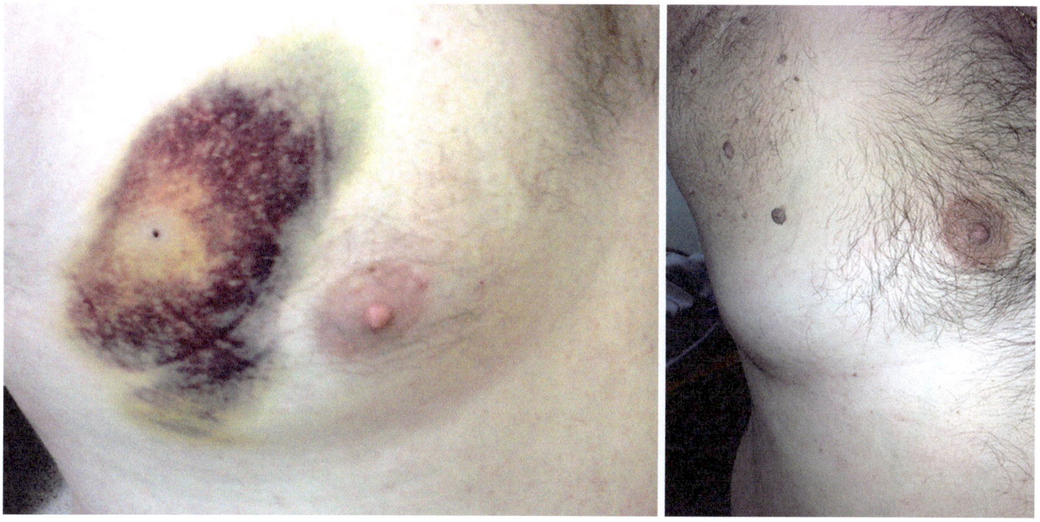

Fig. 9.1 Breast cancer. The view of the male breast after biopsy. Deformation of the breast shape

tive. The rate of metastasis detection is 32–45.8% (Bazhenova et al. 1985).

In this context radiologic imaging techniques should be considered as the golden standard of diagnosis.

Mammography in men as well as in women may be targeted and include screening, axillography, pneumocystography, and ductography. Mammogram is a two-dimensional image of the breast. It permits to analyze thickness, density of glandular tissue, spatial arrangement, shape, margins, and dimensions of the lesions (Fig. 9.2).

Indications for mammography of male mammary glands are listed below:

- Age > 60 years
- Suspicion or clinical features of breast cancer in any age group
- Other chronic breast diseases, especially nodular types (e.g., nodular type of chronic gynecomastia)

Some experts consider mammography to be a method of choice for diagnosis of breast cancer in men, useful for differential diagnosis of gynecomastia and breast cancer. The others find the effectiveness of this method doubtful (Semiglazov 2004, Harchenko and Rozhkova 2005).

Mammographic diagnostic criteria of breast cancer in men and women are the same. The characteristic features of cancer in men are various lesions of increased radiological density, with radiant specular margins and stranded structure with poorly defined edges often containing microcalcifications. Dense spots are located eccentrically in contrast to gynecomastia. Mammography often (but not always) allows to differentiate breast cancer and gynecomastia due to specific location of the latter behind the nipple and relative symmetry of structures and also by the state of regional lymph nodes. Lean breast tissue in men often significantly complicates the performance of mammography, sometimes making it impossible. However, this test can be a useful supplement to preventive medical examination and clinical and instrumental assessment, including US.

Magnetic resonance imaging (MRI) in men (as well as in women) allows to assess the structure of the breast; to detect a lesion; to specify its margins and shape; to identify a capsule, its intactness, or irregularity; to clarify if there is an invasion to the surrounding structures; and to detect lymph nodes (Fig. 9.3).

Men as well as women are referred for **X-ray computed mammography** to specify tumor invasion into the tissues of retromammary space,

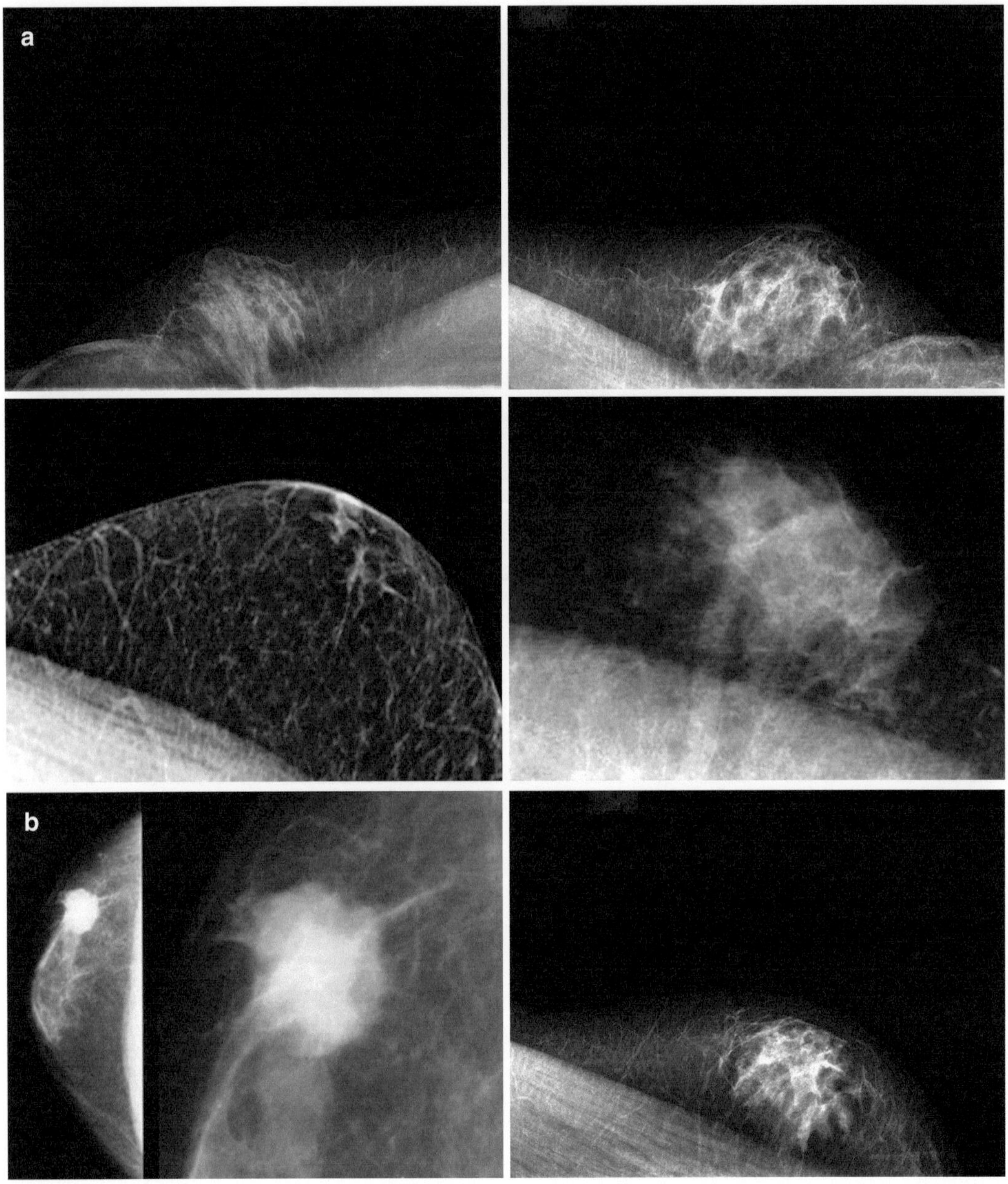

Fig. 9.2 Mammography in men. (**a**) 1–4 Gynecomastia. (**b**) 1–2 Breast cancer

metastases in axillary and infraclavicular lymph nodes, and remote metastases (Fig. 9.4).

Mammoscintigraphy besides general assessment of male breast may specify distribution of radiopharmaceuticals in the targeted area including axillary and other lymph nodes.

In men estrogen and progesterone receptors are often present in the tumors. There are some interesting facts as follows:

- Estrogen receptors are present in malignant tumors of male breast in 65–100%.
- Clinically significant levels are observed in over 85% of cases.
- Comparing to women, the rate of receptor-positive tumors in men do not increase with age.
- There is a correlation between the clinically significant level of estrogen receptors and a response to hormonal therapy.

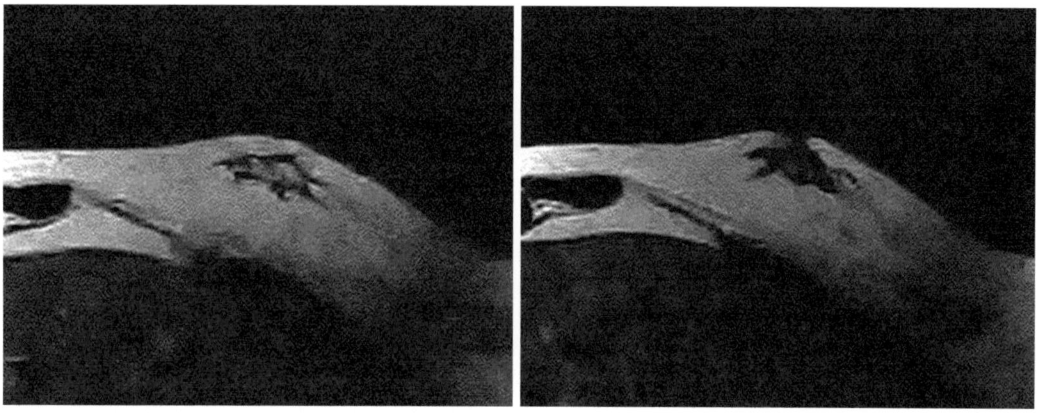

Fig. 9.3 1–2 Magnetic resonance imaging. T2FRFSE. Nodular gynecomastia

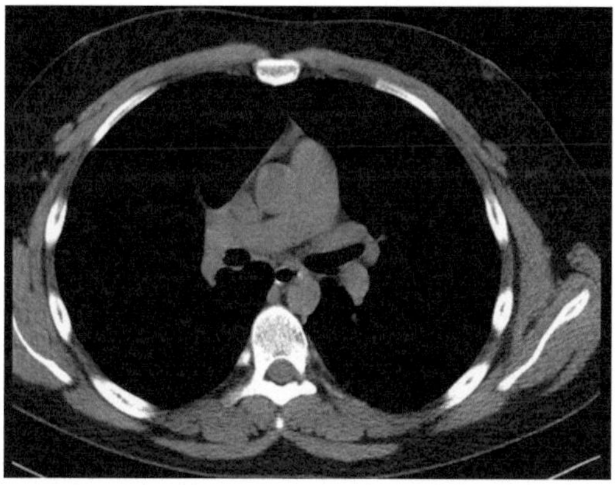

Fig. 9.4 Computed mammography. Breast cancer

Morphologic diagnosis is established after invasive diagnostics and further verification of the breast tumor. When diagnosing breast cancer in men, the sensitivity of fine needle biopsy is 69.5% and core biopsy 94.8%; positive predictive value of fine needle biopsy is 98.3% and core biopsy 98.2% (Nikolayev 2015).

Cytology and histology are the most valuable verifying methods. Usually it is not difficult to receive material for cytology. Real-time ultrasound and doctor's high expertise allow biopsy sampling exactly from the target area.

Ultrasound is now one of the most widespread and affordable imaging methods for diagnosis of breast pathology, early and differential diagnosis of breast masses, and guidance of minimally invasive modalities.

According to Sencha et al. (2015), high efficacy of US in diagnosis of breast carcinoma in men is the result of high sensitivity (86.9%) and specificity (85.3%). US allows assessing the areas, which are inaccessible to mammography, such as retromammary space, regions of lymph drainage, and the relation of a tumor to skin and nipple.

US exhibits the following advantages, as compared to mammography:

- Possibility of inspection of breasts in ectomorphic patients
- In the cases of dense background of the breast in young men
- For assessment of the breast at acute trauma or inflammation
- For examination of postoperative scars and detection of early and late complications and early recurrence of the disease
- Relatively simple and fast method
- No radiation dose applied
- Perfect for repeated examinations to assess dynamic changes
- Supplies unlimited access to examination of regional lymph nodes
- Easy guidance for puncture biopsies

In the first visit, the correct diagnosis of cancer is established in 20–52% of male patients. The most difficult is the diagnostics of breast cancer comorbid to gynecomastia, which is observed in 12–40% of patients.

Epidermal cysts, lipomas, stromal hyperplasia, or intraductal papillomas in retroareolar region in small breasts practically always result in hyperdiagnosis of malignant lesions with mammography. Therefore, US allows to avoid unnecessary puncture biopsies and surgery in men (Fisenko 1999).

According to Bazhenova et al. (1985), diagnostic complex based on clinical data and additional methods (US, mammography and other radiological modalities, cytology, etc.) provides correct diagnosis, including impalpable masses, in 95.5–99% of men.

9.2 Anatomy, Physiology, and Development of the Male Breast

Normal anatomy and individual features of the breast and regional lymph nodes in men are to be considered at the examination. Correct diagnosis and interpretation of ultrasound picture require adherence to the US technique and knowledge of specific features of anatomic structure of male breast.

Male breast is a paired organ, which is located on the front surface of the chest and on the fascia of large pectoral muscle between the parasternal and the front axillary lines at the level of II–IV ribs (Fig. 9.5). The size and the shape of breasts are subject to change with age and vary depending on subcutaneous fat thickness, anatomy, and constitution.

The male nipple is located on the middle clavicular line. Male nipple and the areola zone are small; the height of a nipple is 2–5 mm. Lobules and ducts are short and undeveloped. The nipple consists of muscular and epithelial tissues. It is surrounded by the areola—a pigmented skin area with a big number of sweat glands.

Mammary gland lies between the two split leaves of the superficial thoracic fascia.

Adipose tissue can be observed as subcutaneous fat and fatty lobes, which are surrounded with connective tissue fibers. Breast capsule is formed by connective tissue and fixed to the pectoral fascia.

Male breast (as well as female) receives blood supply from the mammary, subclavian, and intercostal arteries. Their branches form an anastomotic network located mostly subareolarly (Fig. 9.6). Venous network is formed by the homonymous veins.

The lymphatic system is presented by intramammary lymph ducts, efferent ducts, and regional lymph nodes: axillary, supraclavicular, pectoral, and substernal lymph nodes. Intramammary lymph ducts form a complex rete with anastomoses and plexuses.

Breast innervation is provided by the branches of thoracic, brachial, and intercostal nerves. Nipple nerves are rather numerous and end with tactile corpuscles.

Breast in men and women originate from the fourth pair of lactiferous points and similarly develop until puberty. Within the fourth to eighth weeks of gestation, thickening of epithelium

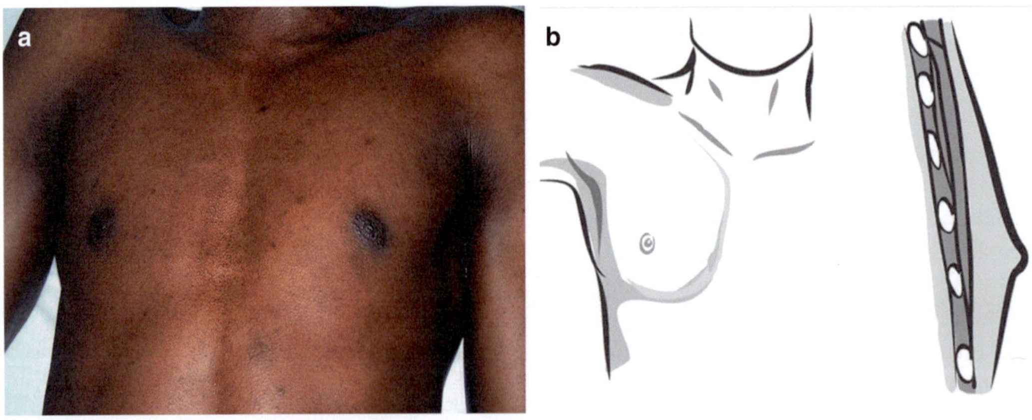

Fig. 9.5 Gross anatomy of normal breast. (**a**) Photo. (**b**) Scheme

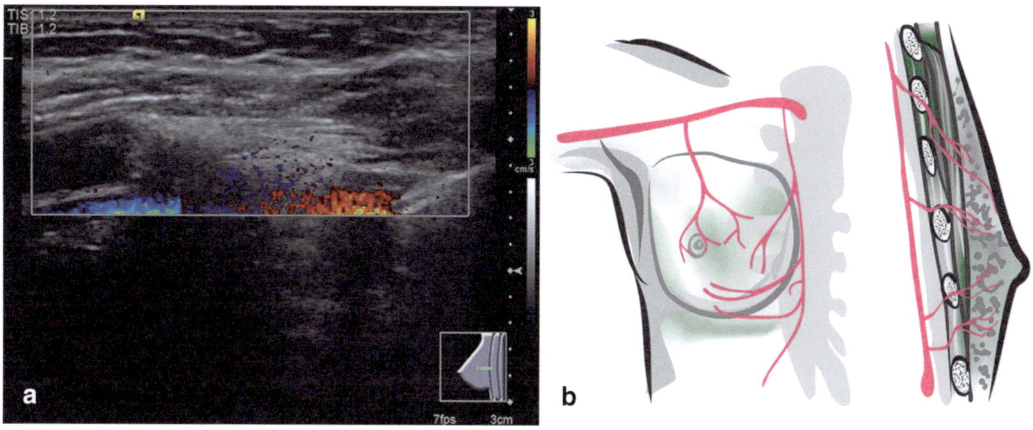

Fig. 9.6 Vascular supply to male breast. (**a**) Echogram. (**b**) Scheme

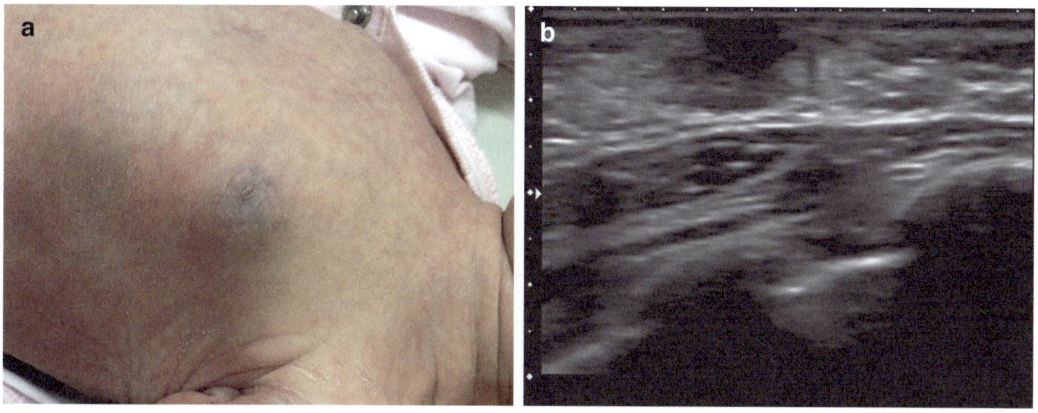

Fig. 9.7 The breast of a newborn boy. (**a**) General appearance of the breast. (**b**) Grayscale US

appears in a form of paired streaks in the middle of which the breast bud is identified (lactiferous streaks). Eight pairs of these streaks are inverted into the cutaneous bud of the connective tissue. Some people have several pairs of glands in the lactiferous streaks of the skin, although most of them remain undeveloped after birth.

Breast tissue at birth is identical in boys and girls (Fig. 9.7a). From birth to puberty, breasts in girls and boys are represented by matrix (fragments of glandular tissue and ducts in germinal status) surrounded by adipose and connective tissues (Fig. 9.7b).

Breast in boys and girls up to 7–8 years old has a similar structure (Fig. 9.8).

At puberty the breasts in boys remain rudimentary, while in girls they start fast development. They differentiate under hormonal influence, when at puberty estrogens start to stimulate proliferation of glandular tissue, while androgens counter this effect. Most of the boys have a 30-fold increase in the level of testosterone and a triple increase in the level of estrogen in this period. At the age of 12–16 years, US may reveal the image identical to the girls at thelarche in the retroareolar area of healthy boys (Fig. 9.9). This reflects natural physiological changes in the teenagers bodies.

During the fast puberty, the transitional proliferation of ducts and stroma finally results in atrophy of ducts and involution of the breast. US in male usually fails to differentiate the elements of mature glandular tissue (Fig. 9.10).

As a result, the breast of an adult man mainly consists of the adipose tissue (subcutaneous fat)

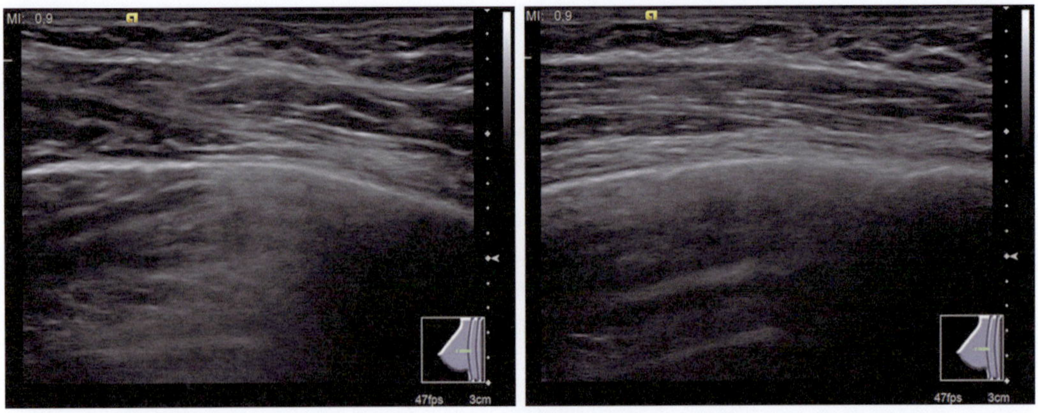

Fig. 9.8 1–2 The breast of an 8-year-old boy. Grayscale US

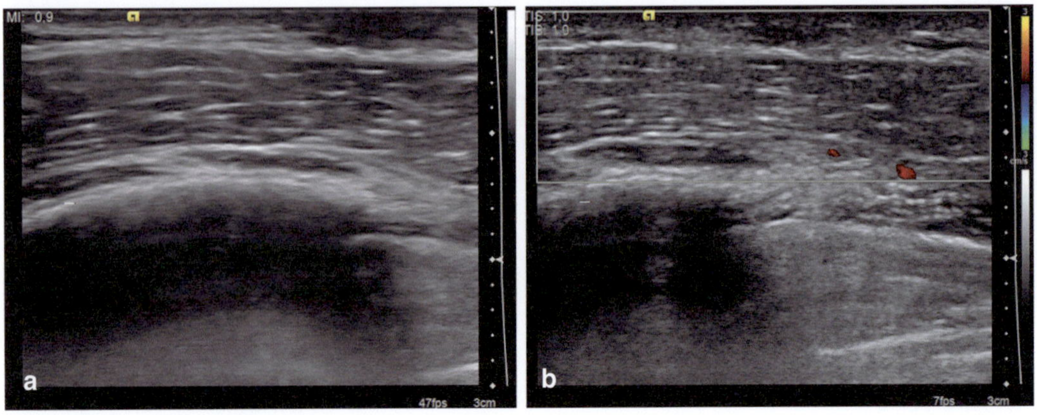

Fig. 9.9 Breast of a 14-year-old boy. (**a**) Grayscale. (**b**) CDI

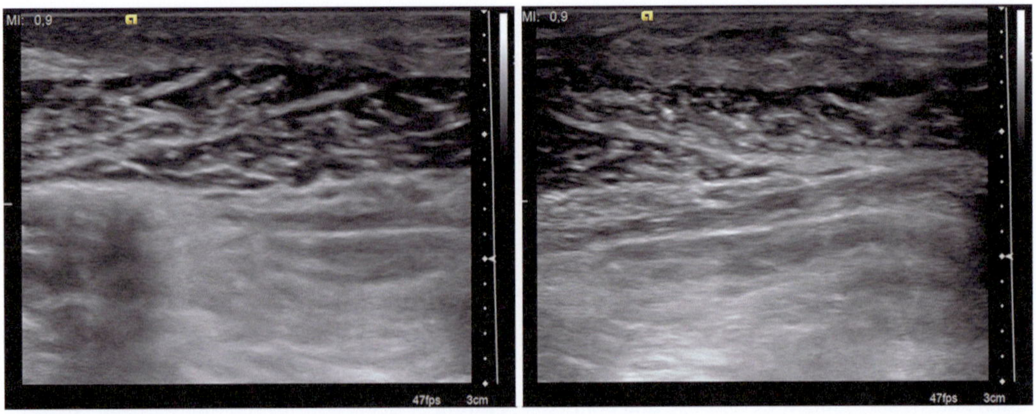

Fig. 9.10 The breast of a 19-year-old man. Grayscale US

with insignificant subareolar residual ducts and the fibrous tissue. Development of breast lobules demands estrogens and progesterone, which are detected in extremely low quantities in men. In rare cases, interstitial lymph nodes may be visualized.

All variants of breast malformations and diseases, which can occur in women (girls), may be detected in men (boys).

9.3 The Technology of Ultrasound of the Male Breast

Breast US in men does not demand special preparation, as opposed to women, the latter having preferable time of examination at certain periods of the menstrual cycle.

Indications for breast US in men are the following:

- Discomfort or pain in the breast area regardless of the detection of any palpable mass
- Breast induration
- Palpable masses within the breast
- Changes of the breast skin, nipple, and areola
- Contralateral breast cancer
- Palpable masses in axillary areas and surrounding zones
- As a screening method in patients with a family history of breast cancer

The results of breast US, which often supplement the data of X-ray mammography, especially in ambiguous cases, are important for:

- Differential diagnostics of lesions initially detected with palpation or mammography
- Examination of breast in children and teenagers
- Examination in the acute period of a breast trauma or inflammation
- US guidance of puncture biopsy of breast lesions
- Detailed assessment of breast infiltrations of uncertain nature

Breast US is performed with linear probes with the frequency 7.5–18 MHz, now more often 7.5–12 MHz.

Breast US is performed in the patient's supine position with hands under the head (Fig. 9.11). In men it is also possible to perform the examination in the sitting or standing position. Since any position does not cause breast displacement, it does not influence the scanning and the image quality.

It is rational to perform multiple projection scanning in the supine position, right and left lateral recumbent position, and seated with hands behind head.

Usually the intact breast is examined first. An US specialist should know that the breast region in men is not limited with the area of the nipple, areola, and retroareolar space. A field about 7–10 cm in diameter should be scanned from periphery to the nipple similar to the female breast.

According to the standard procedure recommended for women, while describing the loca-

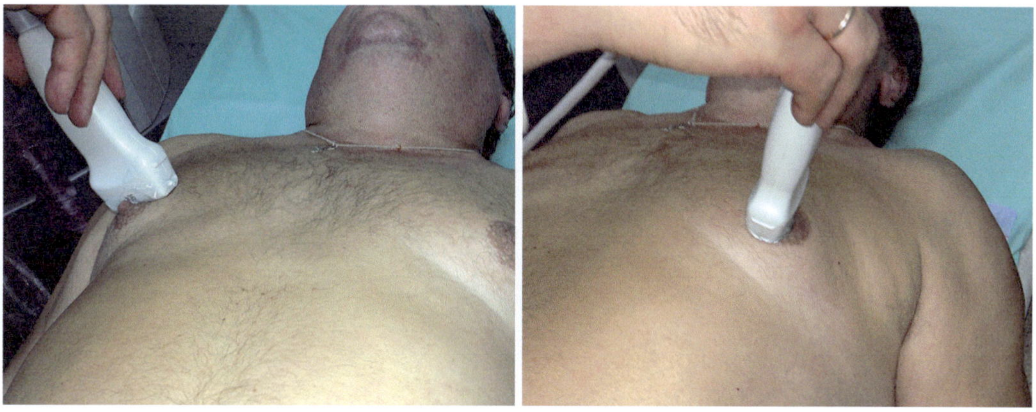

Fig. 9.11 1–2 Breast US in a man. Position of a patient and ultrasound probe

tion and specification of pathological process in men, the breast is conventionally divided into four quadrants: upper(superior)-outer(lateral), upper(superior)-inner(medial), lower(inferior)-inner(medial), and lower(inferior)-outer(lateral). The terminology of "o'clock positions" is appropriate for more accurate indication of the lesion location (see Chap. 2).

The direction of scanning and the sequence of quadrants do not matter. Subareolar zone and nipple are to be scanned especially carefully using fan movements of US probe from different directions, because the acoustic shadow from the nipple can hide various pathological processes. If some area is suspicious for pathological process, it is advised to use other technologies. These may be time-consuming and need additional software. Moderate compression with the probe is applied as well. This aims to assess the mobility of the lesion against the surrounding tissues and to decrease US artifacts resulting from acoustic shadows of connective tissue structures.

It is necessary to assess the status of regional lymph nodes (axillary, sub- and supraclavicular, parasternal).

Intervals between breast US in men are rather arbitrary. Absence of clinical signs and masses in the breast and axillary areas and normal oncomarkers eliminate further US follow-up.

In doubtful case control, US may be recommended to check the changes or distinguish pathologic and physiologic signs (as a rule, ultrasonography once a year and seldom once in 3–6 months).

9.4 Normal Male Breast with Ultrasound

The US image of normal male breast is rather constant and does not depend on age and cyclic physiological features. Small variability of US picture is caused only by constitutional features of a man (subcutaneous fat).

It also depends on the type of the US scanner, US regimes and setup modes, and the specialist's experience.

As a rule, in the process of scanning, the following structures are specified in the male breast (Fig. 9.12):

- Subcutaneous fat
- Anterior fascial leaf
- Elements of lactiferous ducts (if any imaged)
- Posterior fascial leaf, retromammary space
- Nipple and areola
- Regional lymph nodes

The possibility to assess the breast skin depends on the probe frequency and the US scanner class.

Normal **breast skin** in men (as well as in women) is imaged as homogenous hyperechoic 0.5 mm layer. Prior to puberty, the thickness of the skin usually ranges from 2 to 5 mm. It reaches

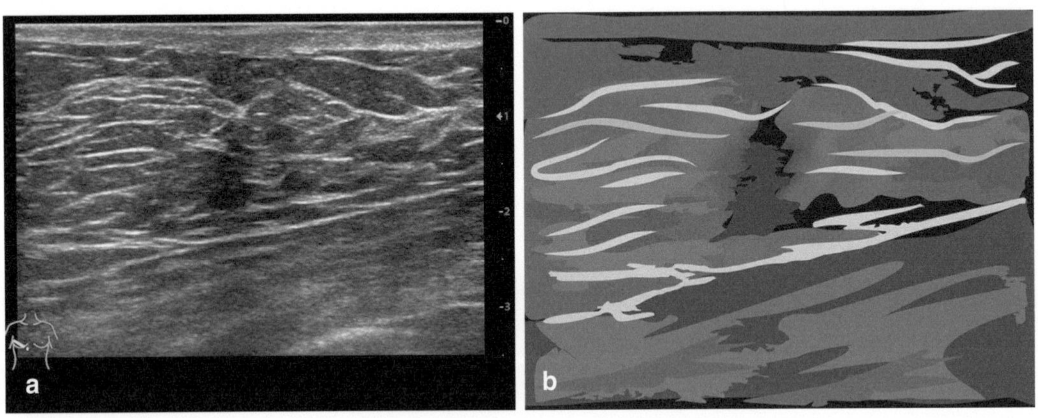

Fig. 9.12 Normal ultrasound anatomy of male breast. (**a**) Grayscale US. (**b**) Scheme

2–4 mm after puberty (Zabolotskaya and Zabolotsky 2005).

Inflammatory process, postradiation therapy status, and postoperative edema are accompanied with thickening and rough echostructure of the skin. The skin may have a heterogeneous structure of varying severity, and it can be visualized as two hyperechoic lines separated by a thin hypoechogenic septa. The margin between the skin and the subcutaneous fat is hardly seen.

Subcutaneous fat. Adipose tissue shows decreased or moderate echodensity and homogeneous structure with linear hyperechoic inclusions, which often exhibit vague acoustic shadows (small amount of elongated structures of decreased echodensity with rare hyperechoic connective tissue bands).

Adipose tissue often looks like round hypoechoic structures arranged in rows. Adipose lobules are often bordered by symmetric lateral acoustic shadows. In excessive adipose layer, repeated lateral acoustic shadows from adjacent fat lobules hinder accurate differentiation of breast echostructure. Compression of the breast with US probe usually reduces this artifact.

The **anterior (superficial) leaf of the fascia** often shows as an echoic line that separates subcutaneous fat from glandular parenchyma.

Imaging of **lactiferous ducts** also depends on male breast development. Normally, lactiferous ducts in men are abortive and short. In the majority, they do not show at ultrasonography.

Cooper's ligaments and glandular tissue in male breast are absent and therefore not detected with US.

The **posterior leaf of the fascia** separates the breast from the retromammary space and shows as thin (about 0.1 cm) hyperechoic linear structure.

The **retromammary space** contains retromammary adipose tissue, large and small pectoralis muscles, intercostal muscles, and pleura. Retromammary fat consists of hypoechoic lobules between the echoic lines of posterior leaf of the fascia and anterior margin of the large pectoralis muscle.

Pectoralis (large and small) and intercostal **muscles** are defined as hypoechoic structures isolated with septa. Identification of muscles ensures that the breast layer is examined completely.

The echostructure of the ribs depends on the amount of osteal and cartilaginous components. Each part of a rib has specific US image. Transverse US scan reveals an osteal part of a rib as an oval structure with increased echodensity on periphery and acoustic shadowing. Cartilaginous part is hypoechoic with accurate anterior and posterior margins and some posterior shadowing. However, some inner structure can be observed in cartilaginous part. Intercostal muscles are defined in intercostal spaces as hypoechoic structures with typical muscular pattern.

The pleura can be detected as an echoic line, which displaces with breathing. It is the deepest structure that can be distinguished at breast US.

Imaging of the structures of retromammary space is not always possible. It substantially depends on the US probe frequency and the US scanner class.

The **nipple and areola** are normally defined as a round structure of moderate or decreased echodensity with comparatively homogeneous structure and distinct even contours. Sometimes there is posterior acoustic shadow behind the nipple, which results from muscular and connective tissue fibers in the area.

There are some specific US features of the breast in men of different age groups.

In boys before puberty, the breast consists of adipose tissue and fibrous stromal component without any glandular tissue. Adipose tissue has low echodensity, relatively homogeneous structure with fine echoic linear inclusions without acoustic shadow. The thickness of the adipose layer is about 0.5–1 cm. Ductal system, which is undeveloped, shows as merging hypoechoic structures in the retroareolar space. The glandular tissue in boys is not defined.

The thickness of adipose tissue mainly depends on the patient's constitution but, as a rule, increases with years.

In early puberty, adipose tissue can be defined with US as a thin layer between the skin and glandular tissue. With years, the thickness of the adipose layer increases along with slight increase in its echodensity. It also becomes more heterogeneous. Connective tissue structures of the breast have high echodensity and are often accompanied with an acoustic shadow. It is necessary to consider this fact during breast US to avoid mistaking of artifacts for pathological changes. It is advised to compare symmetric areas of both breasts for differential diagnosis of a suspected lesion with specific features of unchanged tissue. Further age changes in adipose tissue are characterized by increased heterogeneity of connective tissue, which is defined as echoic linear structures.

Normal US picture of the breast in men of the same age may be different. It depends on several individual factors (anatomical and constitutional features, injuries or surgical interventions, hormonal treatment, etc.).

In elderly men, the skin is visualized as two hyperechoic lines with a thin hypoechoic fat layer in between. The thickness of the skin is different. Almost the entire breast consists of hypoechoic fatty lobules (round hypoechoic structures with a distinct hyperechoic rim).

During ultrasonography, it is necessary to compare the features of the right and left breasts in different regions and quadrants, as well as to assess the dynamics of US pattern over a certain period of time (usually 3–6 months). Complete breast information should take into account age specificities, the history of the patient, the patient's complaints, the results of clinical examination (palpation), functional state of the body, concomitant pathology, and the hormonal status.

Normal breast of an adult man shows at US as adipose tissue containing some residual ducts and fibrous tissue in subareolar area (Fig. 9.13).

The skin is seen as an echoic line of 0.5–1.5 mm. Subcutaneous fat lies under it and is defined as a relatively uniform hyperechoic fat layer of 2–3 cm thick. Normal breast does not contain any cystic or solid lesions at US and mammographic images (Fig. 9.14).

The standard report of breast US should describe the presence of lesions and the areas with abnormal structure, their sectoral location or clock position, dimensions, structure, echogenicity, contours, relationship with surrounding tissues and vascular supply, and local lymph nodes.

An example of US report of a male patient with normal breast

Name, surname. __S__ Age__31__

Outpatient examination. Date____

Patient's record____

US scanner____

The breasts are of masculine type and consist mainly of adipose tissue. Some fibrous tissue is randomly distributed in all regions. Lactiferous ducts are not seen. Cystic and solid lesions are not detected.

Axillary, supraclavicular, and subclavian lymph nodes are not visualized.

Conclusion: Normal breasts.

9.5 Ultrasound Diagnosis of Breast Diseases in Men

Differential diagnosis of focal abnormalities and tumors due to their variety cannot be limited to only one disease. Most of breast conditions occur both in men and women, such as the following examples:

- Benign diseases (gynecomastia, tumors, inflammation)
- Malignancies (sarcoma, breast cancer metastases from other organs)
- Various inflammatory processes
- Various posttraumatic changes

The imaging findings are often crucial for differentiation of breast diseases in men.

9.5.1 Gynecomastia

One common breast abnormality in men is gynecomastia. It demands a complex examination with the use of radiologic (primarily ultrasound) imaging techniques and careful differentiation with a tumor.

The term "gynecomastia" originates from the Greek words: *gyne*, "woman," and *mastos*, "breast." It is a dyshormonal hyperplastic process characterized by a wide range of proliferative and regressive changes in the male breast tissue,

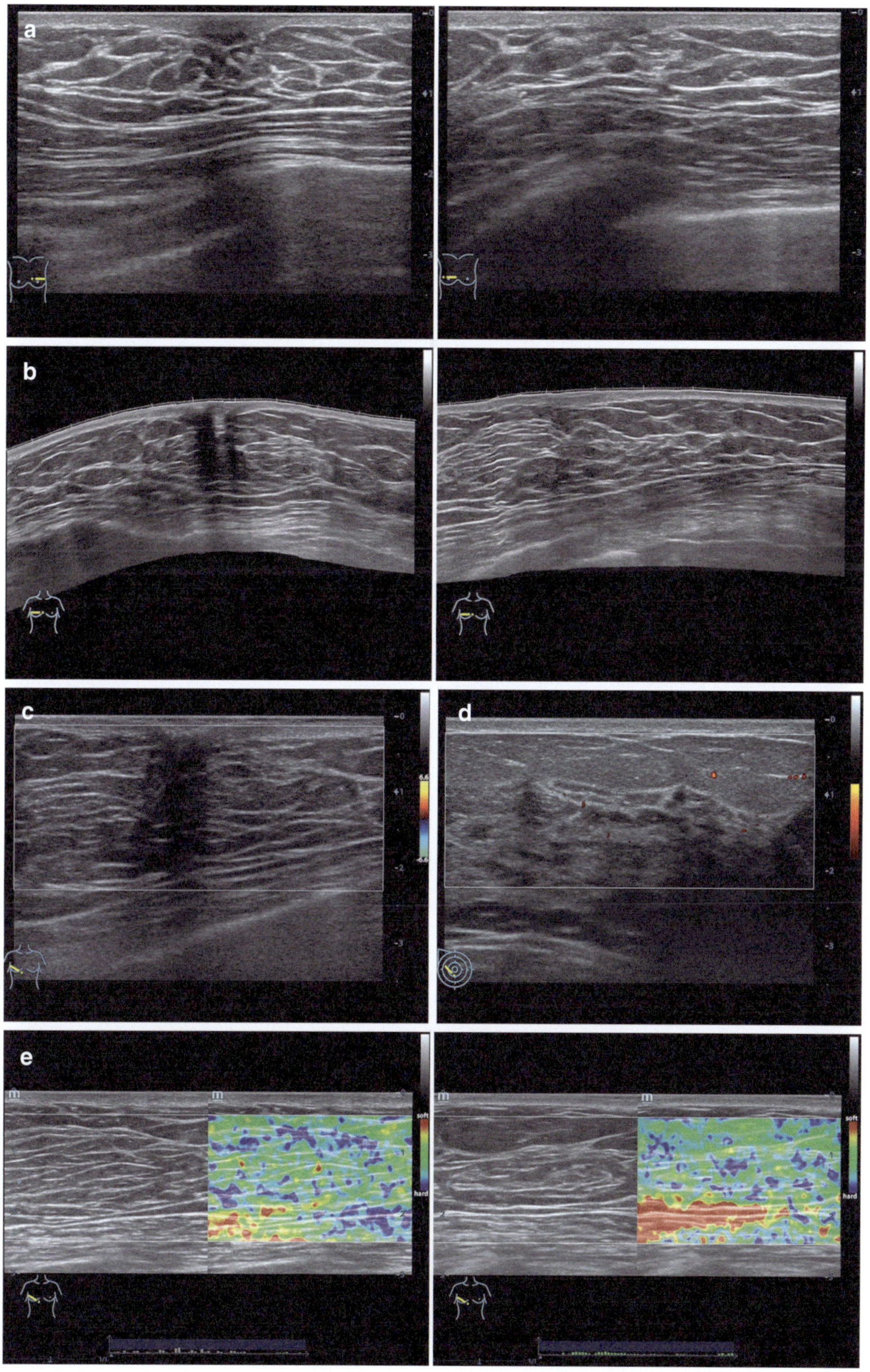

Fig. 9.13 Normal male breast tissue. (**a**) 1–2 Grayscale US. (**b**) 1–2 Panoramic scan. (**c**) CDI. (**d**) PDI. (**e**) 1–2 Compression US elastography

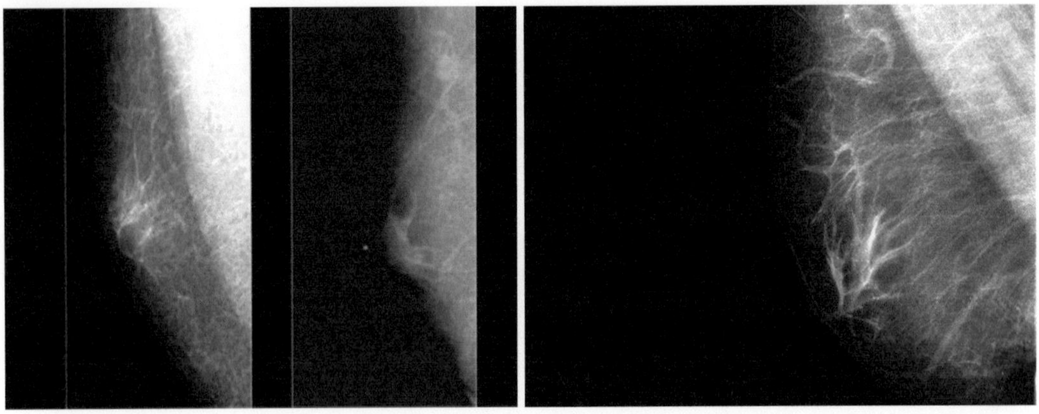

Fig. 9.14 1–2 X-ray mammograms. Normal male breast tissue

which manifest with the enlargement of the mammary gland due to benign intraductal and stromal proliferation.

The incidence is 280–570 per 100,000 healthy men. It is the most common pathologic condition, which accounts for 74% of all processes developing in male breast.

Gynecomastia is progressing as an independent disease in 19% of cases and on the background of other diseases in 81% of cases. In 74% of cases, these diseases are trigger factors for hypertrophy of glandular tissue in boys.

Gynecomastia is an oncologic alert, because this process may be a cancer precursor; cancer incidence is 3–5 times higher than in general population. Most researchers deny the possibility of malignization of gynecomastia and do not consider it a precancerous condition. Some authors have reported a presumed direct transformation of gynecomastia to cancer. In pathological studies of resected breasts, gynecomastia was detected in 26.4% of operated patients; 7.5% of them had bilateral gynecomastia. Symptoms of chronic gynecomastia may mimic breast cancer in men, i.e., the presence of malignant tumors may mask gynecomastia.

The age range of patients with gynecomastia is as wide as 14–75 years, but most commonly it occurs in the fifth to eighth decades of life with maximum prevalence in the fifth decade (27.8%). These data present an indirect evidence in favor of dyshormonal nature of gynecomastia, associated with the involution of sex glands after 50. This changes the balance between androgens and estrogens in favor of the latter. Gynecomastia can be physiological or a consequence of an underlying disease. Twenty-five percent of cases are of idiopathic nature.

Clinically, gynecomastia is characterized with enlargement and induration of the breasts accompanied by discomfort and pain (Fig. 9.15).

Some retraction of the nipple and its fixation may be seen. A typical feature of gynecomastia is its central location under the nipple. Men often do not feel any discomfort and do not notice any pathologic signs. This leads to late diagnosis. One third of male patients with gynecomastia have lesions diffusely distributed within the breast as small fibrous foci in adipose tissue (Fig. 9.16). Sometimes these foci contain cysts of 0.5 cm in size with transparent fluid. About 10% of patients exhibit bilateral changes. In two thirds of patients with gynecomastia, breast infiltrations are focal. They have round shape, elastic or dense elastic texture, and the size of 0.7–8 cm and are centrally located in subareolar area.

There are a large number of classifications mainly based on etiological factors.

Most commonly the following forms are distinguished:

1. Physiological gynecomastia:
   - Neonatal
   - Pubertal
   - Senile
2. True gynecomastia:
   - Idiopathic

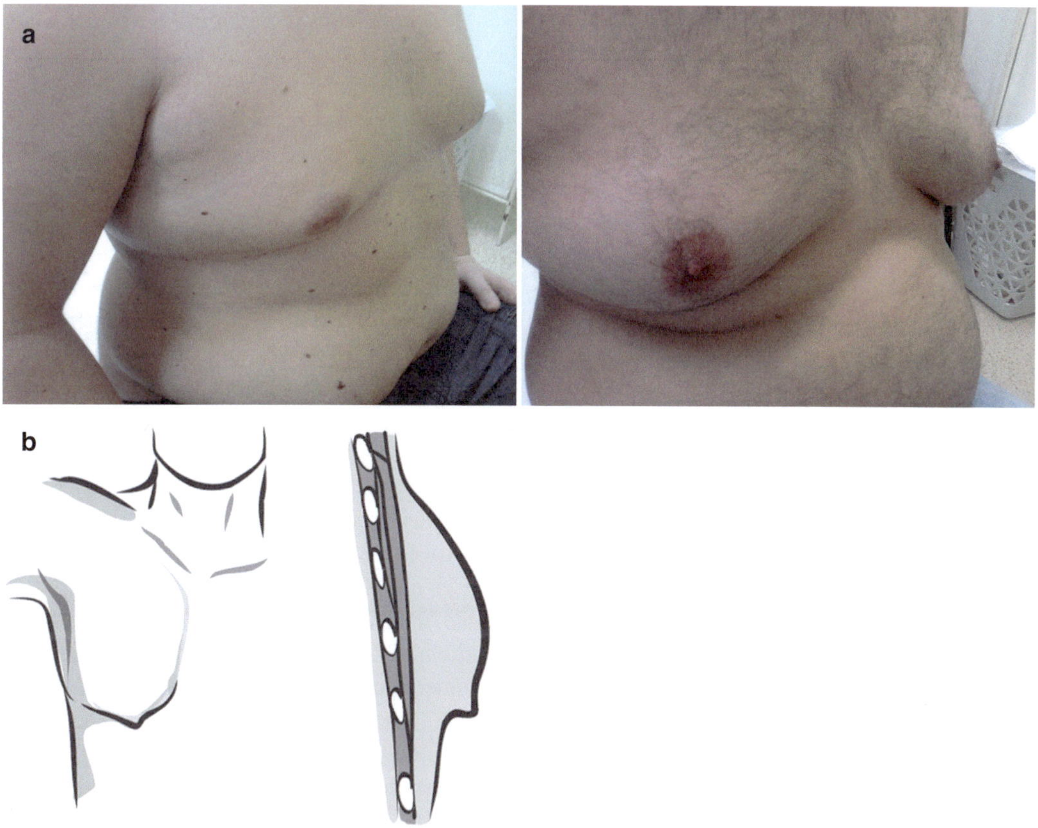

Fig. 9.15 Gynecomastia. (**a**) 1–2 Photo of the breast. (**b**) Scheme

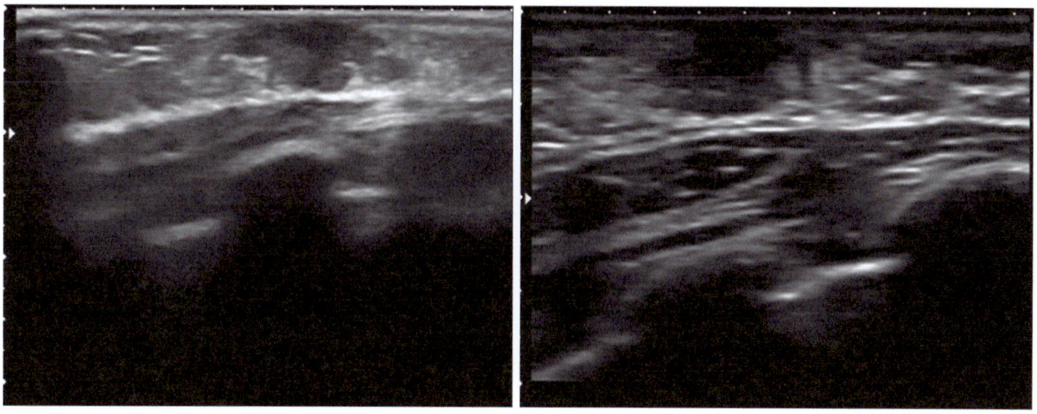

Fig. 9.16 Gynecomastia. Grayscale US

- Persistent pubertal
- Familial

3. Symptomatic gynecomastia
   - In hormone-secreting tumors (e.g., tumors of testicles, tumors of various organs (lung, liver, intestine), which produce chorionic gonadotropin), androsteromas, and adrenal hyperplasia
   - In endocrine diseases, including genetic (e.g., true hermaphroditism, Klinefelter

syndrome, congenital adrenal hyperplasia, Kennedy's disease, Graves' disease, etc.)
   - In primary hypoandrogenism (e.g., infectious, granulomatous orchitis, anorchism, castration)
   - In renal and/or hepatic failure
   - Drug-induced (estrogens, human chorionic gonadotropin, spironolactone, flutamide, cardiac glycosides, tricyclic antidepressants, opiates, cannabis, etc.)
   - False gynecomastia (adipose breast tissue hyperplasia)
4. Breast tumors
   - Malignant (cancer or sarcoma)
   - Benign (adenoma, lipoma, fibroma)

Physiological gynecomastia exhibits three age peaks: in newborn, in puberty, and in senile period.

Four degrees of severity of gynecomastia are suggested:

1. Minimal subareolar nodosity
2. Subareolar mass smaller than the areola
3. The mass equals to the areola
4. The mass larger than the areola

According to the size, gynecomastia is classified as light, moderate, and severe, using the formula: CxH/2, where C is breast circumference (cm) and H is breast height (cm). Light gynecomastia corresponds to a value lower than 6 cm^2 (the incidence is 10.4%); moderate, 6–10 cm^2 (the incidence is 71.4%); and severe, more than 10.0 cm^2 (the incidence is 18%).

Distinguishing nodular, diffuse, and diffuse and nodular mastopatia forms is considered the most practical.

There is a classification based on the persistence of pathological hyperplasia in male breast:

1. Neonatal gynecomastia.
2. Pubertal (transitional) gynecomastia as a physiological phenomenon is observed in 40–90% of boys in puberty and disappears thereafter.
3. Persistent pubertal gynecomastia is considered abnormal. It does not exhibit spontaneous regress.

Gynecomastia of newborns is a secondary disorder related to transplacental transmission of maternal hormones to the fetus. It is observed in 60–90% of all newborns. It is characterized with infiltration in subareolar region, sometimes accompanied with colostrum discharge. It spontaneously resolves within several days or weeks and does not require any medical management.

Gynecomastia in puberty is registered in 4–6% of adolescents. It is usually bilateral and asymptomatic. Physiological gynecomastia occurs in 70% of adolescents in puberty and regresses spontaneously in 6–24 months or several years. In a number of cases, it may be a long-lasting severe condition due to sensitivity of the mammary tissue to estrogen stimulation.

Histologically, features of pubertal gynecomastia are alterations in changes of interstitial tissue with insignificant proliferation of ductal epithelium. It demands conservative or surgical treatment only in severe cases. Pubertal gynecomastia usually spontaneously disappears in 6–18 months. Small enlargement of the breasts does not require any treatment in the majority of teenagers.

Persistent gynecomastia is a pathologic condition. After puberty, the remaining enlargement of the breast demands surgical treatment, if conservative treatment fails to improve the situation. Endocrinologic examination permits to classify persistent gynecomastia into four variants: normopubertal, hypopubertal, hyperpubertal, and feminine pubertal.

Senile (involutory) gynecomastia is often met in men older than 60 years. It occurs in men with excessive body weight due to peripheral steroidogenesis in adipose tissue on the background of age-related decrease in testicular hormones. The diagnosis of involutory gynecomastia is established, if other causes of gynecomastia are excluded.

Drug-induced (iatrogenic) gynecomastia is mostly registered in adult men. More than 120 drug groups can induce gynecomastia, such as estrogens, steroids, glucocorticoids, gonadotropins, etc. This type of gynecomastia is reversible and regresses after the drug cancelation.

Gynecomastia in endocrine and non-endocrine diseases can accompany liver or kidney disorders. It is a consequence of disturbance in metabolism and excretion of steroid hormones and prolactin.

Gynecomastia may periodically accompany diabetes (Sencha et al. 2015). The main causes are considered disturbances in liver and kidney functions. Diffuse diabetic glomerulosclerosis usually appears in 4–5 years after manifestation of diabetes and in 15–20 years from the onset of the disease. It is present in all patients with diabetes. Nodular type of glomerulosclerosis is most common. It starts almost from the very beginning of diabetes and quickly progresses resulting in glomerular microaneurysms, which narrow or completely obstruct the capillaries. In turn, it leads to accumulation of toxic products and disrupted destruction of peptide hormones, which accumulate in blood and affect sexual glands and directly breast tissue promoting the growth of ductal tree and development of gynecomastia.

Gynecomastia in men with prolactinoma may manifest with galactorrhea and hyperprolactinemic hypogonadism. Treatment of a tumor of the pituitary gland, conservative (with dopamine agonists) or adenomectomy, leads to involution of gynecomastia. Gynecomastia in subthalamic dysfunctions is caused by disturbance in regulation of adenohypophysis leading to the change in production of prolactin and other hormones. Gynecomastia can be associated with hyperthyroidism in children and be the first sign of hyperthyroidism in adult men, since thyroid hormones activate steroidogenesis. Hypothyroidism may be also accompanied by gynecomastia, when hyperstimulation of the pituitary gland arises under the influence of excess thyroliberin. This is a characteristic for primary hypothyroidism. Correction of hypothyroidism leads to the regression of gynecomastia. In men with cryptorchism, anorchism, after testicular trauma or autoimmune conditions of testicles with their subsequent atrophy, and poor spermatogenesis and synthesis of testosterone, hormone replacement therapy is an option of gynecomastia treatment and prevention. Gynecomastia appears in genetic diseases associated with endocrinopathies (hyperprolactinemia and hypersensitivity of breast tissues to estrogens at Klinefelter's syndrome, increase in production of estrogens in Reifenstein syndrome and testicular feminization syndrome).

Gynecomastia in non-endocrine diseases often accompanies severe pathology of the liver and kidneys, such as hepatitis, liver cirrhosis, and chronic renal insufficiency. The method of choice for treatment in such cases is surgery, since drug administration can negatively affect the main disease.

Gynecomastia occurs in 10–40% of cases with thyrotoxicosis. With an excess of thyroid hormones, the production of estrogens and estrogen-binding globulin increases. Globulin-bound estradiol, which is eagerly accepted by the target cells, will strongly affect the mammary glands. Hypothyroidism can also be accompanied by gynecomastia. This is due to hyperstimulation of prolactotrophs of the pituitary gland under the influence of excessive thyroliberin production, which is characteristic for primary hypothyroidism.

Kidney disease may cause gynecomastia. Gynecomastia may accompany the so-called uremic hypogonadism, characterized by low secretory activity of Leydig's cells on the background of chronic renal insufficiency caused by suppression of glomerular filtration and increased blood levels of urea and its decay products (guanidine, ammonia, etc.), creatinine, residual nitrogen, urinary acid, and other toxic substances. Kidneys are also the place of degradation of peptide hormones. Their impaired destruction leads to their accumulation in blood, and to adverse effects on testes and the breast tissue, potentiating proliferation of the duct system and development of gynecomastia. Breast enlargement may be observed in men with chronic renal insufficiency on hemodialysis. Gynecomastia often arises within the first weeks of hemodialysis and spontaneously disappears in most cases. Development of this condition does not correlate with hemodialysis duration.

Of special value for understanding of the connection of gynecomastia with prostate diseases are the data about the increase of conversion of testosterone to dihydrotestosterone in the hypertrophic prostate tissue. Close relationship between the prostate and testes in the pathogenesis of gynecomastia is based on interaction of secretory functions of these organs. Cessation of the prostate function is accompanied by testicular atrophy and abnormal spermatogenesis. Enhanced secretory activity of the prostate suppresses the activity of testicles, while reduced activity stimulates their function.

Gynecomastia as a paraneoplastic syndrome can arise in cases of hormone-producing tumors. Bilateral gynecomastia often is the first and single sign of a tumor (lung, pancreatic, liver, kidney, testicular cancer) for a long time. Breast enlargement is induced by ectopic secretion of estrogens or gonadotropins by the tumor. Gynecomastia may be observed in cases of benign hormone-active adrenal tumors (feminizing adrenal or testicular tumors) in any age.

Gynecomastia is idiopathic in 25% of cases, where the cause is left undetermined.

Gynecomastia can be unilateral or bilateral and symmetric or asymmetric.

Obesity in men leads to breast enlargement due to adipose tissue (so-called **lipomastia** or **pseudo-gynecomastia**).

There are several types of gynecomastia, as follows:

- Nodular (round intense homogeneous lesion)
- Treelike (wide dense fibrous branches)
- Diffuse glandular (similar to mastopathy in women)

Diffuse gynecomastia clinically manifests with a painful swelling of one or both breasts, in some cases with nipple discharge, coarse lobularity, and multiple foci of altering character. Gynecomastia is most often bilateral, although the severity and the prevalence of the disease may vary.

In nodular gynecomastia the areas of nodularities more often occurring in one breast become permanent with a tendency to enlargement.

Proliferative and nonproliferative forms of dysplasia are distinguished. It is believed that the risk of developing breast cancer increases depending on the severity of ductal, lobular, or intra-cystic proliferation. Based on the degree of proliferative activity of epithelium, the following types are specified:

- Gynecomastia without proliferation (the risk of development of breast cancer is 1.5 times higher)
- Gynecomastia with epithelial proliferation (the risk of malignancy increases up to 1.9)
- Gynecomastia with atypical epithelial proliferation (3 times risk increase, up to 25 times according to some publications)

According to Sencha et al. (2015), nodular form is detected in 14% of patients with gynecomastia.

US features of the nodular form of true gynecomastia are as follows (Figs. 9.17, 9.18, and 9.19):

- Hypoechoic area or lesion.
- Central retroareolar location.
- Various size (≥5 mm).
- Irregular shape.
- Different degree of homogeneity.
- Distinct or indistinct contours, rough borders.
- Hypo- or avascular at CDI, PDI, and 3DPD.
- Heterogeneous rough-grained and moderate-grained US elastography color pattern similar to the surrounding tissues in all types of gynecomastia.
- Average shear wave velocity 2.4 m/s with ARFI/VTQ and average strain ratio in different areas do not differ from those in normal breast tissues.
- Sometimes gynecomastia is accompanied by enlarged lymph nodes.

According to Sencha et al. (2015), in nodular gynecomastia, US detects a mass over 0.5 cm in size of irregular shape (in 74.6% of cases); hypoechoic, with heterogenous structure (anechoic component shows in 59.7% of patients) with indistinct contours; and hypovascular at

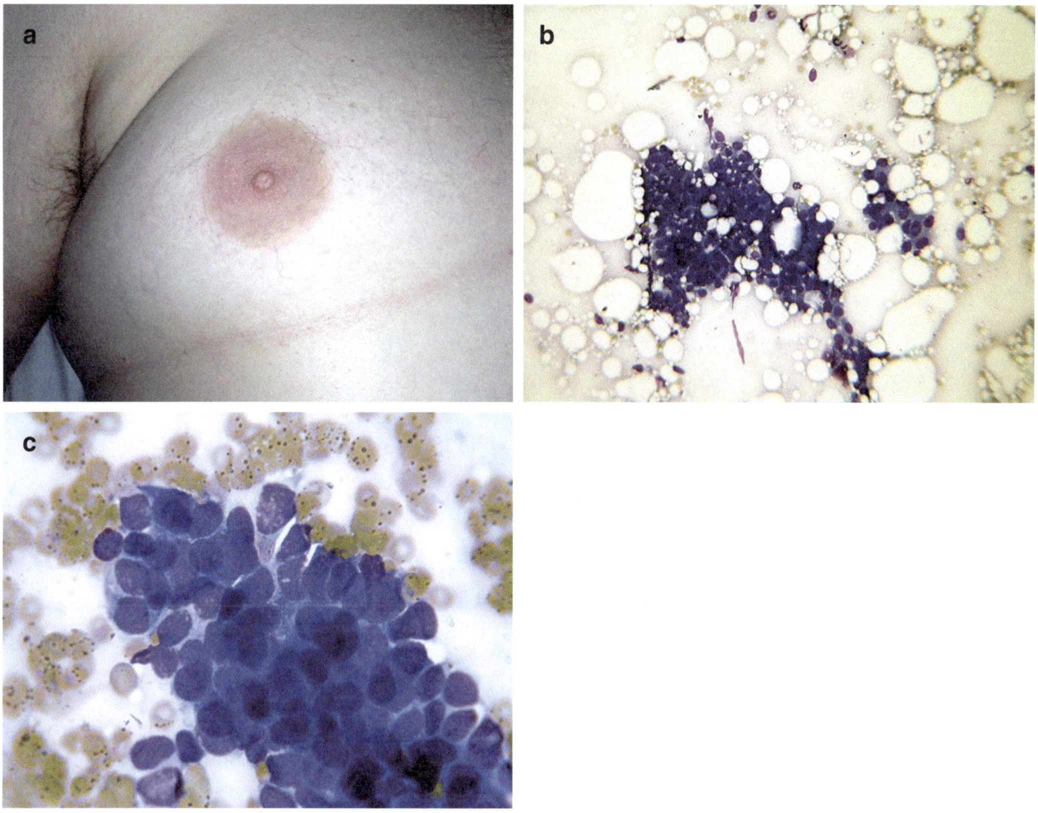

Fig. 9.17 Nodular gynecomastia. (**a**) Breast view. (**b**) Pappenheim-stained image; original magnification, ×200. (**c**) Pappenheim-stained image; original magnification, ×1000

CDI, PDI, and 3DPD (68.4%); rough-grained or moderate-grained compression US elastography color pattern is heterogenous and hardly distinguished from the surrounding glandular parenchyma; average shear wave velocity is 2.4 m/s with ARFI (virtual touch tissue quantification).

The treelike type of gynecomastia, according to Sencha et al. (2015), was revealed in 32.3% of patients. US defined wide dense fibrous linear structures in some breast areas (most often retroareolar) with heterogeneous echostructure (anechoic component was observed in 11.5% of cases), avascular with CDI, PDI, and 3DPD (Fig. 9.19).

Diffuse type of gynecomastia was registered in 53.7% of all men with gynecomastia. At echography, it is more often seen as diffuse changes throughout the structure of the breast, without solid and cystic lesions, avascular with CDI, PDI, and 3DPD (Fig. 9.20).

False gynecomastia exhibits only excess fibroadipose tissue in the breast. Grayscale US reveals hypoechoic breast structure with echoic linear inclusions of connective tissue. Fat forms round hypoechoic spots organized in rows or layers, similar to involutive breast in women. Echoic capsules cover the spots of adipose tissue and form adipose lobes. Sometimes symmetric lateral acoustic shadows may be defined on each side of the adipose lobe. These artifacts completely disappear, when the tissues are compressed with an US probe. The entire breast in false gynecomastia consists of adipose tissue, which is avascular at CDI, PDI, and 3DPD.

Another echographic pattern of gynecomastia is hyperechoic zone with well-contoured filiform hypoechoic ducts, oriented toward the nipple. Often the structure of the tissue (fat lobules) in male breast in moderately expressed gynecomastia does not differ from normal breast tissue.

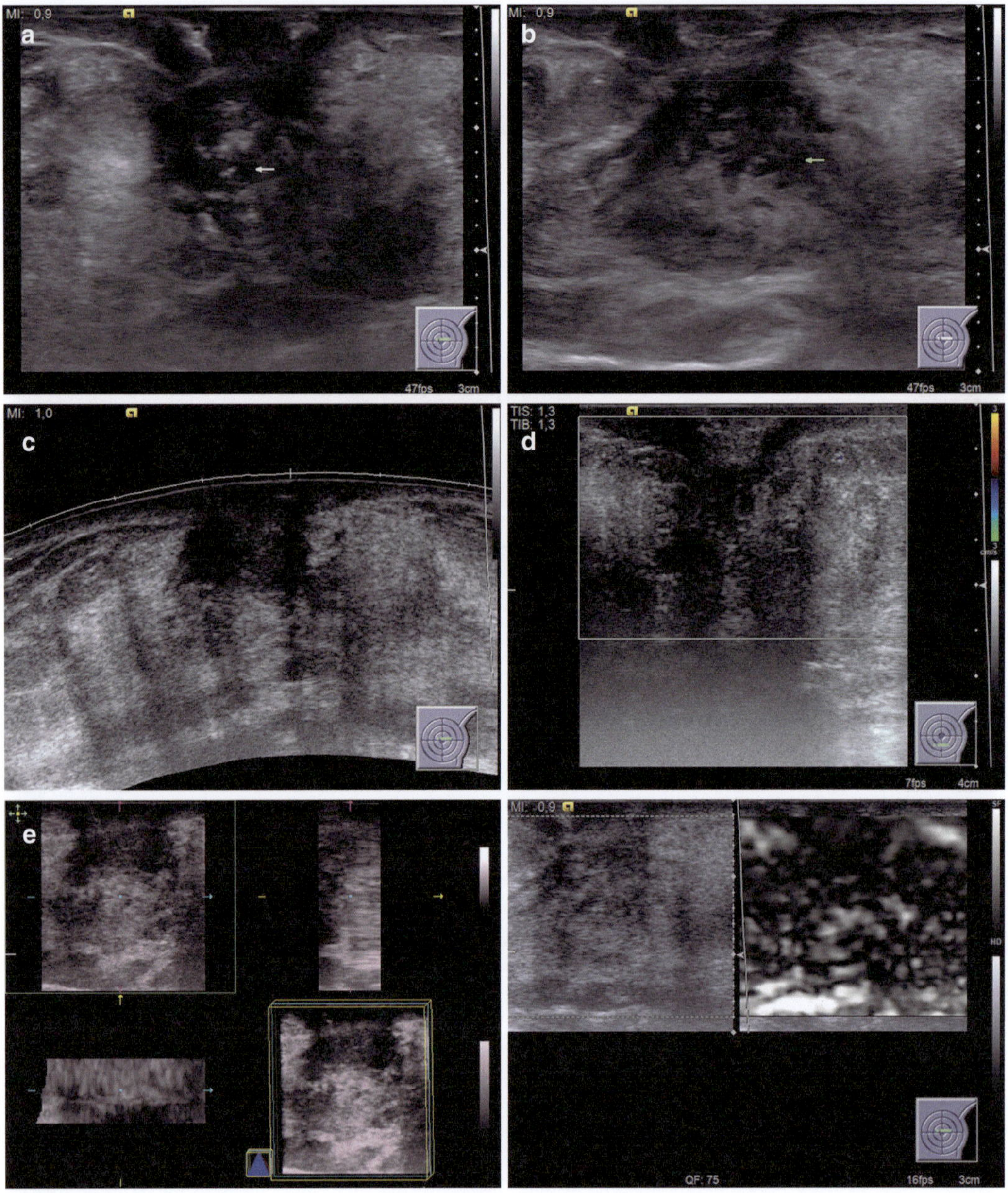

Fig. 9.18 Nodular gynecomastia. (**a**) 1–2 Grayscale. (**b**) Panoramic scan. (**c**) CDI. (**d**) 3D US. (**e**) Compression US elastography

It is rather difficult to differentiate the nodular form of gynecomastia and the breast cancer. Differentiation is provided with the use of contrast agents. In gynecomastia, it reveals only insignificant vascularization (Fig. 9.21) (Sencha et al. 2015 and Kotlyarov et al. 2015). In most cases (60%) on nodular form of gynecomastia, no contrast enhancement appears in the lesion. A peripheral contrast enhancement in nodular gynecomastia is observed less often (40% of patients). It does not contradict the benign nature of the process and is confirmed by histological study.

Gynecomastia develops in three clinical stages: acute, intermediate, and chronic.

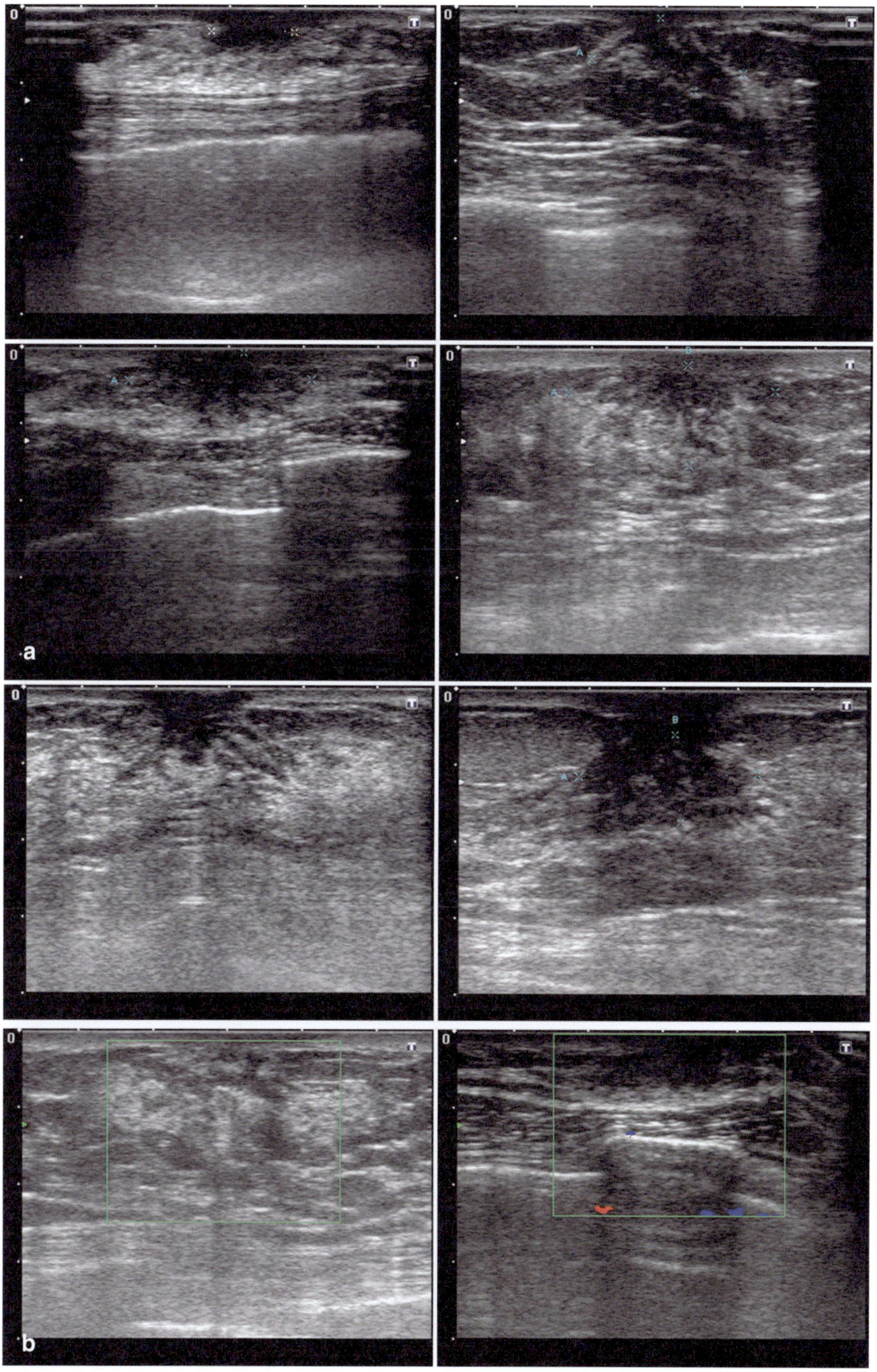

Fig. 9.19 Treelike gynecomastia. (**a**) 1–6 Grayscale US. (**b**) 1–2 CDI

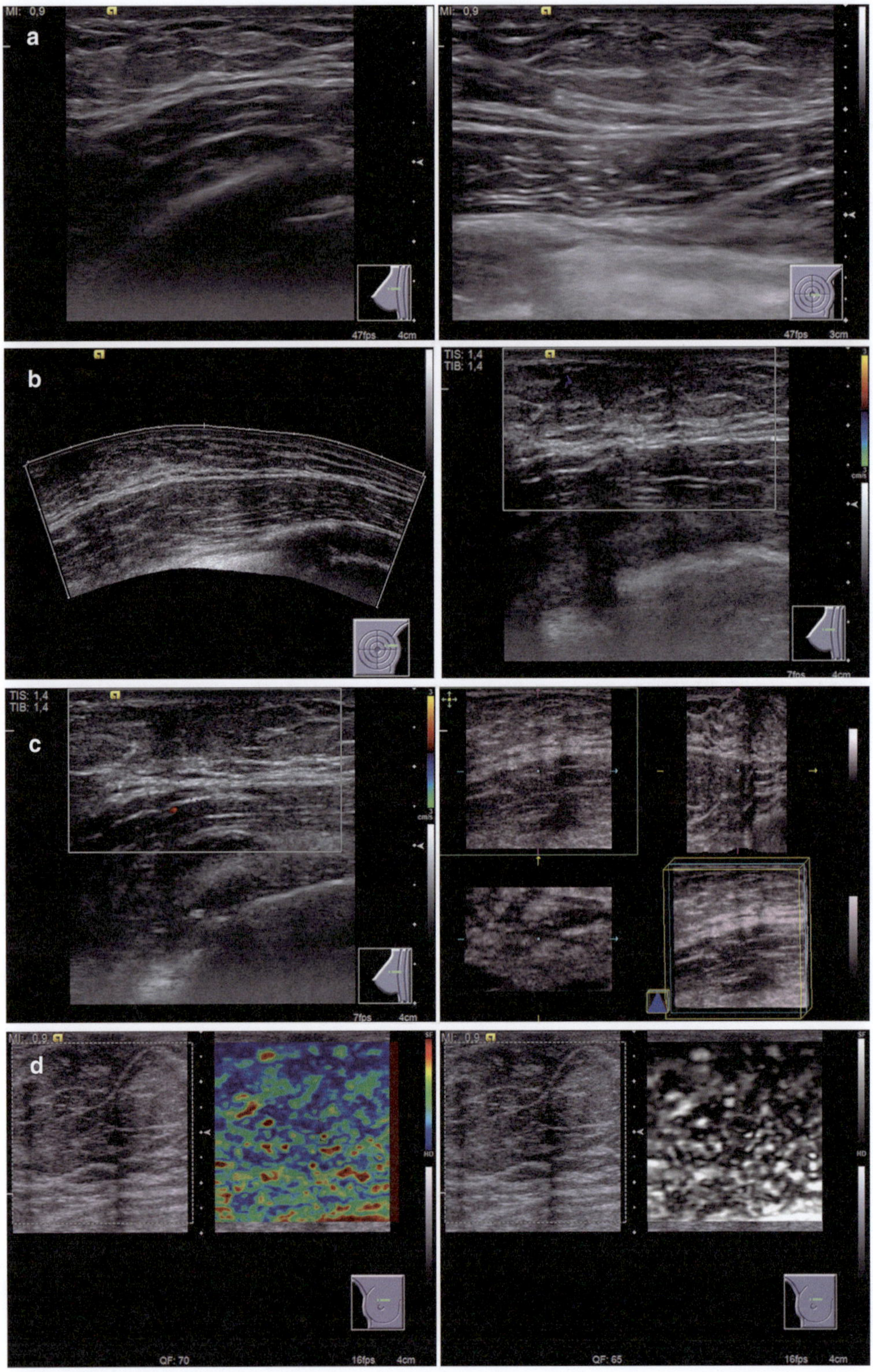

Fig. 9.20 Diffuse glandular gynecomastia. (**a**) 1–2 Grayscale. (**b**) Panoramic scan. (**c**) 1–2 CDI. (**d**) 3D US. (**e**) 1–2 US elastography

Acute, or active, phase of gynecomastia is a consequence of proliferation and hyperplasia of ductal epithelium and myoepithelial tissue. US shows that normal adipose tissue of rudimentary gland under the nipple is substituted by hypoechoic field with rough indistinct contours (Fig. 9.22). The layer of fat is deformed. Such a picture can be similar to a malignant tumor. CDI is not effective in this case, due to low specificity, as the increased vascularization may be of inflammatory origin. Usually vascularization in the area of gynecomastia is scanty; there are 1–2 small twisty vessels in the lesion. At pulsed wave Doppler, monotonous venous blood flow is registered in more than 75% of cases. Arterial blood flow is more often detected in young men and declines with age. True gynecomastia is characterized with high resistance (RI > 0.6) and low velocity (PSV < 10 cm/s) of arterial blood flow. Doppler indicators (the zones of vascular pattern enhancement, of intra- and perinodular vessels) do not correlate with the extent of the disease and the proliferative nodular activity. Differential diagnosis with other nodular breast pathology should not be based only on quantitative Doppler data.

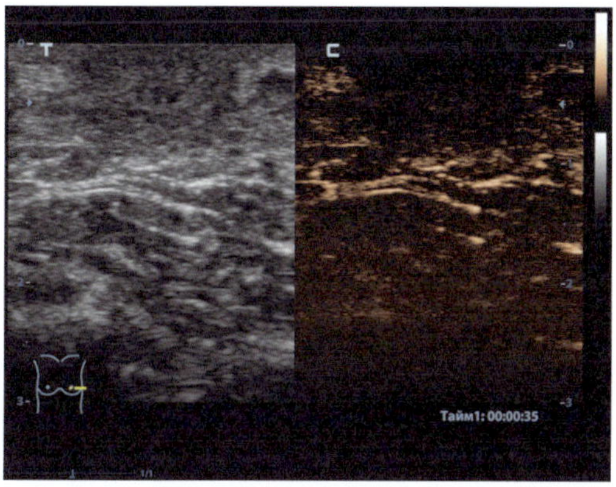

Fig. 9.21 Nodular gynecomastia. Contrast-enhanced US. SonoVue, 2.4 ml. No enhancement in the area of gynecomastia

Intermediate (mixed, transitional) **phase** is histologically characterized with proliferation of ductal epithelium together with moderate fibrosis around the ducts. US reveals hypoechoic area under the nipple and an echoic field of glandular tissue, which is identical to the US image of normal female breast. It is possible to specify subareolar ducts and their branches. Such pattern can be accompanied with posterior shadowing of random character depending on the position of US probe and scan angle. This shadow pattern is different from a shadow behind a malignant tumor (Fig. 9.23).

In the chronic phase, dense fibrous tissue deposits appear around the ducts. US image is similar to the picture of normal female breast. Glandular tissues, less often subareolar ducts and their branches, are well defined (Fig. 9.24).

Fibrosis, which is defined clinically and sonographically, is the principal cause for low probability of gynecomastia involution, if its volume exceeds 70 cm^3 and the disease lasts for more than 1.5 years. Retrospective assessment of the results of histological examinations showed that

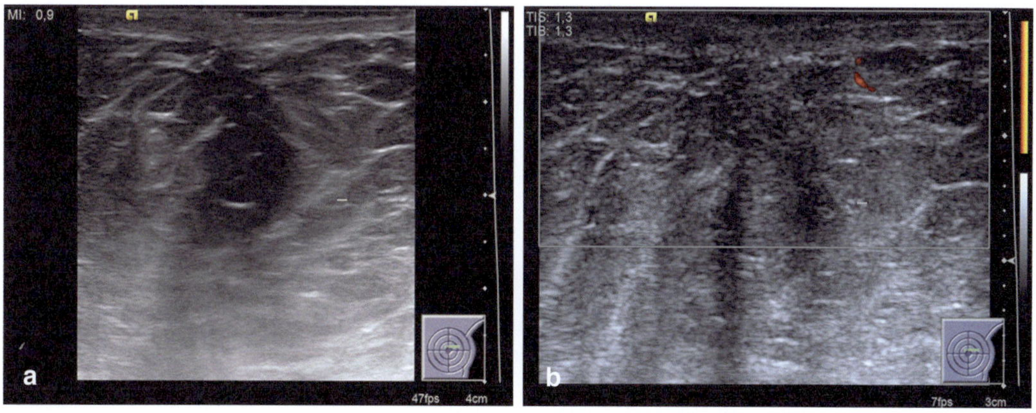

Fig. 9.22 Diffuse glandular gynecomastia. Active phase. (**a**) Grayscale. (**b**) PDI

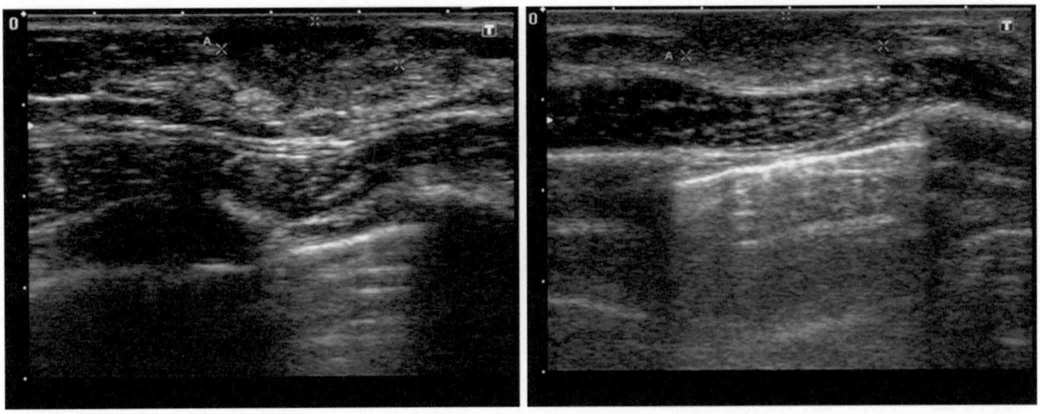

Fig. 9.23 1–2 Diffuse glandular gynecomastia. Intermediate phase. Grayscale US

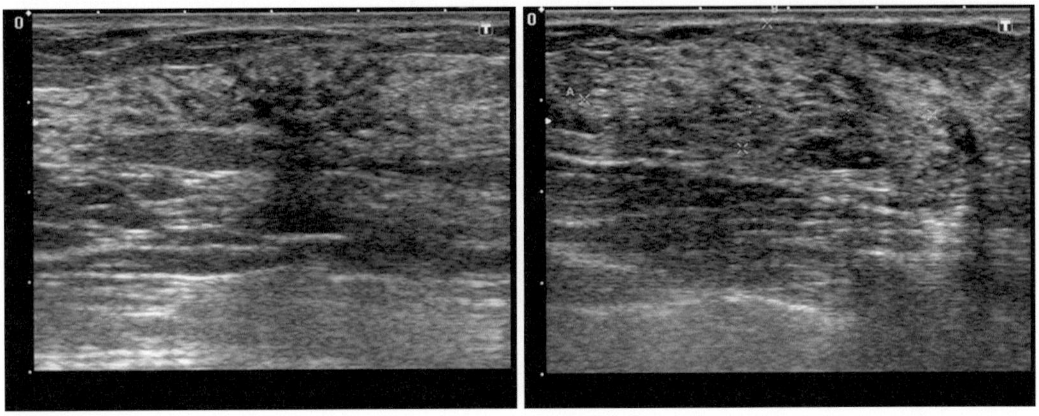

Fig. 9.24 1–2 Diffuse glandular gynecomastia. Chronic phase. Grayscale US

full involution is possible in minor gynecomastia, absence of fibrosis, and short duration of the disease. Partial involution is possible with reduction of the intramammary fat in diffuse and mixed types. Involution of focal gynecomastia is doubtful.

US techniques are highly efficient in differentiation of the density of breast parenchyma and specification of breast lesions in men with gynecomastia. Sensitivity of US for gynecomastia is 86% with specificity of 82% (Sencha et al. 2015).

Dynamic follow-up with breast examinations every half a year is indicated in cases of pubertal gynecomastia with no signs of endocrine or somatic pathology and the lesion not exceeding the diameter of the areola. In cases of gynecomastia larger than the diameter of areola, and/or if gynecomastia arises prior to puberty with no associated endocrine or other pathology, the basic examination should be carried out, including routine blood and urine tests, blood biochemistry, and hormonal profile. If clinical or laboratory signs of endocrine and/or other pathology arise, further radiological examination should be carried out.

An example of US report of a patient with gynecomastia

Name, surname. __S__ Age__33__

Outpatient examination. Date____

Patient's record____

US scanner____

The breasts are of masculine type, mainly presented with adipose tissue, slightly asymmetric in size and shape.

Fibrous tissue is moderately expressed in all regions. A heterogeneous hypoechoic area of

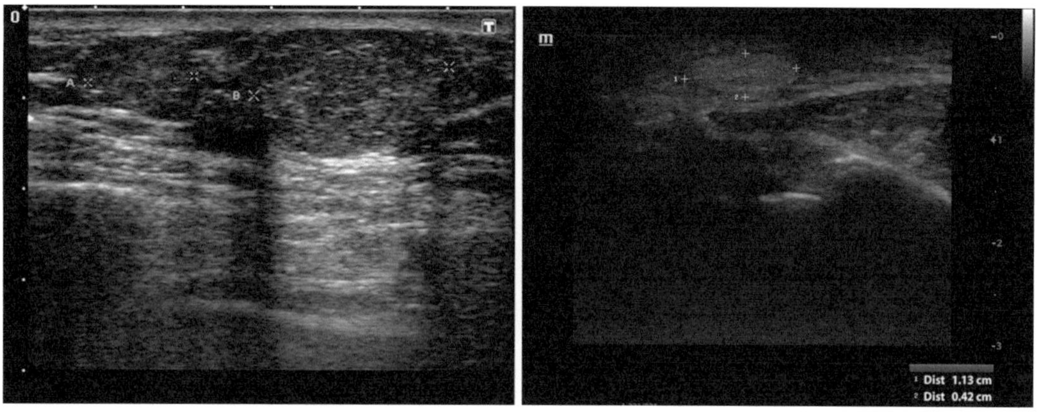

Fig. 9.25 1–2 Male breast lipoma. Grayscale US

12 × 15 mm in size with irregular indistinct margins, avascular at CDI and PDI, irregular at compression US elastography, and moderately painful under compression is detected in retroareolar area of the left breast. The average shear wave velocity with ARFI within the described area is 2.5 m/s. The average strain ratio is 1.3.

Lactiferous ducts are not revealed.

Axillary, supraclavicular, subclavian, and parasternal lymph nodes on both sides are not visualized.

Conclusion: US suggests acute phase of nodular gynecomastia in the left breast.

9.5.2 Benign Breast Pathology in Men

Palpable benign breast masses in men may be represented with tumors (lipoma, fibroadenoma, atheroma, schwannoma, angiolipoma, intraductal papilloma, cyst) or inflammatory lesions (mastitis, subareolar sepsis, abscess, posttraumatic hematoma, adipose necrosis, tuberculosis, syphilis, intramammary lymph nodes, etc.). Newborn boys may develop galactocele. Benign breast tumors in men are rare. They confer about 4.6% of all male breast diseases.

The principal diagnostic feature is detection of a mass within the breast.

Lipoma is a benign tumor originating from adipose tissue. Lipomas and fibroadenomas account for 4.6% of all breast lesions in men. Lipomas in the rudimentary breast of a man can be solitary or multiple. True lipoma consists of mature adipose tissue surrounded with a capsule. It is palpated as a mobile soft lesion of round or oval shape.

As a rule, US diagnosis of breast lipoma is not difficult. US features of lipomas in men are the same as in women.

Lipomas exhibit the following typical sonographic features (Fig. 9.25):

- Moderate echogenicity, comparable to normal adipose tissue.
- Round or oval shape.
- Clearly outlined contours, even borders.
- No dorsal echo amplification or attenuation.
- Sometimes irregular structure (because of fibrous inclusions).
- Easily deformed with compression.
- Always avascular at CDI, PDI, and 3DPD.
- Poorly colored, rather homogenous at compression US elastography.
- Average shear wave velocity with ARFI is 1.9 m/sec; strain ratio is 1.1–1.2 compared to normal surrounding tissues.

Lipoma should be differentiated from liposarcoma. The latter exhibits faster growth, relatively lower echoity, and more density at palpation and pathological vascularization at CDI, PDI, and 3DPD. Biopsy will verify the diagnosis. Morphological confirmation is the decisive factor in diagnosis.

Epidermal cyst (atheroma or seborrheic cyst) is the third in the list of the most common benign lesions of male breast. Most often these cysts arise as a result of occlusion of hair follicles, skin damage, traumas, surgeries, or bites of insects.

US may reveal a hypoechoic lesion of round or irregular shape adjacent to the skin (Fig. 9.26).

True breast cysts in men are rare. Their etiology in men is the same as in women. Cysts may be palpated as single or multiple soft, dense elastic, and easily displaced masses, often painful. US image of cysts is similar in men and women. As a rule, on the background of fatty adipose tissues of male breast, it is possible to clearly differentiate the entire cystic wall. If the cyst is accompanied by inflammation or gynecomastia, part of the cyst contour is not visualized, and therefore there are significant difficulties in differentiation with malignant processes.

Breast cysts exhibit the following US features (Fig. 9.27):

- Anechoic structure
- Predominantly homogenous echostructure
- Round or oval shape
- Easily compressed
- No reflection from the internal content
- Distal echo amplification
- Distinct differentiation of outer and inner contours
- Avascularity at CDI and PDI
- Absence of color pattern at compression US elastography

Up to 95% of breast cysts in men as well as in women have no solid component on the capsule (Korzhenkova 2004). Such cysts are characterized as simple or typical and uncomplicated.

The cysts may be single, multiple (more often), unilateral, bilateral, simple, and com-

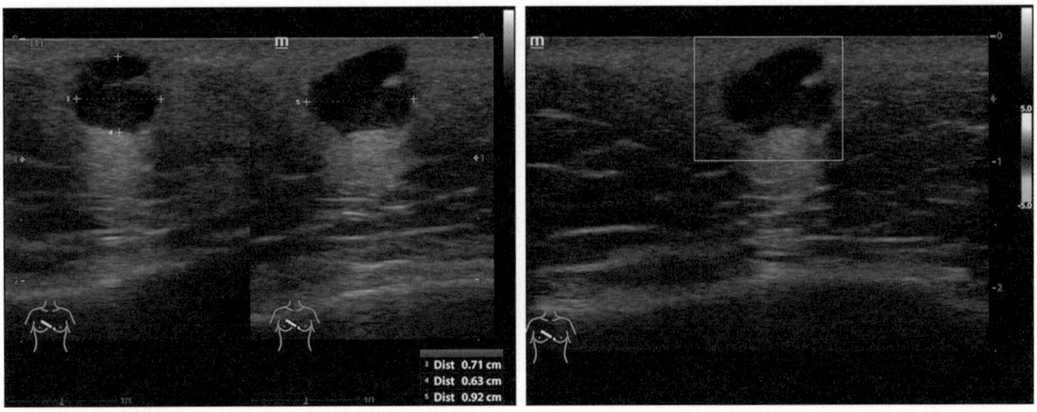

Fig. 9.26 Epidermal breast cyst. (a) Grayscale US. (b) CDI

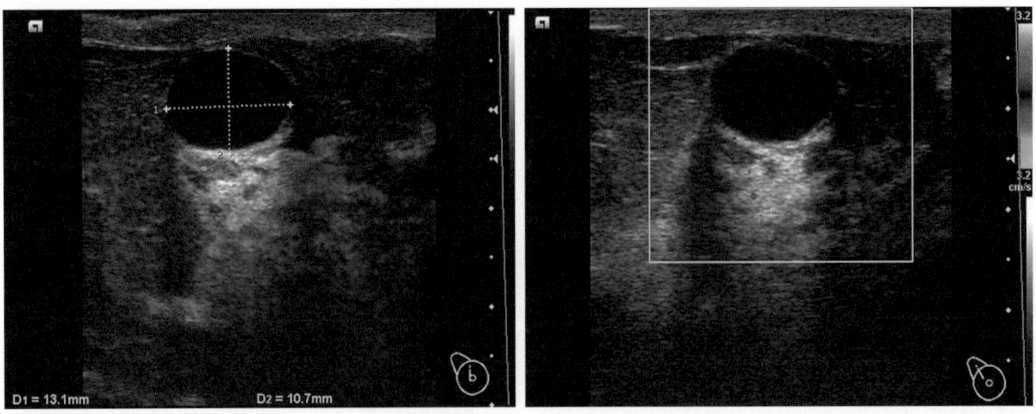

Fig. 9.27 Simple breast cyst in a man. (**a**) Grayscale US. (**b**) CDI

plex. Only US allows 100% diagnosis. Breast microcysts (with the size of 1–2 mm) and macrocysts (simple and multilocular) may occur.

Breast cysts in some cases can show no characteristic posterior echo amplification. This often happens in smaller cysts, the cysts surrounded by dense structures located near the thorax, or in cysts with expressed fibrous capsule.

Atypical cysts may be sometimes noted in men. These are often long-existing, recurrent cysts or cysts with inflammation.

US features of atypical cysts are as follows (Fig. 9.28):

- Thick walls
- Contents with inclusions
- Solid component with different types of vascularization
- Coloring of the walls (especially posterior) and solid component at compression US elastography

Complex cysts are more often of malignant nature (papillary cancer) in men than in women. Atypical US image of a cyst may be due to intracavitary lesions. Any growths along the inner surface of the cystic wall together with vascularization demand a targeted US-guided puncture followed by a cytologic examination and are an indication for breast resection with an urgent histological examination.

Intraductal papilloma (intraductal diffuse papillomatosis) is a benign intraductal epithelial proliferation appearing as a solid lesion that grows within the lumen of a lactiferous duct. This lesion may be solitary or multiple.

Papillomas are often characterized with the following US features (Fig. 9.29):

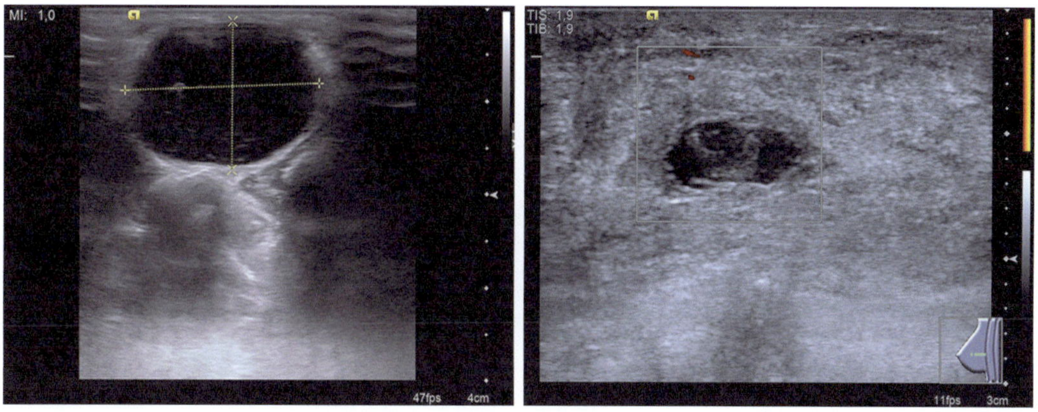

Fig. 9.28 Complex breast cyst in a man. (**a**) Grayscale US. (**b**) PDI

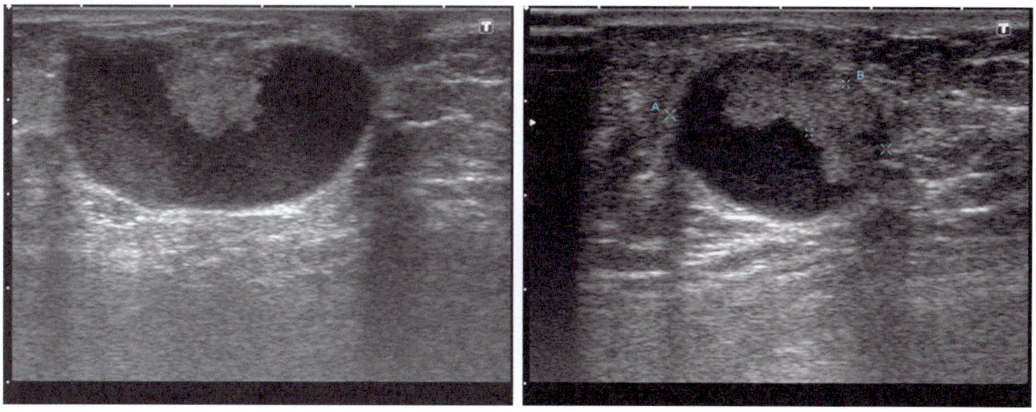

Fig. 9.29 (**a**) Intraductal papilloma in a man. Grayscale US image. (**b**) Cystadenopapilloma in a man. Grayscale US

- Solid papillary structures in the lumen.
- Iso- or hyperechoic, lobular structures with rough borders surrounded by the cystic contents. Ductal papillomas of distal ducts (more than 3 cm from the nipple), accompanied by atypical epithelial hyperplasia (according to FNA with cytology), are always suspicious of ductal cancer (noninvasive or invasive).
- Hypo- or hypervascularization of the solid component, parietal decay, intracystic outgrowths.
- Coloring of the cystic walls (especially, posterior) and of the solid component at compression US elastography.

Fibroadenomas are benign tumors and occur extremely rare in men. Unlike fibroadenomas in women, fibroadenomas in men seldom grow larger than 2 cm.

Fibroadenomas in men usually demonstrate the following US features:

- Solid breast lesion of decreased echogenicity
- Small size (more often)
- Homogenous structure
- Round or oval shape
- Distinct even borders
- A- or hypovascular at CDI and PDI
- Irregular mosaic coloring at compression US elastography different from the surrounding structures

The tumor grows slowly for several years and compresses the surrounding tissues. Hence, it is often possible to define the capsule of the lesion.

Atheroma in men as well as in women is a retention cyst of the skin sebaceous gland, but in some cases it has both clinical and ultrasound signs of a benign breast tumor. Atheroma is characterized with bulging of the overlying skin. At the border of the fusion of the skin layer with the mass, sharp corners are formed. This symptom is definitive for atheroma. In the process of slow growth, the lesion causes pressure on the surrounding tissue. It leads to appearance of the specific rim of "safety" around it.

Atheroma exhibits the following US features in men (Fig. 9.30):

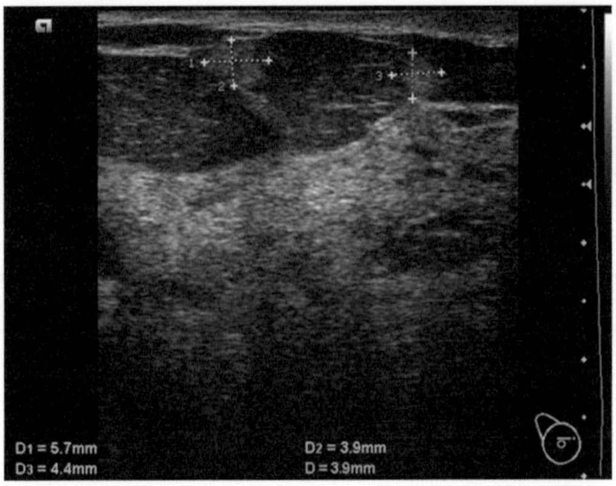

Fig. 9.30 Breast atheromas in a man. Grayscale US

- Superficial lesion.
- Echogenicity, comparable to adipose tissue, more often moderate.
- Various sizes.
- Round shape.
- Distinct even contours.
- Homogenous or heterogenous structure (dependent on fibrous inclusions).
- Avascular at CDI, PDI, and 3DPD.
- Absence of color pattern within the lesion at compression US elastography.
- Average shear wave velocity with ARFI is 1.6 m/sec; strain ratio is 1.1–1.2 compared to normal surrounding tissues.

Benign breast lesions in men should be differentiated from a large group of inflammatory, posttraumatic changes, malignant tumors, and other masses. A wide range of ultrasound technologies and their efficient and consistent use allow timely diagnosis.

9.5.3 Breast Inflammatory Conditions

Nonspecific inflammatory condition (mastitis) in male breast is registered significantly less often than in women. It is the rarest condition (2.6%) among all benign breast diseases in men.

Clinically, the inflammation process has no obvious signs. Examination and local symptoms do not ensure the correct diagnosis. In most cases it is necessary to wait and observe, and such follow-up will provide differential diagnosis and the choice of rational therapy.

As a rule, inflammation appears in young and active men, who may have had trauma of the breast or the anterior thorax, right prior to the onset of the first symptoms.

Practically all cases show with the nipple retraction, local skin edema (with hyperemia in some cases), and enlargement of regional lymph nodes. Often the man feels sick and has abnormal laboratory tests.

The inflammation can be acute or chronic, local, or diffuse. Acute mastitis develops in the following stages: serous inflammation, infiltration, and abscess.

Mastitis in men has the following US features (Fig. 9.31):

- Thickening of the skin over the area of inflammation (compared to the healthy parts and the other breast)
- Increase in echogenicity of subcutaneous fat
- Decreased structural differentiation of parenchymal elements
- Hypoechoic areas of disrupted parenchyma with distinct or indistinct margins within the breast
- Indistinct border between the deep layer of derma and adjacent structures (cellular or glandular tissue)
- Hardening of connective tissue components
- One or several cystic cavities
- Enlargement of axillary lymph nodes

US features directly correlate with clinical symptoms. Acute mastitis exhibits acute onset with severe pain; local edema and hyperemia of the skin, usually in the central part; dense infiltration; fever; and local hyperthermia. With progression of the inflammatory process, serious impregnation is followed by diffuse purulent infiltration of the breast parenchyma and subsequent abscess formation.

Abscessing mastitis, particularly, subareolar mastitis in male breast, is characterized by formation of a local abscess. Sonographically, it shows as a mass of heterogeneous structure due to anechoic necrotic foci and echogenic detritus, which is accurately delineated with echogenic pseudocapsule (Fig. 9.32). Most of abscesses have hypoechoic or anechoic structure. At CDI and PDI, it is often surrounded with a zone of increased vascularity.

The vessels at acute mastitis, as a rule, are shown properly located at PDI. The vessels gradually decrease in diameter and have no lacunar dilatations or protrusions of the walls.

Breast tuberculosis is registered quite seldom and mainly affects women. Men make about 4% of all patients with breast tuberculosis. Nodular, fistulous, ulcerative, and sclerosing types of breast tuberculosis are specified. Nodular type is characterized by dense painful nodules, which merge and form an infiltration, and by the retracted nipple. Axillary lymph nodes are enlarged and dense. Further development of granulomas leads to their destruction, with chronic fistulas and purulent discharge. Ulcerations of the

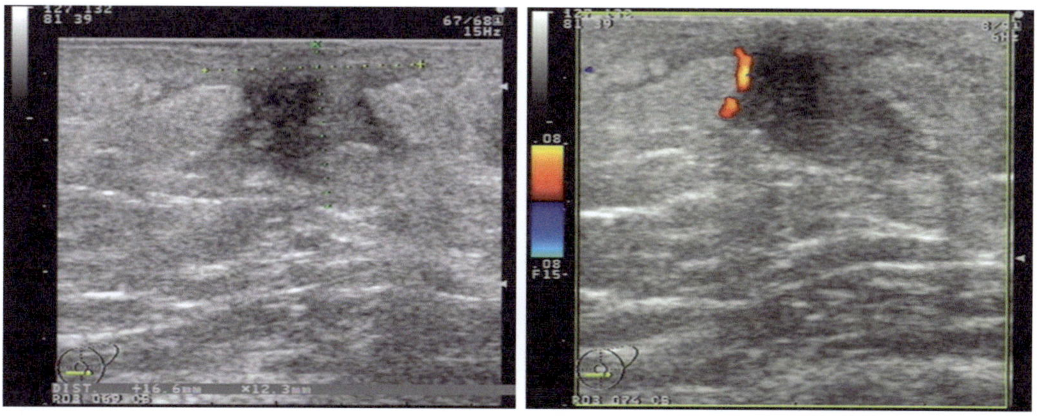

Fig. 9.31 Mastitis in a man. (a) Grayscale US. (b) CDI

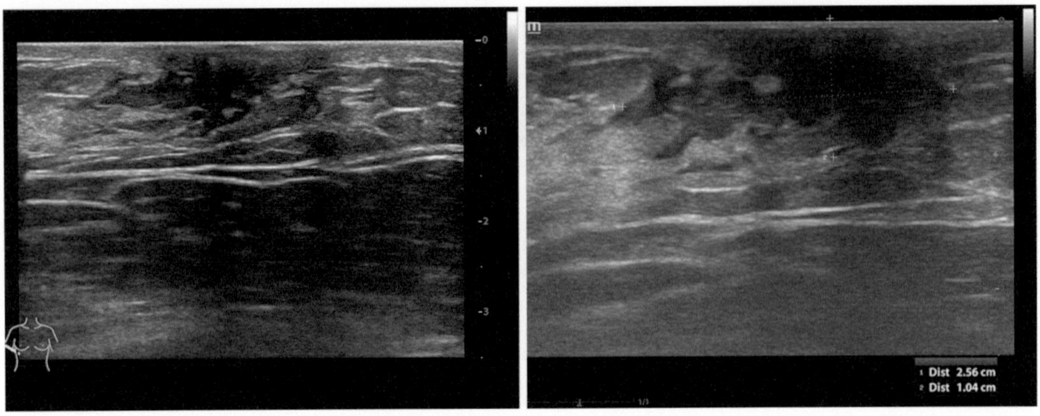

Fig. 9.32 1–2 Subareolar infiltrate, developing breast abscess. Grayscale US

skin over the infiltrations have rough thick edges and poor granulations at the bottom. The ulcers in the nipple and areolar area are similar to Paget's disease. The diagnosis of tuberculosis is based on the history, the results of tuberculin tests, as well as cytological and histological examinations. A combination of tuberculosis and breast cancer with involvement of axillary lymph nodes is possible in men. Differential diagnosis of these diseases is difficult, as in the current context, breast tuberculosis more often has a solitary character. Such comorbidity suggests hematogenous spread from the old foci of tuberculosis.

Puncture biopsy and subsequent cytological examination of the punctate are of great importance in the morphological diagnosis and differential diagnosis of inflammatory processes in male breast. Core needle biopsy is often impossible in case of severe inflammation and uninformative in diffuse breast cancer.

9.5.4 Posttraumatic Changes within Breast

Traumatic injuries and posttraumatic changes (contusions, hematomas) in the breast in men are more common than in women and account for 1–2% of all breast pathologies. They can be closed or open, isolated or combined. Closed injuries include bruises and hematomas of the breast. Open injuries confer cut, stab, gunshot, and bitten wounds. Breast tissues are resistant to direct injuries, but due to good innervation of the body, bruises may be accompanied by traumatic shock, especially if the lesion occurs in the paraareolar or nipple area.

In mild breast contusions, bleeding usually stops spontaneously. Echography shows only a slight swelling of soft tissues of the muscular-aponeurotic layer (Fig. 9.33). Extensive traumas can be combined with injuries of the chest—bruises, broken ribs and sternum, pneumothorax, and hemothorax. Any breast injury can be complicated by bleeding and suppuration. The trauma affects the integrity of the vessels and leads to an obscure hemorrhage.

US is most valuable in breast trauma in men (as well as in women) associated with hemorrhage and breast hematomas. Hematomas require special attention, as these may be a marker or the first clinical manifestation of a malignant tumor, considering the process of neoangiogenesis (tumor vessels do not have a muscular wall; they are fragile and easily damaged).

During the first few days and weeks, hematoma is detected with US as a lesion with the following features (Fig. 9.34):

- Anechoic mass in the breast
- As a rule, located superficially, often retroareolarly
- Usually of round and regular shape, less often of irregular shape
- Avascular at CDI and PDI
- Seldom colored at compression US elastography

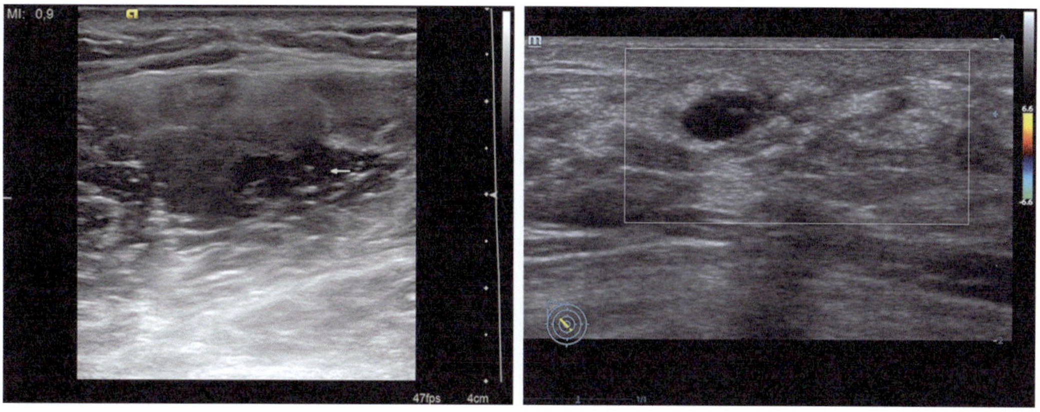

Fig. 9.33 Breast bruise, soft tissues edema. (**a**) Grayscale US. (**b**) CDI

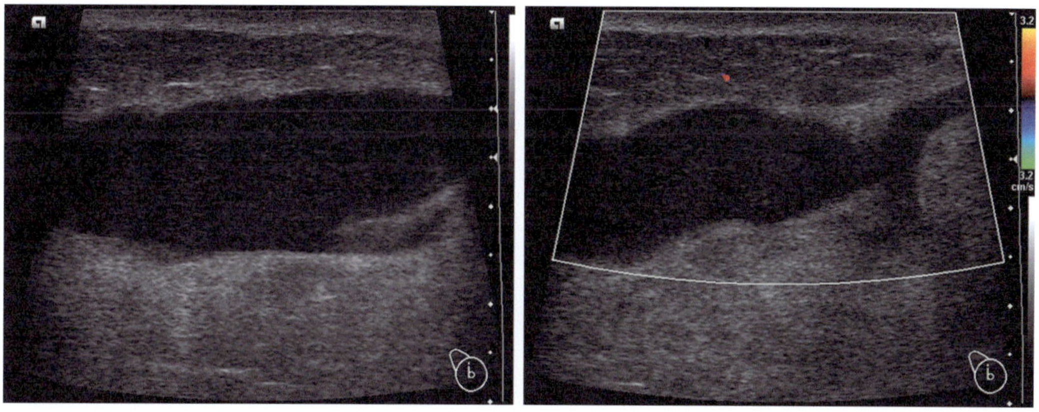

Fig. 9.34 Posttraumatic breast hematoma in a man. (**a**) Grayscale US. (**b**) CDI

Hematoma in men sometimes (less often, than in women) results in oleogranuloma or necrosis. Echographically, adiponecrosis in men (as well as in women) is defined as hypoechoic or hyperechoic irregular areas without distinct contours or, conversely, clearly shaped, often with or without posterior acoustic shadow (Fig. 9.35). Disorganization of the architectonics of the surrounding tissues, and with time, calcifications may occur in oleogranulomas. Past trauma or surgery in the history, specific ultrasound signs, and absence of malignant features at ultrasonography allow to diagnose oleogranuloma, ruling out the breast cancer relapse in the scar.

Cytological examination of the punctate contributes to correct diagnosis. In the most questionable cases, surgical intervention with diagnostic and therapeutic purposes should be considered.

9.5.5 Male Breast Cancer: Capabilities of Multiparametric Ultrasound

Breast cancer in men is a rare disease. With an incidence of 1 per 100,000, it occurs approximately 100 times less than in women. Of all malignant tumors developing in men, breast cancer is 0.2–1.5%. Attention to breast cancer in men is increasing due to growing prevalence of this disease.

There is evidence that the incidence is slightly higher in black men than among white, regardless of the age: the prevalence of the disease among white men is 1.1 cases per 100,000 population, whereas among the black is 1.8 cases per 100,000. On the contrary, morbidity

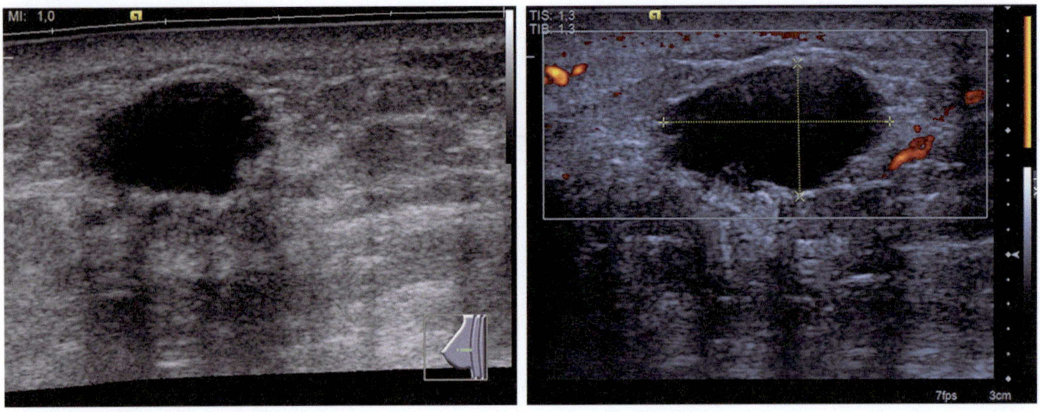

Fig. 9.35 Posttraumatic oleogranuloma in a man. (**a**) Grayscale US. (**b**) PDI

rate among black women is lower than that in white women excluding those younger than 40 years old.

The majority of publications on breast cancer in men are based on relatively scarce clinical material. Very few deal with more than 100 observations.

Until present, the mechanisms of male breast cancer development remain unclear. The major risk factors are as follows:

- Age—the sixth and the seventh decades of life
- Absolute or relative increase of estrogens levels, diseases of male reproductive system (tumoral or non-tumoral), adrenal tumors
- Hypogonadism or Klinefelter's syndrome
- Hermaphroditism
- Gynecomastia
- Long hormonal treatment with female hormones
- Chronic liver diseases
- Family history of male breast cancer (in father or brothers)
- Breast exposure to radiation at young age
- Breast traumas
- Presence of female sex chromatin and 47 chromosomes sets due to extra X chromosome

The most frequent risk factors for breast cancer in men are obesity grade II–III (46%), prostatic diseases (28%), testicular pathology (11%), and family history (8%).

Six percent to thirty percent of patients link the onset of breast cancer with trauma. Some researchers believe that the breast traumas lead or contribute to cancer development, while the others argue that there is no relationship. Single or repeated trauma can induce hemorrhage leading to enlargement of the breast. After a while, in some cases of trauma, fat necrosis and fibrosis may develop, which are sometimes difficult to distinguish from a tumor.

The family history of breast cancer is noted in 7–27% of cases (closest relatives). About 10% of men with breast cancer are genetically predisposed. Breast cancer may be associated with true hermaphroditism.

There are few genetic studies devoted to correlations of BRCA genes with the incidence of breast carcinoma in men. At present, one of the most important morphological factors in male breast cancer is the expression of Her2/neu and Ki-67, as the course of the disease is similar to that in women but more aggressive.

Breast cancer in men in most cases (81%) occurs on the normal background. Less often (9–30%), elements of gynecomastia can be observed along with breast cancer.

As well as in women, the risk of breast cancer development in men increases with age. The disease can occur at any age. According to Sencha (2015), the average age of patients with breast cancer is 65.8 ± 8.6 years. The average age of men who died from breast cancer was 74.3 years.

Male breast cancer is usually unilateral. Bilateral synchronous or metachronous lesions develop only in 5% of cases. Analysis of publications of 1927–1971 demonstrated that bilateral cancer was registered in 1.4% of men. Later publications reported higher incidence (up to 12%).

Malignant breast neoplasms often exhibit eccentric location around the areola that distinguishes them from benign lesions. Location of the tumor behind the nipple results in nipple retraction. Fixed skin over the tumor is observed in 1/3 of cases of breast cancer in men. If the tumor invades retromammary space, it becomes adherent to the large pectoralis muscle. The majority of breast pathologies in men initially develop from rudimentary lactiferous ducts, which are mainly located behind the nipple. Hence, the pathological process, whatever it is, a cancer or a nodular gynecomastia, is more often localized in retroareolar area. Eccentric localization is possible in both diseases, however, is more often observed in breast cancer than in gynecomastia with the ratio 4:1.

The average duration of the disease history in men is 6–18 months. Breast cancer in men is usually asymptomatic. Usually, the first event in the disease history is detection of the tumor by the patient himself (44.2%). The most frequent sign of this disease is retraction of the nipple—64.3% of cases. The other early symptoms (pain, skin ulceration, breast deformation, discharge from the nipple, etc.) are much less frequent. In 30% of cases, there is a thickening of the skin, its retraction, and ulceration. In 10% of cases, bloody discharge from the nipple is detected. Due to the small volume of the parenchyma of male breast and its proximity to the skin, the appearance of the tumor can be defined already at early stages (Fig. 9.36). Fifty-three percent of men with primary treatment for breast cancer are initially diagnosed with stage II; 46.8% of these patients have locally advanced disease.

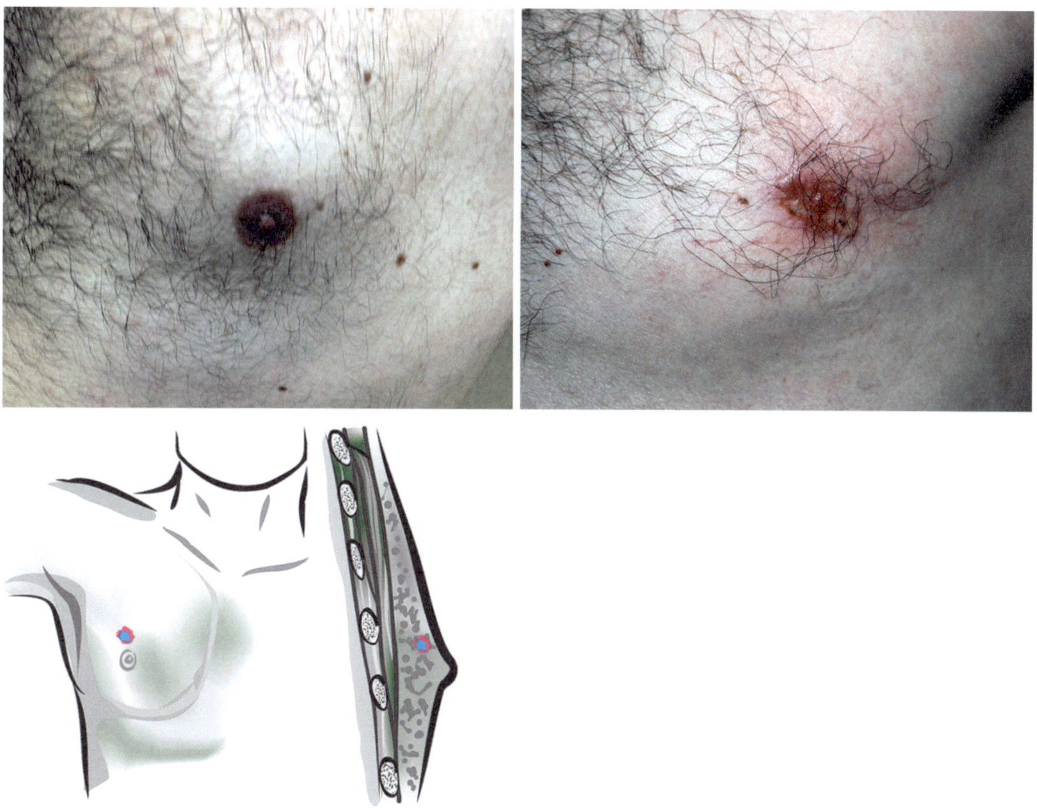

Fig. 9.36 Male breast cancer. Breast view. (**a**) 1–2 Photo. (**b**) Scheme

Despite the characteristic clinical picture, only 1/3 of men with breast cancer address to a doctor within 1 month after positive X-ray mammography, while the majority do not visit a doctor for many months and sometimes for years. Twenty-one percent of patients address a doctor with a breast ulcer. By now, the terms of first appointment have significantly decreased (from 14–21 to 1–8 months). However, neglected cases of breast cancer in men are associated not only with the patients' neglect to their health but also with low oncologic alertness of health practitioners. Approximately in 20% of cases, the diagnosis of breast cancer in men is not established at the first visit to a doctor.

The main complaints and clinical manifestations in men with breast cancer are as follows (Sencha et al. 2015): a mass at the echogram (81.5%), eccentrical localization (69.7%), discomfort in the breast (69.7%), deformation of the breast (nipple-areolar region) (65.6%), retraction of the nipple (64.75%), pain (34.4%), thickening and/or ulceration of the skin (34.4%), swelling (34.4%), discharge from the nipple (19.7%), masses in the axillary region (48.3%), and absence of complaints (3.3%).

Subcutaneous fat in men is lean compared to women. The proximity of the gland to the skin and to the underlying tissues is the reason why the tumor very early becomes immobile against the anterior chest wall and the skin over the tumor becomes fixed and wrinkled. Even with superficial palpation, it is possible to find solid cartilaginous mass with irregular contours, which is centrally located behind the nipple or areola or near them. Examining the nipples and the areolas, it is necessary to pay attention to the thickening of the areola fold (Krause symptom) and the presence or absence of nipple discharge and to identify possible symptoms of retraction or the symptom of "orange peel." Skin ulceration over of the tumor in men occurs much earlier than in women.

More frequently, the tumor occurs in the left breast with the ratio 1.07–1.63:1. The ratio is similar to the female breast, but there is no explanation for this fact in the literature.

The average diameter of the detected tumor is usually 2–4 cm, but it can vary from 0.5 to 12.5 cm.

Invasive ductal cancer is the most common type of breast cancer in men, as well as in women (80.2% and 82% of all breast cancers, respectively). Intraductal cancer in men and in women is detected with almost equal frequency (1.3–2.3%, respectively). Specific histological types of cancer in men are found in 20% of cases and in women in 13%. The following malignant breast tumors are also described in men: inflammatory cancer, lobular carcinoma, papillary cancer, ductal carcinoma in situ, atypical ductal hyperplasia of the breast epithelium, and tubular breast cancer. Single cases of breast sarcoma in men are described. The histological structure of breast sarcomas is quite heterogeneous: fibro-, leiomyo-, neuro-, reticulo-, lympho-, and carcinosarcomas are found.

The clinical picture of Paget's disease of the breast, which is described in detail in women, is about the same in men. The incidence of this disease in women with breast cancer is 0.5–3.8%, on the average about 2%. In men, Paget's disease occurs significantly less often. There was reported that the incidence of this disease is 1% of all breast cancer cases in men. The average age is 56, which is 6 years more than the average age of women with the same pathology. An average duration of the disease history from the first symptoms to the first visit to a doctor is 8 months.

Inflammatory (edematous) types of breast cancer in men are extremely rare and have very unfavorable course. Perhaps not all authors distinguish this form of cancer when describing their own observations.

Carcinomas in men are less differentiated compared to similar tumors in women. The breast cancer in men has a worse prognosis (5-year survival is 20–30%); it progresses rapidly and metastasizes early.

Ultrasonographic features of breast cancer in men. Today, ultrasonography is a highly effective and mandatory method of examination, along with X-ray methods, clinical examination, and palpation, in the diagnosis of breast pathology both in women and in men.

All histological types of breast cancer observed in women occur in men almost with the same frequency. According to Sencha et al. (2015), the results of the morphological analysis of the biopsy and surgical material reveal various forms of breast cancer: ductal invasive carcinoma was found in 40.2% of cases, lobular invasive carcinoma in 9.9%, tubular adenocarcinoma in 4.1%, solid adenocarcinoma in 4.1%, moderately differentiated adenocarcinoma in 3.3%, serous adenocarcinoma serous in 1.6%, keratinizing squamous cell carcinoma in 1.6%, leiomyosarcoma in 0.8%, and unspecified carcinoma in 34.4%. 18.9 of patients have T1 stage of breast cancer according to TNM classification; T2, 44.3%; T3, 25.4%; and T4, 11.4%.

More than half of the patients were diagnosed with local progression of cancer; metastatic lymph nodes were observed in 48.3% of patients (Sencha et al. 2015). The severity of clinical manifestations of breast cancer is largely dependent on the severity and extent of the tumor.

Breast cancer in men, as well as in women, may occur in a nodular or diffuse (edematous-infiltrative) forms.

Nodular breast cancer is characterized, first of all, by the presence of a mass with grayscale US.

Grayscale mode allows to obtain comprehensive information (up to 75–95% of all signs) about the nature of the pathological process, minimizing the unspecified diagnosis. Breast cancer in men basically has the same ultrasound signs as in women.

The most characteristic ultrasound signs of focal changes in male breast, suggesting their malignant nature, are as follows (Figs. 9.37 and 9.38):

- Irregular shape
- Hypoechogenicity of a mass
- Eccentric localization
- Heterogenous structure
- Hyperechoic calcificated inclusions
- Anechoic component
- Tuberous margins
- Indistinct contours
- Avascularity at CDI
- Hypervascularity
- Irregular distribution of blood vessels in the nodular structure; chaotic, disorganized vascular pattern, and pathological transformation of blood vessels
- Altered elasticity; intensive color pattern (red or blue), different from surrounding structures; homogeneity of coloring within the lesion at compression US elastography
- Average shear wave velocity with ARFI 4.2 ± 0.032 m/sec and average strain ratio 2.8 ± 0.013 compared to normal surrounding tissues
- Positive axillary lymph nodes

Sencha 2015 reports the following most characteristic ultrasound signs of breast cancer in men (n = 122): hypoechogenicity of a mass (95.1%); heterogeneity of the structure (70.5%); eccentric localization (69.7%); tuberous margins (69.7%); irregular shape (60.65%); indistinct contours (56.55%); hyperechoic microcalcificated inclusions (15.6%); anechoic component (11.5%); avascularity at CDI (55.7%); irregular distribution of blood vessels in the node structure, chaotic, disorganized vascular pattern, and their pathological transformation (13.1%); altered elasticity at compression US elastography, intensive color pattern (red or blue) different from surrounding structures (84.6%); homogeneity of the node coloring (88.5%); and positive axillary lymph nodes (75.4%).

A large spectrum of modes, technologies and ultrasound scanning frequencies greatly facilitates daily work of a diagnostician and provides detalization of the breast structure and surrounding tissues. High spatial-contrast resolution, integrated analysis of the obtained results allow to collect more information at different depths of the target zones with less efforts and for a shorter period of time. Localization of a palpable breast tumor in male differs from its location in women. For example, in almost 50% of women with breast cancer, the tumors are located in the upper-external quadrant, 15% in the upper-internal, up to 10% in the lower-external, up to 5% in the lower-internal, and up to 17% in the central breast compartments, whereas in 59.7% of men, the central, subareolar zone is most often affected.

Due to anatomic features of male breast, the most frequent location of cancer is subareolar area. Tumors can be located under the nipple and merge into the skin. However, more often they

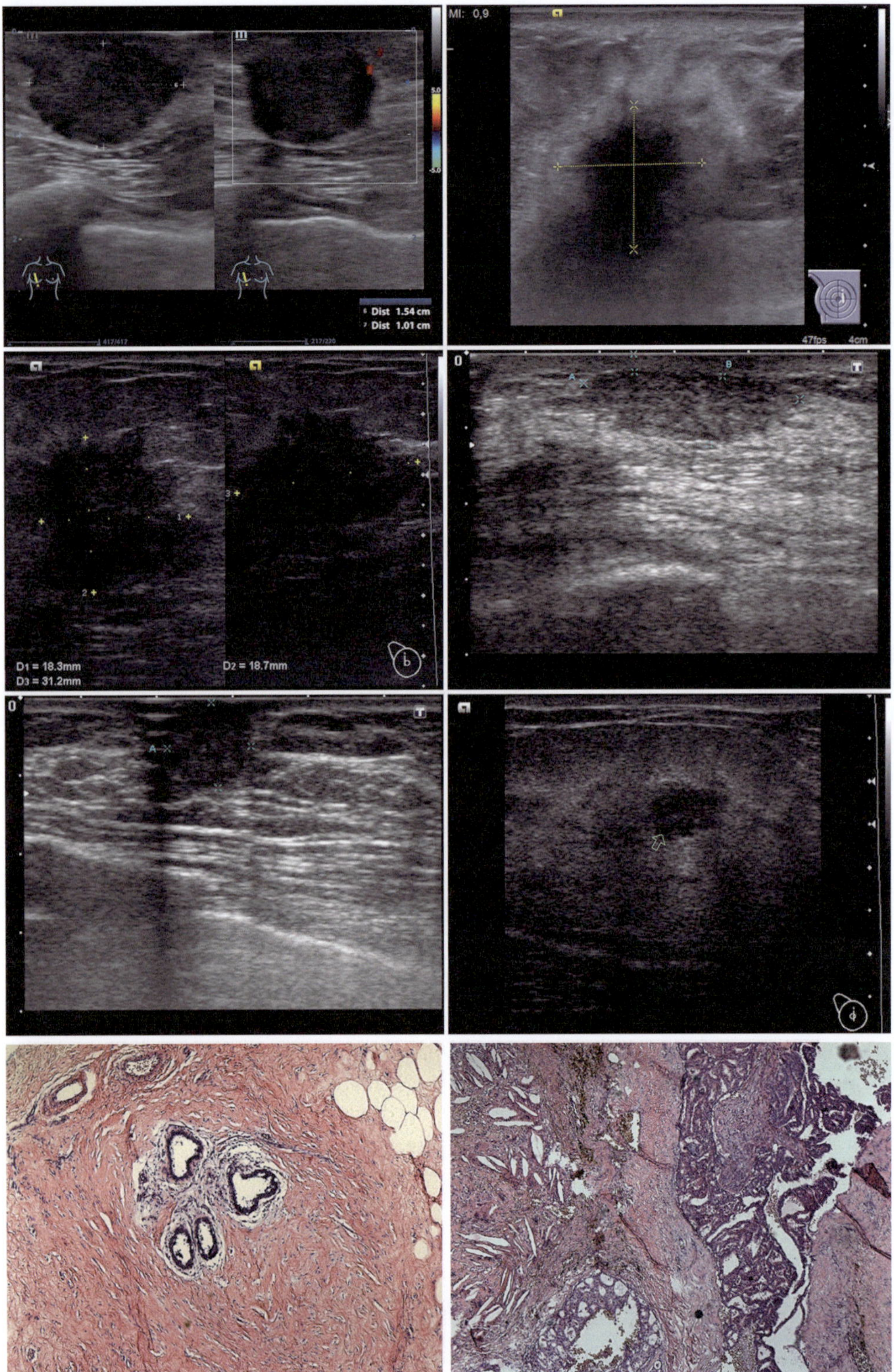

Fig. 9.37 Male breast cancer. (**a**) 1–6 Grayscale US. (**b**) Microscopy. Azure-eosin stained image; original magnification, ×20. (**c**) Microscopy. Azure-eosin stained image; original magnification, ×100

have slightly eccentric location. The last variant can be accompanied by an umbrella-shaped extrusion on the skin surface. It is very important to carefully examine the backside of the lesion to assess its relation to pectoral muscle, because this is important for surgery and planning of postoperative treatment.

Invasive masses usually disrupt the normal arrangement of fatty and connective tissue. Malignant tumors may be slightly hypoechoic and have rather distinct contours. In the presence of calcification and heterogeneous echostructure with a spotted posterior shadow, the probability of a malignant tumor increases.

At present, there is no universal point of view concerning the microcalcifications in male breast cancer and their significance for diagnostics. Absence of hormone-dependent cyclic changes in men possibly explains why no calcifications are observed in the vessels, ducts, gynecomastia, and benign breast tumors. Breast calcifications on mammographic images are an extremely dangerous sign. It should be noted that calcifications in men, unlike in women, are always found against a clearly defined tumor mass.

Breast cancer may be unilateral or bilateral (3–15% of cases), synchronous or metachronous. Cancer in one breast can develop simultaneously with a tumor in another breast or occur 10 or more years later (Rozhkova 1993). According to this author, synchronous lesions in the other breast were noted in 43% of cases. Multicentric tumor growth in breast cancer was noted in 18% of women. Multiple tumors are found in men with similar incidence.

The grayscale image of breast cancer in men may resemble gynecomastia without typical malignant signs (Sencha et al. 2011). Some other authors consider that tumors of male breast cannot be effectively differentiated from true gynecomastia with ultrasonography. If the benign nature of the breast mass is doubtful, biopsy is necessary.

Ultrasound diagnostics have limited value in detection of masses on the background of fatty involution of breast tissue and of assessment of the duct tumors extent. Especially this refers to men, who have been operated for gynecomastia. Breast tumors localized in retromammary space, as well as lesions smaller than 1 cm in diameter, often remain unidentified. An essential limitation of the method is its dependence on the type of the scanner and the operator's skills.

Inflammatory breast cancer in men occurs very rarely. It is noticed in 1.6% of patients.

Absence of a solid nodular mass often causes difficulties in differentiation of edematous-infiltrative type of breast cancer in men (as well as in women).

At **CDI and PDI**, normal vascular pattern of breast tissue in men, as well as in women, is scanty. As a rule, a color pattern shows as single color spots (points), which are evenly or unevenly distributed throughout the breast (Fisenko 1999; Harchenko et al. 1993, Sandrikov and Fisenko 1998). According to Folkman (1995), one of the significant signs of breast cancer is the vascular asymmetry of the breast.

Tumor growth often depends on the formation of new minor vessels along with development of tumor vasculature. According to Sencha (2015), nodular type of breast cancer is more often avascular at CDI (55.7% cases). Hypovascularization was detected in 24.6% of patients with breast cancer and hypervascularization (two and more color spots) in 19.7% of patients. The vascular pattern of neoangiogenesis in men with malignant lesions is much more poor than in women with similar pathology. As a rule, even one vascular spot in the structure of a mass is considered to be an unfavorable sign (Fig. 9.38).

In men, as well as in women, there are no specific values of velocity parameters and blood flow indices with **PW Doppler**.

3D image reconstruction in breast cancer in men, as well as in women, allows to assess the number and the structure of the lesions, to specify their location in relation to surrounding structures; to reveal indistinct tuberous margins, calcified areas, multiple nodes, and the tumor growth; and to assume the volume of affected and intact breast tissue (Fig. 9.39).

3D reconstruction of US image in **3DPD vascular mode,** in contrast to 2D CDI and PDI,

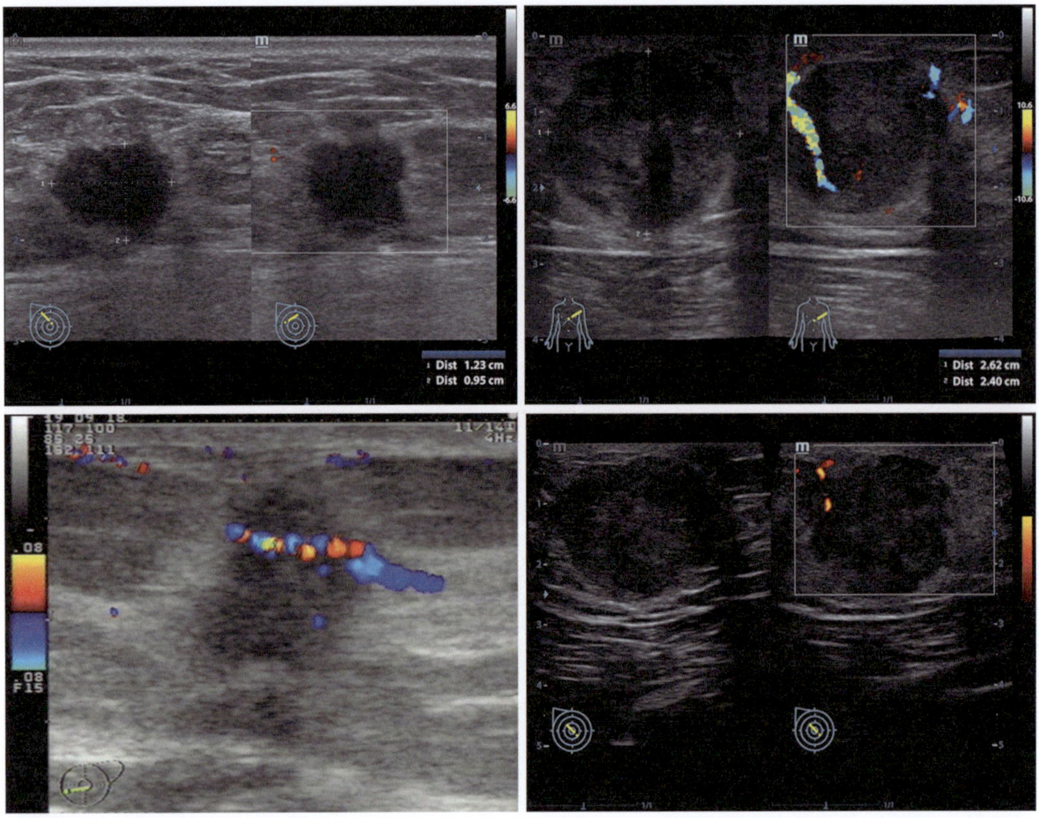

Fig. 9.38 Breast cancer in a man. (**a**) 1–3 CDI. (**b**) PDI

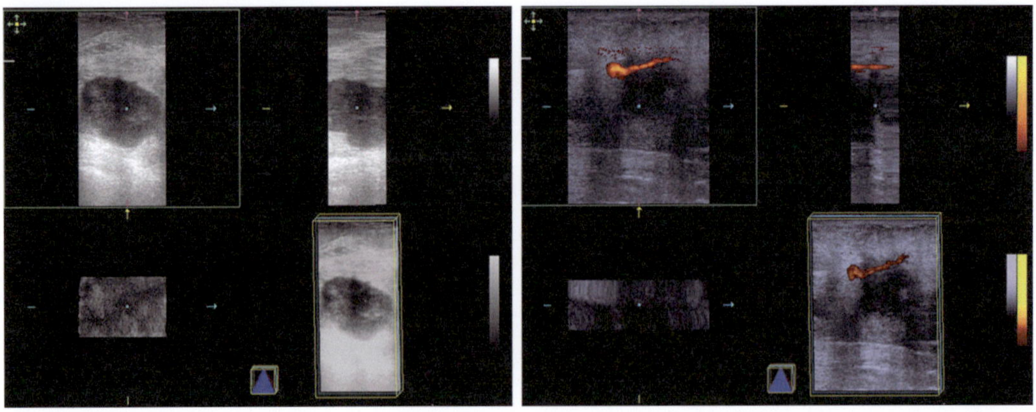

Fig. 9.39 Breast cancer in a man. (**a**) 3D. (**b**) 3DPD

allows more precise assessment of pathological transformation of vessels within a malignant mass, their density, and chaotic nature. 3D reconstruction is valuable not only for assessment of vascularity but also for the guidance of puncture biopsy.

Ultrasound elastography is an effective technology for visualizing the tissues of superficial organs, including differentiation of breast pathology in men. In 81.3% of cases, breast masses show as intensive, well-shaped color patterns (blue or other color depending on the scan-

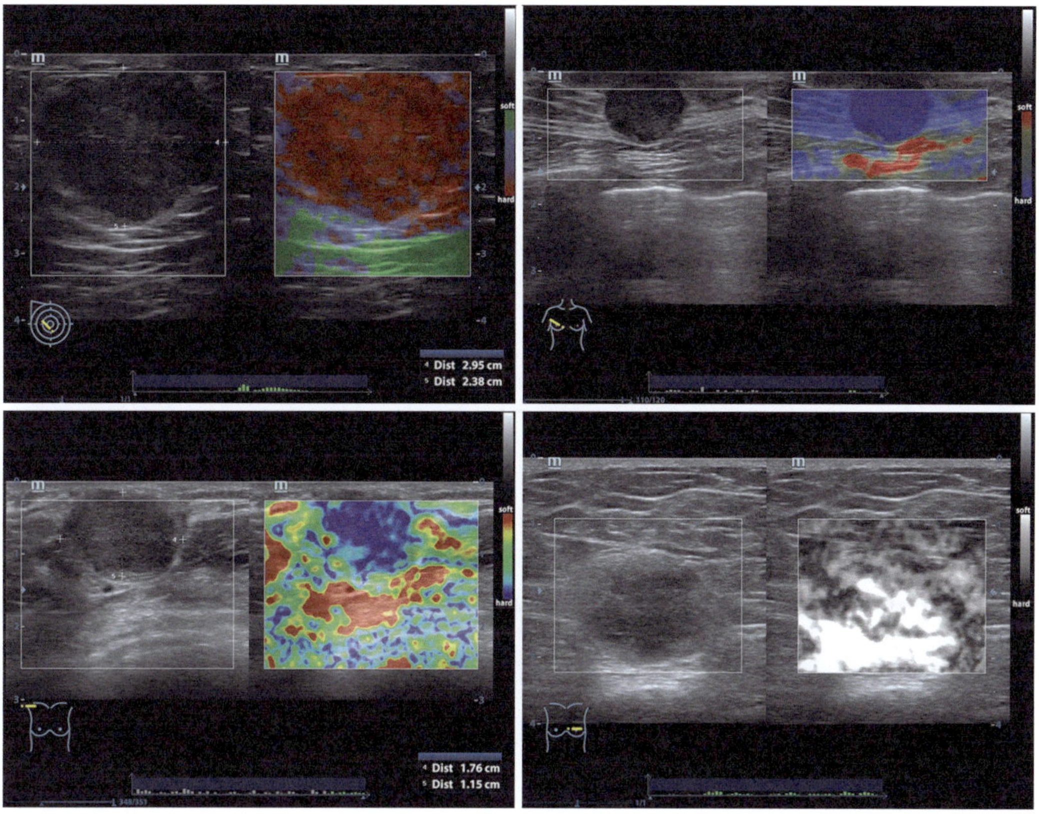

Fig. 9.40 Breast cancer in a man. 1–4 compression US elastography. Intensive "hard" color of breast tumor

ner setting) with compression US elastography (Fig. 9.40) (Sencha 2015).

In 81.8% of patients, coloring of breast masses with compression elastography is uneven. Differences in sizes of masses are often defined with grayscale US and compression US elastography (Sencha 2015). The average strain ratio in the malignant mass of the male breast is more than 2.3 in relation to the unchanged parenchyma (Fig. 9.41).

In recent years, the technology based on the algorithms for calculation of shear wave velocity to assess the stiffness of the tissue has been developed. The more dense is the tissue (which is more specific for a malignant tumor), the higher is the shear wave velocity generated through the tissue (Piscaglia et al. 2011). The average shear wave velocity in a malignant node in the male breast is 2.7 m/s with ARFI (virtual touch tissue quantification).

At **contrast-enhanced echography**, malignant breast pathology in men is characterized by heterogeneous, intense contrast enhancement. The vessels are often located asymmetrically and unevenly in the structure of tumor. They are often pathologically transformed and deformed (Fig. 9.42).

Breast sarcoma is also a rare disease in men. It accounts for 2–5% of all malignant breast tumors in men and 0.6–1% in women. Men with breast sarcoma are 10–20 years younger than men with breast cancer. Sarcoma exhibits fast enlargement of a solitary or multiple nodules of the tumor. The skin over the tumor becomes stretched, thin, glittering reddish and bluish and exhibits vasculature. Fibrosarcoma in men, as well as in women, is the most often histological type.

Ultrasound elastography significantly increases capability of ultrasound for breast

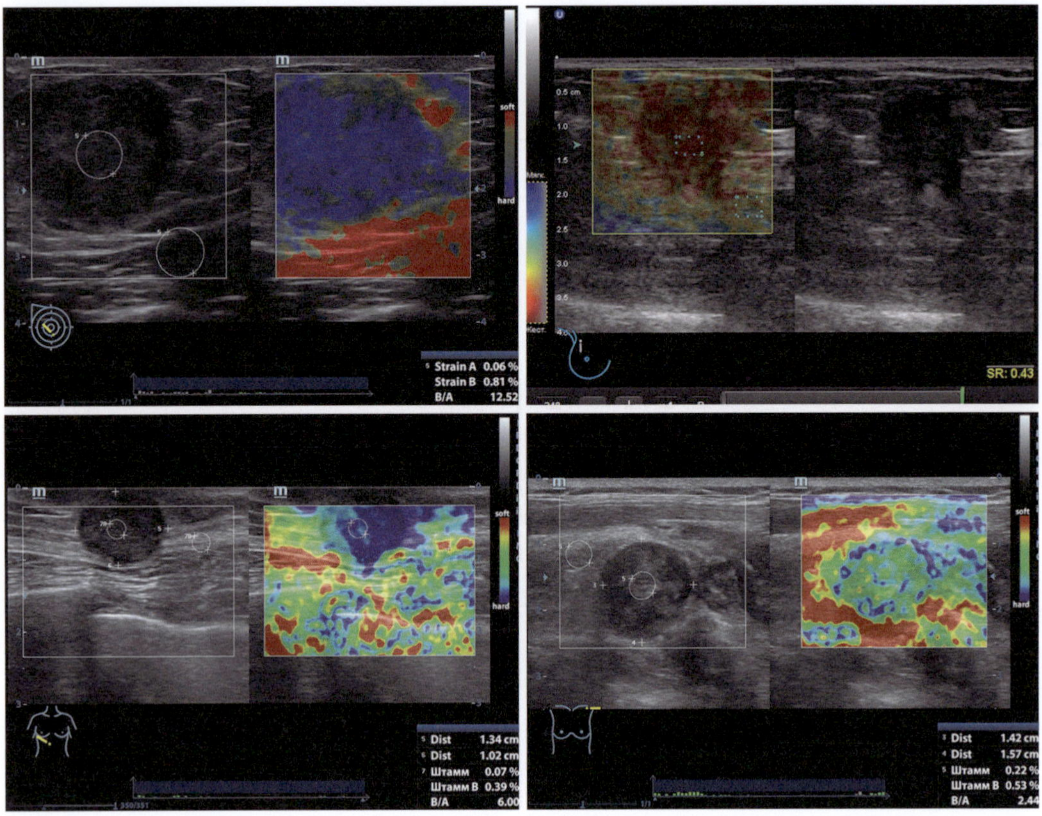

Fig. 9.41 Breast cancer in a man. 1–4 compression US elastography. Strain ratio

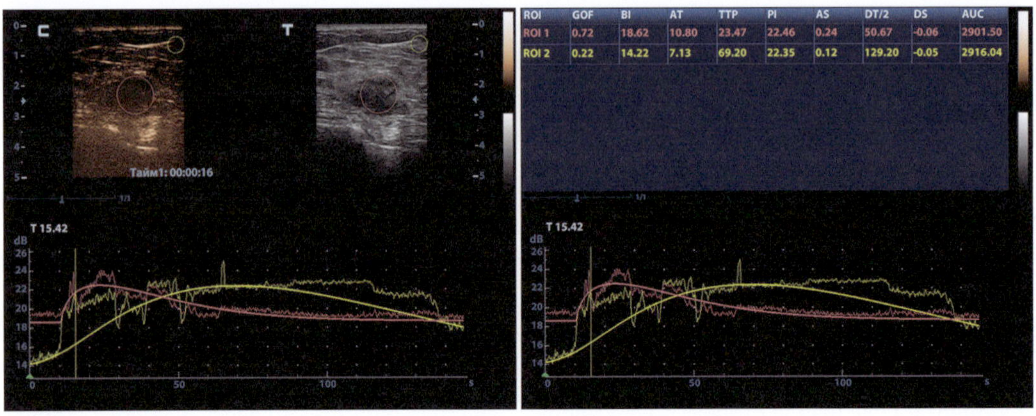

Fig. 9.42 Breast cancer in a man. CEUS. SonoVue 2.4 mL. 1–2. Echograms. Significant asymmetric intranodular contrast enhancement, different quantitative indices in the tumor and normal breast tissue

masses. Diagnostic values of US elastography for malignant masses of male breast are as follows: sensitivity, 96%; specificity, 99%; positive prognostic value, 97%; and negative prognostic value, 99% (Sencha 2015).

Awareness of the population and medical stuff about male breast cancer may be of great importance in identifying the disease at early stages and, as a result, providing a more successful treatment. Late diagnosis is also caused by patients' neglect to the symptoms, by untimely referral for medical care, as well as by ignorance of general practitioners.

The algorithm for examination in men with breast cancer should include, first of all, mammography or breast ultrasound, chest CT, and, if available, PET/CT with 18-FDH. High qualification of diagnosticians, collaboration of doctors of different specialties at all stages of diagnostics, adherence to the principles of continuity of care, and optimal use of diagnostic equipment and new technologies are of benefit for the patient.

Timely ultrasound and X-ray diagnosis, reinforced with modern techniques and technologies, and analysis of the entire set of signs allow to evaluate the condition of breast in men in full scope, the nature of the lesion, and extent of the disease and to assess the condition of surrounding structures and lymphatic nodes. Dynamic ultrasound allows precise follow-up of the patient after treatment.

An example of US report of a patient with male breast cancer

Name, surname. __S__ Age__41__

Outpatient examination. Date____

Patient's record____

US scanner____

The breasts are of masculine type, mainly presented with adipose tissue. Fibrous tissue is moderately expressed in all areas	
Right breast	Left breast
A mass of low echogenicity (1.6 × 1.5 × 1.3 cm in size; irregular stellar shape, with indistinct, uneven contours; heterogenous; hypervascular at CDI and PDI, moderately painful) is detected in the lower-external quadrant. It is intensively, heterogeneously colored in compression US elastography. The average shear wave velocity in ARFI is 3.9 m/s. The average strain ratio in the mass against the unchanged areas is 3.7	Cystic and solid lesions are not revealed

On the right side, there are several axillary lymph nodes, 0.8–2.6 cm in size. They are hypoechoic, heterogenous, poorly differentiated, and hypovascular.

Left axillary lymph nodes and supra- and subclavicular, parasternal nodes at both sides are not visualized.

Conclusion Right breast mass. Echographic signs of cancer. Metastases in right axillary lymph nodes.

Ultrasound of Regional Lymph Nodes in Breast Cancer

10

Yury Patrunov, Alexander N. Sencha, Ekaterina Sencha, and Ella Penyaeva

Abstract

Regional lymph nodes are a barrier, preventing the spread of both the infection and cancer cells from the nearby organs and systems. Up to 55% of sonographically detected abnormal lymph nodes are impalpable. Lymph nodes have morphologic zones, each with specific features of structure and function. Usually, two main components of lymph node are well distinguishable—the cortical and medullar layers. The main sonographic features of lymph nodes are the size, shape, structure, and vascularization. Vascular pattern of lymph nodes may be classified into four categories: "hiliar," activated "hiliar" (central), peripheral, and mixed type. Reactive changes of lymph nodes may result from various pathological processes (an inflammatory process, vaccination, injections, etc.). The incidence of breast cancer metastases in regional lymph nodes in women and men is 19–80%. About 7% of tumors simultaneously metastasize to two regions. The sensitivity of ultrasound in the detection of affected lymph nodes in breast cancer is 70–99% with specificity of 83–97%. Currently, grayscale ultrasound is the principal method for differential diagnosis of the pathology in the axillary area. Sentinel lymph node biopsy is an alternative to lymphodissection in patients with early stages of breast cancer with no clinical signs of metastatic lesions in axillary lymph nodes.

Y. Patrunov (✉) · E. Penyaeva
Department of Ultrasound Diagnostics of Radiology Center, Yaroslavl Railway Clinic, Yaroslavl, Russia

A. N. Sencha
Division of Visual Diagnostics, National Medical Research Center for Obstetrics, Gynecology and Perinatology named after Academician V.I. Kulakov of Ministry of Healthcare of Russian Federation, Moscow, Russia

E. Sencha
Department of Ultrasound Diagnostics, Federal State Budget Hospital "9 Treatment and Diagnostic Center" of the Ministry of Defense of the Russian Federation, Moscow, Russia

Lymph node is a peripheral organ of the lymphatic system, which acts as a biological filter through which lymph flows from the organs and parts of the body.

Regional lymph nodes are a barrier, preventing the spread of both the infection and cancer cells from the nearby organs and systems. Lymph nodes are located along lymphatic vessels and form groups (aggregations) at places of their confluences. The amount of lymph nodes in each region is individual and variable.

Lymph nodes have morphologic zones, each with specific features of structure and function. Usually four zones are specified: cortex, paracortex, medulla, and hilum (gate) (Fig. 10.1).

G. T. Sukhikh, A. N. Sencha (eds.), *Multiparametric Ultrasound Diagnosis of Breast Diseases*,
https://doi.org/10.1007/978-3-319-75034-7_10

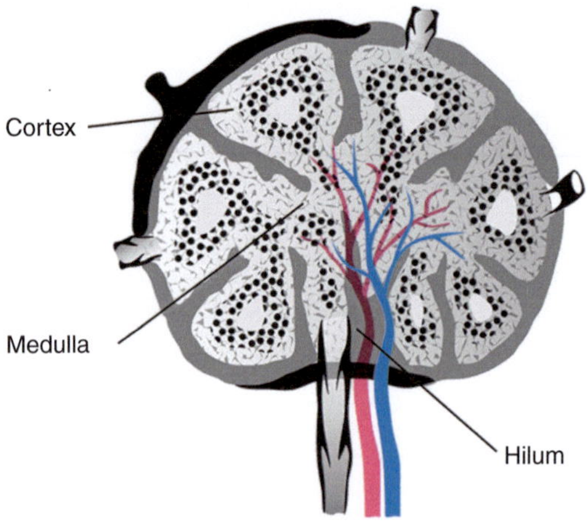

Fig. 10.1 Lymph nodes structure. Scheme

The cortical zone consists of a large number of lymph nodules which produce the immune cells. The paracortical zone is located in the middle part of lymph nodes. It consists of cells, which resemble macrophages by their structure, with the processes on the outer membrane. Communicating with each other, they form a barrier against penetration of foreign proteins and microorganisms into the lymph nodes. Maturation of lymphatic cells that take part in antiviral protection occurs in the paracortical zone of the lymph nodes. The medulla is located in the very center of the node and divided with septa bearing vascular plexuses. It produces immune cells that take part not only in protecting the body from infections but also stimulate hematopoiesis in the red bone marrow.

The study of regional lymph nodes, primarily axillary, is mandatory in breast ultrasound, as the lymph from the breast goes to the axillary collector. In some cases, metastatic enlarged neck lymph nodes are the first clinical manifestation of breast cancer.

Physical examination and palpation of axillary lymph nodes are not always informative and have a low sensitivity (50–88%), since deep lymph nodes are often not accessible (Frolov 1996 and Harchenko et al. 1996).

In 1975 ultrasound was suggested for assessment of lymph nodes. Until the mid-1990s it was thought that the structure of normal lymph nodes is not visible at ultrasonography. Normal lymph nodes could not be distinguished from the surrounding adipose tissue, especially when the size was <5 mm (Trofimova 2000). This was due to low resolution of the equipment used at that time. Latest ultrasound technologies and scanners allow not only to detect lesions <5 mm but also to visualize unchanged nodes <10 mm.

In some cases, enlarged metastatic (primarily axillary) lymph nodes are the first clinical manifestation of breast cancer. However, enlarged lymph nodes may be a consequence of other breast diseases. At the age of 30, about 80% of cases of lymphadenopathy are benign, while only 40% in patients over 50 years.

US of lymph nodes is performed in a standard supine position of a patient for breast scanning (Fig. 10.2). For the study of axillary lymph nodes, the patient consequently raises the right and the left arm.

Axillary, supraclavicular, subclavian, substernal, and pectoral groups of lymph nodes demand high-frequency 7.5–18 MHz US linear probes (Fig. 10.3).

Provisional margins for ultrasound examination of lymph nodes are as follows: in the axillary region, the lateral border of the small pectoral muscle and the lateral edge of the latissimus muscle of the back; in the supraclavicular region, the upper edge of the clavicle and the medial margin of the digastric muscle; in the subclavian area, the projection of the subclavian vessels and surrounding loose tissue; and in the parasternal region, intercostal spaces along the edges of the sternum from the base to manubrium.

Axillary lymph nodes accessible for ultrasound include the following groups:

- Nodes located medially to the pectoralis minor muscle
- Nodes located along the axillary vessels
- Nodes located between the pectoralis major and minor muscles

Axillary lymph nodes can be classified into the following levels:

- Level 1 (inferior axillary) lymph nodes located laterally to the lateral border of the pectoralis minor muscle.
- Level 2 (middle axillary) lymph nodes located between the medial and lateral edges of the

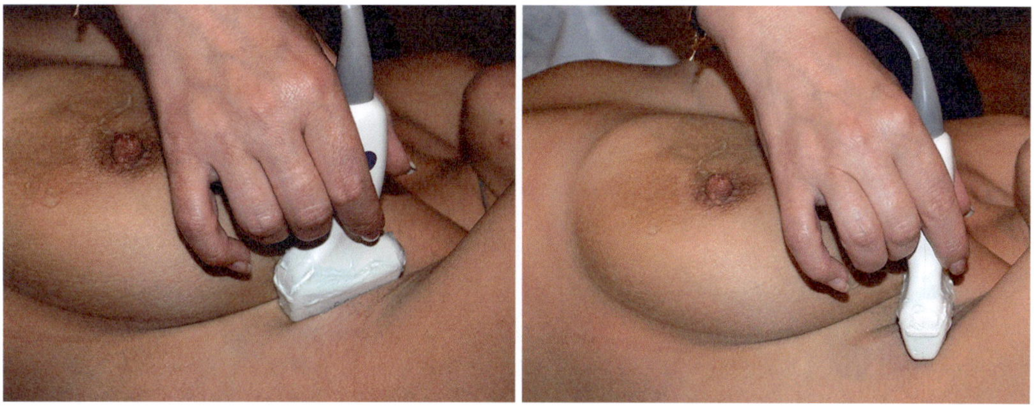

Fig. 10.2 1–2 Patients position. Probe location for US of axillary lymph nodes

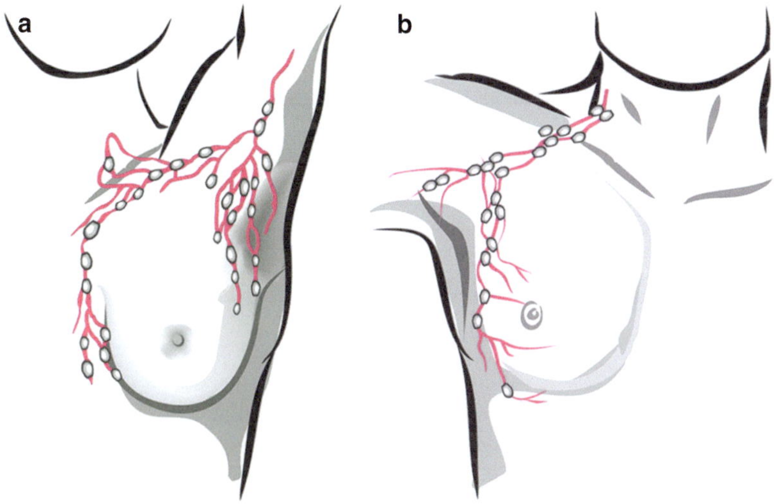

Fig. 10.3 Scheme. Location of main lymph nodes affected in breast pathology. (**a**) In women. (**b**) In men

pectoralis minor muscle and interpectoral (Rotter's) lymph nodes.

- Level 3 (apical axillary) lymph nodes located medially to medial edge of the pectoralis minor muscle including subclavian and apical lymph nodes.
- Intramammary lymph nodes are classified as axillary (subclavian) lymph nodes.

The following criteria are accepted for ultrasound evaluation of the lymphatic system and lymph nodes:

- Extent of lymph node lesions by groups (areas)
- Number of lymph nodes
- Dimensions (3D)
- Anterior-posterior and transverse diameter ratio
- Uniformity of changes
- Shape (flat, oval, spherical, or irregular)
- Echogenicity of lymph nodes in general (high, medium, or low)
- Differentiation of lymph node components (is present, is not present)
- Differentiation of hilum (is present, is not present)
- Echogenicity of the core (high, low, or isoechoic)
- Mobility of lymph nodes under compression
- Elasticity at compression US elastography
- Vascularity

The main sonographic features of lymph nodes are the size, shape, structure, and vascularization.

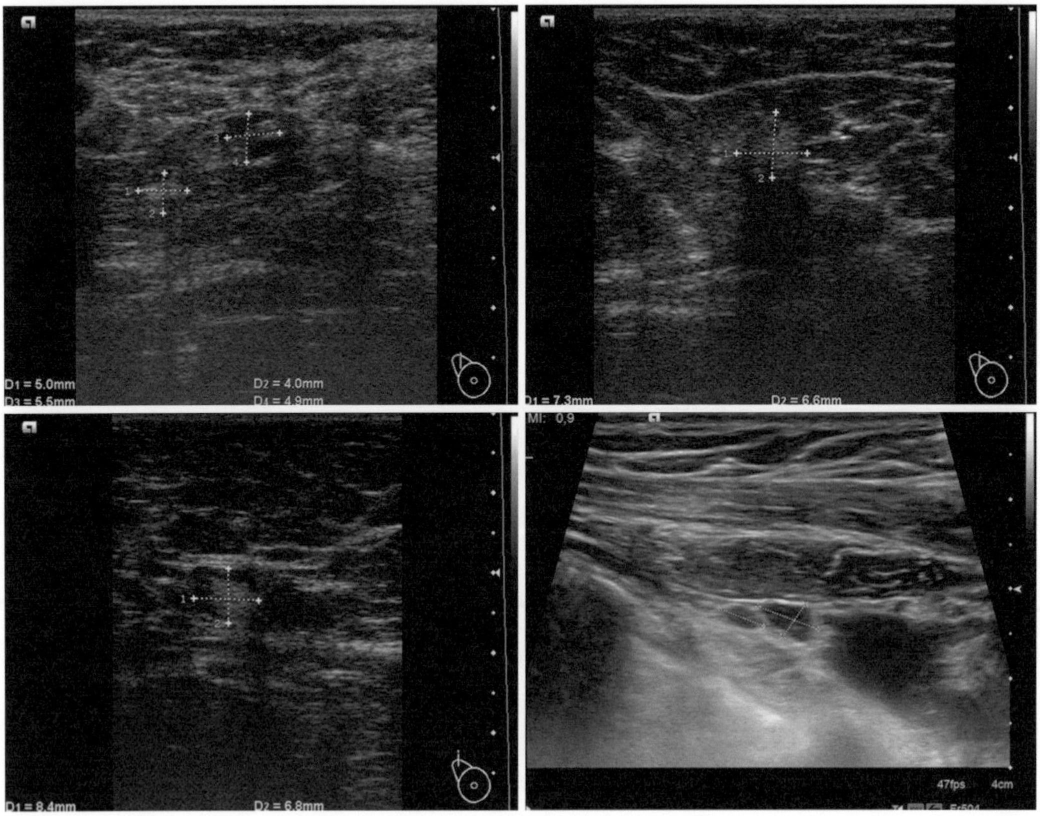

Fig. 10.4 1–4 Normal axillary lymph nodes. Grayscale US

Normal axillary lymph nodes demonstrate the following sonographic features (Fig. 10.4):

- Oval (rarely bean-shaped, ribbon-shaped)
- Length < 10 mm
- Mixed echogenicity, usually hypo- or isoechoic marginal part and hyperechoic central part
- Heterogeneous echostructure
- Even borders, distinct contours
- Painless, relatively mobile when compressed with an US probe
- Often hypo- or avascular pattern in the hilum at DPI, CDI, and 3DPD
- No coloring at compression US elastography

Usually, two main components of lymph node are well distinguishable—the cortical and medullar layers. Their proportion and echogenicity depend on many factors, such as age, localization, medical history, etc. Normally, the cortical layer of a lymph node is thin and is practically undetectable. Stimulation with antigens leads to thickening and decrease in echodensity of the cortical layer or to increased overall echogenicity of the lymph node, facilitating its visualization.

The Solbiati index, which is the ratio of the largest to the smallest diameter of a lymph node, is normally 2.9 ± 0.13 cm in adults and 2.4 ± 0.05 cm in children (Solbiati and Rissato 1995).

Assessment of vascularity with CDI and PDI provides additional data for differential diagnosis of the causes for lymph nodes enlargement (Fig. 10.5). Vessels, if any detected in normal or reactively enlarged lymph nodes, are usually located within the hilum. In large benign hyperplastic lymph nodes, the vascular pattern remains regular. Vessels (arteries) are normally observed along the capsule and radially from the hilum to the periphery.

Vascular pattern of lymph nodes may be classified into the following categories:

1. “Hilum” type: the vessels are visualized in the hilar region as single arterial and/or venous fragments without spreading to the lymph node parenchyma and without branching.

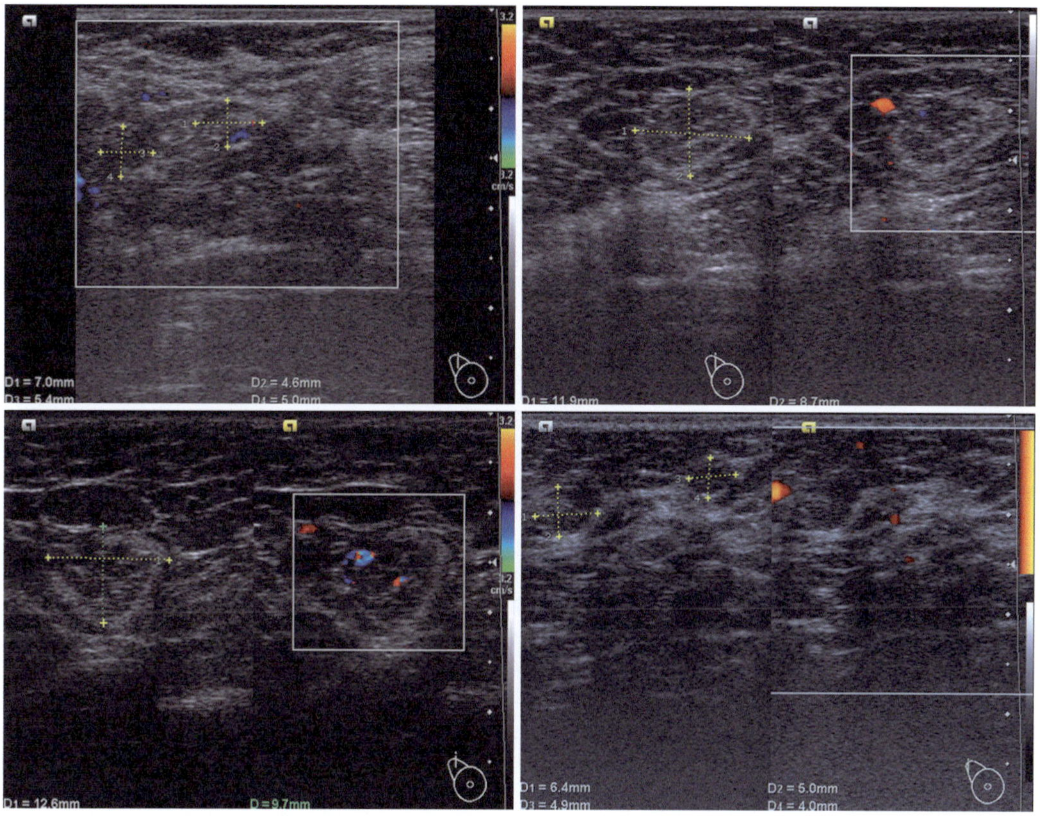

Fig. 10.5 1–4 Normal axillary lymph nodes. Echograms. CDI and PDI

2. Activated "hilum" type (central): venous and arterial vessels are visualized in hilum and medulla in a treelike shape with branches.
3. Peripheral type: perinodular vascular rete corresponds to the vascular fragments localized along the periphery of lymph nodes, in the cortex, mainly in the subcapsular areas.
4. Mixed type: blood supply is presented with color spots both in central and peripheral area:
   - One larger artery in the hilum and single color dots from small vessels
   - Fragment of afferent artery and chaotic vessels within the solid component of the lymph node in otherwise unchanged lymph nodes

PW Doppler does not contribute to differential diagnosis of enlarged lymph nodes. According to Sinyukova et al. (2007), normal lymph nodes exhibit single vessels in 58% of cases. In cases of multiple vessels, their distribution within the lymph node is homogenous.

Neck lymph nodes may be enlarged due to several aspects, such as the following:

- Inflammatory changes in the head and neck (specific and nonspecific)
- Neck lymph node metastasis
- Primary diseases of lymph nodes in hemoblastoses: hemosarcoma (lymphogranulomatosis, lymphosarcoma, reticulosarcoma) and leukemia (lymphocytic leukemia, myeloid leukemia)

Reactive changes of lymph nodes may result from various pathological processes (an inflammatory process, vaccination, injections, etc.). Lymph nodes, which are close to a tumor, can also show nonspecific reaction of inflammatory character.

Nonspecific types of lymphadenitis are classified as follows:

1. According to disease severity
   - Acute
   - Subacute
   - Chronic
2. According to localization
   - Isolated
   - Regionary (groups)

- Extensive
- Generalized

Individual lymph nodes and conglomerates may be present.

Hyperplastic lymph nodes usually exhibit the following US features (Sinyukova et al. 2007) (Fig. 10.6):

- Enlarged size (>1 cm)
- Oval shape
- Iso- or hypoechogenicity
- Heterogeneous echostructure, thickening of the cortical layer
- Even borders, often with distinct contours
- Avascularity or hypovascularity at CDI, PDI, and 3DPD (Figs. 10.5 and 10.6)
- Low values of PSV, EDV, and RI in PW Doppler
- No difference in color pattern compared with the surrounding tissues at compression US elastography

Inflammatory lymph nodes show fast dynamics. They often become invisible in 5–7 days without any therapy and in 3–5 days if treated. Usually these terms are longer and may last for to 30–60 days. Treatment speeds up the lymph nodes involution, resulting in the restoration of the oval shape and distinct margins of the node, the increase in overall echodensity with the recovery of corticomedullary differentiation, and the decrease in blood flow and tenderness under compression with US probe.

The incidence of breast cancer metastases in regional lymph nodes in women and men is 19–80% (Sinyukova et al. 2007 and Trufanov et al. 2009).

Palpation of axillary lymph nodes in advanced stages is quite informative (Fig. 10.7).

A comprehensive imaging based on malignancy criteria is more likely to detect metastasis even in the lymph nodes of normal size (Zabolotskaya and Zabolotsky 2000). The sensitivity of US in detection of affected lymph nodes in breast cancer is 70–99% with specificity of 83–97%. It largely depends on the quality of the equipment, skills, and experience of the examiner (Cosgrove et al. 1990; Svensson et al. 2000; Drincovic 2002). Palpable axillary lymph nodes sometimes are the primary and the only symptom of breast cancer. Usually, this type of cancer is classified as hidden, occult, or axillary form. According to reported data, this form is relatively rare in women, ranging from 0.19 to 2% (Bazhenova et al. 1985). There are few reports of latent breast cancer in men.

According to Sencha et al. (2011), US reveals metastases in axillary lymph nodes in women with breast cancer were in 37.5% of patients. In 13.6% of cases, combined lesions of axillary and other groups of lymph nodes (primarily supraclavicular and subclavian, jugular, parasternal) were defined. In addition to metastases in axillary lymph nodes (up to 75%), malignant cells may be found in paraglandular (6–8%), parasternal (20–28%), and interpectoral (2%) lymph nodes. About 7% of tumors simultaneously metastasize to two regions.

Main US signs of metastatic breast cancer (Figs. 10.8, 10.9, and 10.10) are as follows:

- >10 mm in size.
- Oval or irregular shape.
- Uneven borders; indistinct contours (seldom in normal nodes).
- Low echogenicity.
- Heterogeneous echostructure with thick cortex.
- Pathological hyperechoic inclusions.
- Abnormal anechoic components (due to necrosis).
- Displacement, deformation, or unclear image of the hilum.
- Formation of conglomerates with limited mobility.
- Vascularity at CDI, PDI, and 3DPD may vary.
- No color pattern at US elastography.

There is no clear connection between the location of metastases and possible location of the primary breast tumor. In 40% of cases, the number of lymph nodes is more than three.

According to Sencha et al. (2011), the main ultrasound signs of breast cancer metastases in lymph nodes ($n = 131$) are lymph nodes >10 mm in size (19.1 ± 2.1 cm); decreased echogenicity (94.2%); heterogeneity of the echostructure

(87.5%); rough borders (55%); oval (50%) or irregular (46%) shape; displacement, deformation, and unclear image in the hilum (39.4%); anechoic component (34%); pathological hyperechoic inclusions (5%); formation of conglomerates, their low mobility under pressure with US probe; different vascularization at CDI, PDI, and 3DPD (hypovascularity in 58% of cases, hypervascularity in 27.5%); and at US elastography, no coloring in 75.6% of cases.

Currently, grayscale US is the principal method for differential diagnosis of the pathology

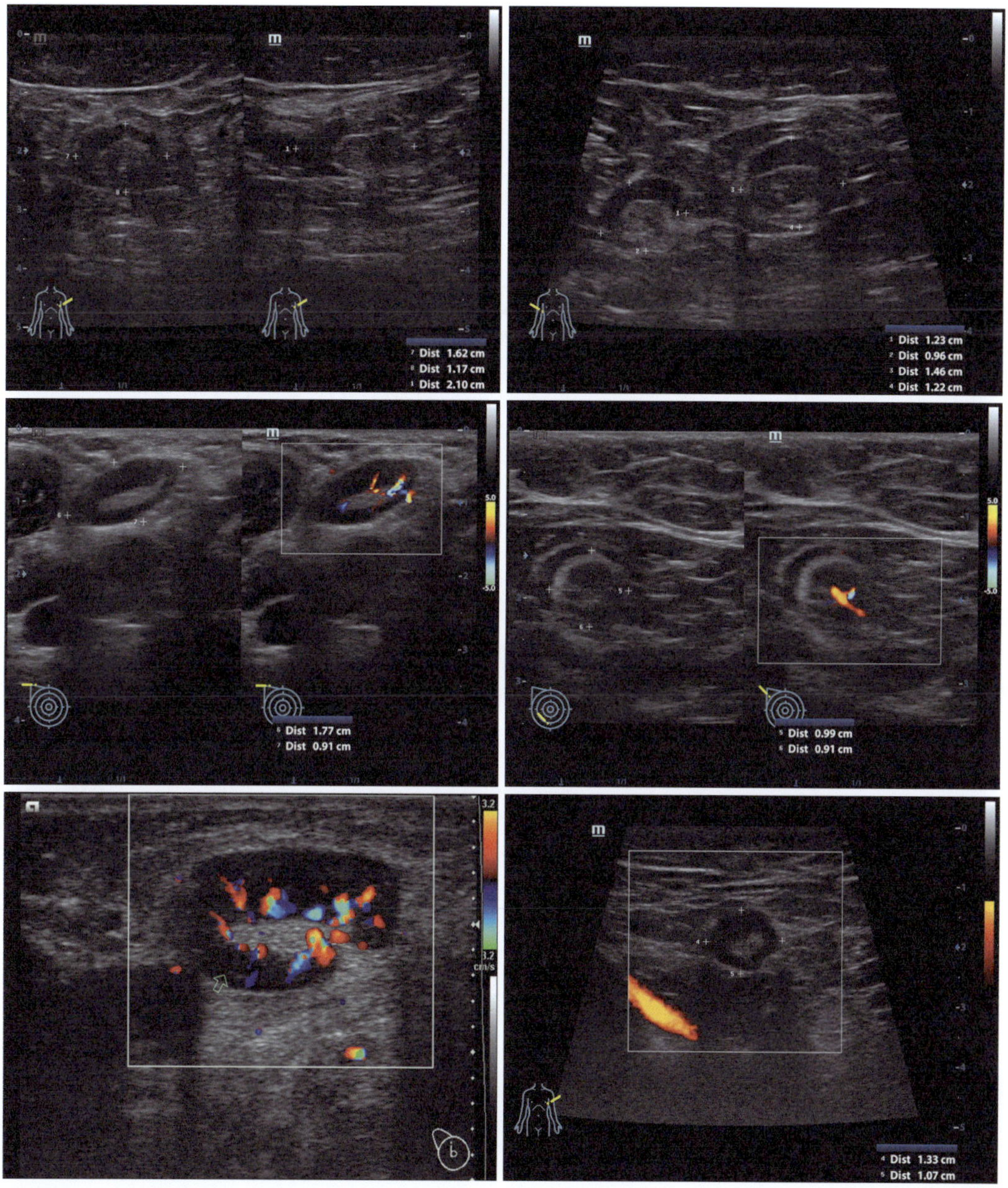

Fig. 10.6 1–8 Reactive hyperplasia of axillary lymph nodes. 9–14 Reactive hyperplasia of intramammary located lymph nodes. Grayscale, CDI, PDI, and US elastography

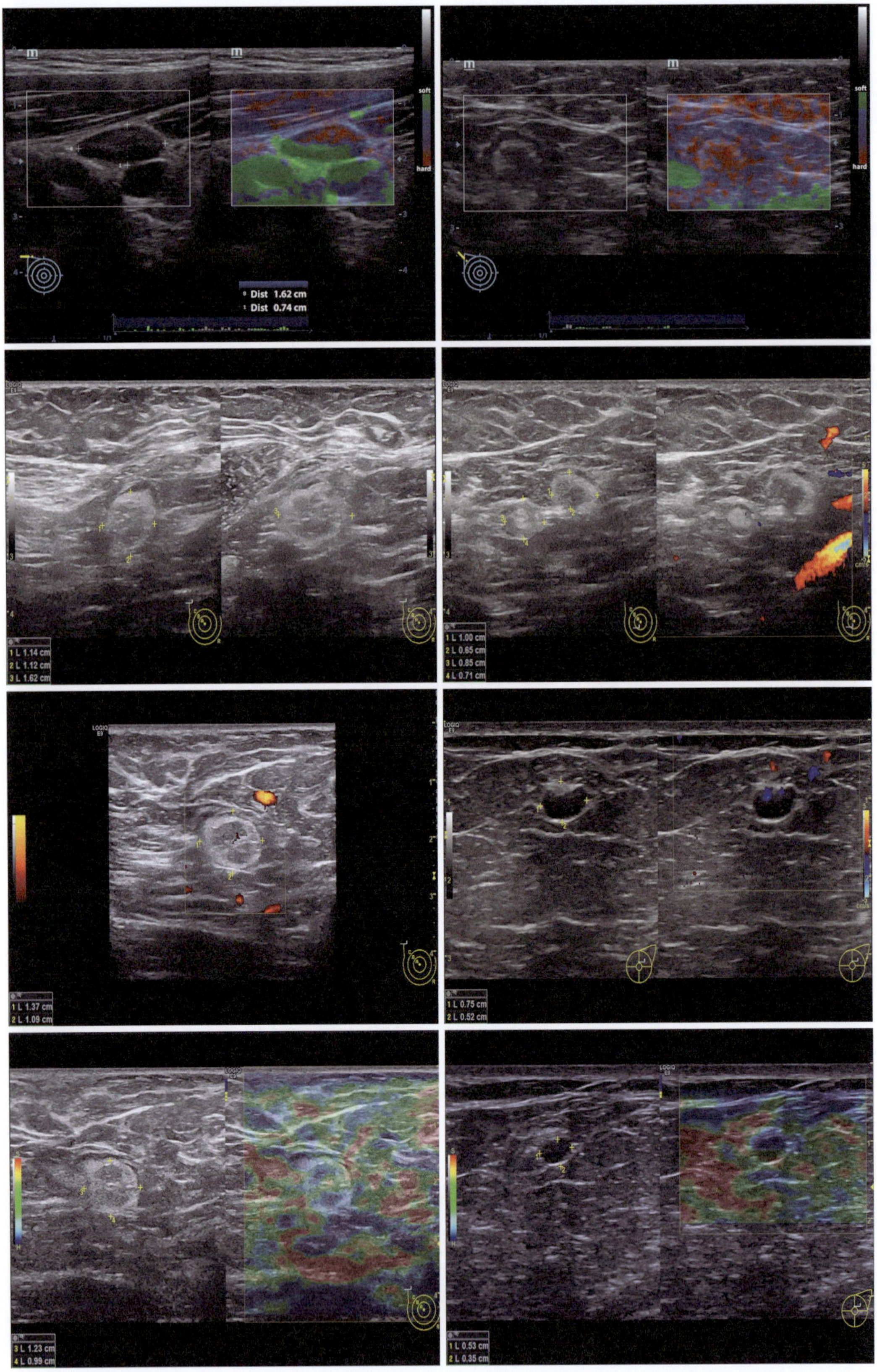

Fig. 10.6 (continued)

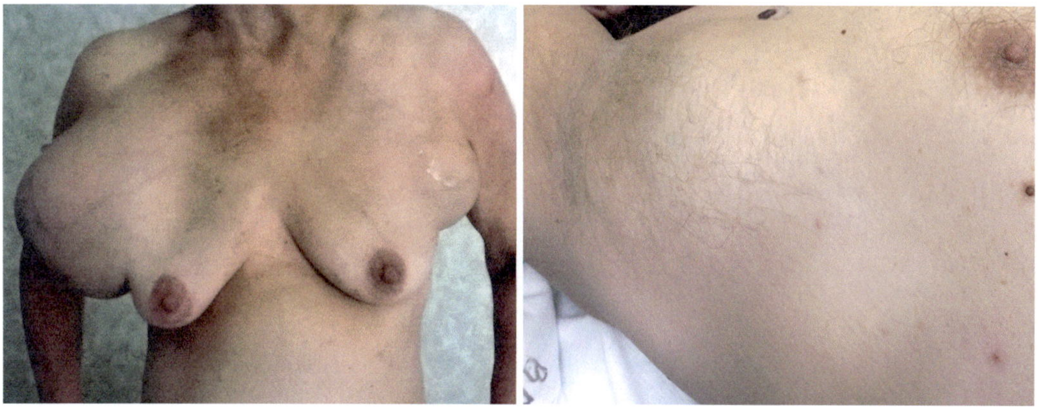

Fig. 10.7 1–2 Breast cancer with metastatic axillary lymph nodes. Photo. Patient's general appearance. Enlargement of axillary lymph nodes

in the axillary area. It is much more informative than palpation and mammography in defining the nature of enlarged lymph nodes. Up to 55% of sonographically detected abnormal lymph nodes are impalpable.

According to Trufanov et al. (2009), metastatic axillary lymph nodes are characterized by multiple "chain" nodes involvement (>2), only on the breast cancer side, oval shape, heterogeneous echostructure, rough contours, and irregular thickening of the margins, sometimes with formation of conglomerates and compression of nearby structures and vessels.

Rough indistinct margins of a lymph node at grayscale echogram are, as a rule, a consequence of capsule invasion. Heterogeneity of echostructure, presence of anechoic inclusions, and calcifications are signs of necrosis and fibrosis within the affected lymph node. Echogenicity of a metastatic lymph node is associated with morphological structure of the primary tumor and the proportion of lymphoid and tumoral tissue. Along with the decrease in normal elements within the lymph node, its structure becomes more homogeneous and hypoechoic (Kharchenko and Rozhkova 2005). According to Trufanov et al. (2009), metastatically changed supra- and subclavicular expansion and neck lymph nodes are of round or irregular shape. They are hypoechoic with distinct and uneven contours. As a rule, parasternal and interpectoral lymph nodes preserve their inner differentiation and color pattern (in 40% of cases). Many researchers believe that narrowing or absence of the hilum in combination with thickened cortical layer denotes malignant changes.

The risk of metastases in regional lymph nodes depends on the size of the primary tumor. Breast cancer of stages T1–T3 metastasizes in axillary lymph nodes in 3%, 7%, and 15% of cases, respectively. Metastatic progression leads to expansion of the tumor outside the lymph nodes to the surrounding fat. Lymph node metastases with extracapsular expansion and infiltration of surrounding tissues often merge and involve the surrounding organs and structures (subcutaneous adipose tissue and muscles).

Color coded modes are now widely used. They help to assess angioarchitectonics and blood supply of lymph nodes (Kharchenko et al. 1993; Smirnova 1995; Cosgrove et al. 1990; Madjar et al. 1995). CDI detects vascularization in 93% of metastatically changed lymph nodes. Blood vessels are often of irregular caliber, twisty, and chaotically distributed. When analyzing vascular patterns of lymph nodes with CDI and PDI, it is necessary to compare affected and normal sides. The state of feeding arteries and intraparenchymal vessels is conveniently assessed with 3D spatial imaging. Spatial reconstruction allows to assess visual characteristics of vascular structures: spatial symmetry of a vessel and its branches, asymmetric dilations, and narrowings.

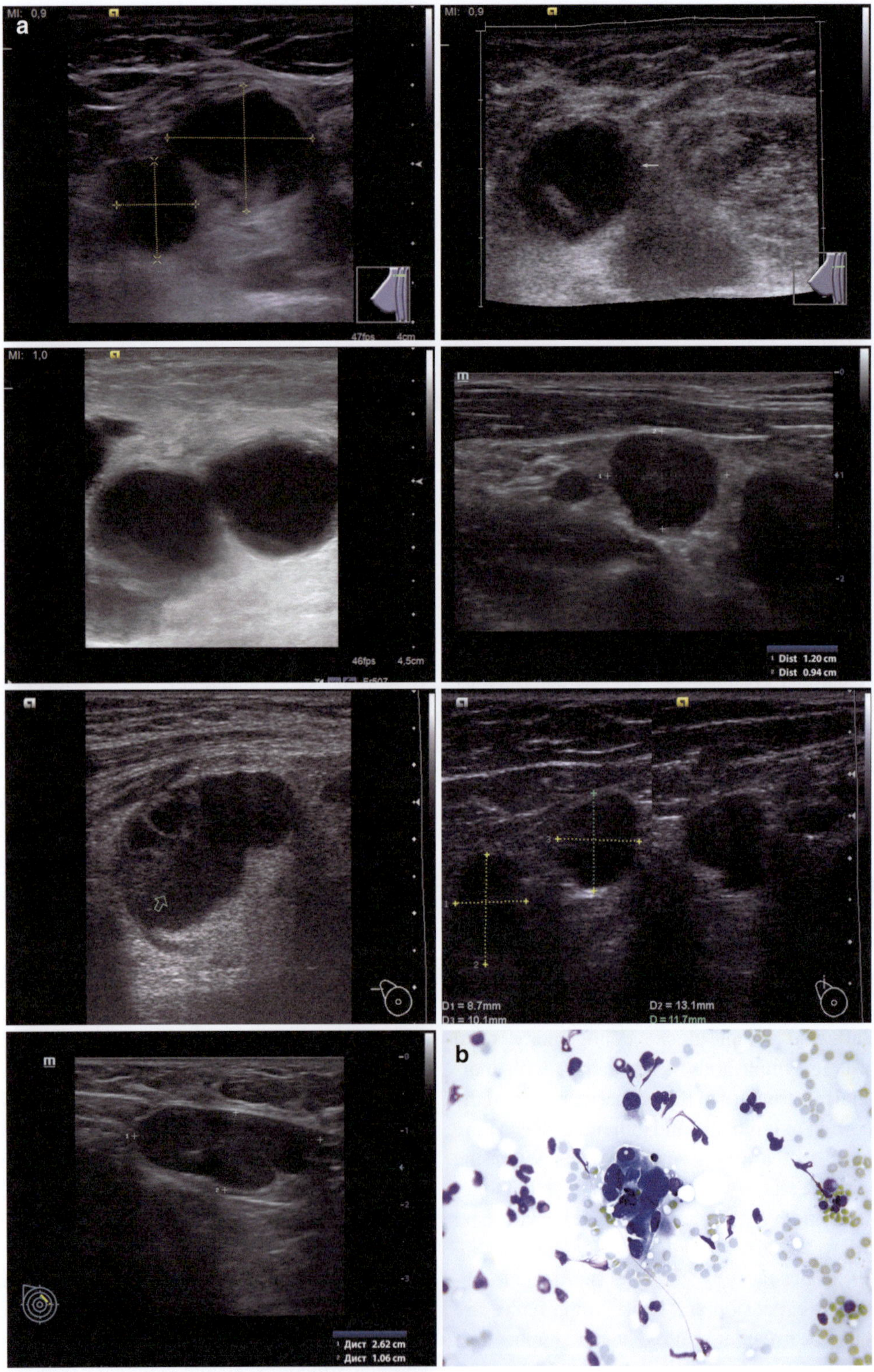

Fig. 10.8 Breast cancer metastases in the axillary and subclavian lymph nodes. (**a**) 1–7 Grayscale echograms. (**b**) Metastasis of medullar breast cancer in the axillary lymph node. H&E-stained image of a section; original magnification, ×400

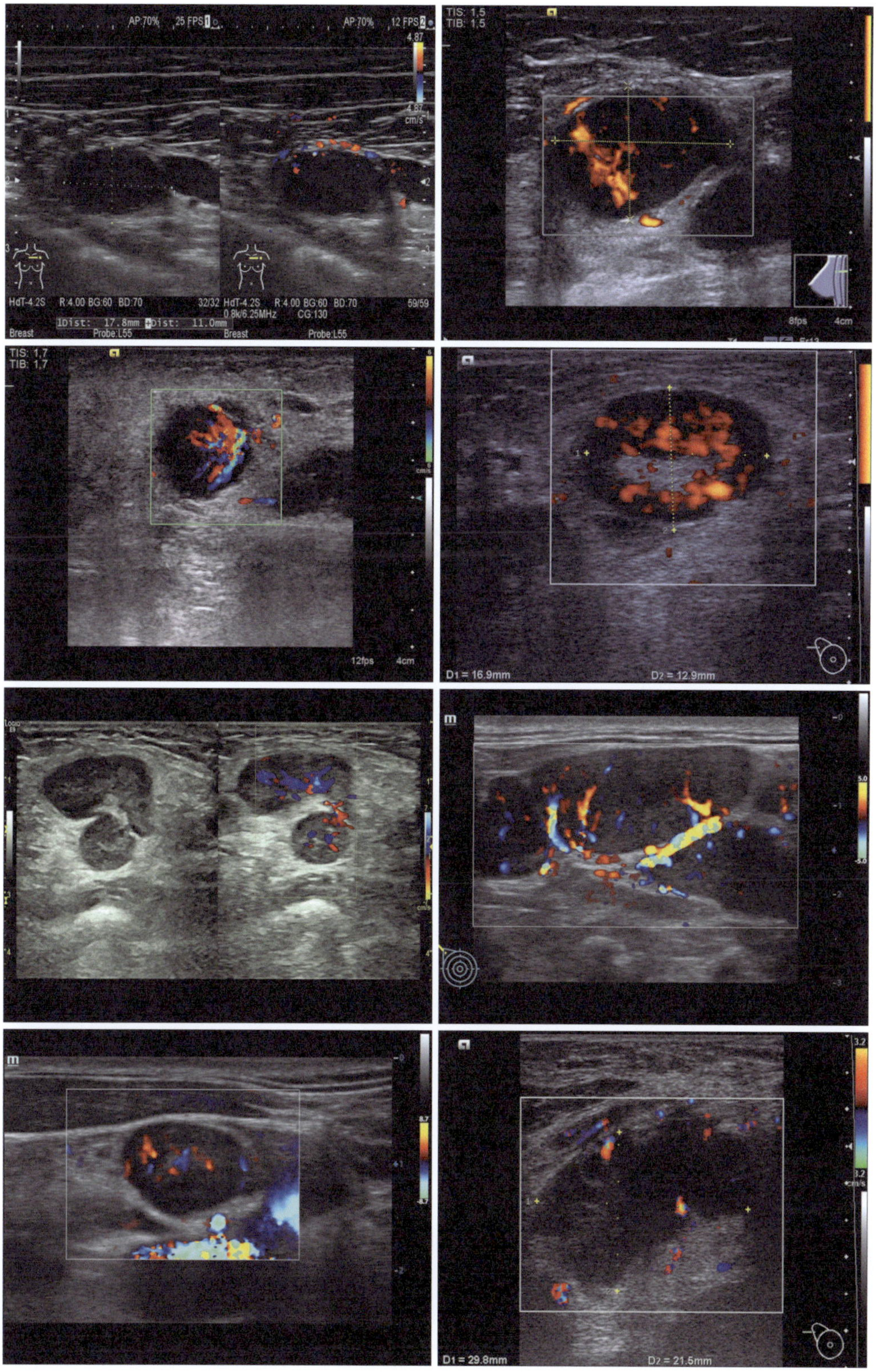

Fig. 10.9 1–8 Metastases of breast cancer in axillary lymph nodes. CDI and PDI

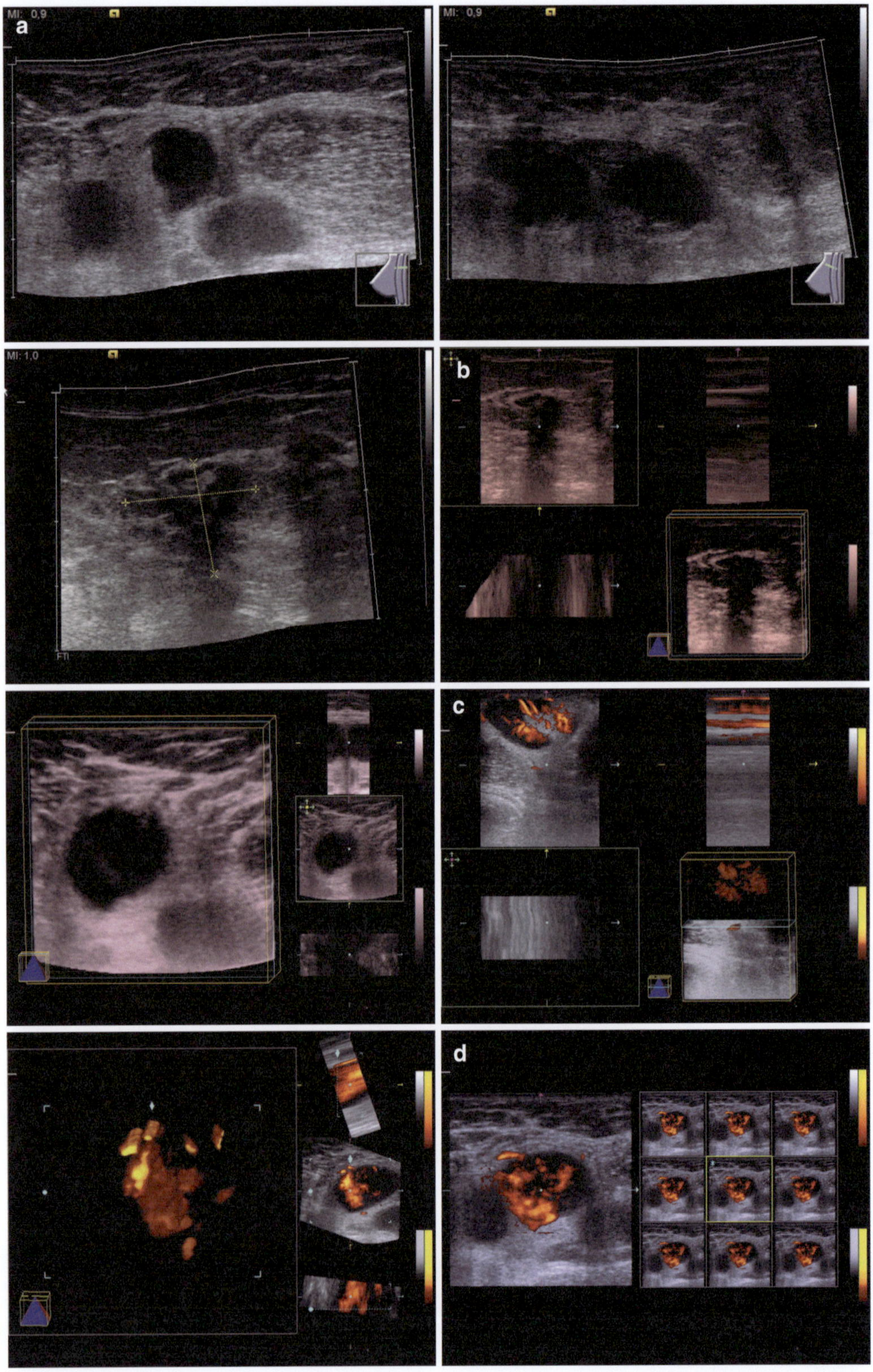

Fig. 10.10 Metastasis of breast cancer in axillary and subclavian lymph nodes. (**a**) 1–3 Panoramic scan. (**b**) 1–2 3D US. (**c**) 1–2 3DPD. (**d**) Multislicing

Metastatic changes in lymph nodes are often characterized by a moderate or high degree of vascularity. According to Trufanov et al. 2009, lymph nodes may appear avascular or exhibit single color signals in the central part or along the periphery of the node. The average indices of blood flow in these lymph nodes are PSV, 42.8 ± 2.5 cm/s; EDV, 10.5 ± 0.8 cm/s; RI, 0.75 ± 0.01; and PI, 1.6 ± 0.06. Some authors suggest EDV can be used to differentiate metastatic and reactive lymph nodes. Meanwhile, high indices of PW Doppler are sometimes found in lymph node hyperplasia. Some researchers believe that a significant increase of RI > 0.9 (others indicate >0.73) or RI decrease is a criterion for malignancy. Difficulties in assessment of lymph nodes with PW Doppler are caused by tortuous, multidirectional blood vessels within lymph nodes, which prevents from correct measurements and is time-consuming.

Compression US elastography does not always correctly image abnormal lymph nodes (Fig. 10.11). Strain ratio below 3.28 is likely to be associated with reactive lymph nodes (88.9%). Compression elastography allows to assess the class of BI-RADS lymph nodes, which is statistically and clinically significant for further management of the patient (metastatic lymph nodes refer to class 4 BI-RADS, while reactive lymph nodes refer to class 2 BI-RADS).

The sensitivity of compression US elastography in diagnosis of metastatic breast cancer is 84% with specificity of 83.3%.

Metastases induce distortion of vascular pattern of affected lymph nodes including hilar blood vessels. Tumor infiltration of the cortex is associated with neoangiogenesis and an increase in the number of capsular vessels. It leads to peripheral hypervascularization with twisty and aberrant vessels feeding the periphery of the tumor lesions. These changes can be observed with contrast-enhanced ultrasonography (Fig. 10.12).

CEUS is a very accurate method for evaluation of axillary lymph nodes and detection of metastatic lesions in breast cancer. Its diagnostic value is similar to sentinel lymph node biopsy: sensitivity, specificity, and accuracy are 100%, 82%, and 92%, respectively.

Sentinel lymph node biopsy (SLNB) as an alternative to lymphodissection in patients with early stages of breast cancer with no clinical signs of metastatic lesions in axillary lymph nodes. The first nodes (1–3), into which lymph fluid flows from the breast are considered sentinel. SLNB is currently a "gold standard" of surgical intervention in areas of regional metastasis in patients with early breast cancer with no clinical signs of axillary lymph nodes lesions. Patients with micrometastases (<0.2 mm), or solitary tumor cells in sentinel lymph nodes, or with a limited number of lesions in sentinel lymph nodes (1–2) do not need full axillary lymphadenectomy, provided that postoperative radiotherapy and adjuvant systemic therapy will be performed (Lyman et al. 2017). In this regard, it is extremely important to find reliable tools that allow to suspect metastatic lesions of regional lymph nodes before surgery. In the publication of Verheuvel et al. (2015), it was demonstrated that patients with axillary metastases detected by ultrasound had larger tumor sizes ($p < 0.001$), worse prognosis, higher degree of malignancy ($p = 0.001$), presence of lymphovascular invasion ($p = 0.035$), HER2-positive status ($p = 0.006$), absence of expression of hormonal receptors ($p = 0.003$), macrometastases ($p < 0.001$), extranodal spread ($p < 0.001$), and level 3 of lymph node lesion ($p < 0.001$) in comparison with patients, in whom the axillary lymph node metastases were diagnosed with SLNB. Accordingly, the patients with metastases in regional lymph nodes, who were diagnosed with ultrasound, had a lower 5-year recurrence-free and a 5-year overall survival rates in comparison with the patients from the SLNB group (72.6% vs. 87.7% and 73.0% vs. 82.4%, respectively, $p < 0.001$). Therefore, an increase in the sensitivity of ultrasound will allow to diagnose metastases in axillary lymph nodes prior to surgery, and thus will decrease the number of patients subject to SLNB, and, unfortunately, increase the number of patients, who will undergo axillary lymphadenectomy in full volume. This will lead to the increase of postoperative complications, such as

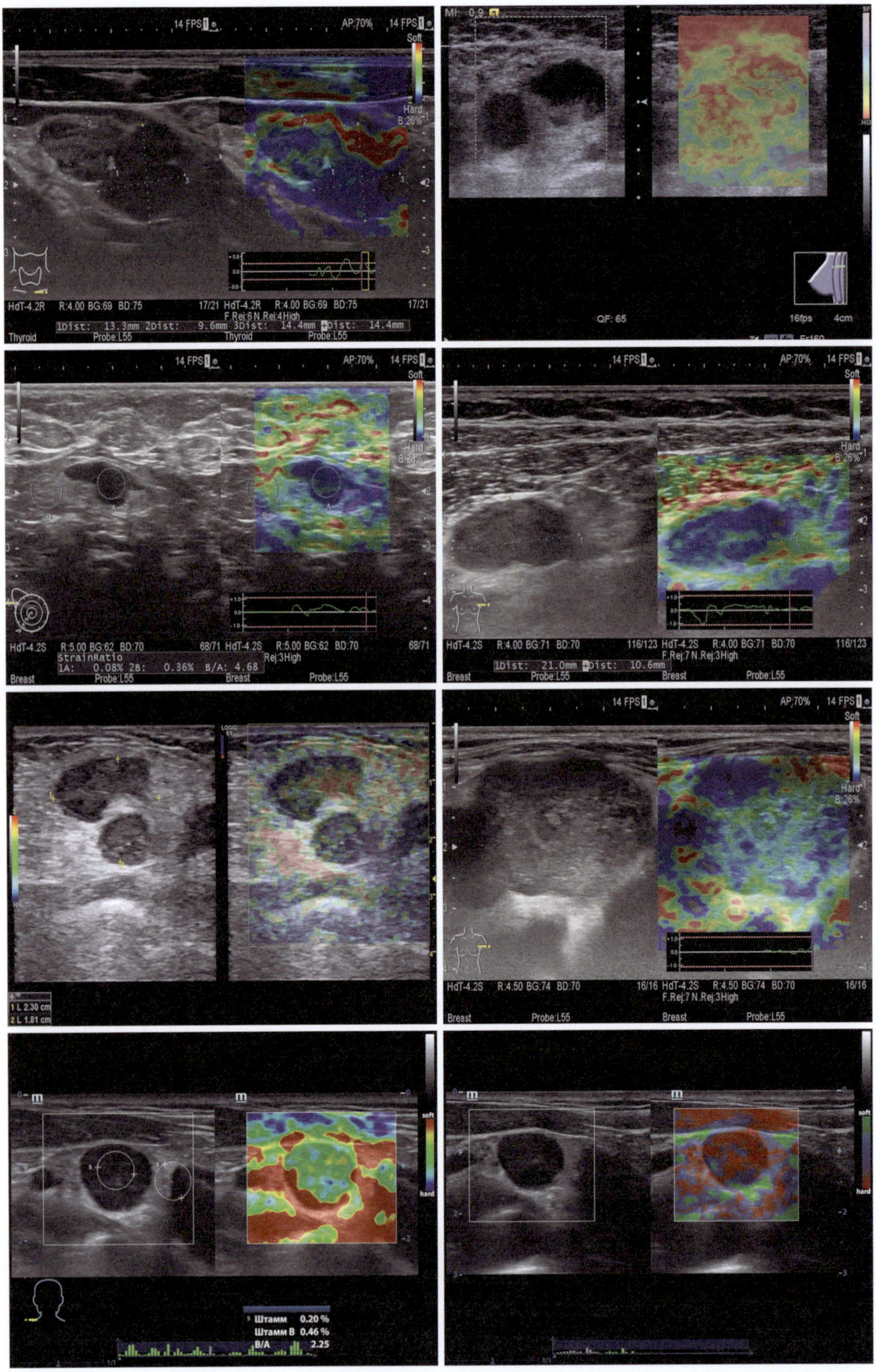

Fig. 10.11 1–8 Metastases of breast cancer in axillary and subclavian lymph nodes. Compression US elastography. Various coloring modes

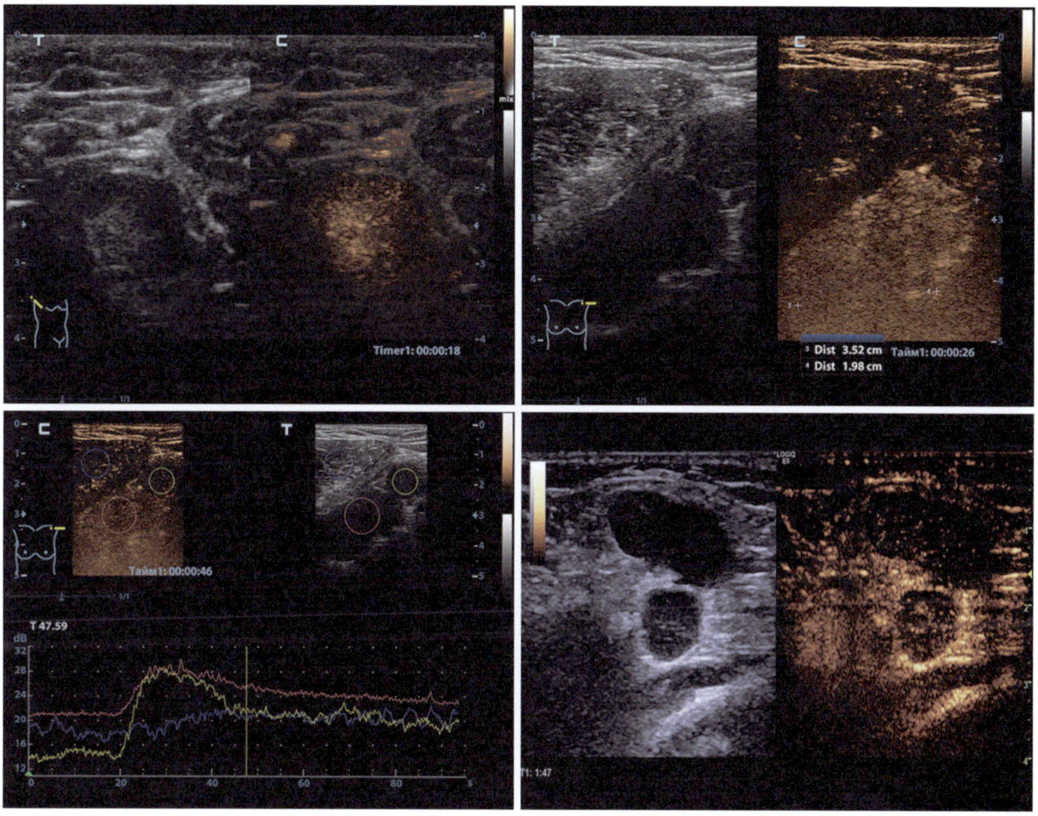

Fig. 10.12 1–4 Metastatic axillary lymph node. Contrast-enhanced ultrasonography. SonoVue, 2.4 mL. Echograms. Deformation of the hilum of lymph nodes

pain, movement restriction, and edema of the upper limb. Thus, a paradoxical situation arises: the better is ultrasound diagnosis of metastases in regional lymph nodes, the greater is the likelihood of developing serious postsurgery complications in patients with breast cancer.

Given that breast cancer in men is more aggressive than in women, metastatic changes in regional lymph nodes are found in men earlier, primarily in axillary lymph nodes. Only 34% of patients apply for medical care with primary manifestations of the disease; in 46.8% significant local spread is found at the first visit. Early affection of regional lymph nodes is associated with both anatomical features of male breast and with active contractions of the muscles of the anterior chest, resulting in increased local lympho- and blood circulation. That is why the enlargement and density of axillary lymph nodes may be one of the first signs of the disease. Approximately every second patient with breast cancer has enlarged axillary lymph nodes at his first address to the doctor. However, the reliability of clinical assessment of the axillary zone is not high. False positive results range from 8% to 50%. Ultrasound characteristics of metastatic lymph nodes in male breast cancer do not differ from those in women. The volume and severity of changes often depend on the nature and extent of the tumor.

Ultrasonography does not allow to determine the morphological characteristics of the lymph nodes. However, it identifies indirect signs that assist a clinician in further diagnostics. Incorrect assessment of regional lymph nodes may lead to disruption of treatment or inadequate surgical interventions. This worsens the prognosis and the quality of patients' lives. Finally, the question of the nature of abnormal lymph nodes is often solved with US-guided FNAB followed by cytology. Biopsy of regional lymph nodes is still a standard staging procedure. FNAB allows to increase the ultrasound sensitivity in detection of axillary lymphadenopathy up to 96%, the specificity up to 94%, and the diagnostic accuracy up to 88%.

Distant metastases are observed in 6–55.5% of patients with breast cancer. They are detected mainly in the peripheral parts of the lungs (29.4–62.5%), in pleura, bones (5.2–31.4%), mediastinal lymph nodes (7.5%), the liver, brain, ovaries, or neck lymph nodes (Rozhkova 1993). Less often breast cancer metastasizes to the thyroid gland, pancreas, retroperitoneal or submandibular lymph nodes, anterior abdominal wall, or soft tissues of the extremities (Sinyukova et al. 2007) (Fig. 10.13).

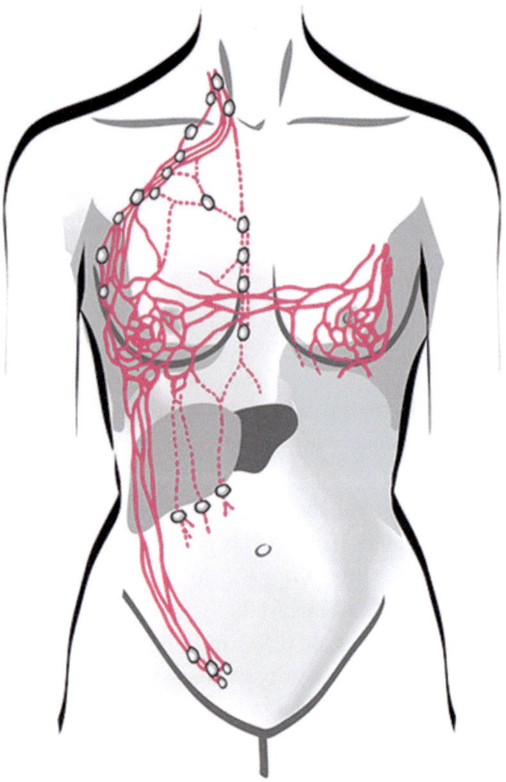

Fig. 10.13 Lymphatic spread of breast cancer. Scheme

Up to 20% of men with breast cancer have distant metastases at the first visit, while 18–54% of patients develop distant metastases after treatment of a local disease. Early metastatic dissemination of breast cancer in the lungs is often multiple (78.3% of cases), while late metastases appear multiple only in 38.6% of cases.

Metastases of breast cancer in men are more often detected in the interval of 4 months–9 years after the primary treatment. The highest incidence of metastasis (50%) occurs in the first 3 years, in the next 2 years another 25% evolve, and 25% are found in 6–9 years. These data confirm the need for not only effective integrated systemic treatment at early stages of breast cancer in men but also the development of effective therapy at the later stages of the disease.

Other radiological methods can be used for detection of distant metastases: X-ray, CT, MRI, and scintigraphy.

Ultrasonography should be used to detect the lesions of the abdominal organs (first of all, the liver), pelvic organs, retroperitoneal space, thyroid gland, soft tissues, the pleura, inguinal, and other superficially located lymph nodes to specify the extent of the disease and to rule out distant metastasis (Figs. 10.14, 10.15, and 10.16).

Less often, breast may be the site for metastatic lesion of malignant tumors of other localizations, for example, in melanoma, colorectal cancer, and kidney tumors (Fig. 10.17). Such metastases to male breast are also extremely rare. There are only few publications on metastatic lesions of the breast in men with prostate, pancreatic, and thyroid cancer. Diagnostic mistakes are expectable in such cases. Specification of the lesions bases on the results of fine or core needle biopsy with morphological study.

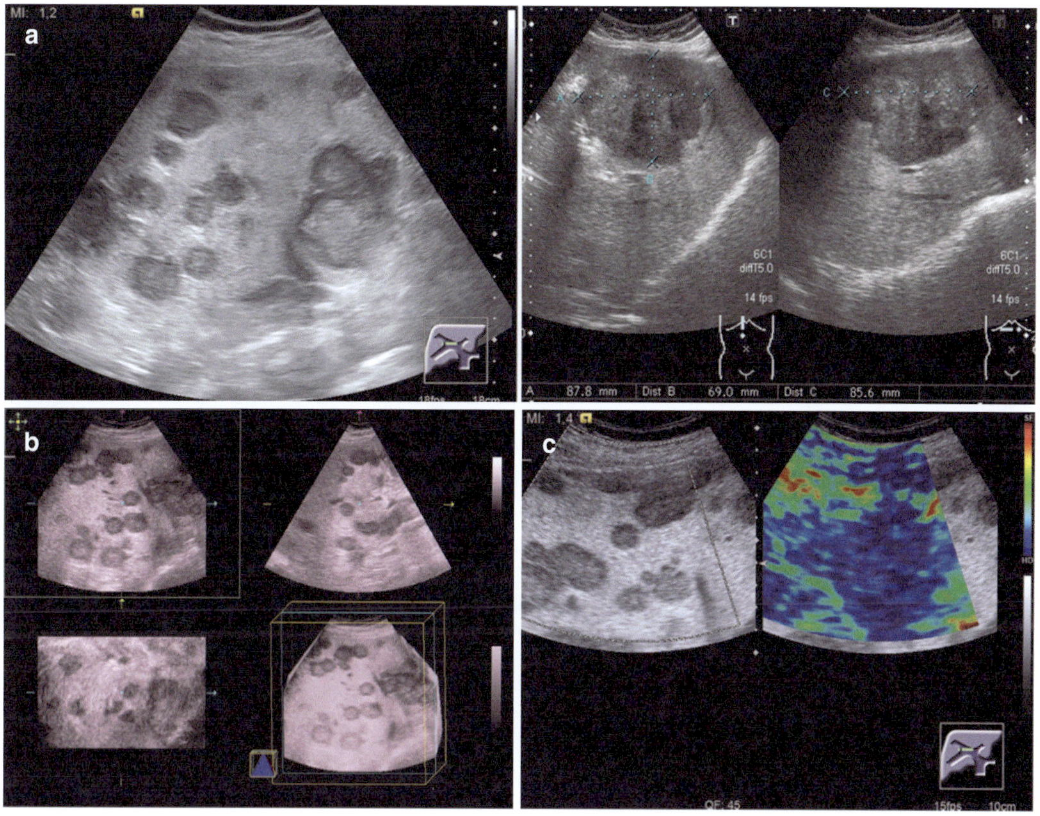

Fig. 10.14 Metastases of breast cancer in the liver. (**a**) 1–2 Grayscale US. (**b**) 3D. (**c**) Compression US elastography

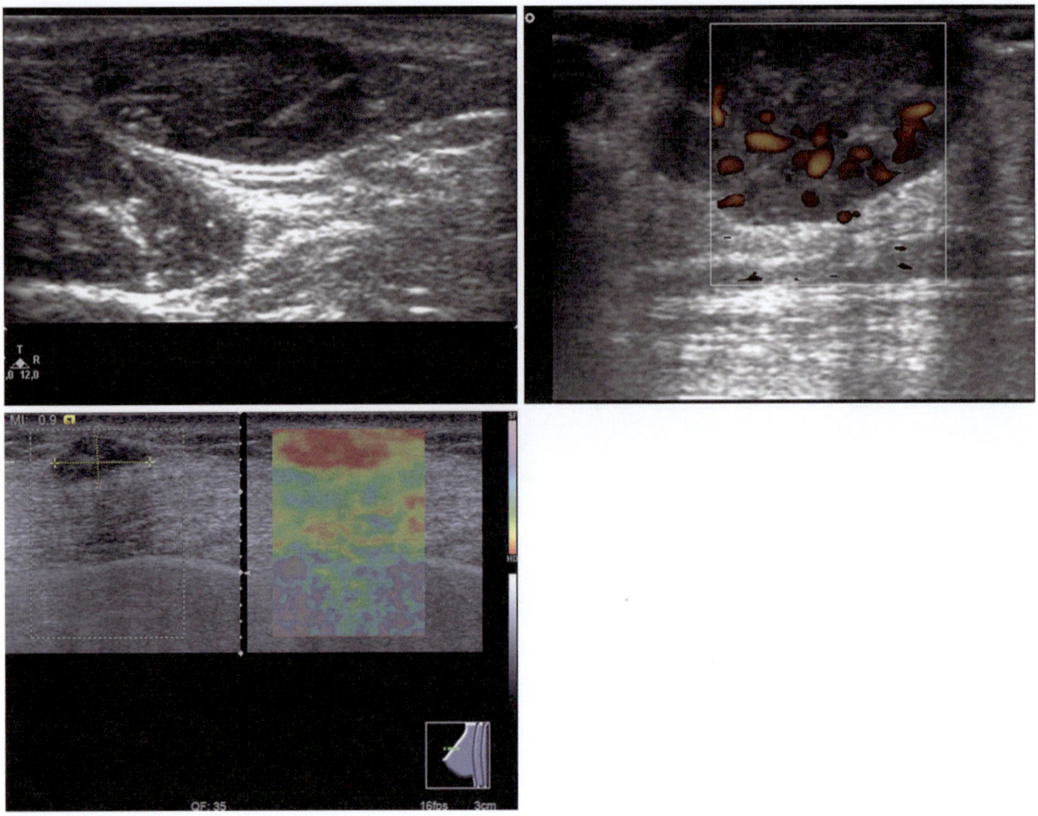

Fig. 10.15 Metastases of breast cancer in soft tissues. (**a**) Grayscale US. (**b**) PDI. (**c**) Compression US elastography

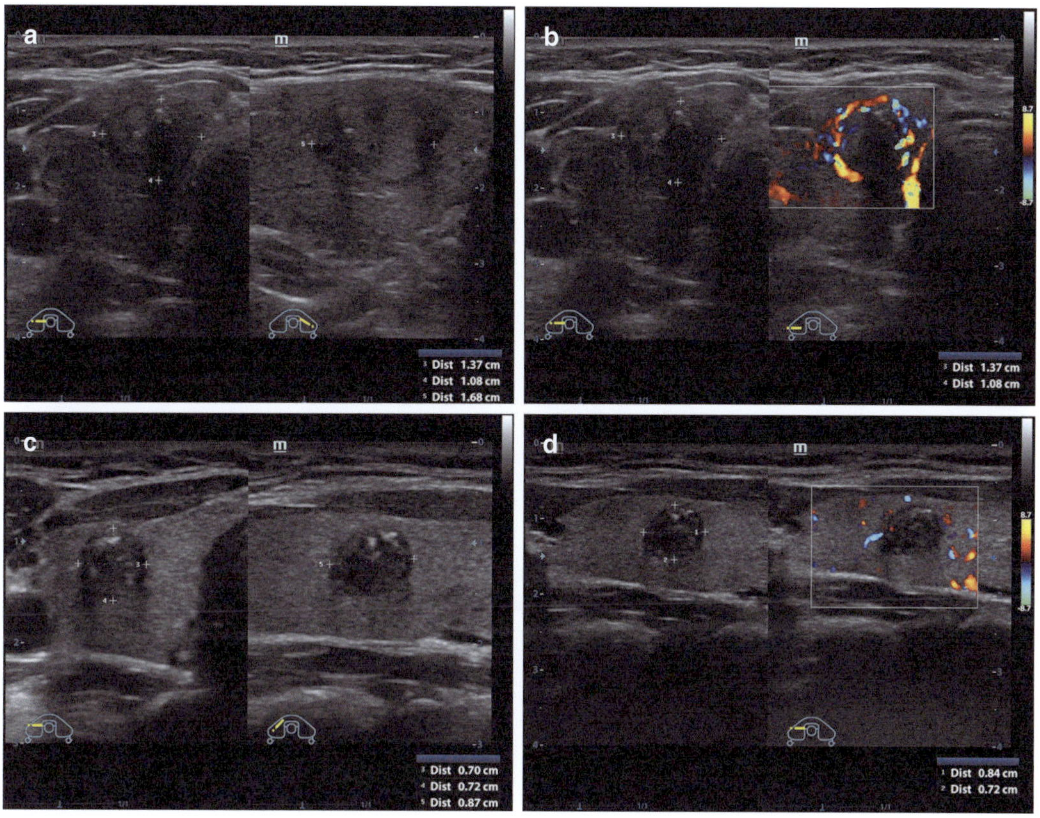

Fig. 10.16 Metastasis of breast cancer in thyroid parenchyma. (**a**, **c**) Grayscale US. (**b**, **d**) CDI

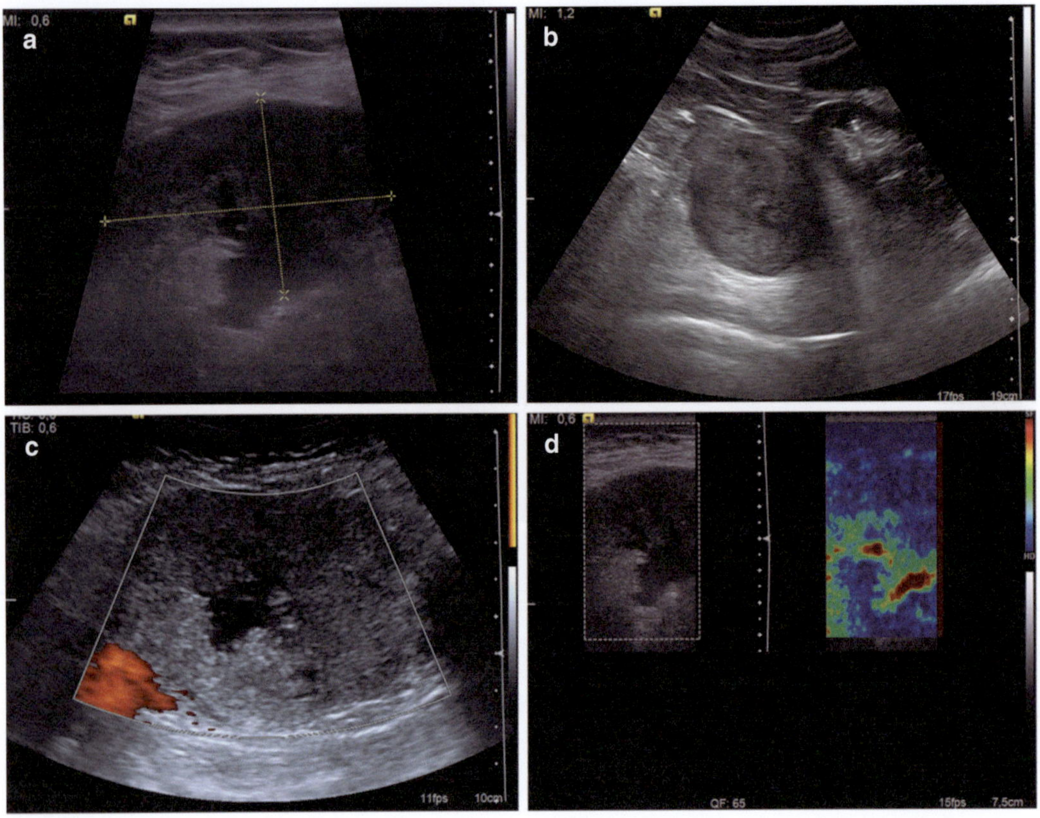

Fig. 10.17 Metastasis of skin melanoma in the breast. (**a**, **b**) Grayscale US. (**c**) CDI. (**d**) Compression US elastography

11 Ultrasound of Postoperative Breast

Valeriy Rodionov and Alexander N. Sencha

Abstract

Today, 60–80% of newly diagnosed breast cancer cases are treated with breast-sparing surgery. Breast-sparing procedures (tumorectomy, radical resection) include extensive tumor excision with simultaneous one-stage axillary lymphadenectomy. To reduce the volume of axillary lymphadenectomy and the risk of early (formation of lymphatic cysts and infections) and late (postmastectomic syndrome) complications, sentinel lymph nodes biopsy is used. Most common postsurgical complications are bleeding, hematomas, lymphorrhea, seromas, infectious complications, lipogranulomas, and complications due to implants. Depending on the terms, surgical complications are divided into early, which occur in the nearest 6 weeks after surgery, and late, which occur later. Breast reconstruction means only aesthetic restoration. The goal of breast reconstruction includes restoration of breast volume, creation of its aesthetic shape, and restoration of the skin, nipple-areolar complex, and symmetry. Breast reconstruction with an implant (silicone) or with patient's own tissues may be used. Different authors report breast cancer recurrence after radical resection or radical mastectomy in 2.8–71%. Puncture biopsy of solid lesions in postoperative breast or its bed and postsurgical scars is mandatory and often a key aspect for differentiation and verification of tumor recurrence.

V. Rodionov (✉)
Department of Breast Diseases, National Medical Research Center for Obstetrics, Gynecology and Perinatology named after Academician V.I. Kulakov of Ministry of Healthcare of Russian Federation, Moscow, Russia

A. N. Sencha
Division of Visual Diagnostics, National Medical Research Center for Obstetrics, Gynecology and Perinatology named after Academician V.I. Kulakov of Ministry of Healthcare of Russian Federation, Moscow, Russia

11.1 Breast Condition After Surgery: Ultrasound Follow-Up

Present-day advances in the treatment of breast cancer have significantly influenced the course of the disease and life expectancy. A few decades ago, the diagnosis of disseminated breast cancer practically was a sentence, and the main treatment task was to relieve the symptoms of the disease. The average life expectancy of patients did not exceed 12–15 months; 15% of patients survived for more than 3 years, only 10% for more than 5 years. Today, the average life expectancy of such patients is 51 months. Three- and 5-year overall survival in some cancer types (metastasis in bones and soft tissue) is 61% and 40%, respectively (Semiglazov 2001). In some cases,

G. T. Sukhikh, A. N. Sencha (eds.), *Multiparametric Ultrasound Diagnosis of Breast Diseases*,
https://doi.org/10.1007/978-3-319-75034-7_11

aggressive treatment for both the primary tumor and metastases allows to prolong the patients' life up to 15 years and longer in more than 25% of cases. The need for the revisal of the treatment strategy and the tactics in patients with newly diagnosed, disseminated, and so-called oligometastatic breast cancer does really exist, as modern technologies help to detect the minimal signs of distant metastases that quite recently were left behind. The number of patients with detected disease at stage IV is increasing. They are 7% of the total number of newly diagnosed breast cancer.

In treatment of patients with breast cancer, a comprehensive approach is used, which includes both local (surgery and radiation therapy) and systemic (chemotherapy, hormonal therapy, etc.) impacts on the primary tumor. Treatment of patients with breast cancer should be implemented by a multidisciplinary team, including a surgeon-oncologist, chemotherapist, radiotherapist, oncomorphologist, and radiologist. Treatment tactics should be based on clinical characteristics (the size and location of the primary tumor, the degree of lymph nodes involvement) and the biological features of the tumor (pathomorphological characteristics, including biomarkers and gene expression). It also depends on the age, general health condition, and preferences of a patient.

The standard treatment option for early breast cancer is surgery with subsequent adjuvant systemic treatment. This approach improves the indices of both recurrence-free and the overall survival. In a local advanced (inoperable) process, the neoadjuvant treatment has been used for several decades, which leads to the disease downstage allowing to perform surgery in most patients. Currently, the neoadjuvant treatment is used not only for inoperable but also for operable tumors, both with the purpose to ensure for organ-sparing treatment instead of radical mastectomy and to determine sensitivity to systemic therapy.

Surgery is the main treatment option and, when applicable, is carried out as the first step depending on the local status of the tumor. Presurgery treatment can reduce the mass of the primary tumor and suppress the probable micrometastases present by the time of diagnosis. Despite the large number of globally conducted clinical trials on the effectiveness of various therapeutic schemes, there is no strong evidence about the combinations with best results. After removal of the primary tumor, relative risk of death is reduced by 39%. Three-year survival rate is 35% in patients after surgery with "clean" resection margins, 26% in the group with the residual disease in the resection margins, and 17.3% in unoperated patients.

The type and volume of surgical intervention is determined primarily by the nature and extent of breast pathology, as well as the extent of the surrounding tissues involvement.

In this regard, there are the following types of surgery:

1. Surgery for inflammatory breast diseases (acute and chronic mastitis) by opening and draining of an abscess
2. Surgery for benign and malignant breast tumors (e.g., fibroadenoma, breast cancer, nodular fibrocystic breast disease, etc.)

   The following operations can be performed:
   - Total breast tumor biopsy
   - Sector resection
   - Radical resection
   - Mastectomy
   - Axillary dissection
1. Plastic procedures:
   - Augmentation mammoplasty with silicone implants
   - Reduction mammoplasty
   - Mastopexy
   - Breast reconstruction (including single-stage breast reconstruction) after subtotal subcutaneous mastectomy

Classical radical Halsted-Meyer mastectomy involves removal of the breast, including the skin, breast tissue, areola, and nipple, major and minor pectoral muscles, as well as bloc axillary dissection. Classical radical mastectomy is often complicated by postmastectomy syndrome—pain and limited mobility in shoulder joint and upper limb lymphedema.

Sparing Patey-Dyson mastectomy preserving the large pectoral muscle includes removal of the breast and small pectoral muscle and axillary lymph node dissection. In Madden mastectomy, both pectoral muscles are preserved. Sparing mastectomies are accompanied by less postsurgical complications in comparison with classical mastectomy.

Skin-sparing mastectomy is a technique comprising removal of the breast tissue with preservation of the entire skin envelope, and in some cases the nipple-areolar complex. This type of mastectomy allows to minimize the scar area and to preserve the natural breast contours for the purpose of its further reconstruction.

At present, the indications for mastectomy are as follows: large tumor size (relative to the breast size), impossibility to achieve negative margins of resection, previous radiotherapy on the chest wall/breast or other contraindications to radiation therapy, or patient's choice. In other cases, preference should be given to breast-sparing treatment.

Today, 60–80% of newly diagnosed breast cancer cases are treated with breast-sparing surgery. Breast-sparing procedures (tumorectomy, radical resection) include extensive tumor excision with simultaneous one-stage axillary lymphadenectomy. Absolute contraindications for breast-sparing surgery are pregnancy, when radiation therapy is necessary, diffuse "suspicious" microcalcifications on mammograms, and extensive tumor spread, when tumor removal with a single incision and good cosmetic outcome are not possible. Relative contraindications are previous radiation therapy on the chest or breast, systemic diseases with skin lesions (especially scleroderma and systemic lupus erythematosus), a tumor >5 cm, and positive resection margins. Currently, surgical margin is assessed with staining of invasive tumor or ductal carcinoma in situ (DCIS). At least 2 mm tumor-free margin is considered negative. For patients, who underwent breast-sparing treatment, the cosmetic outcome is very important. To achieve this, oncoplastic transplantation is used. Oncoplastic approaches may lead to better cosmetic results, especially in patients with large breast, unfavorable tumor-breast proportion, or cosmetically disadvantageous tumor location in the breast (in the central zone or in the lower hemisphere).

To reduce the volume of axillary lymphadenectomy and the risk of early (formation of lymphatic cysts and infections) and late (postmastectomic syndrome) complications, sentinel lymph nodes biopsy is used. Sentinel lymph nodes are those first (1–3) lymph nodes in the chain of lymphatic drainage of the breast. Sentinel lymph nodes can be visualized with the use of contrast-enhanced, radionuclide, and fluorescent imaging. Double mapping technique (administration of radiocolloid + methylene blue dye), or use of indocyanine green fluorescence after SLNB, allows to identify sentinel lymph nodes in >97% of cases. Sentinel lymph nodes biopsy, in contrast to total axillary lymphadenectomy, is now accepted as a standard for surgical staging of regional lymph nodes in early breast cancer in the absence of clinical evidence of metastasis. Besides, all patients with micrometastases or isolated tumor cells (<0.2 mm) in sentinel lymph nodes with minimal number of affected lymph nodes (1–2) in cases of applied postsurgical radiotherapy and adjuvant systemic therapy do not need total axillary lymph node dissection (Lyman et al. 2017).

Breast reconstruction means only aesthetic restoration. The goal of breast reconstruction includes restoration of breast volume, creation of its aesthetic shape, and restoration of the skin, nipple-areolar complex, and symmetry.

There is no optimal method of reconstruction, which could be applied to all patients with equal success. Currently the following techniques are used:

- Breast reconstruction with an implant (silicone)
- Breast reconstruction with patient's own tissues (latissimus dorsi muscle flap—LD-flap), lower transverse rectus abdominis musculocutaneous flap (TRAM-flap), deep inferior epigastric perforator flap surgery (DIEP-flap), superior gluteal artery perforator flap (S-GAP-flap) surgery
- Combined reconstruction using both methods

Both a simultaneous and a delayed breast reconstructions are possible. Restoration of symmetry is necessary for achievement of good results. Therefore, in order to comply with these conditions, as well as to improve the appearance of the breast, surgical interventions on the contralateral breast are often necessary. These may be:

- Reduction mammoplasty
- Augmentation mammoplasty
- Mastopexy
- Preventive mastectomy

The best variant of reconstruction for each patient should be discussed individually, taking into account anatomical features, treatment, prognosis of the disease, and the patient's preferences.

New techniques of surgical treatment and wide application of breast-sparing procedures demand corresponding diagnosis. New diagnostic algorithms that allow to plan the most adequate surgical treatment, to predict and effectively detect early and late complications, and to diagnose early signs of tumor recurrence after surgery are necessary. The role of ultrasound, the integrated application of the latest and innovative technologies in this regard, is absolutely crucial.

Most common postsurgical complications are:

- Bleeding, hematomas
- Lymphorrhea, seromas
- Infectious complications
- Lipogranulomas
- Complications due to implants

Depending on the terms, surgical complications are divided into early, which occur in the nearest 6 weeks after surgery, and late, which occur later.

Ultrasound in early postoperative period aims to diagnose the complications caused by accumulation of the blood or lymph under the skin flaps, when drainage is abnormal. With increased lymphorrhea, the fluid accumulates in the tissues subcutaneously and in interfascial spaces and is visualized as homogeneous anechoic regions of various sizes with uneven margins. They form so-called seromas and lymphocele. With the increase in fluid volume in the tissues, accompanied by fever and worsening of general health condition, targeted punctures are performed under ultrasound control with fluid aspiration.

Hematoma is diagnosed as an anechoic or hypoechoic heterogeneous mass with linear echogenic inclusions (clots), of regular (less often irregular) shape, and with clear even contours, avascular at CDI, PDI, and 3DPD (Fig. 11.1). Hematoma is sometimes difficult to differentiate with seroma, which is often a finding on the background of postoperative tissue changes. Both seromas and hematomas are avascular with color Doppler and CEUS.

Increased echogenicity of the skin and underlying tissues, often with small fluid inclusions among the fat lobules, indicates the lymphatic edema—local lymphostasis in the postsurgical area (Fig. 11.2).

In case of large hematoma, an US-guided puncture or surgical drainage is performed.

The features of tissues that form the scar after mastectomy (collagen fibers, loose connective tissue, fibrosis), the severity of edema, and aseptic inflammation provide a variety of ultrasound images in the scar area. Sometimes ultrasound fails to show any signs of the scar or just notes some structural deformations of reduced or increased echogenicity, heterogeneous echostructure, and linear (sometimes irregular) shape, less often with posterior acoustic shadows; avascular at CDI, PDI, and 3DPD; and moderately heterogeneously colored at compression US elastography (Figs. 11.3 and 11.4).

Despite the fact that reconstruction of breast with the use of the patient's own tissues is a very sophisticated technique and very traumatic procedure for the patient, it allows to attain good aesthetic outcome in the majority of patients (Fig. 11.5).

Lipogranulomas (oleogranulomas) are often found after oncoplastic breast-sparing surgery and breast reconstruction with patients' own tissues. Lipogranulomas are a consequence of adipose tissue necrosis and often exhibit a palpable mass with indistinct contours, skin hyperemia or cyanosis, local edema, skin dimpling over the mass, or retraction of the nipple.

With ultrasound, the manifestations of fat necrosis vary from solid hypoechoic mass with dense acoustic shadow to complex cystic masses that decrease in size with time. This histologically corresponds to involution of fat necrosis. Cystic masses may have hyperechoic inclusions or a parietal component. Solid masses can have clear or indistinct borders on the background of the distorted architectonics of breast parenchyma. A specific US feature of fat necrosis is the mobility of hyperechoic inclusions within the cystic content, when the patient changes the position.

Hyperechoic masses, which may be the signs of necrosis, usually are not oncologically worrisome, as hyperechoic lesions account for less than 0.8% of cancers. Despite the low incidence, differential diagnosis should be made with invasive ductal and lobular cancer, lymphoma, and angio- or liposarcoma. Basic ultrasound characteristics (margins, shape, abnormal blood flow) justify a fine needle or core biopsy of the mass or follow-up.

The use of implants in breast reconstruction is the most common technology. According to the

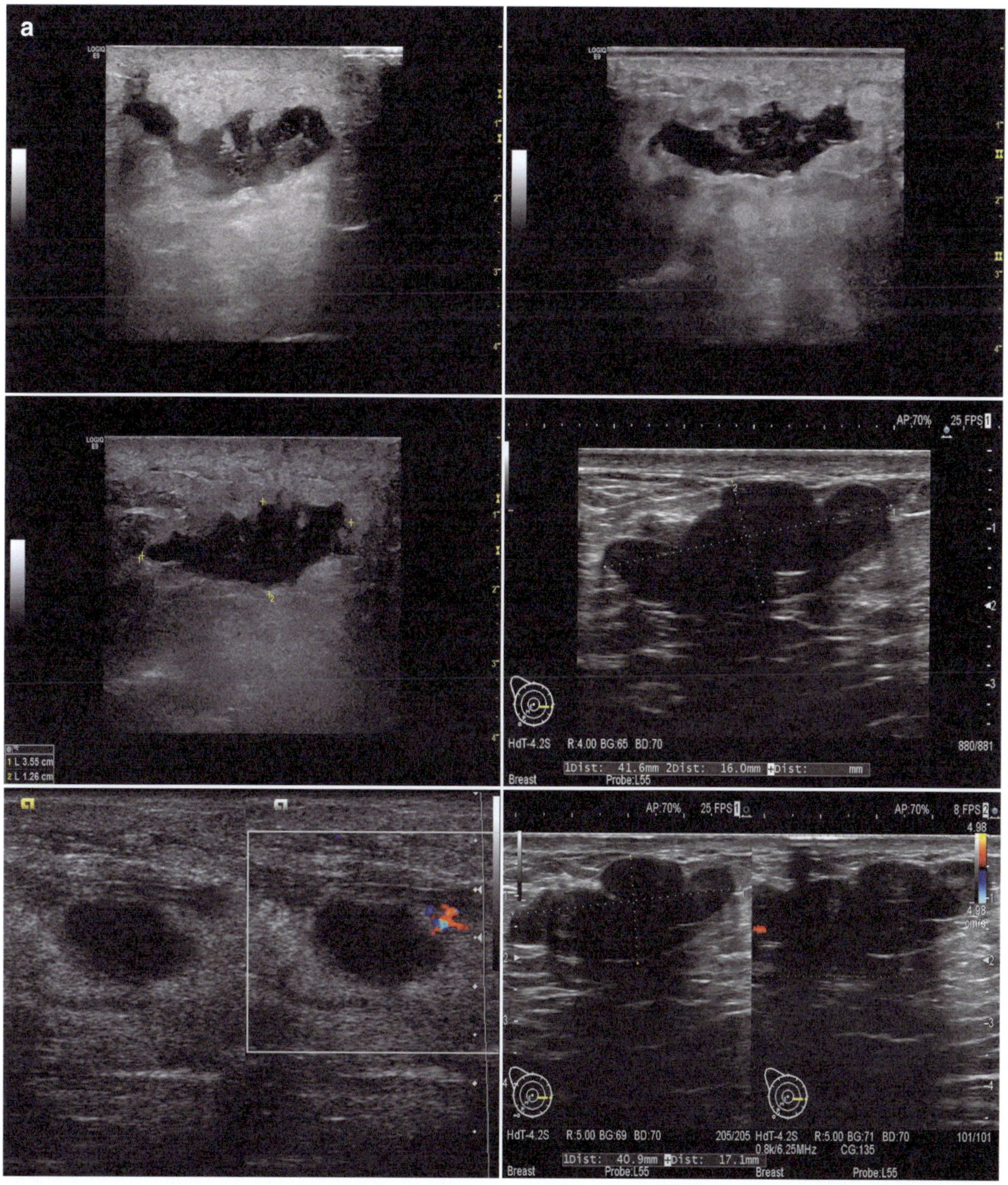

Fig. 11.1 State after breast sector resection. (**a**) Hematomas of postsurgical scar. 1–4 Grayscale US, 5–6 CDI. (**b**) Seroma of postsurgical scar. 1–2 Grayscale US. 3–4 CDI. 5–6 CEUS

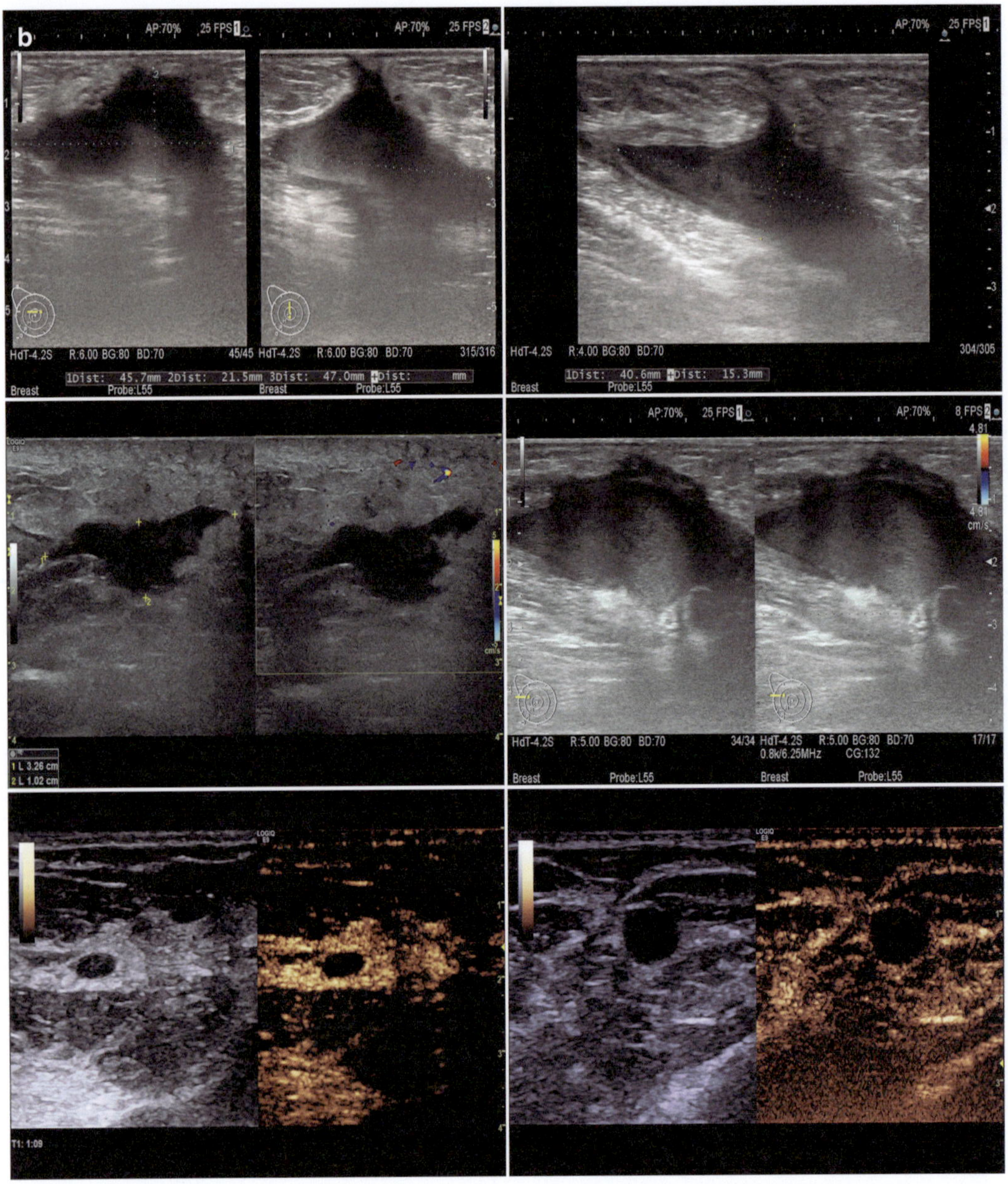

Fig. 11.1 (continued)

American Society of Plastic Surgeons, there has been an annual increase in the number of plastic surgeries. The total number of interventions in 2011 was 1,579,079. More than 200,000 procedures are performed annually in the United States and more than 130,000 in the UK. The main advantages of this technology are fast and simple surgical procedure, insignificant blood loss, and no need for donor tissues. Such reconstruction is performed using three variants of implants:

- Endoprosthesis filled with silicone gel or isotonic NaCl solution
- Tissue expander, which is used to stretch the tissues with subsequent replacement with an endoprosthesis
- Permanent expander, combining the possibilities of stretching, but which is not replaceable

Modern prostheses have multilayer barrier shells to prevent rupture of the implant and gel

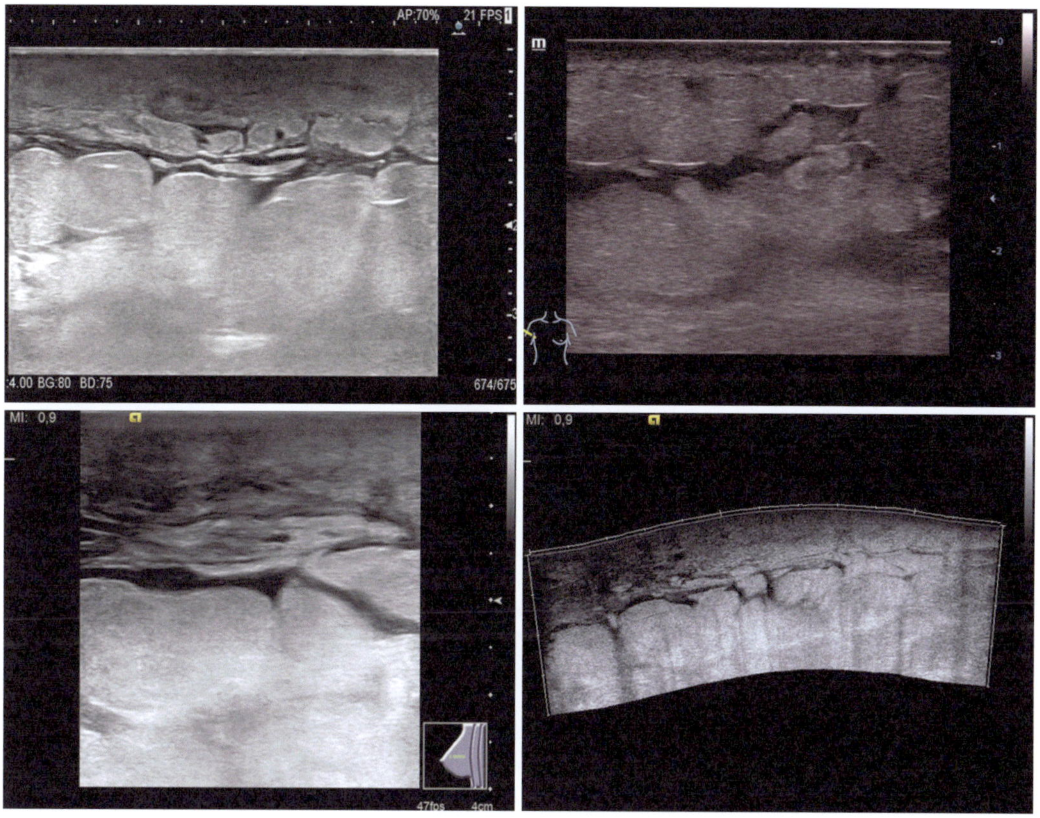

Fig. 11.2 State after radical breast resection. Lymphostasis. 1–4 Grayscale US and panoramic scan

contamination. The texturized surface, as well as the micro-polyurethane coating of the implants, solves the problem of capsular contracture, not allowing the myofibroblasts to form linear structures, which may constrict the capsule.

Understanding of possible implant positions in the anterior thorax greatly facilitates and systematizes ultrasound imaging.

Breast reconstruction comprises development of the space under the large pectoral muscle, which is separated from the place of its attachment in the lower and lateral parts, and subsequent implant placement. The lateral and inferior areas of the implant are covered with the mobilized anterior pectinate muscle together with the subcutaneous flap of the upper epigastric region or part of the fascia of the rectus abdominis muscle.

When performing augmentation mammoplasty, there are several options for implant placement, which are usually well defined basing on the echography data, such as the following:

- Under breast tissue
- Under the fascia of the pectoralis major muscle
- In two areas: the lower part of the implant (large)—under the breast tissue, the upper part—and under the pectoralis major muscle
- Completely under the muscle

Breast ultrasound in the presence of endoprosthesis allows to specify:

- Its location
- Size (thickness, dimensions, gel volume)
- Integrity of the implant
- Its structure, degree of homogeneity
- Its borders, contours
- Condition of the tissues surrounding the implant, normal breast parenchyma, and regional lymph nodes

After mammoplasty, ultrasound usually detects anechoic silicone endoprosthesis of

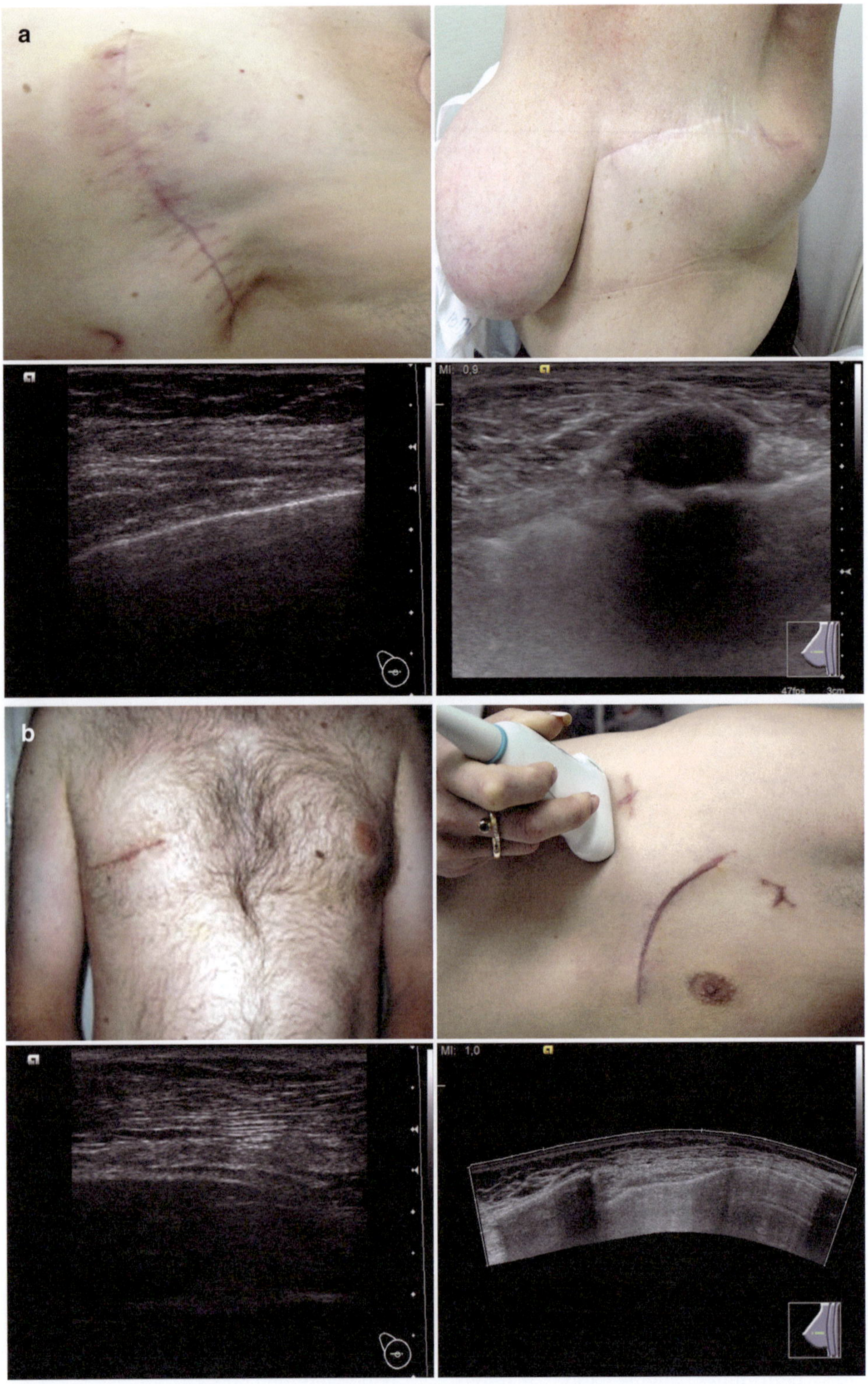

Fig. 11.3 State after mastectomy. Bed of the breast. (**a**) 1–2 View of a woman after surgery. 3–4 Grayscale US. (**b**) 1–2 View of a man after surgery. 3–4 Grayscale US and panoramic scan

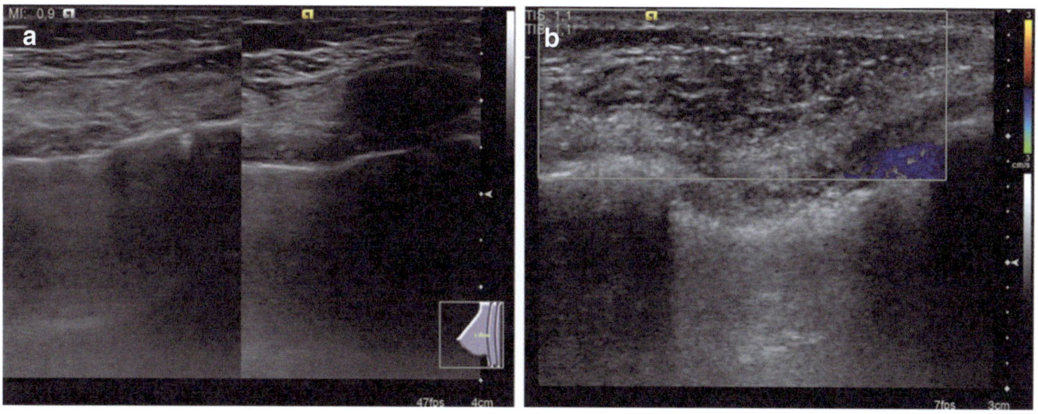

Fig. 11.4 Status after mastectomy. Local fibrosis in the bed of the breast. (**a**) Grayscale US. (**b**) CDI

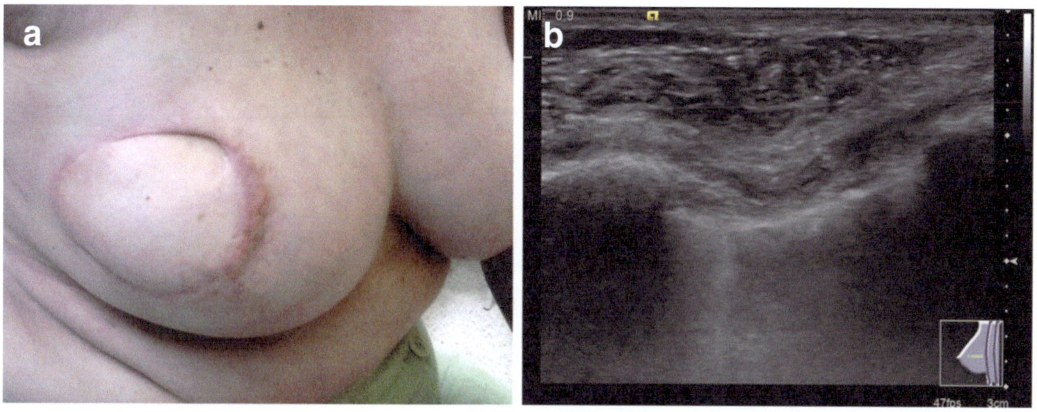

Fig. 11.5 State after mastectomy. Breast reconstruction with a flap. (**a**) View of the breast. (**b**) Grayscale US

regular round-oval shape. Its envelope is visualized as one or more parallel echoic lines (Fig. 11.6). Formation of a periprosthetic fibrous capsule is a normal physiological reaction of breast tissue to a silicone implant, as fibrotic changes are formed around any foreign body. The capsule isolates the prosthesis from the surrounding tissues. The fibrous capsule is visualized as two parallel echoic lines located superficially to the implant shell. The capsule may have even contours but more often looks wavy with radial folds that extend from the periphery to the center of the implant. If the implant is set retroglandularly, the breast tissue is seen in front and adjacent to the capsule of the prosthesis, while the pectoralis major muscle is located behind the implant. In retropectoral placement, the implant is located behind the pectoralis major muscle.

Despite the successful development of plastic surgery, the ratio of postsurgical complications after aesthetic breast surgery remains rather high—6–28.6%, depending on the type of surgical intervention (Shumakova et al. 2011). Unsatisfactory aesthetic outcomes, both early and delayed, are observed in 18–60% of patients. Breast endoprosthetics is the safest type of augmentation mammoplasty, still causing complications in 28.6% of cases. Gel injection mammoplasty causes complications in 90–100% of cases.

Echography (often in combination with X-ray mammography) is capable to detect the following early postsurgical complications (up to 6.9%): disruption of surgical wound, local inflammatory complications (1–53%), bleeding, hematoma (5.6%), and seroma (11.1%). It detects the fol-

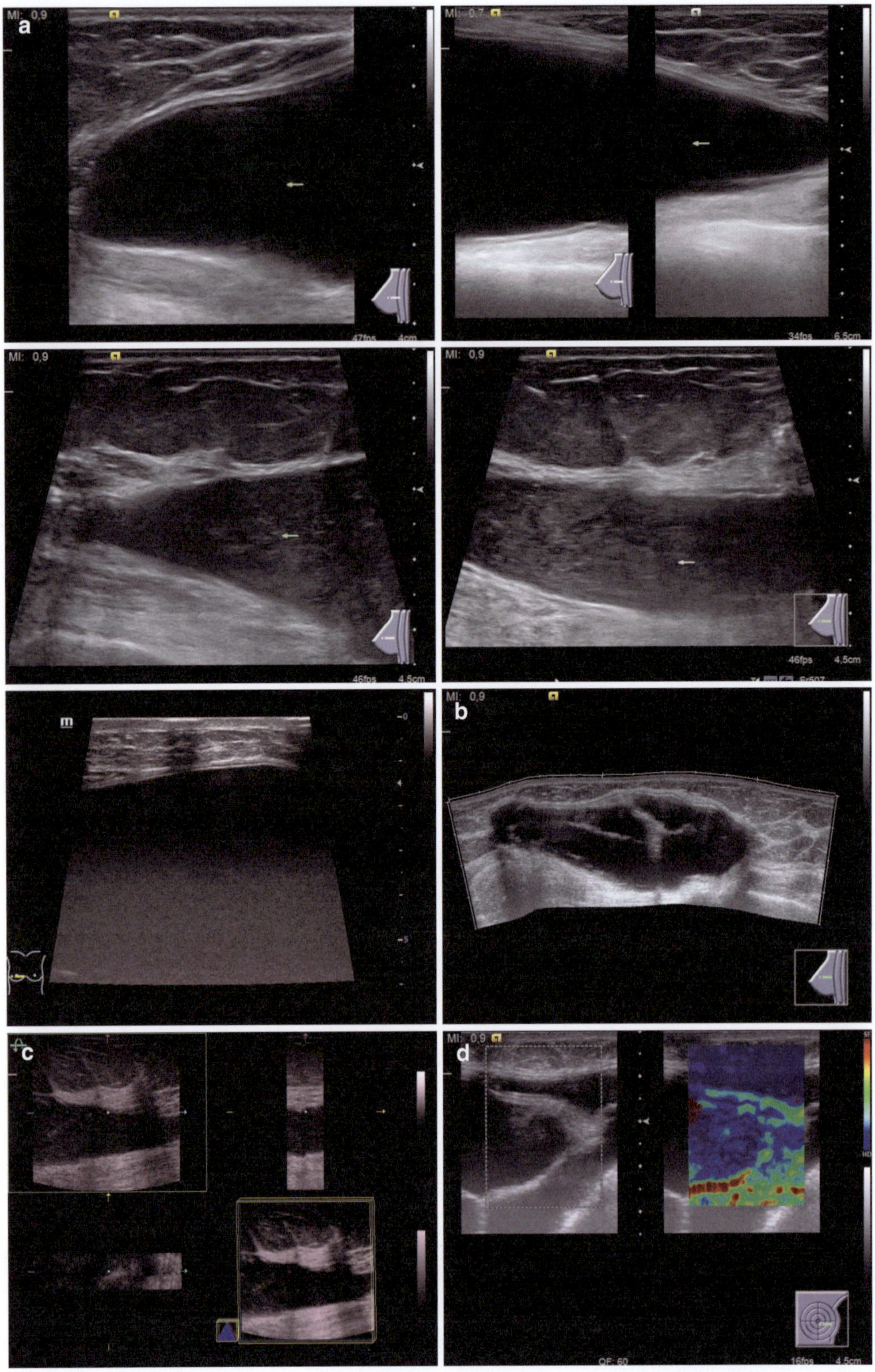

Fig. 11.6 Status after breast reconstruction with endoprosthesis. (**a**) 1–5 Grayscale. (**b**) Panoramic scan, (**c**) 3D. (**d**) Compression US elastography

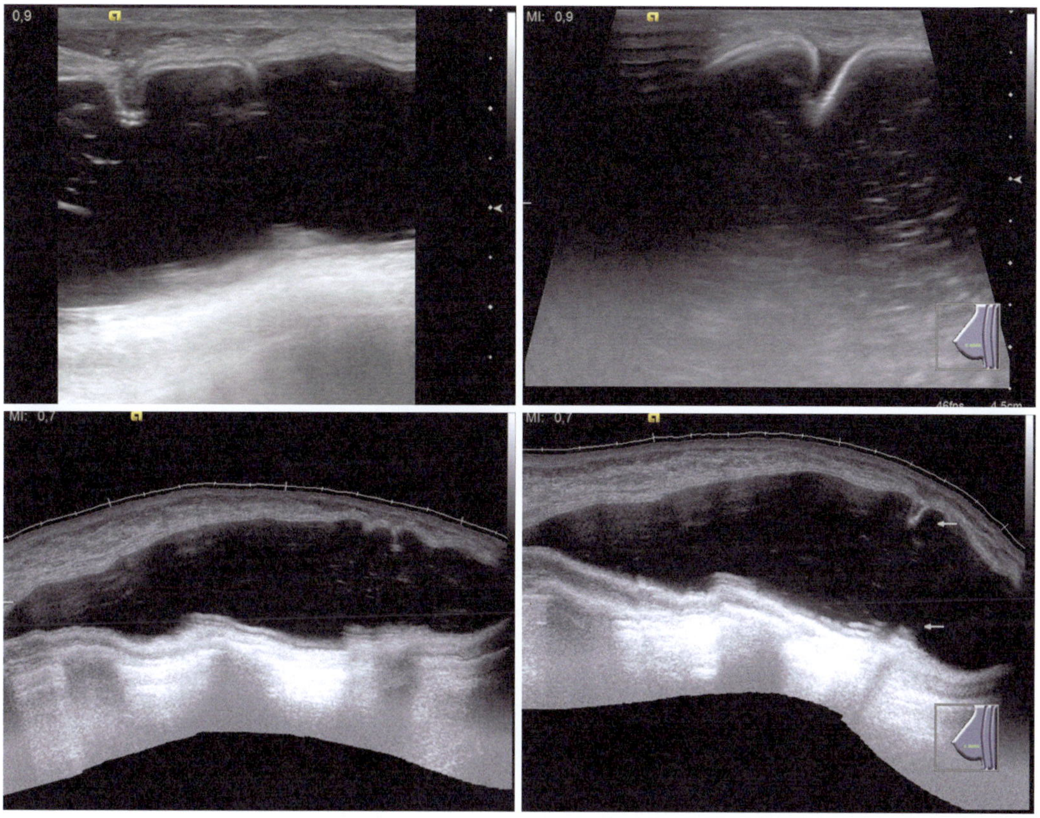

Fig. 11.7 State after mammoplasty with implant. Fibrous capsular contracture of the implant. (**a**) 1–2 Grayscale US. (**b**) 1–2 Panoramic scan

lowing late complications (up to 65.3%): prosthesis rupture (31.9%), pseudotumor, silicone, deep folds, prosthetic hernia (4.2%), fibrous capsular contracture (95.8%), seroma (1–2%), irregular breast volume, and migration and rotation of endoprosthesis (Shumakova et al. 2011).

Imaging after mammoplasty allows early detection, specification of breast and implant changes, dynamic follow-up, and adequate treatment choice. Sensitivity and specificity of imaging methods in mammoplasty complications are as follows: mammography, 37.3–71.3%; ultrasound, 74.7–91.3%; MRI, 81–95%, respectively.

Fibrous capsular contracture is the formation of pathological fibrous capsule around the implant, associated with excessive connective tissue and contraction. Clinically, fibrous capsular contracture manifests with breast induration and subsequent deformation, often accompanied with severe pain. Capsular hypertrophy occurs in 50% of patients with the smooth-shell breast implants and less often in women with textured implants.

The below-listed indirect US signs allow to judge about the development of fibrous capsular contracture after endoprosthetic surgery (Fig. 11.7):

- Change of the shape of implant
- Change of the proportion of implant dimensions
- Increase of the angle between anterior and posterior walls (more than 60°)
- The appearance of deep fixed folds
- Fluid accumulation (seroma) in the implant's capsule

Ultrasound is an effective method of measurement of the depth of peripheral implant's folds, as well as of assessment of the condition of the surrounding breast tissues and their reaction to the implant folds. Deep folds that cause seroma have depth of more than 30 mm. They do not disappear with change in patient's position or breast massage. Seromas are visualized as an anechoic zone between the prosthesis shell and the periprosthetic fibrous capsule.

Implant rupture is the most dangerous complication of endoprosthetics. Implant rupture may be caused by trauma but more often occur spontaneously. The incidence of ruptures is increased with the implant's "age" and reaches its peak 10–15 years after the surgery. Probability for implants' integrity within 5 and 10 years after their installation is 98% and 85%, respectively. Clinically, it is extremely difficult to suspect a rupture of endoprosthesis, as manifestations are nonspecific. The following symptoms may be registered: deformation of the contour (44%), implant displacement (20%), heterogeneity of soft tissues (17%), pain (13%), and inflammation (3%). However, in 50% of cases, physical examination is not reliable. This complication can be diagnosed with ultrasound with sensitivity of 50–70% and specificity of 25–30%. The sensitivity of mammography in detection of implant rupture does not exceed 25–30%. At the same time, the possibilities of ultrasound are limited in assessment of the integrity of the implant's posterior wall and the tissues behind it. The two categories of breast implant rupture are intracapsular implant rupture and extracapsular implant rupture.

Intracapsular implant rupture involves disruption of the integrity of the prosthesis shell and migration of the gel into a cavity bounded by fibrous capsule. Intracapsular ruptures account for 77–89% of all implant damages. This complication shows at ultrasound a "stepladder sign" characterized with multiple horizontal and curved parallel transverse lines inside the implant. Sometimes a small amount of anechoic silicone between the prosthesis shell and the fibrous capsule can be noticed.

Extracapsular rupture is a type of rupture where the integrity of not only implant membrane but also of fibrous capsule is disrupted and silicone gel leaks out to the surrounding tissues. With ultrasound, large aggregates of silicone appear as anechoic or hypoechoic masses, which are difficult to distinguish from cysts. Free silicone is represented as an echoic mass with distinct anterior margin and acoustic shadow—so-called snowstorm sign. Silicone can migrate to axillary lymph nodes, thorax, and abdominal cavity.

Ultrasound often detects heterogeneity of the ruptured implants with hyperechoic linear inclusions (endoprosthesis fragments in silicone) (Fig. 11.8).

Women with breast implants may develop diffuse and focal pathologic conditions similar to those without mammoplasty. According to Shumakova et al. (2011), after augmentation mammoplasty with silicone gel implants, the following breast diseases may occur: mastopathy (88.9%), fibroadenoma (3.5%), mastitis (5.6%), and breast cancer (1.1%) (Figs. 11.9 and 11.10). In recent years, there has been an increase of the incidence of cancer in women with breast implants due to progressing number of plastic surgeries and the use of silicone implants for a long period (more than 20 years). Echography is a crucial method in early and differential diagnosis of breast pathology in the presence of implants. Changes in the breast with implants, especially focal changes (cysts, fibroadenomas, tumors), often do not differ echographically from the breast without implants. The sensitivity of ultrasound in the diagnosis of breast cancer after mammoplasty is 71.4%, specificity 85.7%.

Breast augmentation with gel injection without shell is now less often used than at the end of the twentieth century. This technique often results in severe complications, especially after injection of polyacrylamide gel, which undergoes destruction, dehydration, and fragmentation with subsequent migration of its fragments from the injection site, either under its own gravity or due to muscle contraction. In such cases, gel fragments and gel-impregnated breast are surrounded with a capsule and forms geleoma.

Geleoma is a focus of chronic aseptic lymphocytic inflammation comprising conglomerates and fragments of injected gel (or gel from endoprosthesis), the elements of fibrous deformed breast tissue, capsule, and surrounding tissues. Geleoma may be single or multiple and can be located next or remote to an implant (Fisenko 2014).

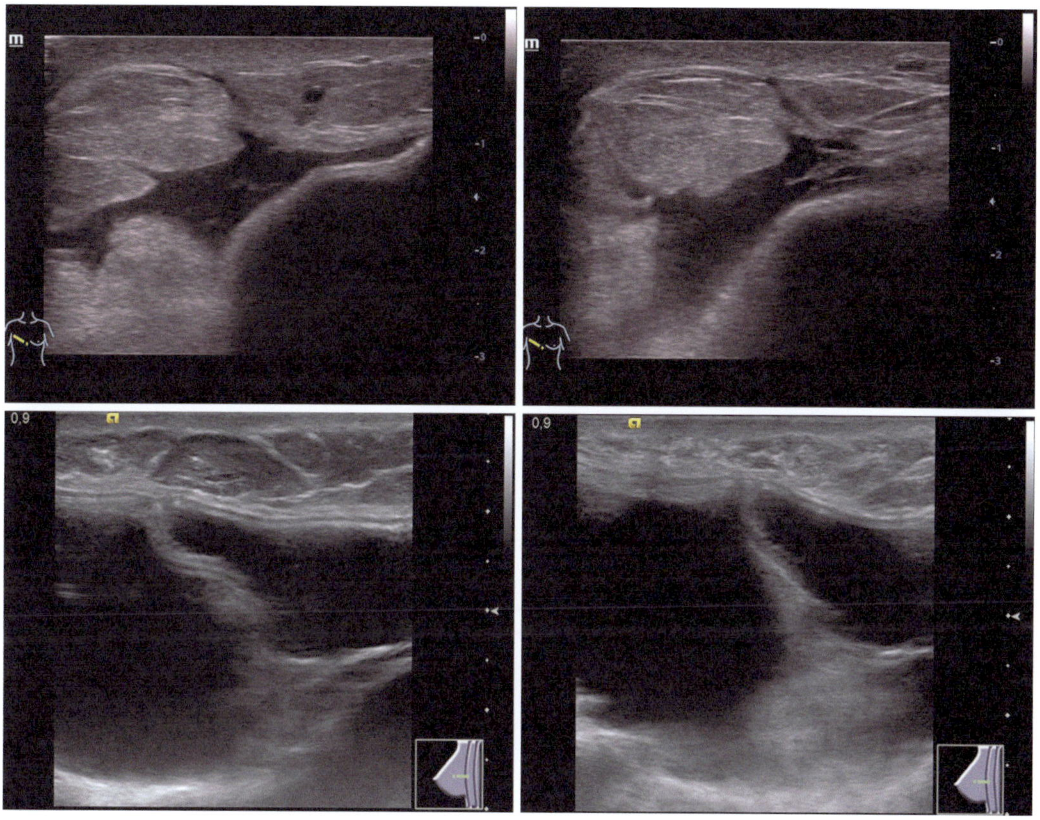

Fig. 11.8 1–4 State after mammoplasty: breast endoprosthesis. Rupture of endoprosthesis. Grayscale US

Geleomas may mimic fibroadenoma or breast cancer with US. According to Fisenko (2014), after breast augmentation mammoplasty, geleomas migrate in a fan-shaped pattern from retromammary space to breast tissue and the surrounding soft tissues, up to the axillary, subclavian, and parasternal areas, and less often down to the iliac region (4.8%).

Ultrasonographic features of geleoma are listed below (Fig. 11.11):

- Low echogenicity
- Regular or irregular shape, uneven thickness
- Heterogeneous echostructure, sometimes with fluid component, hyperechoic inclusions, and septa
- Hyperechoic capsule
- Distinct contours
- Even borders
- The effect of posterior echo enhancement
- Avascular with CDI, PDI, and 3DPD

According to Svensson (1997), there are three types of breast geleomas: cystic (46–56%), sclerotic (3%), and mixed (42–51%).

In color-coded Doppler images, single vessels can be found in large geleomas. This causes difficulties in differentiation with breast cancer. However, the parameters of arterial blood flow in geleomas do not significantly differ from those in the surrounding soft tissues. As a rule, geleomas are classified in the category BI-RADS 4. All geleomas should be punctured and morphologically accessed.

Ultrasound is an available and highly informative method for the assessment of breast condition after mammoplasty, detection of early and late complications, specification of concomitant diseases, and guidance of breast puncture.

Optimal combination of imaging modalities significantly improves the diagnosis of complications and breast diseases after mammoplasty.

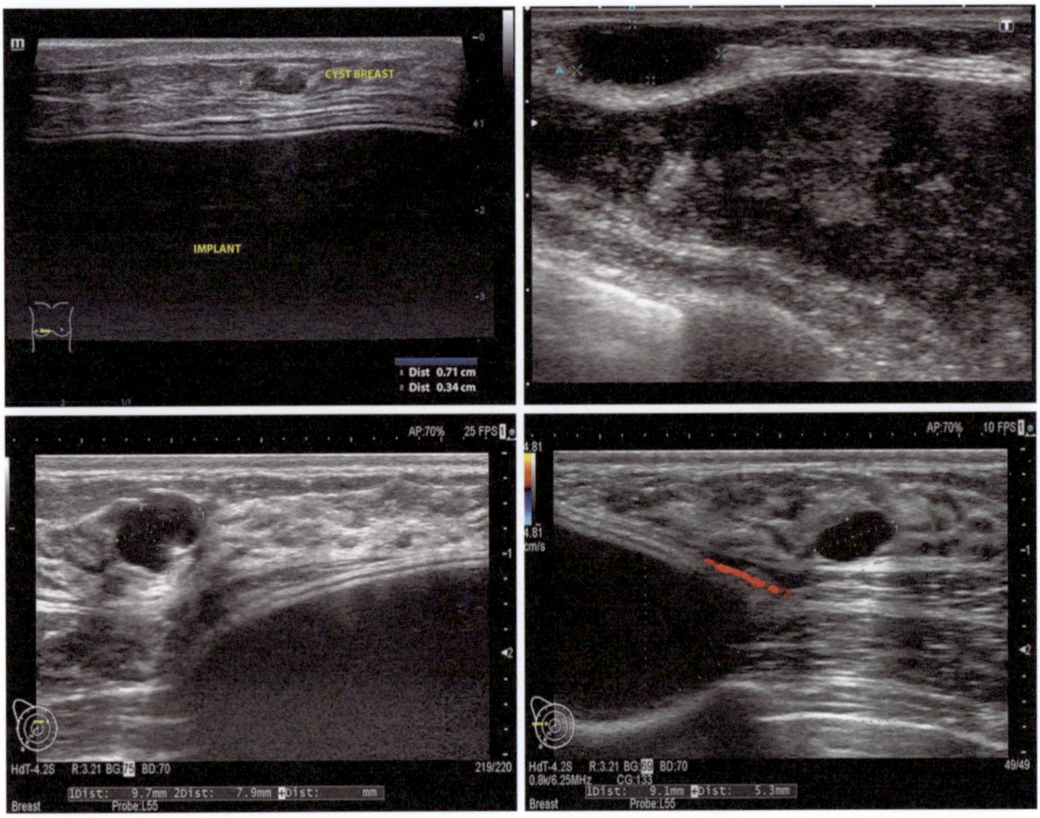

Fig. 11.9 1–4 Status after radical breast resection, breast reconstruction with endoprosthesis. Breast cyst. Grayscale US and CDI

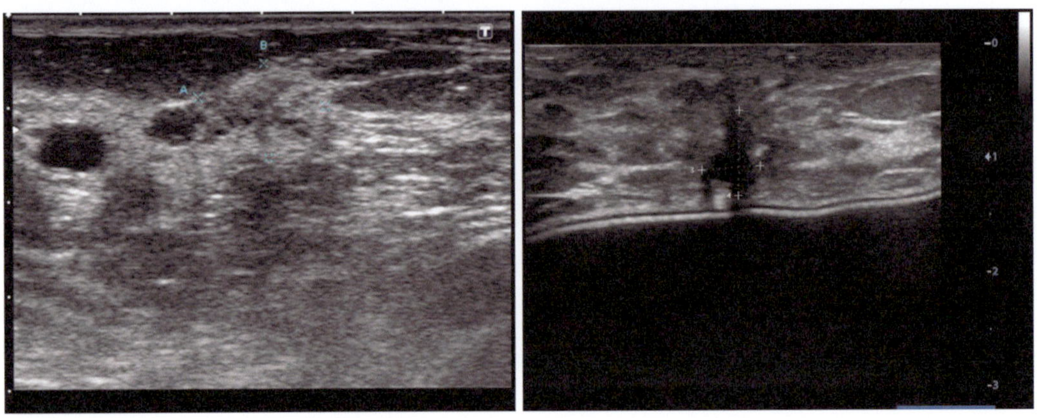

Fig. 11.10 1–2 Status after mammoplasty. Recurrent breast cancer. Grayscale US

MRI is the most informative method for diagnosing endoprosthesis ruptures. MRI helps to clarify the nature of changes in the breast and implants that are detected with ultrasound. The sensitivity of MRI in the diagnosis of implants rupture is 91.9% with specificity of 97.2% (Shumakova et al. 2011). Mammography clearly defines extracapsular ruptures of implants but is poorly informative in the diagnosis of intracapsular ruptures. The sensitivity and specificity of mammography

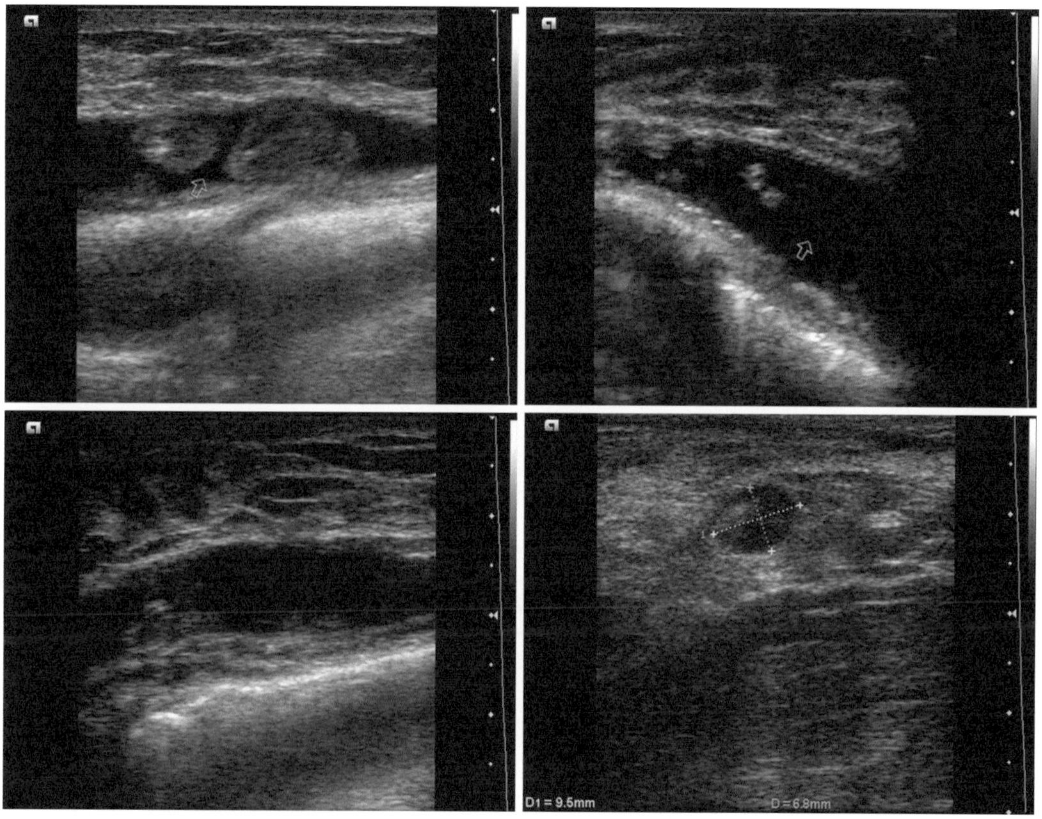

Fig. 11.11 1–4 Status after breast reconstruction. Breast geleomas. Grayscale US

in the diagnosis of breast implants ruptures are 28.4 and 88.3%, respectively. It is advisable to use ultrasound as the first-line imaging method in the breast study after augmentation mammoplasty with silicone implants. The sensitivity of ultrasound in the diagnosis of breast implants ruptures is 77% with the specificity of 91.7%.

Annual US is strongly recommended to control the condition of breast tissues and the implant.

11.2 Diagnosis of Recurrent Breast Cancer

Early detection of recurrent malignant tumors is one of the main problems of present-day oncology. Despite the integrated and combined approaches to the treatment of patients with breast cancer, in 40–50% of women, the process disseminates over a 5-year period after radical treatment. Local disease recurrence takes a special place in the course of the disease. Local recurrence is a tumor similar to the primary one by its morphological structure. It occurs in the same place after radical surgery (radical mastectomy or breast-sparing surgery). Regional recurrence implicates metastatic regional lymph nodes, regardless of the volume of lymphatic dissection (standard axillary lymphadenectomy or SLNB).

The majority of authors do not divide these recurrences into local and regional, believing that the term "local recurrence" means all recurrences, which occur in the surgery area. This creates difficulties not only for determination of the incidence of recurrence and their clinical and morphological characteristics but also for assessment of treatment possibilities and disease prognosis.

Different authors report breast cancer recurrence after radical resection or radical mastectomy in 2.8–71%. Even in the cases, when patients do not have metastases in regional lymph nodes, the recurrence of the disease reaches 25–30% (Ciatto et al. 1994). The highest risk of breast cancer recurrence is within the first 5 years, but nevertheless, it may persist for 15–20 years after surgery.

There are some publications about correlation of certain clinical signs with the incidence of breast cancer recurrence. The results of numerous studies testify a high risk of recurrent breast cancer in young women, especially in those who had undergone breast-sparing surgery. Local recurrence occurs in 40% of patients under 35 years of age and only in 13% over the age of 50 years. In 20–40% of cases, isolated local recurrence results in the dissemination of tumor process.

There is some evidence of increased incidence of local recurrence with enlargement of the primary tumor lesion and the regional prevalence of the process. The size of a breast tumor >5 cm is often associated with positive resection margins, which significantly increases the risk of local recurrence, provided that up to 80% of such recurrences occur in the chest wall. However, with carcinoma in situ, local recurrences have also been described. The incidence of local recurrence within 5 years after surgery was 20.9% in patients with carcinoma in situ, who had undergone a breast-sparing surgery, and 10.4% with additional postsurgical radiotherapy. Detection of tumor cells at the resection margins is an essential evidence of inadequate surgery, and this doubles the risk of local recurrence.

Multicentric growth of breast tumor increases the risk of recurrence. Local recurrence rate increases in patients with metastases in lymph nodes. It significantly increases with the increase in the number of tumor-affected lymph nodes.

Morphological factors as risk criteria of recurrent breast cancer are very important. Often, lobular breast cancer is associated with high incidence of local recurrences. According to a number of publications, this is due to high incidence of bilateral disease, high rate of multicentric growth, clinically latent lymph node lesions, and positive resection margin. At the same time, some retrospective studies did not show any significant difference in the long-term treatment outcomes in patients with invasive lobular carcinoma after surgical treatment of different volume.

The spread of breast cancer cells beyond the main tumor can go along adjacent ducts and lobules, as well as through blood and lymphatic vessels. With intraductal cancer and cancer with predominance of the intraductal component, the breast lesion is often noted far beyond the initial one. Incomplete removal of cancer mass is the basis for recurrence. Local recurrence in the remaining breast increases within 5 years by 15%. Tumor dissemination through lymphatic clefts (lymphovascular invasion) is often associated with lymph nodes metastases and is an unfavorable risk factor not only for local recurrence but also for distant metastases.

Probability of local recurrence depends on the grade of malignancy of the tumor. In malignancy grade III, the rate of local recurrence is 12.1%, while in combination of malignancy grade III with lymphovascular invasion, the recurrence increases up to 21.2%.

In recent years, there is the increased evidence that tumor biology plays a key role in the development of local recurrence in patients with breast cancer. Large studies have noted the lowest risk of local recurrence after breast-sparing treatment in luminal subtypes of cancer (1.5–9.4%) and the highest in triple-negative (8.8–14.2%) and especially in HER2-positive (7.6–18.8%) subtypes. Moreover, this pattern is also observed in patients, who underwent radical mastectomy—the incidence of local recurrence was 8%, 14.3%, and 16.2% in the groups of luminal A, HER2-positive, and triple-negative breast cancer, respectively.

There are also genetic risk factors for local recurrence in patients with breast cancer. The local recurrence was higher (21.8%) among the patients with breast cancer CA1/2 mutations than in the sporadic cancer group (12.1%). The majority of recurrences of BRCA-associated breast cancer occur in early intervals after surgery.

Recurrences in regional lymph nodes are less often in 1–3% of patients at early stages of breast cancer and in 1.7–15.9% of patients at any stage. These recurrences are associated with poor prognosis. In 1/3 of patients with recurrences in the axillary and in supraclavicular lymph nodes, distant metastases are diagnosed. Isolated regional recurrences in breast cancer patients can be treated quite effectively, but it is difficult to diagnose them due to a number of reasons. First, there are no screening methods to assess axillary and supraclavicular areas. X-ray mammography is not adequate for these purposes, because only the lower part of the axillary region can be imaged with this technique. Second, the false-negative results of the physical examination of the axilla reach 40%, because it is extremely difficult to palpate lymph nodes of small size among adipose and scar tissue. Only in 15.4% with regional recurrence of the metastases in the axillary and supraclavicular lymph nodes were detected by palpation. On the contrary, false-negative results of echography were only 23%.

US is a universal and available method for early detection of breast cancer recurrence. Integrated use of various basic and advanced technologies permits monitoring of the therapy (Evseeva et al. 2011). In general, the sensitivity, specificity, and diagnostic accuracy of US in the diagnosis of regional breast cancer recurrence in patients is 76.9%, 98.7% and 98.2%, respectively. However, the interpretation of the ultrasound results is often difficult. Especially this applies to patients, who were operated for cancer and/or had received radiation therapy, as they often exhibit fibrosis of the breast tissues and the structures of the anterior chest wall. This significantly complicates early detection of recurrent breast cancer in the zone of primary surgical intervention and its differential diagnosis with various postsurgical and/or post-radiotherapy changes.

The following ultrasound signs characterize local recurrence of breast cancer in the area of radical resection or radical mastectomy (Sencha et al. 2011) (Fig. 11.12):

- A small solid mass (usually 1–2 cm)
- Decreased intensity of ultrasound signal
- Usually homogeneous structure
- Irregular or round shape
- Uneven borders
- Indistinct (less often distinct) contours
- Intranodular blood flow at CDI, PDI, and 3DPD
- Intense coloring at compression US elastography, different from the surrounding parenchyma
- Average value of strain ratio >3.8

In late postoperative period (3–6 months and later), with any kind of surgical intervention, oleogranulomas or fat necrosis may arise as a response to traumatic effects during surgery. Fat necrosis may also develop at any age in women and men with collagenoses, diabetes, less often idiopathically (without a clear cause) or after trauma. It is detected as a painful, dense mass.

According to US, in postoperative period (as well as after traumas), oleogranulomas show along the postsurgical scars as regular round masses of various echogenicity (an-, hypo-, hyperechoic) and various size (usually up to 10 mm), with distinct borders, homogeneous (or heterogeneous) echostructure, and avascular with CDI, PDI and 3DPD (Fig. 11.13).

Calcifications with acoustic shadows are characteristic for oleogranulomas. The surrounding tissues may be intact or demonstrate the signs of lymphostasis. It is very difficult to perform differential diagnosis of fat necrosis or oleogranulomas with recurrent breast cancer in the chest wall scars and in the remaining part of the breast after breast-sparing and breast reconstruction surgeries. Recurrent tumors that are small in size may have similar echogenicity, echostructure, shape, contours, and boundaries and be avascular like oleogranulomas in Doppler modes.

To verify oleogranulomas FNB is not appropriate, as there is very little cellular material (often no material). Treatment is indicated depending on the result of core needle biopsy. In case of negative data, subsequent follow-up and ultrasound monitoring are recommended.

Decreased intensity and strand structure are often specific for local fibrosis and for oleogranuloma moderate echogenicity, heterogeneous structure, and inclusions of calcifications and liquid zones (Fig. 11.14).

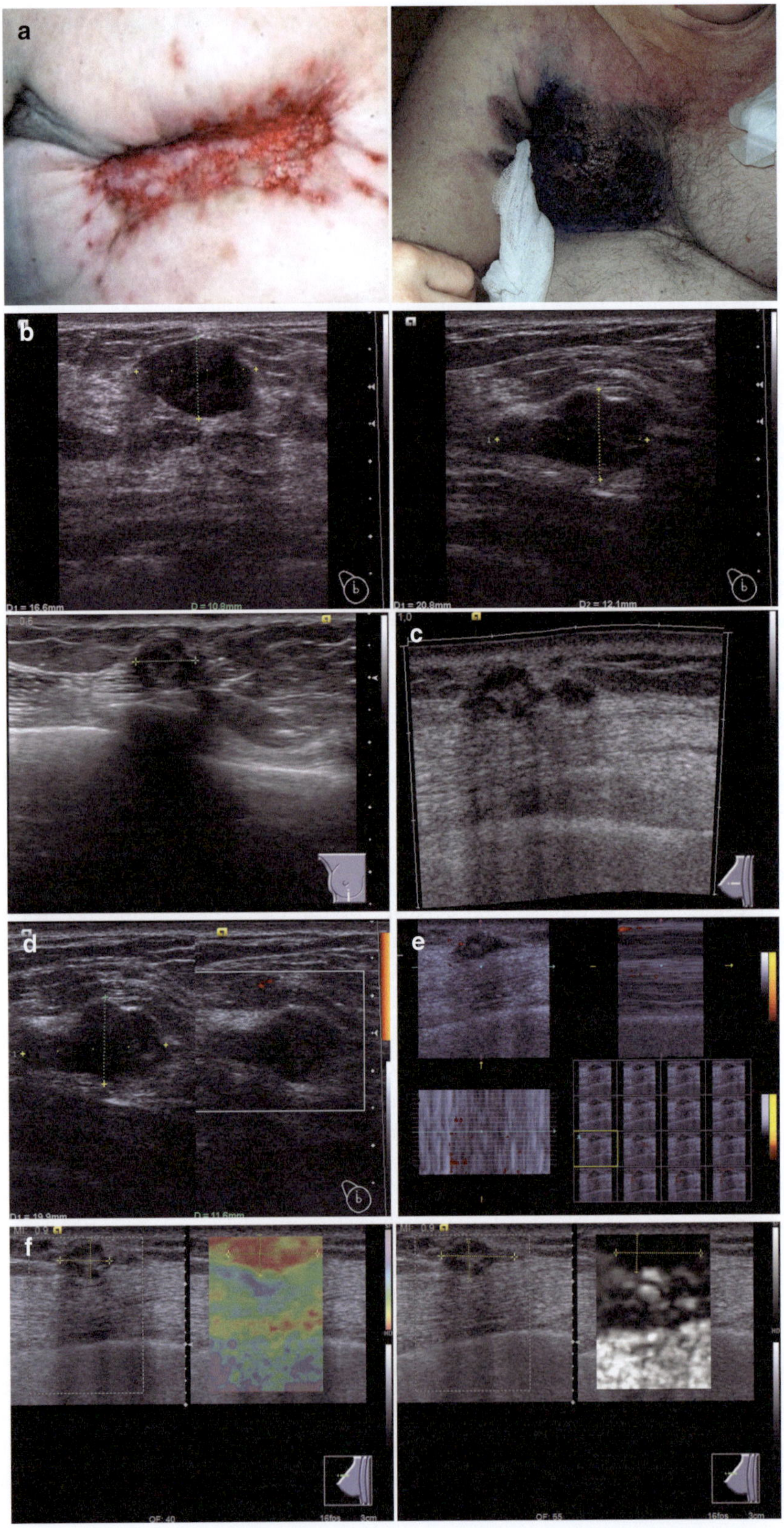

Fig. 11.12 State after radical breast resection. Recurrent breast cancer in a man. (**a**) 1–2 Appearance of the patient. (**b**) 1–3 Grayscale US. (**c**) Panoramic scan. (**d**) CDI. (**e**) Multislice. (**f**) 1–2 Compression US elastography

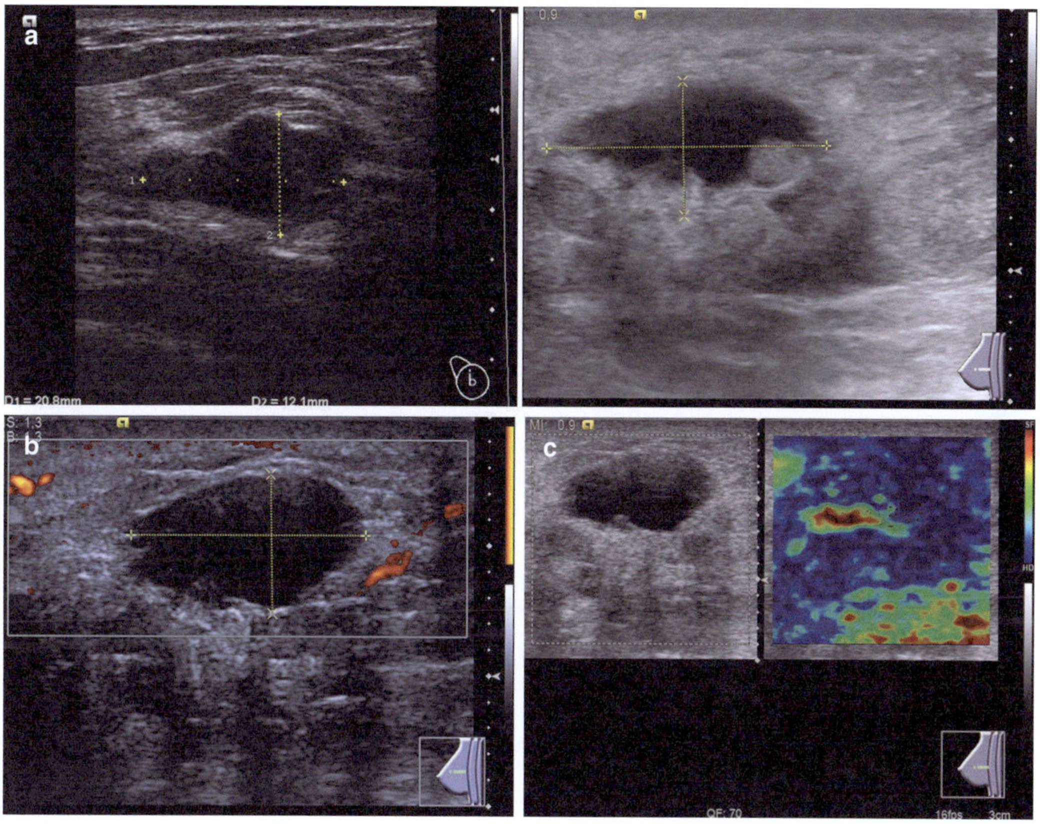

Fig. 11.13 Status after radical breast resection. Oleogranuloma. (**a**) 1–2 Grayscale US. (**b**) PDI. (**c**) Compression US elastography

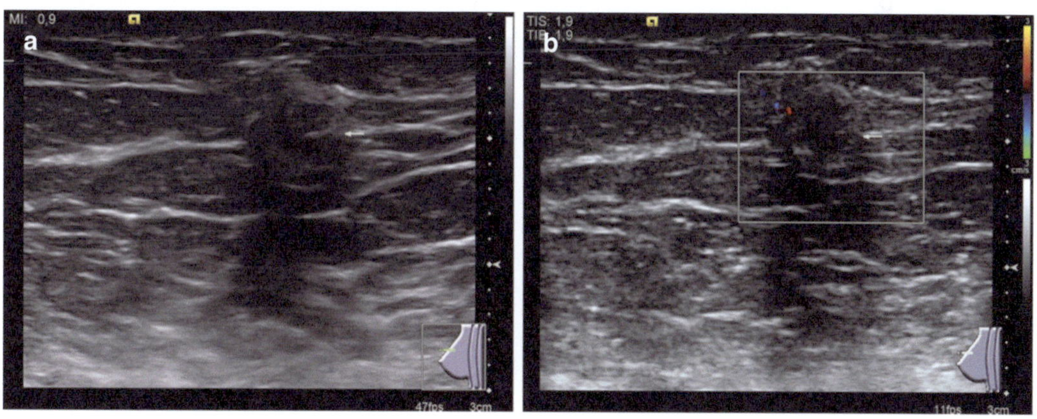

Fig. 11.14 Status after radical breast resection. Local fibrosis. (**a**) Grayscale US. (**b**) CDI

Doppler sonography determines blood flow in 82.8% of recurrent breast cancers. As a rule, oleogranulomas, local fibrosis, and cystic lesions are avascular with CDI, PDI, and 3DPD.

US and mammography are complementary methods for the diagnosis of local breast cancer recurrence. Ultrasound is practically the only widely available and cost-effective diagnostic method for recurrences in the area of radical mastectomy. Its sensitivity in the diagnosis of local breast cancer recurrence in the area of radical resection is 91.1%, specificity 96%, and accuracy 94.3%. The corresponding figures for mammography are 86.7%, 84%, and 85.7%, respectively. The corresponding indices for recurrences in the zone of radical mastectomy are 98%, 86.5%, and 93.5%, respectively (Sencha et al. 2011).

Puncture biopsy of solid lesions in postoperative breast or its bed and postsurgical scars are mandatory and often a key aspect for differentiation and verification of tumor recurrence.

12 Ultrasound-Guided Invasive Methods in the Diagnosis of Breast Diseases

Alexander N. Sencha, Yury Patrunov, Valeriy Rodionov, and Ekaterina Sencha

Abstract

The main invasive diagnostic manipulations for breast examination conducted with imaging guidance (ultrasound or X-ray) are core needle biopsy, vacuum biopsy, fine needle aspiration biopsy (FNAB), and ductography. Core needle biopsy of mammary gland lesions is carried out with stereotactic X-ray accessory and special tools—a biopsy gun and guillotine needles for precise sampling sufficient for pathology. Puncture of breast masses under the control of echography, in combination with X-ray mammography, increases the detectability of cancer to 95–98%. FNAB with cytology is the least invasive and highly feasible method. It is the leading modality among the invasive diagnostic interventions for benign breast diseases. Ductography is the technology of X-ray imaging of artificially contrasted lactiferous ducts. Treatment of the breast cyst by puncture is sufficient in most cases. If the cyst is filled with fluid again, the procedure can be repeated or enhanced by one of the variants of sclerotherapy (destruction). Laser ablation, cryoablation, and other ablative procedures for solid breast masses have limited indications. Invasive interventions on mammary glands are highly effective and well tolerated by patients; nevertheless, they require certain indications, respect of contraindications, and strict adherence to the intervention technique.

A. N. Sencha (✉)
Division of Visual Diagnostics, National Medical Research Center for Obstetrics, Gynecology and Perinatology named after Academician V.I. Kulakov of Ministry of Healthcare of Russian Federation, Moscow, Russia

Y. Patrunov
Department of Ultrasound Diagnostics of Radiology Center, Yaroslavl Railway Clinic, Yaroslavl, Russia

V. Rodionov
Department of Breast Diseases, National Medical Research Center for Obstetrics, Gynecology and Perinatology named after Academician V.I. Kulakov of Ministry of Healthcare of Russian Federation, Moscow, Russia

E. Sencha
Department of Ultrasound Diagnostics, Federal State Budget Hospital “9 Treatment and Diagnostic Center” of the Ministry of Defense of the Russian Federation, Moscow, Russia

A morphological conclusion on the structure of breast tumors is possible after invasive sampling and pathological study or cytology. Only morphological verification allows to plan specific treatment.

All invasive technologies are divided into the following groups according to the aim of the procedure:

- Diagnostic
- Treatment
- Both diagnostic and therapeutic (“diapeutic”)

G. T. Sukhikh, A. N. Sencha (eds.), *Multiparametric Ultrasound Diagnosis of Breast Diseases*,
https://doi.org/10.1007/978-3-319-75034-7_12

The main invasive diagnostic manipulations for breast examination conducted under radiologic guidance (ultrasound or X-ray) are:

- Core needle biopsy
- Vacuum biopsy
- Fine needle aspiration biopsy (FNAB)
- Ductography (ductoscopy)

General contraindications for invasive manipulations are:

1. Absolute:
   - Decompensated coagulopathies, irreversible disorders of the hemostasis
   - Inadequacy of the patient, mental and mood disorders
   - Lack of informed consent for the intervention, patient's refusal to undergo the procedure
2. Relative:
   - Health problems (severe disease, intoxication, hyperthermia, cephalgia, general weakness, hypertension, etc.)
   - Certain laboratory and instrumental tests data (e.g., hemostasis indicators beyond the reference level)
   - Poor visualization of the target lesion

Prior to any invasive procedure, a medical and surgical history of the patient is reviewed. The patient is informed on the purpose, technology of the manipulation, and possible adverse effects and complications and offered to sign a written informed consent.

Invasive manipulations demand strict adherence to aseptic and antiseptic rules. The procedures are carried out in special premises such as a small operating room equipped with a first aid kit and medical devices for resuscitation. Ultrasound probe and working surfaces of the X-ray are pretreated with disinfectants based on chlorhexidine solution, alcohol, and other disinfectants; a sterile set of disposables is used.

Core needle biopsy (CNB) of mammary gland lesions is carried out with stereotactic X-ray accessory and special tools—a biopsy gun and guillotine needles for precise sampling sufficient for pathology (Fig. 12.1).

Indications for breast CNB are listed below:

- Suspected malignancy or neoplasms of unknown origin (BI-RADS categories 4, 5)
- Impalpable breast tumors
- Calcifications (pathological, suspicious, uncertain)
- Asymmetric local fibrosis

Methods of neoplasm puncture:

- Blind puncture (without imaging control).
- With preliminary ultrasonographic marking. Marks are applied on the skin over the lesion, which is imaged with US, to specify the location, depth, etc., prior to the puncture.
- With ultrasound guidance: visual control of the direction and movement of the puncture needle ensures the targeted sampling (Fig. 12.2).

Steps of manipulation:

- Basic ultrasound study.
- Target echography for navigation in the zone of interest.

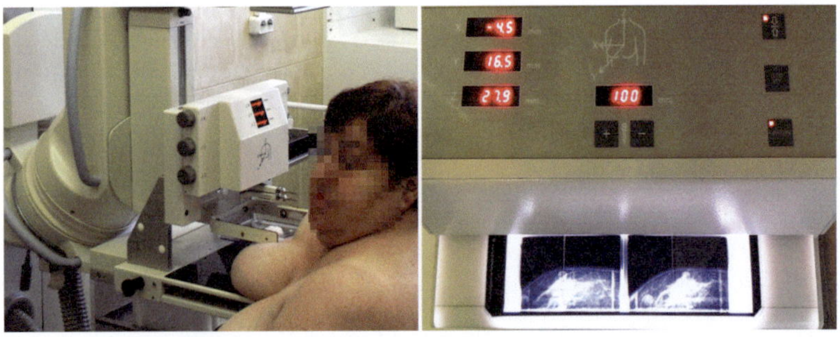

Fig. 12.1 1–2 Core needle biopsy of the breast. X-ray stereopairs with tumor coordinates

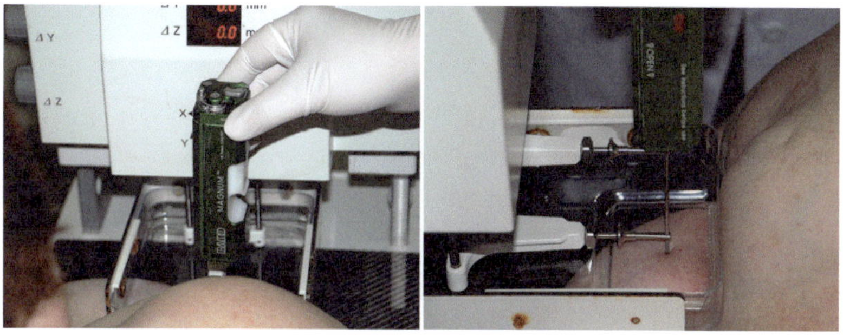

Fig. 12.2 1–2 CNB of breast cancer

- Targeting the biopsy needle close to the tumor.
- Visual control of the needle location and direction: the needle should be parallel to the structures of the anterior thoracic wall to avoid their injury, with a distance of at least 2 cm from the tumor to the adjacent structures.
- Obtaining material (3–6 tissue samples).
- Placement of samples (3–6) 15–22 mm long on a slide and then into special disposable transport cartridges immersed in containers with 10% neutral formalin solution.

Guillotine type 14–18G needles are widely used in mammology due to their capacity to obtain tissue bars of 100–300 mg. These needles have an extended groove, which fills with tissue sample. When the needle cannula slides, the tissue sample is cut off from its main mass (the "guillotine principle") providing a histological specimen. The following types of needles are distinguished:

- Mechanical—both the groove and the cutting cannula movements are operated manually, through the successive actions of the operator.
- Semiautomatic—the groove is moved manually, while the activation of the cannula is carried out automatically by a spring-loaded trigger mechanism.
- Automatic—automatic reusable biopsy gun and a disposable biopsy needle. Only the bringing of the needle to the biopsy site is performed manually, while the groove is put forward and the cutting cannula is activated automatically by pressing the trigger of the gun.

The advantages of semiautomatic needles include their greater maneuverability and delicacy (and, therefore, safety) when taking a biopsy from the foci located close to the important anatomical structures (vessels, cavities, etc.). After the spring system of the automatic needle's gun is activated, no further control over the progress of the needle is possible. One disadvantage of a semiautomatic needle is possible unintended deviation of its axis when the groove is manually put forward into dense histological structures. At the same time, prompt insertion of the automatic needle groove ensures high-quality sampling of dense tissues. The rather high cost of such instruments requires visual (ultrasound or stereoradiographic) control, which enhances diagnostic value in 96–100% of cases.

Because of the larger diameter of the needle and not so well tolerated technique (compared to aspiration), it is preferable to perform a biopsy under local anesthesia, avoiding infiltration of the mass, which is clearly visible under ultrasound guidance.

Stereotactic percutaneous core needle biopsy under radiologic control with a needle of the guillotine type is an invasive procedure, which is performed in an outpatient facility, takes 10–15 min, and does not require any preliminary preparation of a patient, except for cancellation of anticoagulant therapy 3–5 days prior to biopsy.

The size of the tissue sample depends on the diameter of the needle (14, 16 G) and the length of the cutting surface (15, 22 mm). The optimal number of samples (3–6) ensures the repeatability of the material (multiple repetition of the material on the slices demonstrates the prevailing pathology from one sample to the next).

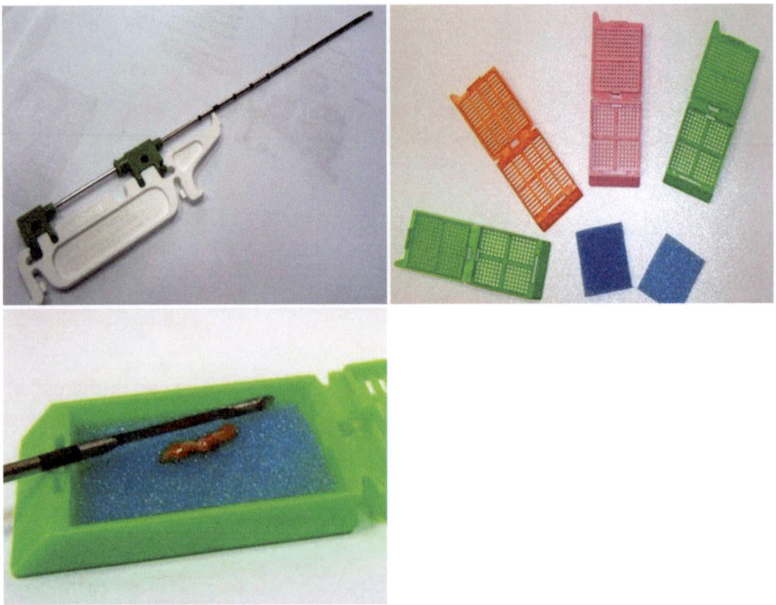

Fig. 12.3 1–3 Equipment for CNB

Moreover, the diagnosis of calcifications in the parenchyma requires more samples than in the cases of tumors (6–10 samples).

High-quality equipment should be used to process and transport material without destruction and loss (Fig. 12.3).

Samples obtained from a tumor are sufficient to determine the most important indicators and prognostic factors, such as invasion, degree of malignancy, hormonal receptors, expression of Her2/neu, etc.

Histological examination is extremely important not only for diagnosis of malignant tumors but also fibrocystic breast disease (FBD). Only morphological investigation allows to differentiate nodular mastopathy from breast cancer, to clarify the degree of severity of proliferative processes, and to state the indications for sector resection.

Nodular mastopathy is obviously a precancerous disease. However, the risk of breast cancer increases only in patients with proliferative fibroadenomatosis and reaches the maximum (4–5 times) in cases of hyperplasia associated with cellular atypia. In these cases sectoral breast resection is recommended in order to prevent development of a malignant tumor in the future. Diagnostic efficacy of an adequate CNB is equal to sector breast resection.

The main tasks of US during the invasive diagnostic manipulations on the mammary gland are mentioned below:

Prior to the manipulation:

- Preliminary conclusion about the structure of the mass, its location, vascularity, elasticity, and state of surrounding tissues and organs
- Selection of an optimal minimally invasive technique and specification of the manipulation in a particular patient (together with a mammologist, oncologist, surgeon)
- Determination of the puncture vector and needle pathway
- An assessment of the probability of potential adverse effects and complications during and after manipulation

During the invasive manipulation:

- Guidance of the needle insertion according to the previously chosen optimal path
- Absolute control over the needle's tip position in the examined mass
- Monitoring of the state of the surrounding structures
- Monitoring over the manipulation, judgment on its effectiveness
- Detection of adverse effects and complications

After the manipulation:

- Evaluation of the effectiveness of manipulation
- Assessment of the surrounding organs and tissues
- Detection of early (up to 30 min) and delayed (up to 3–4 weeks) complications
- Dynamic monitoring of changes of ultrasound parameters

According to Mazo et al. (2015), the sensitivity and specificity of ultrasound-guided core needle biopsy for breast masses smaller than 1 cm is 94% and 100% and of X-ray-guided CN, 97% and 100%, respectively. For masses over 1 cm in size, CNB is informative in 100% of cases.

CNB provides material for morphological and histological verification and immunohistochemical analysis.

Immunohistochemistry (IHC) is a method of staining of biological material with preserved cell morphology. It is used to determine the location of a specific antigen in tumor tissues or cell structures with the use of specific antibodies and sensitive detection systems.

The results are evaluated qualitatively and quantitatively with a light microscope. The material for the study is bioplates, specially processed and formed in paraffined blocks (Fig. 12.4). The main indicators that allow to plan target therapy in cases of breast cancer are the expression of estrogen and progesterone receptors, proliferative activity factor Ki-67 and oncoprotein C-erbB-2 (Human Epidermal Growth Factor Receptor 2—Her2).

In oncologic practice, IHC allows to reveal the molecular structures of tumor cells associated with the degree of differentiation, the ability to invade and metastasize, the sensitivity to chemotherapy, and the course and the prognosis of the disease in a particular patient. IHC analysis should be performed when it is otherwise impossible to define tumor histogenesis and for immunophenotyping of malignant lymphomas. However, the IHC, which is widely used in clinical practice, has a number of disadvantages:

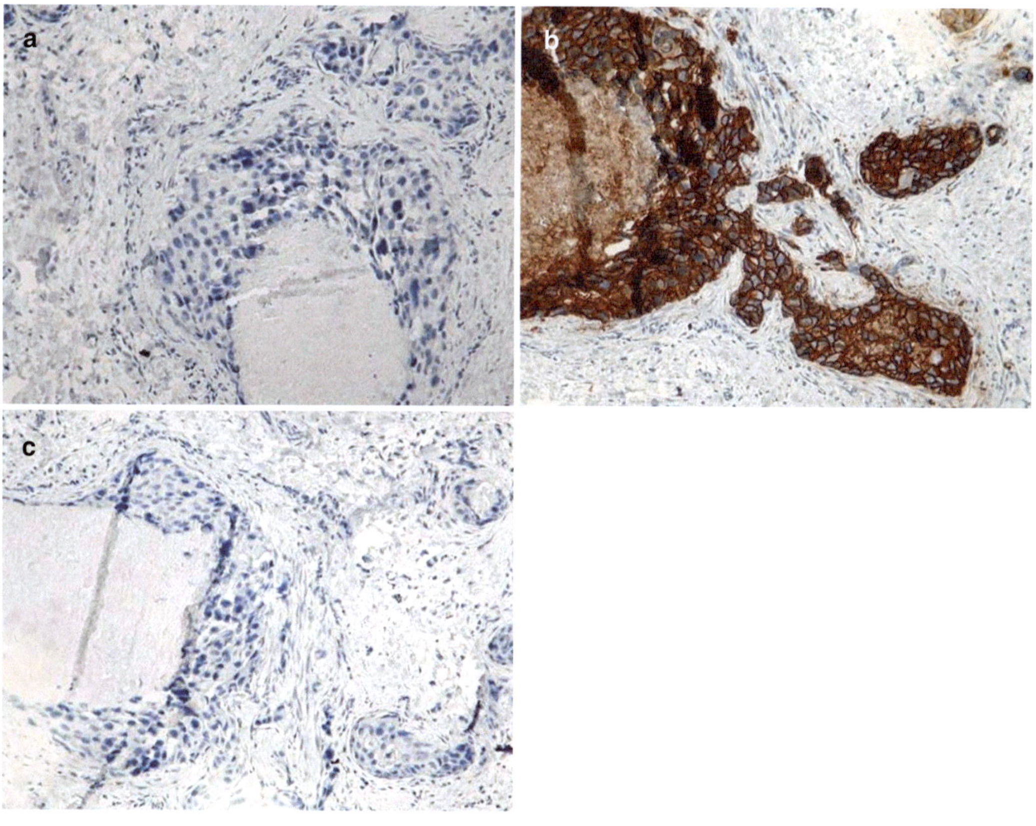

Fig. 12.4 Immunohistochemistry of breast cancer. (**a**) ER. (**b**) C-erbB-2. (**c**) PR

- Loss or masking of an antigen
- Long procession of a specimen

Assessment of the expression of molecular markers at the cell level—**immunocytochemistry** (ICC)—can be an alternative to IHC in some aspects. The material for the study is obtained with conventional FNAB, which is simple, minimally traumatic, and provides sufficient cell material. With small and impalpable masses, this type of biopsy is carried out under ultrasound or X-ray navigation. ICC does not require a lot of time. The expression of molecular markers defined with ICC or IHC concurs in 61–92% of cases. Membrane and cytoplasmic markers are more often positively stained in cytological than in histological preparations. This can be due to more delicate processing of cytopreparations, the absence of loss, and the masking of antigens during wiring and dewaxing of the material with aggressive chemical reagents.

IHC should be performed at least in 96% of all CNB. The biopsy material of early breast cancer does not need IHC, since this investigation will be performed later with the surgical specimen (Table 12.1).

Factors that limit the biopsy value may be related to the localization of a mass, in particular, in the region of the transition fold, in the retroareolar region, or in the scar. These are adjacent to the chest wall and subject to trauma (pain shock, pneumothorax, bleeding). US guidance of the biopsy is of particular importance in the cases of cystic cancer or cancer with cystic component, edematous-infiltrative cancer, and X-ray-negative breast cancer, where the possibilities of stereotactic CNB under the radiologic control are limited. In such cases, US-guided fine needle aspiration biopsy is used.

Table 12.1 Various breast conditions and CNB rate

Breast conditions	Number of biopsies (n = 1503)	%
Impalpable lesions with signs of malignancy	383	25,4
Asymmetric local fibrosis	32	2,1
Pathological calcifications	27	1,9
Malignant neoplasms (BI-RADS 5)	1019	67,8
Suspicious neoplasms (BI-RADS 4)	42	2,8
Total	**1503**	**100**

Stereotactic biopsy is often the definite and final step of diagnosis. Its sensitivity in the diagnosis of breast cancer is 97.6%; specificity, 100%; and diagnostic accuracy, 98% (Kuplevatskaya 2004).

Vacuum biopsy (VACB—vacuum-assisted core biopsy) of breast lesions is an ergonomic and highly effective method of obtaining cell material for tumor verification, providing a variety of tissue samples by a single needle insertion under the control of ultrasound navigation or stereoradiography. A special device based on a vacuum aspirator is used for this procedure.

The principle of vacuum biopsy units is the same as of the techniques applying guillotine biopsy needles. A biopsy needle with a size of 8, 9, or 11 G is fixed in the vacuum-assisted handle of the device. Vacuum facilitates more tissue aspiration through the fine aperture of the biopsy needle; after this, sample is cut and captured by the blade rotating around the aperture. Vacuum aspiration draws the sample into a container. The entire biopsy (except for driving the needle to the lesion) is fully automatic, controlled by electronic settings.

The technique can be performed not only for diagnostic but also for therapeutic purposes. Ultrasound control, high qualification, and experience of an ultrasonographist allow to take material straight from the area of interest, display the position of the needle in the lesion, and activate the vacuum in real-time mode (Fig. 12.5).

Samples of tissues obtained with vacuum biopsy are eight times larger than the samples obtained by the guillotine needle 14G. Multiple sampling from a single focus of the breast can completely eliminate the signs of a mass at an echo- or mammogram; this is especially important in case of benign lesions.

The disadvantages of the technique include the risk of hematoma in the zone of intervention, especially with multiple sampling. The risk is

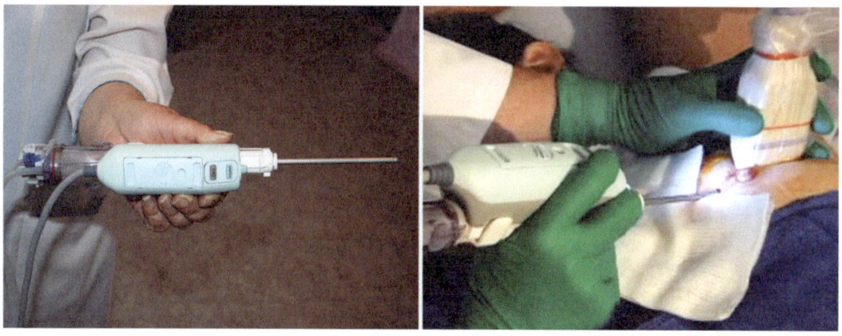

Fig. 12.5 1–2 Vacuum biopsy of a breast tumor

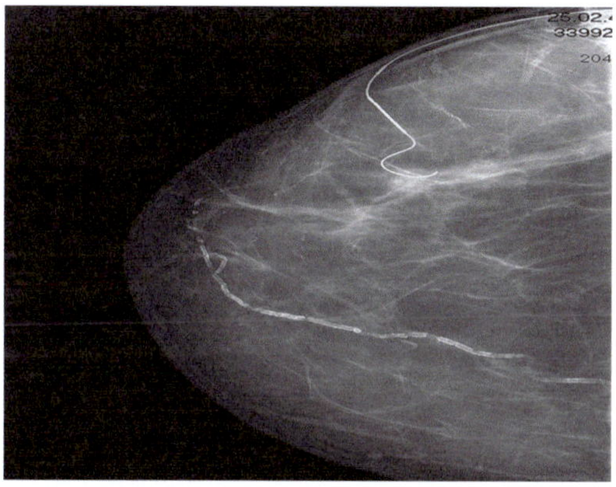

Fig. 12.6 Impalpable breast cancer. Radiogram. 1. Preoperative labeling

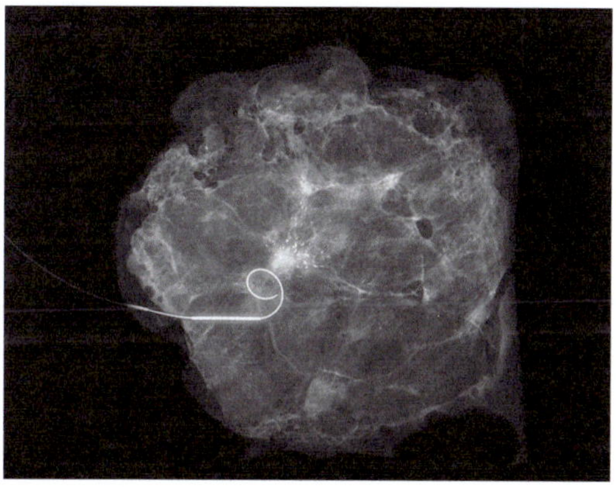

Fig. 12.7 Sectography. Impalpable breast cancer with microcalcinates

secured to some extent by a possibility to bring the hemostatics directly to the biopsy site.

Vacuum biopsy is more expensive and less safe than conventional puncture biopsy, but it is more effective and better tolerated by patients.

The detected impalpable masses can be **preoperatively labeled** to ensure their removal during breast-sparing procedures or pathohistological study in the removed breast. Ultrasound-positive tumors are labeled under the control of echography. To mark X-ray-positive tumors, a stereotactic technique is used. At the final step, an "anchor" marking needle is installed in the lesion (Fig. 12.6). The accuracy of the "anchor" location should be checked with X-ray.

In order to ensure complete removal of calcifications or impalpable tumors, an X-ray of the removed specimen—**sectorography**—can be performed (Fig. 12.7). A part of the removed breast, marked, for example, in methylene blue, is sent to the pathomorphology laboratory for extraction of material for tumor verification.

Labeling of impalpable breast lesions with anchor needles prior to surgery and sectorography of the removed part became important due to growing incidence of preclinical forms of malignant neoplasms and other breast diseases detected at screening. These techniques contribute to the accuracy of removal of the lesions and facilitate their subsequent histological examination.

Wide application of echography as a method of navigation and control ensures high efficiency of **fine needle aspiration biopsy** (FNAB) for obtaining informative material from a pathological focus (Fig. 12.8). The subsequent **cytological study** allows to clarify the morphology and to carry out differential diagnosis. The method of imaging plays the leading role in improving the diagnostic value of FNAB. Blind biopsy of palpable masses brings sufficient material in 50–60% of cases, stereotactic technique in 60–70%, and US-guided technique up to 85%. According to Sinyukova et al. (2007), puncture of breast masses under the control of echography, in

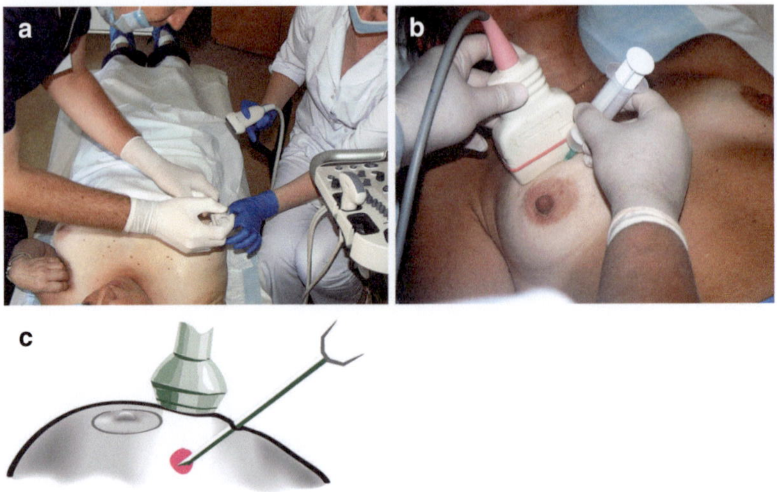

Fig. 12.8 US-guided FNAB of a breast lesion. (**a**) The position of the medical personnel. (**b**) The position of the probe and needle. (**c**) Scheme

combination with X-ray mammography, increases the detectability of cancer to 95–98%. According to Mazo et al. (2015), the sensitivity, specificity, and accuracy of US-guided FNAB of breast masses smaller than 1 cm in size and of 1–2 cm are 67% and 86%, 93% and 99%, and 85% and 95.5%, respectively. If the size of a mass is more than 2 cm, the sensitivity and specificity of FNAB is 100%.

US-assisted FNAB is useful in the following cases:

- Impalpable X-ray-negative breast masses
- Puncture biopsy of cysts
- Nodules in the scar
- Breast implants
- Lesions in the retromammary space
- Heterogeneous breast masses (for precise selection of the zone of diagnostic interest)
- Enlargement and lesions of regional lymph nodes

FNAB is the least invasive and highly feasible method. It is the leading modality among the invasive diagnostic interventions for benign breast diseases. To perform a minimally invasive procedure, strict adherence to aseptic and antiseptic rules is necessary. The procedures are carried out in specially equipped rooms—dressing or small operating room. The probe is cleaned with disinfectants based on chlorhexidine or alcohol.

The techniques of US-assisted FNAB are as follows:

1. A "free-hand" technique is often used in large masses. Advantages of the technique are flexibility of manipulations and good visualization of the needle.
2. A technique with the use of a special puncture probe allows to preliminarily evaluate the needle pathway. However, during manipulation, the needle is often poorly visualized, and the flexibility of manipulation is limited due to the rigidity of the device. The procedure requires special needles.
3. A technique with the use of special adaptors provides good needle imaging with a certain restriction of manipulations due to the rigidity of the device, and the number of biopsies is limited by the set of sterile instruments.
4. Technique is based on the ultrasound-assisted GPS navigation.

Some devices significantly facilitate FNAB. Special biopsy needles are long (10–20 cm) and have a modified echoic tip, which allows precise localization of its position. Outer distance marks and movable limiters permit control of the depth of needle insertion. Mandrins prevent clogging of the needle lumen on its way to the lesion. The disadvantage that hinders use of such needles is their relatively high cost. The

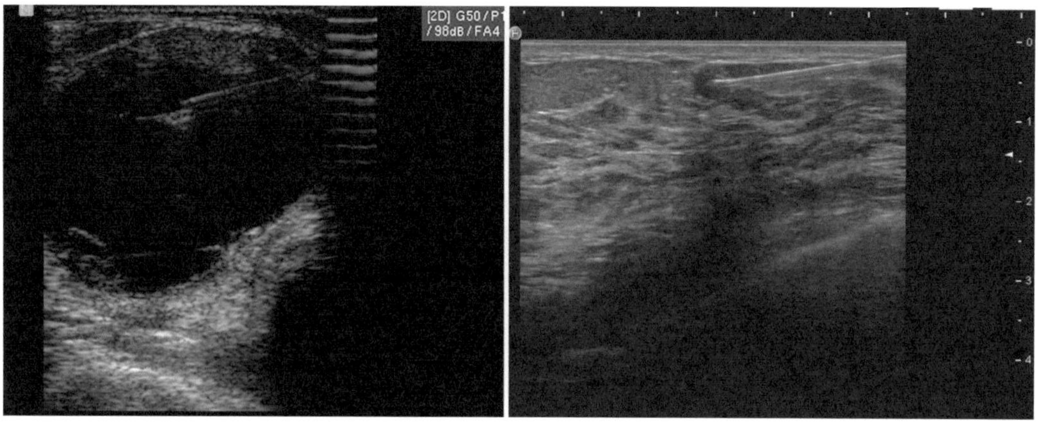

Fig. 12.9 1–2 Fine needle aspiration biopsy. Grayscale ultrasound image of the needle

use of biopsy accessories facilitates puncture biopsy, allowing to mark and follow the needle route. Coaxial needle conductors and special "holders" facilitate aspiration and increase the vacuum in the syringe.

FNAB of breast masses is most often performed with "free-hand" technique. Guidance and puncture may be performed by one or two specialists: an ultrasonographist together with a surgeon, oncologist, or mammologist. The team approach is preferable. Ultrasound probes with a frequency of 7.5–18 MHz are recommended for ultrasound guidance of FNAB.

No special patient preparation to FNAB is necessary. The patient lies supine with the arms along the body. Anesthesia is not recommended, since novocaine injection compromises ultrasound image and affects the cells. Moreover, the procedure of local anesthesia can be as painful as the biopsy itself. The skin is disinfected with a 70% solution of alcohol, and sterile ultrasound gel is applied. Puncture is performed with a disposable syringe of 5–10 mL bearing a 40 mm needle with a diameter of 0.8 mm. All needle movements and all manipulations are registered on the screen. The direction and depth of needle insertion are adjusted if necessary. The needle is visualized as a hyperechoic point (at transverse scan) or a hyperechoic line (at longitudinal scan), which changes its position with the needle movements. If there is any doubt about the true location of the needle, it is advisable to change angle of the needle or of the ultrasound probe or to change the settings of the ultrasound device. The image of the needle will not change then, while the artifacts will weaken or disappear (Fig. 12.9).

After the needle is brought to the lesion, the samples are taken by aspiration of at least from three sites. To create negative pressure, the syringe pump is pulled back, and the material is aspirated into the needle. After aspiration the syringe with the needle is removed. When a mass has a heterogenous echostructure, the material is taken from the most suspicious parts in the center and periphery and in cases of cysts with solid component, from the less vascularized areas with CDI. After the biopsy, the puncture site is treated with 70% alcohol and compressed with a sterile cloth for 10–15 min to prevent hematoma.

For subsequent cytological study, the smears on slides are stained routinely according to the Pappenheim method (Fig. 12.10).

Ultrasound imaging may identify cysts with parietal vegetations. Targeted US-guided puncture of the solid component in the cyst may confirm mural breast cancer (20% of atypical cysts) and cystadenopapilloma (75%).

The main advantages of US biopsy guidance are as follows:

- Real-time monitoring, fast procedure
- Targeted sampling
- Absence of ionizing radiation, safety for the patient and medical personnel

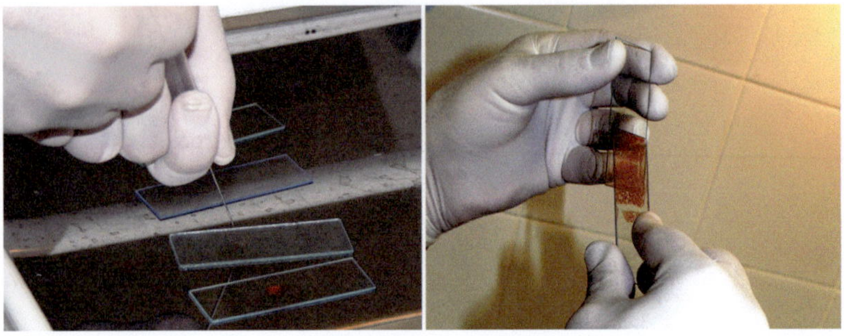

Fig. 12.10 (**a**) FNAB-obtained material on a slide. (**b**) Smears performance

- High resolution, largely depending on the class of equipment
- The possibility to store the images on video, thermal film, and digital media

Ultrasound control during biopsy has the following disadvantages:

- Dependence on the class of equipment
- Dependence on the experience and skills of an ultrasonographist
- Dependence on the image quality, related to local features (such as tissue density, structure and location of the lesion, patient position and health, and the adequacy of behavior during manipulation)

FNAB has some limitations in differentiation of breast pathology. The diagnostic value of FNAB is significantly influenced by the skills of the specialist who performs the puncture, the accuracy of needle insertion, the amount of material obtained, the quality of slides, and the skills of the cytologist. In 10.8–25% of cases, the amount of cells obtained with FNAB does not allow confident report (Semiglazov 2001). Often this is due to technical difficulties (67.5%), such as insufficient visualization of the needle tip, scarce cell substrate in the samples, or specific features of the morphological structure of the breast tumor (32.5%). Aspiration biopsy does not allow to differentiate invasive cancer from cancer in situ and does not provide prognostically important histological and immunochemical information on the tumor.

FNAB with ultrasound guidance provides informative cell material, which makes the cytological analysis accurate up to 96%. US-guided biopsy contributes to morphological diagnosis based on the results of cytological analysis in the shortest possible time (the day of patient's referral), clarification of indications, and timely planning of surgical treatment. This is the reason for its wide use in daily practice.

When FNAB is applied to a typical (simple) breast cyst, the diagnostic aspect is perfectly complemented by therapeutic effect: complete US-controlled cyst evacuation leads to cyst obliteration in 80% of cases.

Ductography (galactography) is the technology of X-ray imaging of artificially contrasted lactiferous ducts. This method is a kind of mammography of the lactiferous ducts with the introduction of a contrast agent.

After preparation of the nipple, areola, and surrounding skin with 70% alcohol solution, 1–2 mL of 1% novocaine is injected into the base of the nipple, thereby producing anesthesia and relaxation of the lactiferous ducts. Then the nipple is slightly compressed to determine the lactiferous duct, which produces the discharge. A thin, flexible catheter is carefully inserted into this duct. Water solution of contrast agent is injected through the catheter in the volume of 0.25–0.5 mL (up to 8 mL). The breast is placed on a mammogram stand and compressed with a plate. This allows to distribute the contrast evenly along the duct. For more complete distribution of the contrast, manual massage of the mammary gland can be done. X-ray scans after the introduction of contrast agent are performed in two projections (direct and oblique). Contrast agent is removed from the duct after the procedure is finished. Usually 1–2 ducts are examined. This technique

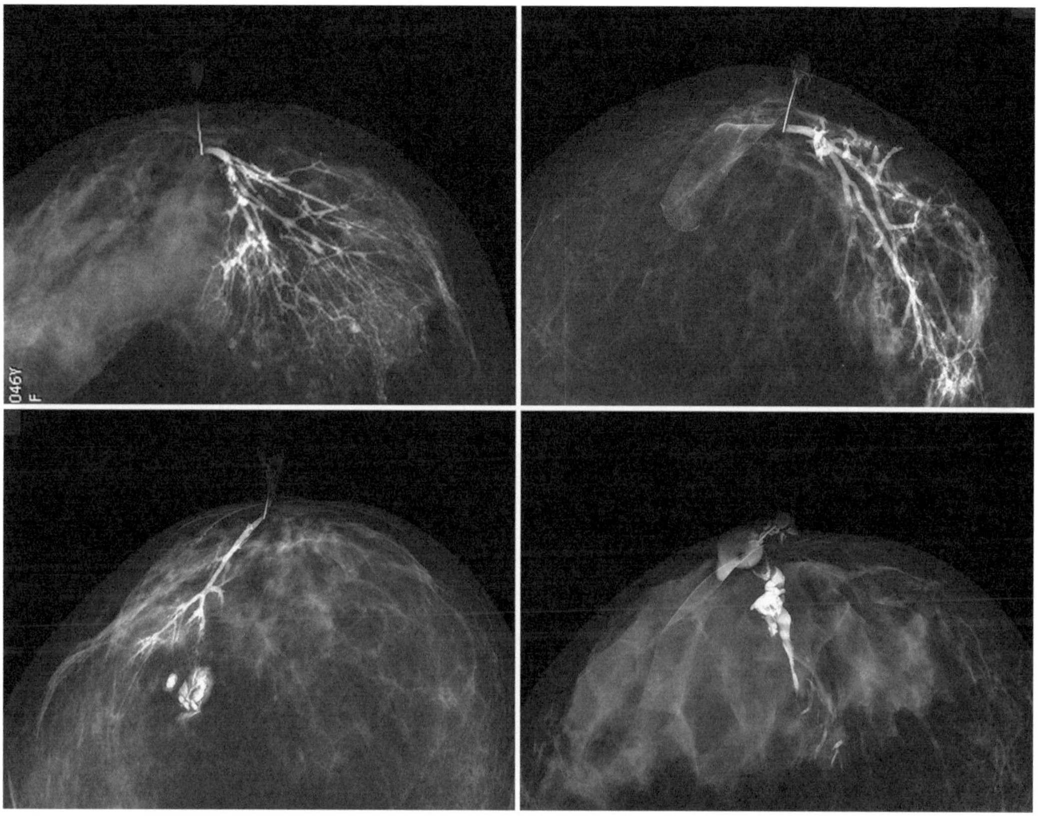

Fig. 12.11 1–4 Ductography. Intraductal carcinoma

allows to examine the lactiferous ducts in detail—the type, structure, lumen, and contours—to detect intraductal masses, and to study the location, size, and shape of the tumor (Fig. 12.11).

Indications for ductography are listed below:

- Abnormal nipple discharge (bloody or brown)
- Suspected ductal papilloma (papillomatosis)
- Suspected intraductal cancer
- Breast adenoma
- Complex breast cyst and suspected epithelioma of the cystic wall
- Nodular or diffuse mastopathy

Contraindications to ductography are as follows:

- Iodine intolerance (the contrast agent contains iodine)
- Acute inflammation of the breast (mastitis, abscess, purulent inflammation of the nipple, etc.)
- Breastfeeding
- Presence of atypical cells in the cytological study of smears of nipple discharge
- Scarred nipple

According to Rozhkova (1993), 92–96% ductographies define the cause of abnormal discharge and specify the location of the mass and the extent of the disease. Ductography may cause therapeutic effect. Abnormal discharge from the nipple may stop after ductography in 40% of cases due to washing of the duct system with iodine-containing contrast agents.

Ductoscopy is an endoscopic study of lactiferous ducts. It is performed with or without local anesthesia and includes dilatation of the ducts up to 0.5 mm in diameter and introduction of a silicone fibroscope with an outer diameter up to 0.4 mm. Next, the duct is washed with saline and blown with air. The technique allows to determine the sites of tumor-like strands and intraductal papillomas. Tissue biopsy from the suspicious site is possible. This method is especially useful for early diagnosis of intraductal breast cancer. In comparison with contrast X-ray mammography, this method is more informative, although it is expensive due to the complexity of performance and high costs for diagnostic equipment.

Pneumocystography—introduction of gas (air) into the cyst after aspiration of its contents, followed by radiography in two projections. The technique was previously widely used for the analysis of cystic lumen. Currently it is almost completely replaced with ultrasonography.

Minimally invasive diagnostic techniques allow obtaining histological samples and specification of the following features:

- Histological type of the tumor
- The degree of malignancy (grading system is based on the degree of structural and cellular polymorphism, as well as on the severity of proliferative processes)
- The most complete biological characteristic of the specific breast cancer (in accordance with the specific set of tissue markers)

Optimal selection of diagnostic techniques (primarily including imaging and navigation) often allows to determine the patient management with the following aspects:

- Predict an outcome of the disease.
- Foresee probable response to treatment.
- Evaluate the degree of therapeutic pathomorphosis of the tumor at the stage of chemoradiotherapy and adjust (if necessary) the treatment regimens.
- Determine the appropriate volume of surgery.
- Analyze further prognosis, options for rehabilitation, and prevention of disease recurrence.

Minimally invasive modality (MIM) is a procedure that causes less damage in the body than the open intervention used for the same purpose.

Ultrasound guidance is a necessary component of MIM at all stages. US is used before, during, and after MIM. Many aspects (including ultrasound) of MIM in the treatment of breast diseases have not been fully studied, many questions are disputable, and some data are contradictory. Most of them are in the stage of analysis, generalization, justification, and general recognition by surgeons, endocrinologists, and specialists in ultrasound diagnostics.

MIM treatment of breast diseases is a promising high-tech trend of mammology. Their greatest advantage is the selective destruction of pathological foci with no (or minor) damage to the surrounding tissues. The other benefits are feasibility, low cost, minimal trauma, no need for general or local anesthesia, low risk and severity of possible complications and adverse effects, and, consequently, shortened hospital stay, treatment, and effective labor, household, and social rehabilitation. MIM is often the only possible method of treatment, as it can be used in severe and debilitated (previously considered inoperable) patients.

These technologies are simple and can be used in any surgical hospital, which dramatically increases the accessibility to this type of treatment. Significant progress has been achieved in the field of interventional radiology due to the use of minimally invasive technologies in combination with imaging methods. These interventions are performed with fluoroscopic, ultrasound, or X-ray assistance or with a combination of these methods.

In recent years, new technologies for minimally invasive treatment of benign breast diseases, primarily cysts and fibroadenomas, have been developed. These do not affect the volume, shape, and function of the mammary gland. Many authors report the successful use of various MIM (RFA, HIFU, laser, cryoablation) of breast cancer with low rate of side effects.

Diagnostic/therapeutic manipulations on the mammary gland:

1. For fibrocystic mastopathy and breast cysts:
    - Aspiration of the cystic contents
    - Air injection into the cyst after aspiration
    - Ethanol injection
    - Air and ethanol injection (pneumoethanol degradation)
    - Ozone-oxygen mixture injection
    - Vacuum aspiration-resection biopsy

2. For fibroadenomas:
   - Step-by-step or one-step destruction (enucleation) with a mammotome (vacuum total biopsy)
   - Laser ablation
   - MRI- or HIFU-guided focused ultrasound pyrotherapy
   - Cryodestruction (cryoablation)
   - Electrochemical lysis of benign tumors
   - Radiofrequency ablation (RFA)
3. For mastitis:
   - Puncture of an abscess, often with subsequent draining
4. For atheromas:
   - Radiofrequency ablation (RFA)

The general contraindications for MIM are listed below:

1. Absolute:
   - Decompensated coagulopathies, irreversible disorders of the coagulation system
   - Inadequacy of the patient, mental or psycho-emotional disorders
   - Lack of informed consent for the MIM procedure or patient's refusal
2. Relative:
   - Patient's bad health condition (severe disease, intoxication, hyperthermia, cephalgia, general weakness, hypertension, etc.)
   - Test results
   - Poor visualization of the target organ, zone (site, focus), or the lesion

In most cases, treatment of the breast cyst by puncture is sufficient. If the cyst is filled with fluid again, the procedure can be repeated or enhanced by one of the variants of sclerotherapy (destruction).

Ablation of breast cyst implicates aspiration of its contents and introduction of air or sclerosing agents (96% ethyl alcohol, synthetic glue compositions, ozone-oxygen mixture, etc.). This is the most popular and effective method of minimally invasive treatment. Under ultrasound control, the contents of the cyst are evacuated with a 5–10 mL syringe leaving 1–2 mL in the cavity. The contents of the cyst are sent for cytological study. After this, without removing the needle from the cystic cavity, 1–1.5 mL of sclerosing agent is injected through the same needle. Ninety-five percent alcohol is utilized most often. In cases of large cysts, an alcohol-air mixture may be applied. After the exposure (1–2 min, as a rule), complete reaspiration is necessary. The needle is pulled out and the cyst is compressed. Cystic walls adhere to each other, and in most cases the fluid can no longer accumulate.

If ozonotherapy is applied, the cavity is washed with novocaine after complete aspiration of the contents of the cyst. Ozone-oxygen mixture in the volume of 2–3 cm^3 is slowly injected.

In the opinion of Harchenko et al. (1999), percutaneous sclerotherapy of breast cysts allows to avoid surgery in 70% of cases. However, ablation is difficult in multiple, deep cysts and is contraindicated in cases of proliferation and atypia of cystic epithelium, multiple cysts, polycystic glands, and the history of breast cancer. If the cyst is recurrent for more than five times after the puncture and ablation, sector resection is recommended.

Laser ablation, cryoablation, and other ablative procedures for solid breast masses should be preceded by a standard clinical examination followed by ultrasonography and an US-guided puncture of the mass. Prior to the procedure, ultrasound is performed in order to assess the size, structure, and blood supply of the mass, as well as its characteristics (location, relationship with vessels, etc.). In benign lesions (e.g., breast fibroadenoma) of small size without progressive growth, the patient may be offered one of the minimally invasive image-guided procedures.

Electrochemical lysis on breast cancer is reported to be effective in breast cancer and metastases in the liver, if the lesion size is below 4 cm. Benign breast tumors, when exposed to electrochemical lysis, develop necrosis. The use of optimal lysis regimes allows to achieve adequate destruction of a benign tumor up to 2 cm in diameter with minimal side effects. Percutaneous electrochemical lysis of benign breast masses up to 2 cm allows to reduce surgical aggression and achieve better cosmetic results in comparison with traditional methods.

Interstitial laser photocoagulation (laser ablation) is a minimally invasive technology for treating benign breast masses by local thermal destruction with laser radiation. The technique is an alternative to conservative management of patients with benign breast masses.

Cryoablation is a minimally invasive method of deep freezing of breast fibroadenoma under ultrasound control by application of special probes. Freezing induces the decrease in the tumor functional activity, reduction in size, and destruction. Electronic devices, usually in automatic mode, calculate dosage and exposure of refrigerant (more often argon). Ultrasound navigation provides accurate imaging of the probe in real time. Cryodestruction, as a rule, is a less traumatic and painful procedure in comparison, for example, with radiofrequency ablation and other thermal and radiation methods of minimally invasive treatment of breast masses.

The main factors that influence the effectiveness of laser ablation and other types of destruction are the structure, size, and vascularization of the lesion.

Ultrasound guidance is a guarantee of safety and generally determines the effectiveness of treatment. Ultrasound features registered during laser ablation and other methods of destruction are an integral part of the procedure and should be used to ensure maximum effectiveness, safety, and comfort for the patient. The ultrasound features and artifacts in the grayscale and color-coded modes can differ depending on the MIM and the settings of ultrasound equipment.

Recently, a **total vacuum biopsy** of benign masses with US guidance has become widely introduced. It is a low-traumatic outpatient operation, which sometimes allows to totally remove the breast mass, making it equal to sector resection and lumpectomy. It has a number of advantages, such as short time and low cost of treatment, minimal trauma, and best cosmetic results. Benign masses of small size (usually up to 1.2–2.0 cm) with a capsule or pseudocapsule (fibroadenomas, lipomas, cysts) are subject to total biopsy. Possible complications may be edema or hematoma in surrounding tissues. With a size of more than 1.2 cm, preference is often given to sector resection. Confirmed breast cancer is a contraindication for total vacuum biopsy.

Neoadjuvant systemic therapy is increasingly used in the treatment of breast cancer patients. This treatment allows to reduce the size of the primary tumor and perform an organ-sparing operation, to evaluate the individual sensitivity of the tumor, and to achieve a complete response. It is thought that the complete morphological regression of the primary tumor and regional metastases are markers of a favorable prognosis. The proportion of patients who are achieving complete tumor response to the ongoing effective drug treatment is steadily increasing and reaches 30–60%. At the same time, the achievement of complete morphological regression of the breast tumor may confuse planning surgery. Organ-sparing procedures may be hindered by poor visualization of the tumor. Certain difficulties also arise at the stage of morphological evaluation of therapeutic pathomorphosis due to the absence of a macroscopic tumor node. Therefore, a radiocontrast marker installed in the tumor prior to the start of systemic therapy is a necessary reference point for the entire multidisciplinary team—radiotherapist, surgeon, and morphologist. A radiocontrast biologically inert metallic marker (gold or titanium) is usually introduced using a metal conductor.

Insertion of a marker into the primary tumor is performed in aseptic conditions under the control of mammography and ultrasound. The puncture needle is inserted into the center of the tumor; an interstitial marker made of titanium nickelide (or gold) wire that takes the form of a rod (preferably 5–10 mm in length) is set in the lumen of the needle and is pushed into the tumor under ultrasound control. The interstitial marker comes fixed in the tumor and remains there for the entire course of neoadjuvant chemotherapy.

Sentinel lymph node biopsy (SLNB) in breast cancer is one of the most dynamically developing methods of radiologic medicine (Krivorotko et al. 2017). Important are those first (1–3) nodes, into which lymph flows from the

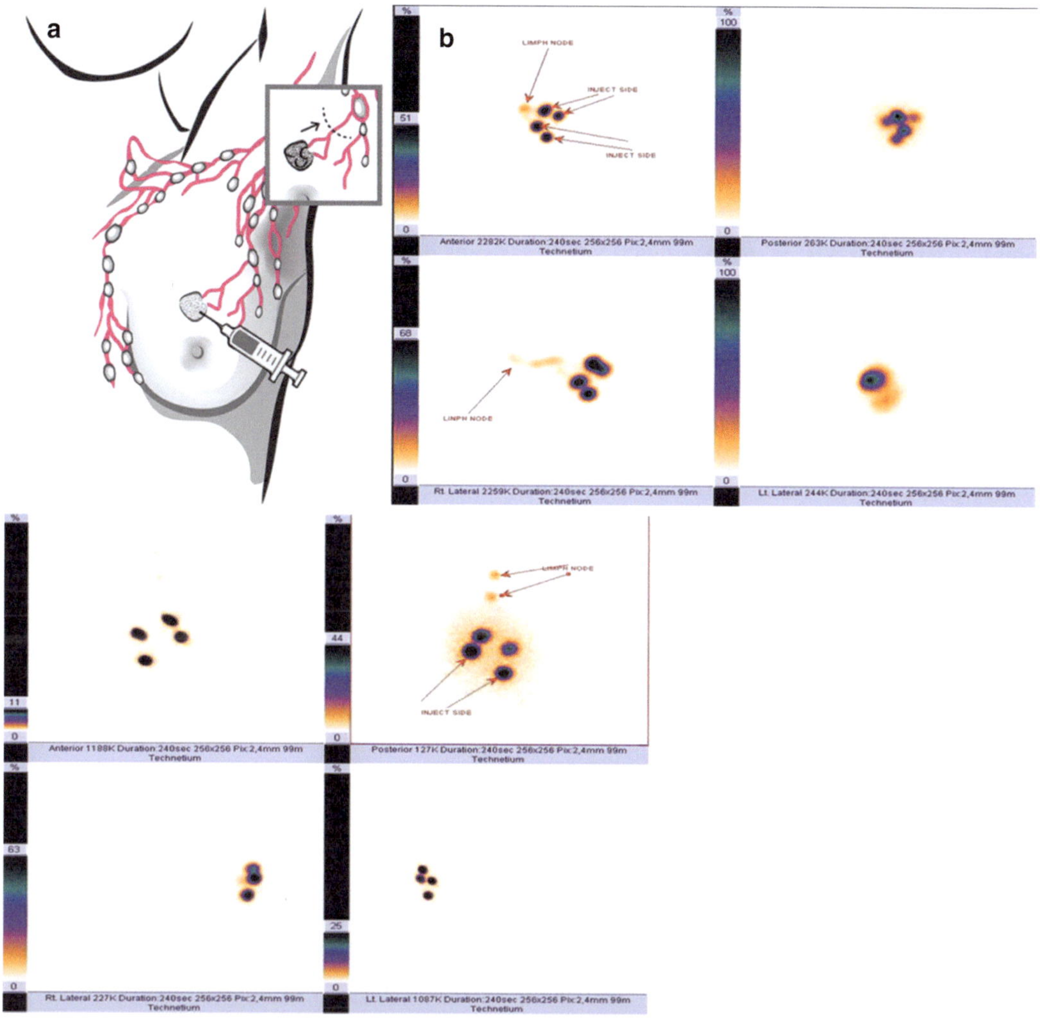

Fig. 12.12 SLNB. (**a**) Scheme. (**b**) Lymphoscintigraphy of the “sentinel” lymph nodes in breast cancer. Technefit, ^{99m}Tc, 4*20 MBq intradermally

breast. SLNB is currently the “gold standard” of surgical intervention in the areas of regional metastasis in patients with early breast cancer with metastasis-free axillary lymph nodes.

With preoperative marking of sentinel nodes, a radiopharmaceutical (e.g., Technefit, ^{99m}Tc) is usually injected intradermally (intratumoral, peritumoral, or subareolar administration is also possible) in the tumor projection. In the initial scintigrams (as a rule, 20 min after the injection), the accumulation of radiocontrast preparation at the injection sites is registered. Later, the foci of the radiopharmaceutical accumulation in the projection of axillary (or other) lymph nodes are noted and documented (Fig. 12.12).

According to Krivorotko et al. (2017), the survival rate of patients with unaffected and affected sentinel lymph nodes reaches 100% and 97.4%, respectively. The threshold number of affected lymph nodes that influences the prognosis was more than 1 (p = 0.0187); the survival rate of patients with 0–1 affected nodes was 99.7% and with more than one affected node, 95.7%.

SLNB has high diagnostic accuracy and low rate of false-positive results. Surgical treatment of patients with radioisotope detection and intraoperative histological examination of sentinel lymph nodes allows accurate staging of breast cancer. SLNB in patients with breast cancer can prevent unjustified disabling axillary lymphadenectomy.

Assessment of regional lymph nodes before systemic therapy is necessary for adequate staging of breast cancer and for further evaluation of treatment efficacy. In addition, a complete pathomorphologic response from metastatically affected regional lymph nodes may eliminate lymphodissection in favor of SLNB and therefore reduce the number of postoperative complications. However, identification of sentinel lymph nodes after neoadjuvant therapy is difficult because the treatment induces a blockade of lymphatic vessels and fibrosis of lymph nodes. This results in high probability of false-negative results of SLNB that reach 15%. A possible solution of this problem is marking of metastatic lymph nodes before the start of therapy with an ultrasound-guided marker (the technique is similar to the marking of the primary tumor) for its subsequent accurate visualization during surgical treatment. Based on the results of a large prospective study ACOSOG Z1071 (American College of Surgeons Oncology Group), the marking of metastatic lymph nodes allowed to reduce the number of false-negative results of SLNB by two times (from 13.4% to 6.8%), according to Boughey et al. (2016).

The main tasks of US during MIM are given below.

Before the manipulation:

- Preliminary conclusion about the structure of the mass, its location, vascularization, elasticity, and the state of surrounding tissues and organs
- Selection of the optimal method of MIM and specification of the manipulation in a particular patient (together with a surgeon, mammologist, oncologist)

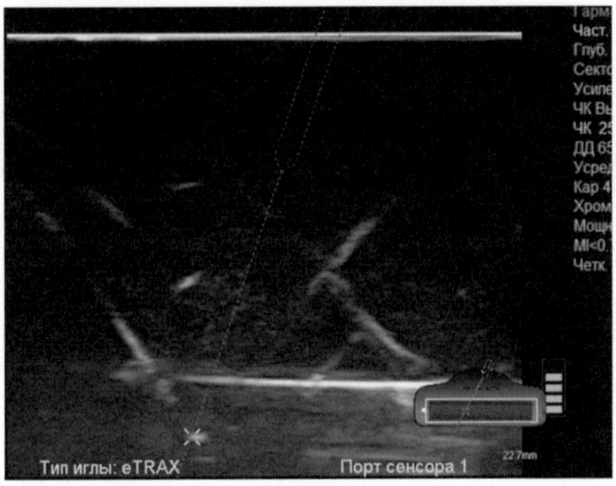

Fig. 12.13 FNAB. Ultrasound GPS navigation of the puncture

- Determination of the optimal puncture vector and needle pathway
- Assessment of the probability of potential adverse effects and complications during and after MIM

During MIM:

- Guidance of the needle insertion according to the previously chosen optimal pathway
- Absolute control over the tip of the needle position in the examined mass
- Monitoring of the state of the surrounding structures
- Dynamic monitoring of the manipulation, judgment on its effectiveness
- Detection of adverse effects and complications during MIM

After MIM:

- Evaluation of the effectiveness of manipulation in the zone of interest
- Assessment of the tissues surrounding the mass
- Detection of early (up to 30 min) and delayed (up to 3–4 weeks) complications
- Analysis of the structure and vascularity of the mass in the short-term (3–4 weeks) and long-term (more than 1 month) periods and follow-up of the changes in ultrasound parameters

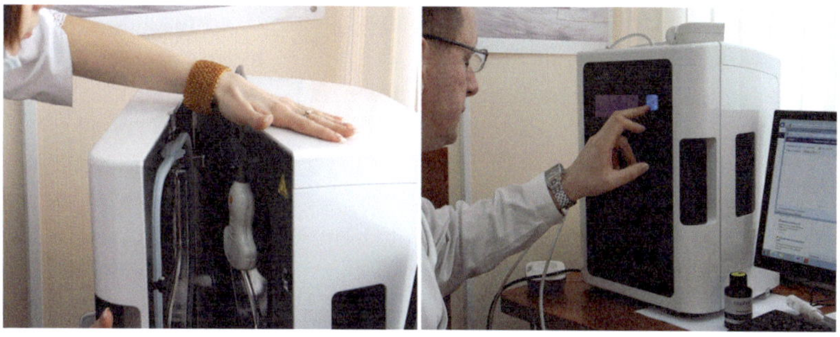

Fig. 12.14 1–2 Sterilization of an ultrasound probe in "Trophon" system

Ultrasound GPS navigation of the puncture needle is a promising technology (Fig. 12.13) built into some ultrasound devices of the latest generation. The technology allows real-time monitoring of the puncture needle through its positioning in the electromagnetic field.

At MIM, the rules of aseptics and antiseptics must be strictly followed. The procedures are carried out in specially equipped premises—dressing or small operating room—and the probe is disinfected with chlorhexidine solution or alcohol. Ultrasound probe can be sterilized in the "Trophon"-type apparatus (Nanosonics Ltd., Australia) that is compatible with any ultrasound probes (Fig. 12.14). One of its advantages is safety for the personnel and US probe with high degree of sterilization of working surfaces. The processing of probes in the apparatus is based on low-temperature plasma sterilization due to nano-splitting of 35% hydrogen peroxide.

The rate of complications of MIM on the mammary gland depends on the experience and teamwork of mammologist (oncologist, surgeon) and radiologist and on the image quality. Side effects and complications may be local (pain, inflammation, etc.) and general (discomfort, sickness, nausea, sweating, vascular spasm, etc.). The most common are cervicalgia, hemorrhage, and subcutaneous hematoma. The rate of complications and side effects of vacuum biopsy is 1–7%. Complications of FNAB with a 14G needle occur in approximately 2% of observations.

Pain at the puncture site can be caused both directly by tissue damage and by the development of hematoma. Local complications such as subcapsular, interfacial, intermuscular, or subcutaneous hematoma are the results of vessel injury.

The risk of pneumothorax is high when the procedure is performed by an inexperienced specialist, patient's lean body constitution, and peripheral breast masses.

Special attention is required in diagnostic invasive procedures in patients with breast implants. There are certain risks associated with possible damage of the implant and with poor visualization of the tumors adjacent to the prostheses.

Complications of FNAB associated with inappropriate aseptics (inflammatory infiltrates, abscesses) are rare.

After the diagnostic puncture, an appropriate record of the manipulation is made in the patient's history. After US-guided puncture, patient's condition, as a rule, does not require dynamic observation.

Invasive interventions on mammary glands are highly effective and well tolerated by patients; nevertheless, they require certain indications, respect of contraindications, and strict adherence to the intervention technique.

An example of US report of FNAB:

Name, surname. __S__ Age__31__.

Outpatient examination. Date____.

Patient's record____.

US scanner____.

In sterile conditions, a puncture of a mass measuring 2.0–2.2 cm in the lower-external quadrant of the right breast (8 o'clock position, 2 cm below and lateral to the nipple), was performed. The mass was heterogenous with fluid component, avascular in the CDI and PDI modes.

Visualization during the procedure was satisfactory. Samples from the three sites of the lesion (central, posterior, and anterior peripheral) were sent for cytological study.

An aseptic bandage was applied, compression recommended for 7–10 min.

The patient's condition during the procedure was satisfactory.

Mammologist (oncologist):

Ultrasonographist (radiologist):

An example of US-guided core needle biopsy report:

Name, surname. __S__ Age__31__.

Outpatient examination. Date____.

Patient's record____.

US scanner____.

Local anesthesia of biopsy site was performed by subcutaneous injection of 2–4 mL 0.5% novocaine solution.

Ultrasound-assisted core needle biopsy of a hypoechoic lesion of 2.2 × 3.5 × 2.8 cm in the upper-outer quadrant (10 o'clock position, 2 cm above and lateral to the nipple) of the right breast was performed; four samples of tumor tissue were obtained.

Samples of tissue were sent for pathological and immunohistochemical examination.

An aseptic bandage was applied, compression recommended for 7–10 min.

The patient's condition during the procedure was satisfactory.

Mammologist (oncologist):

Ultrasonographist (radiologist):

Preliminary conclusion: cancer of the right breast.

Conclusion

Difficulties in the diagnosis of breast diseases in women and men are due to the variety of nosology, clinical features of diseases, aggressiveness of cancer, and sometimes low efficacy of modern diagnostic methods.

Timely breast US reinforced with up-to-date techniques and technologies allows full evaluation of the condition of the mammary gland, the nature of lesions, the extent of the disease, and assessment of the surrounding structures and lymph nodes. The use of contrast agents significantly helps to detail the structure, vascularization, and extent of tumors. Dynamic ultrasound allows to assess the effectiveness of medical and surgical treatment of various breast diseases.

A structured system based on oncological alertness of general practitioners and the community-targeted mammographic screening allow to optimize early diagnosis of breast pathology, to effectively differentiate breast lesions, and, respectively, to increase life expectancy and life quality of patients.

G. T. Sukhikh, A. N. Sencha (eds.), *Multiparametric Ultrasound Diagnosis of Breast Diseases*,
https://doi.org/10.1007/978-3-319-75034-7

References

Adamyan LV, Orazvaliyeva DG, Burdina LM et al (1989) Condition of mammary glands and endometrium in patients with benign tumors and tumor-like ovarian lesions. Akusherstvo i ginecologiya 4:21–24. (Article in Russian)

Adamyan LV, Kulakov VI, Andreeva EN (2006) Endometriosis. Medicina, Moscow. (Book in Russian)

Balassanian R et al (2016) Invasive Breast Cancer Version 1. 2016, NCCN Clinical Practice Guidelines in Oncology. J Natl Compr Canc Netw 14(3):324–354

Bazhenova AP, Ostrovtsev LD, Hahanashvili GN (1985) Breast cancer. Medicina, Moscow. (Book in Russian)

Bebyakin VG (1974) Primary-multiple tumors on the data of Bashkirian oncological health center. PhD thesis. Ufa (Book in Russian)

Berg WA (2009) Tailored supplemental screening for breast cancer: what now and what next? Am J Roentgenol 192(2):390–399

Borsukov AV, Amosov VN, Bus'ko EA et al (2016) Guidelines 2016 on standardized method of compression elastography of the mammary gland, the thyroid gland, regional lymph nodes, extraorgan lesions and in endosonography. Smolensk (Book in Russian)

Boughey JC, Ballman KV, Le-Petross HT et al (2016) Identification and resection of clipped node decreases the false-negative rate of sentinel lymph node surgery in patients presenting with node-positive breast cancer (T0-T4, N1-N2) who receive neoadjuvant chemotherapy: results from ACOSOG Z1071 (Alliance). Ann Surg 263(4):802–807

Ciatto S, Rosselli del Turco M, Catarzi S et al (1994) The diagnostic role of breast echography. Radiol Med Torino 88(3):221–224

Cosgrove DO, Bamber JC, Davey YB et al (1990) Color doppler signals from breast tumors. Radiology 176: 175–180

Cosgrove DO, Kedar RP, Bamber JC et al (1993) Breast diseases: color Doppler US in differential diagnosis. Radiology 189(1):99–104

De Albertis P, Oliveri M, Quadri P et al (1995) Retrospective analysis of color Doppler ultrasonography and flowmetry findings in solid nodular pathology of the breast. Radiol Med 89(1–2):28–35. (Article in Italian)

Drincovic I (2002) Color doppler in diagnosis of breast diseases. International Breast Ultrasound Seminar, Warsaw, pp 5–7

Evans A, Whelehan P, Thomson K et al (2010) Quantitative shear wave ultrasound elastography: initial experience in solid breast masses. Breast Cancer Res 12(6):R104

Evseeva EV (2015) Optimization of the system of complex clinical-radiological screening of breast diseases. PhD thesis. Moscow (Book in Russian)

Evseeva EV, Senin AN, Sencha AN et al (2011) Ultrasound in early diagnosis of breast carcinoma. Official Proceedings of the 13th Congress of the World Federation for Ultrasound in Medicine and Biology, Vienna, p S101

Faden H (2005) Mastitis in children from birth to 17 years. Pediatr Infect Dis J 24(12):1113

Fiedler V, Neubauer KD, Schneiders A, Herzig P (1996) Ranking of color-coded duplex ultrasonography (CCDU) in the staging of breast tumors. RöFo 165(2):159–165. (Article in German)

Fisenko EP (1999) Ultrasound diagnosis of tumoral lesions of the breast in surgical clinic. PhD thesis. Moscow (Book in Russian)

Fisenko EP (2014) Ultrasound diagnosis of geleomas of soft tissues and mammary glands. Ultrazvukovaya i Funccionalnaya Diagnostic 5:58–68. (Article in Russian)

Fisenko EP, Sandrikov VA (1998) Results of complex ultrasound examination of breast lesions. Ultrazvukivaya Diagnostica 3:39–43. (Article in Russian)

Folkman J (1995) Tumor, angiogenesis. J Adv Cancer Res 43:175–200

Fowble B (1997) Postmastectomy radiation: then and now. Oncology 11:213–239

Frolov IM (1996) Possibilities of various methods of diagnosis in revealing of metastatic lymph nodes of axillary area at breast cancer. Materials of the Conference "Questions of oncologic aid at a stage of reformation of public health services", Yekaterinburg, pp 83–84. (Article in Russian)

Gromov AI, Kubova SY (2004) Possibilities of use of twinkling-artifact at calcifications of various organs. Materials of the 1st Conference "Radiological diagnosis and therapy in clinical medicine", Moscow, pp 35–36. (Article in Russian)

G. T. Sukhikh, A. N. Sencha (eds.), *Multiparametric Ultrasound Diagnosis of Breast Diseases*,
https://doi.org/10.1007/978-3-319-75034-7

Harchenko VP, Rozhkova NI (2005) Clinical mammology. The thematic collection, 1st edn. Strom, Moscow. (Book in Russian)

Harchenko VP, Rozhkova NI, Zubovsky GA, Medvedeva NA (1993) A method of color dopplerography in the diagnosis of breast diseases. Visualizaciya v Clinicke 1(3):33–43. (Article in Russian)

Harchenko VP, Rozhkova NI, Yacob LV (1995) Complex approach to the diagnosis of nodular mastopathy. A review. Mammologiya 1:22–28. (Article in Russian)

Harchenko VP, Frolov IM, Rozhkova NI et al (1996) Possibilityies of various diagnostic methods in assessment of the status of axillary lymph nodes in breast cancer. Vestnik Roentgenologii i Radiologii 1:20–24. (Article in Russian)

Harchenko VP, Rozhkova NI, Frolov IM (1999) Interventional examination procedures in breast diseases. Vestnik Roentgenologii i Radiologii 3:26–30. (Article in Russian)

Haylenko VA, Komova DV, Bogatiryov VN (2005) Diagnosis of breast cancer. Medical Information Agency, Moscow. (Book in Russian)

Holcombe C, Pugh N, Lyons K et al (1995) Blood flow in breast cancer and fibroadenoma estimated by colour Doppler ultrasonography. Br J Surg 82(6):787–788

Kaprin AD, Starinsky VV, Petrova GV eds. (2017) The state of oncologic health care in Russia in 2016. Moscow (Book in Russian)

Kharchenko VP, Rozhkova NI (eds) (2005) Clinical mammology. The thematic collection, 1st edn. Strom, Moscow. (Book in Russian)

Kharchenko VP, Rozhkova NI, Zubovsky GA, Medvedeva NA (1993) A method of color dopplerography in the diagnosis of breast diseases. Visualizaciya V Clin 1(3):33–43. (Article in Russian)

Kolesnik AY, Shershneva MA, Meskih EV et al (2014) New approaches to the diagnostic algorithm of odematous-infiltrative type of breast cancer (literature review). Medicinskaya Visualizaciya 5:124–129. (Article in Russian)

Komarova LE (2006) Mammographic screening and its role in decrease of mortality from breast cancer. Mammologiya 6:5–10. (Article in Russian)

Korzhenevsky AV (2003) Electroimpedance tomography system for three-dimensional visualization of breast tissues. Biomedicinckiye Technologii i Radioelectronica 8:5–10. (Article in Russian)

Korzhenkova GP (2004) Complex X-ray and sonographic diagnosis of breast diseases. Strom, Moscow. (Book in Russian)

Korzhenkova GP, Lukyanchenko AB, Zernov DI (2006) Possibilities of magnetic resonance tomography in algorithm of examination of patients with breast diseases. Mammologiya 1:39–45. (Article in Russian)

Kotlyarov PM, Sencha AN, Kashmanova AV et al (2015) Contrast enhanced ultrasound in the diagnosis of breast lesions in women and men. Medicinskaya Visualizaciya 2:120–128. (Article in Russian)

Krivorotko PV, Tabagua TT, Komyahov AV et al (2017) Byopsy of signal lymph nodes in early breast cancer: experience of scientific-investigation institute named after N.N. Petrov. Voprosi Oncologii 2(63):267–273. (Article in Russian)

Kuplevatskaya DI (2004) Possibilities of X-ray guided stereotactic biopsy in the diagnosis of impalpable breast cancer. PhD thesis. Saint-Petersburg (Book in Russian)

Lee SK, Lee I, Lee KR et al (1995) Evaluation of breast tumors with color Doppler imaging: a comparison with image directed Doppler ultrasound. Clin Ultrasound 23:367–373

Lelyuk VG, Lelyuk SE (2007) Ultrasound angiology. Realnoye Vremya, Moscow. (Book in Russian)

Lyman GH, Somerfield MR, Bosserman LD et al (2017) Sentinel lymph node biopsy for patients with early-stage breast cancer: American Society of Clinical Oncology clinical practice guideline update. J Clin Oncol 35(5):561–564

Madjar H, Prompeler HJ, Sauerbrei W et al (1995) Differential diagnosis of breast lesions by color Doppler. Ultrasound Obstet Gynecol 6(3):199–204

Marquet KL, Funk A, Handt S et al (1995) Displacement margins and edge contour: informative criteria of tumor dignity in ultrasound mammography. Geburtshilfe Frauenheilkd 55:548–552

Mazo ML, Rozhkova NI, Prokopenko SP et al (2015) Invasive radiological diagnostics of breast cancer. Fine needle biopsy or core needle biopsy? Medicinskaya Visualizaciya 4:79–86. (Article in Russian)

Mihaylov SA, Skrynnik EB (1997) Influence of histological structure of tumors on the value of ultrasound diagnosis of breast neoplasms. Materials of the Conference "Modern radiological diagnostics and therapy", Chelyabinsk, pp 131–132. (Article in Russian)

Mitkov VV, Huako SA, Ampilogova ER, Mitkova MD (2011) Assessment of reproducibility of the results of quantitative ultrasound elastography. Ultrazvukovaya i Functionalnaya Diagnostica 2:115–121. (Article in Russian)

Mitkov VV, Chubarova KA, Zabolotskaya NV, Mitkova MD (2013) Possobilities of share-wave elastography in differential diagnosis of focal types of malignant and benign breast tumors. Ultrazvukovaya i Functionalnaya Diagnostica 6:27–38. (Article in Russian)

Mitkov VV, Chubarova KA, Zabolotskaya NV et al (2014) Value of share-wave elastography in the diagnosis of breast cancer. Ultrazvukovaya i Functionalnaya Diagnostica 1:11–24. (Article in Russian)

Mitkov VV, Chubarova KA, Zabolotskaya NV et al (2015) Share-wave elastography in multiparametric ultrasound diagnostics of various size malignant tumors of mammary glands. Ultrazvukovaya i Functionalnaya Diagnostica 2:9–18. (Article in Russian)

Moertel CG (1977) Multiple primary malignant neoplasms: historical perspectives. Cancer 40(4 Suppl):1786–1792

National Comprehensive Cancer Network (2016) Clinical Practice Guidelines in Oncology. Breast Cancer. Version 1.2016. National Comprehensive Cancer Network. NCCN Guidelines. Clinical Guidelines in Oncology

Nikolayev KS (2015) Diagnosis and treatment of breast cancer in men. PhD thesis. Moscow (Book in Russian)
Otto RC (1993) Diseases of the female breast: scrinning, mammography, ultrasound. Ther Umsch 5:323–333
Piscaglia F, Salvatore V, Di Donato R et al (2011) Accuracy of virtual touch acoustic radiation force impulse (ARFI) imaging for the diagnosis of cirrhosis during liver ultrasonography. Ultraschall Med 32(2):167–175
Possover M, Morawski A, Muller E, Hettenbach A (1994) New perspectives in color ultrasound in breast diagnosis. Geburtshilfe Frauenheilkd 54(8): 432–436
Postnova NM, Vasilyev AY, Zykin BI et al (2011) Possibilities of sonoelastography of shift wave in differential diagnosis of breast diseases. Diagn Interv Radiol 5(2):324–325. (Article in Russian)
Radzinsky VE, Ordiyants IM, Maslennikova MN, Pavlova EA (2016) Mammary glands and gynecological diseases: from common pathogenesis to practical solutions. Possibilities of health improvement in women with combination of uterine myoma and benign breast dysplasia. Zdorovye zhenshiny 6:104–109. (Article in Russian)
Rasskazova EA, Rozhkova NI (2014) Screening in early diagnosis of breast cancer. Issledovaniya i Practica v Medicine 1(1):45–49. (Article in Russian)
Rozhkova NI (1993) X-ray diagnosis of breast diseases. Medicina, Moscow. (Book in Russian)
Rozhkova NI, Reshetzova GV, Zapirova SB (2008) About the possibilities of digital mammographic tomosynthesis. Radiologiya-Practica 6:19–23. (Article in Russian)
Rozhkova NI, Zubarev AV, Zapirova SB, Churkina SO, Hohlova EA (2010) New technology—sonoelastography in mammology. Medicinskaya Visualizaciya 4:89–99. (Article in Russian)
Rozhkova NI, Hohlova EA, Zubarev AV, Budanov MV (2011) Possibilities of new ultrasound technology—sonoelastography—in the diagnosis of benign and malignant breast diseases. Luchevaya diagnostic i therapiya 2:56–68. (Article in Russian)
Rybnikova EI, Popov SV, Min'ko BA, Petrosyan SL (2017) To the issue of organization of ultrasound screening of breast pathology. Medicus 3(15):73–75. (Article in Russian)
Sandrikov VA, Fisenko EP (1998) Assessment of blood flow velosities in breast vessels at its tumoral pathology. Vestnik Rossiyskoy, Academii Medicinskih nauk, pp 49–52. (Article in Russian)
Savello VE, Shumakova TA (2014) Radiological diagnosis of breast cancer after augmentation mammoplasty. Thesis of the Congress of Russian Association of Radiologists, Moscow, pp 305–307. (Article in Russian)
Semiglazov VF (2001) Tumors of the breast (treatment and preventive maintenance). Almaty (Book in Russian)
Semiglazov VF (2004) Surgical treatment of breast cancer. Practicheskaya Oncologiya. pp 6–12 (Article in Russian)
Sencha AN (ed) (2015) Imaging of male breast cancer. Springer, Berlin, Heidelberg
Sencha AN, Sergeeva ED, Shmelev DM (2009) Sonoelastography in complex diagnosis of breast lesions. Ultrazvukovaya i Functionalnaya Diagnostica 4:99. (Article in Russian)
Sencha AN, Evseeva EV, Petrovsky DA et al (2011) Methods of ultrasound examination in diagnosis of breast cancer. Vidar, Moscow. (Book in Russian)
Sencha AN, Evseeva EV, Mogutov MS, Patrunov YN (2013) Breast ultrasound. Springer, Berlin, Heidelberg
Sencha AN, Mogutov MS, Patrunov YN et al (2015) Ultrasound examination with use of contrast agents. Vidar-M, Moscow. (Book in Russian)
Sencha AN, Fazylova SA, evseeva EV, Gus AI (2017) Ultrasound multiparametric examination of mammary glands. Geotar-Media, Moscow. (Book in Russian)
Serebryakova SV, Trufanov GE, Fokin VA (2011) MRI-semiotics of breast lesions. Voprosy Oncologii 1: 92–98. (Article in Russian)
Serebryakova SV, Yukhno EA, Shumakova TA (2015) Possibilities of application of descriptive system BI-RADS in MR-mammography. Nevsky radiologichesky forum-2015, book of abstracts. Elbi-SPb, Saint-Petersburg, pp 617–619. (Article in Russian)
Serov VA, Sukhikh GT (2014) Obstetrics and gynecology. Clinical guidelines. GEOTAR-Media, Moscow. (Book in Russian)
Shevchenko EP (1997) X-ray and ultrasound diagnosis of impalpable breast lesions. PhD thesis. Moscow (Book in Russian)
Shevchenko EP (1999) Color Doppler mapping in examination of breast neoplasms. SonoAce International 4:72–76. (Article in Russian)
Shumakova TA, Savello VE, Tihova KE (2011) Diagnosis of complications and diseases of the breasts after augmentation mammoplasty with silicone gel implants. Materials of "Neva radiological forum", Saint-Petersburg, p 271. (Article in Russian)
Sinyukova GT, Korzhenkova GP, Danzanova TY (2007) Ultrasound examination of breasts in oncology. Strom, Moscow. (Book in Russian)
Slinchak SM (1968) Множественные злокачественные опухоли. Здоров'я, Киев
Smirnova NA (1995) Possibilities color doppler in complex diagnosis of breast diseases. PhD thesis. Moscow (Book in Russian)
Sobin LH, Gospodarowicz MK, Wittekind CH (eds) (2010) International Union against Cancer. TNM classification of malignant tumours. 7th ed. Chichester, West Sussex, UK; Hoboken, NJ: Wiley
Sohn C, Thiel C, Bandendistel A et al (1997) Degree of blood supply defined by ultrasound new prognostic factor? Mammoligy 2:7–10
Solbiati L, Rissato G (1995) Ultrasound of superficial structures. High frequencies, Doppler and interventional procedures. Churchill Livingstone, Edinburgh, Hong-Kong, London, Madrid, Melbourn, New York, Tokyo
Svensson WE (1997) A review of the current status of breast ultrasound. Eur J Ultrasound 6(2):77–101

Svensson W, Hashimoto H, Forouhi P et al (2000) Differences of vascular pattern demonstrated by color Doppler ultrasound allow differentiation of fibroadenomas from cancers in the breast. Eur J Ultrasound 11(1):5–6

Tavassoéli FA, Devilee P (eds) (2003) World Health Organization: Tumours of the Breast and Female Genital Organs (Who/IARC Classification of Tumours) (IARC WHO Classification of Tumours)

The Cancer Genome Atlas Network (2012) Comprehensive molecular portraits of human breast tumors. Nature 490:61–70

Trofimova EY (2000) Ultrasound dopplerography in breast cancer. Ultrazvukovaya Diagnostica 2:26–29. (Article in Russian)

Trofimova EY (2002) Ultrasound diagnosis of breast diseases. Visualizaciya v Clinicke 6:44–50. (Article in Russian)

Trohanova OV (2010) Early differential diagnosis of dishormonal breast diseases and control after efficiency of treatment with electroimpedance technologies. PhD thesis (Book in Russian)

Trufanov GE, Ryazanov VV, Ivanov LI (2009) Ultrasound in mammology. ELBI-S-pb, Saint Petersburg. (Book in Russian)

Tyurin IE (2011) Radiological diagnosis in Russian Federation. Radiology 1:6–11. (Article in Russian)

Tyutin LA, Stanzhevsky AA (2003) Radiology in oncologic practice. A review. Voprosy Oncologii 49(5): 543–544. (Article in Russian)

Ueno E (1996) Breast ultrasound. Gan To Kagaku Ryoho 23(1):14–23

US Preventive Services Task Force (2009) Screening for breast cancer: U.S. preventive services task force recommendation statement. Ann Intern Med 151:716–726

Valeur NS, Rahbar H, Chapman T (2015) Ultrasound of pediatric breast masses: what to do with lumps and bumps. Pediatr Radiol 45(11):1584–1559

Verheuvel NC, van den Hoven I, Ooms HWA et al (2015) The role of ultrasound-guided lymph node biopsy in axillary staging of invasive breast cancer in the post-FCOSOG Z0011 trial era. Ann Surg Oncol 22(2):409–415

Vetshev PS, Smiths NS, Beltsevich DG, Ozerov SK (1997) Possibilities of US examination in differential diagnosis of benign lesions and breast cancer. Surgery 6:25–27. (Article in Russian)

Wild JJ, Neal D (1951) Use of high-frequency ultrasonic waves for detecting changes of texture in living tissues. Lancet 6656(1):655–657

Wild JJ, Reid JM (1952) Further pilot echographic studies on the histologic structure of tumors of the living intact human breast. Am J Pathol 28(5):839–861

Yang WT, Ahuja AT, Tang A et al (1996) High frequency ultrasound detection of axillary lymph node metastases in breast cancer. J Ultrasound Med 15(3): 241–246

Yemelyanov VD, Vidyukov VI, Mustafin CK (2011) Relative assessment of radiometric and ultrasound methods in diagnosis of malignant breast lesions. Materials of the "Neva radiological forum", Saint-Petersburg, p 75. (Article in Russian)

Youssefzadeh S, Eibenberger K, Helbich T et al (1996) Use of resistance index for the diagnosis of breast tumors. Clin Radiol 51(6):418–420

Zabolotskaya NV, Gavrilenko NB (2015) Echographic image of various stages of formation of mammary glands in girls of 5-11 years. Ultrazvukovaya i Functionalnaya Diagnostica 3:13–18. (Article in Russian)

Zabolotskaya NV, Zabolotsky VS (1997) Ultrasound mammography. Strom, Moscow. (Book in Russian)

Zabolotskaya NV, Zabolotsky VS (2000) Complex ultrasound examination of breasts. Sonoace International 6:86–92. (Article in Russian)

Zabolotskaya NV, Zabolotsky VS (2005) New technologies in ultrasound mammography. Strom, Moscow. (Book in Russian)

Zhang Y, Jiang Q, Zhang Y et al (2013) Diagnostic value of contrast-enhanced ultrasound parametric imaging in breast tumors. J Breast Cancer 16(2):208–213

Zubarev AV (2009) Elastography—an innovative method of the search of cancers of various localizations. Polyclinica 4:32–37. (Article in Russian)

MIX
Papier aus verantwortungsvollen Quellen
Paper from responsible sources
FSC® C105338

If you have any concerns about our products,
you can contact us on
ProductSafety@springernature.com

In case Publisher is established outside the EU,
the EU authorized representative is:
Springer Nature Customer Service Center GmbH
Europaplatz 3, 69115 Heidelberg, Germany

Printed by Libri Plureos GmbH
in Hamburg, Germany